BMA

The British
Medical Association

CONCISE GUIDE TO
MEDICINES
AND DRUGS

D1178503

BMA

The British
Medical Association

CONCISE GUIDE TO
MEDICINES
AND DRUGS

Chief Medical Editor

PROFESSOR JOHN A. HENRY MB FRCP

St Mary's Hospital, London

Dorling Kindersley

LONDON, NEW YORK, SYDNEY, DELHI,
PARIS, MUNICH, AND JOHANNESBURG

Project Editor Teresa Pritlove
Editorial assistance Joanna Benwell

Senior Managing Editor Martyn Page
Managing Art Editor Louise Dick

DTP Designers Rachel Symons, Julian Dams
Production Controller Rita Sinha
Indexer Julie Rimington

The British Medical Association Concise Guide to Medicines and Drugs provides
information on a wide range of medicines and drugs. The book is not a substitute
for expert medical advice, however, and you are advised always to consult your doctor
for specific information on personal health matters. The naming of any product
or organization in this book does not imply BMA endorsement;
the omission of any such names does not indicate BMA disapproval.

First UK Edition 2001
Reprinted with corrections 2002
The British Medical Association Concise Guide to Medicines and Drugs is based on
The British Medical Association New Guide to Medicines and Drugs (5th edition)

2 4 6 8 10 9 7 5 3 1

Published in the United Kingdom by Dorling Kindersley Limited,
80 Strand, London,WC2R 0RL

A CIP catalogue record for this book is available from the British Library

ISBN 0-7513-0466-2

Printed and bound in Great Britain by Clays Ltd. St Ives plc

see our complete catalogue at
www.dk.com

CONTENTS

INTRODUCTION......6

PART 1
Major drug groups   7–124

BRAIN AND NERVOUS SYSTEM......8
RESPIRATORY SYSTEM......23
HEART AND CIRCULATION......27
GASTROINTESTINAL TRACT......39
MUSCLES, BONES, AND JOINTS......48
ALLERGY......56
INFECTIONS AND INFESTATIONS......59
HORMONES AND ENDOCRINE SYSTEM......78
NUTRITION......88
MALIGNANT AND IMMUNE DISEASE......93
REPRODUCTIVE AND URINARY TRACTS......99
EYES AND EARS......110
SKIN......114

PART 2
A–Z of drugs   125–404

PART 3
Drug finder index   405–464

INTRODUCTION

The British Medical Association Concise Guide to Medicines and Drugs provides clear information and practical advice on drugs and medicines that can be readily understood by a non-medical reader. The text reflects current medical knowledge and standard medical practice in this country. It is intended to complement and reinforce the advice of your doctor.

The book is divided into three parts. The first part covers the major groups of drugs. The second part gives detailed information about 247 individual drugs, arranged alphabetically. The third part consists of the drug finder index.

PART 1: MAJOR DRUG GROUPS

This part of the book is subdivided into sections on each body system or major disease grouping. It contains descriptions of the principal drug groups and information on the uses, actions, effects, and risks associated with each. Common drugs in each group are listed to allow cross-reference to Part 2.

A–Z OF DRUGS

This part consists of profiles of 247 key drugs. Each profile gives detailed information and practical advice and is intended to provide reference and guidance for non-medical readers taking drug treatment. It is impossible, however, to take into account every variation in individual circumstances; readers should always follow a doctor's or pharmacist's instructions where they differ from the advice in this section.

The drugs have been selected to provide representative coverage of the principal classes of drugs in medical use today. For some disorders, a number of drugs are available and the most commonly used drugs have been chosen. Emphasis has also been placed on the drugs likely to be used in the home, although in a few cases drugs administered only in hospital have been included when the drug has been judged to be of sufficient general interest.

HOW TO UNDERSTAND THE PROFILES

For ease of reference, the information on each drug is arranged in a consistent format under standard headings.

Drug name Tells you the drug's generic name, brand names under which the drug is marketed, and combined preparations that contain the drug.

Quick reference Summarizes important facts regarding the drug.

General information Gives a brief summary of the drug's important characteristics.

Information for users Practical information on how and when to take the drug, the usual recommended dosage, how soon it takes effect, how long it is active, and advice on diet, storage, and missed doses.

Overdose action Indicates the symptoms that may occur if an overdose has been taken and tells you what immediate action is required.

Possible adverse effects Indicates adverse effects that may be experienced with the drug.

Interactions Tells you how the drug may interact with other drugs or substances taken at the same time.

Special precautions Describes circumstances in which the drug should be taken with special caution or in which it might not be suitable.

Prolonged use Tells you what effects the drug may have when taken long term and what monitoring may be advised.

PART 3: DRUG FINDER INDEX

The drug finder index provides basic information on over 2,500 generic and brand-name drugs and drug groups, and also directs you to further information about them throughout the book.

PART 1

MAJOR DRUG GROUPS

Subdivided into sections dealing with each body system (e.g., heart and circulation) or major disease grouping (e.g., malignant and immune disease), this part of the book contains descriptions of the principal classes of drugs (e.g., corticosteroids), with information on the uses, actions, effects, and risks associated with each group of drugs. Individual drugs common to each group are listed to allow cross-reference to Part 2.

BRAIN AND NERVOUS SYSTEM

The human brain contains over 100 billion nerve cells (neurons). These nerve cells receive electro-chemical impulses from everywhere in the body. They interpret these impulses and send responsive signals back to various glands and muscles. The brain functions continuously as a switchboard for the human communications system. At the same time, it serves as the seat of emotions and mood, of memory, personality, and thought. Extending from the brain is an additional cluster of nerve cells that forms the spinal cord. Together, these two elements comprise the central nervous system.

Radiating from the central nervous system is the peripheral nervous system, which has three parts. One part branches off the spinal cord and extends to skin and muscles throughout the body. Another, in the head, links the brain to the eyes, ears, nose, and taste buds. The third is a semi-independent network called the autonomic, or involuntary, nervous system. This is the part of the nervous system that controls unconscious body functions such as breathing and digestion (see right).

Signals traverse the nervous system by electrical and chemical means. Electrical impulses carry signals from one end of a neuron to the other. To cross the gap between neurons, chemical neurotransmitters are released from one cell to bind to the receptor sites of nearby cells. Excitatory transmitters stimulate action; inhibitory transmitters reduce it.

WHAT CAN GO WRONG

Disorders of the brain and nervous system may manifest themselves as physical impairments, such as epilepsy or strokes, or as mental and emotional impairments (e.g., schizophrenia or depression).

Illnesses causing physical impairments can result from different types of disorder of the brain and nervous system. Death of nerve cells resulting from poor circulation can result in paralysis, while electrical disturbances of certain nerve cells cause the fits of epilepsy. Temporary changes in blood circulation within and around the brain are thought to

cause migraine. Parkinson's disease is caused by a lack of dopamine, a neurotransmitter produced by specialized brain cells.

The causes of disorders that trigger mental and emotional impairment are not known, but these illnesses have been linked with the defective functioning of nerve cells and neurotransmitters. The nerve cells may be under- or overactive, or poorly coordinated. Alternatively, mental and emotional impairment may be due to too much or too little neurotransmitter in one area of the brain.

WHY DRUGS ARE USED

By and large, the drugs that are described in this section do not eliminate nervous system disorders. Their function is to correct or modify the communication of the signals that traverse the nervous system. By doing so, they can improve symptoms or return functioning and behaviour towards normal. In some cases, such as anxiety and insomnia, drugs are used to lower the level of activity in the brain. In other disorders – depression, for example – drugs encourage the opposite effect, increasing the level of activity.

Drugs that act on the nervous system are also used for conditions that outwardly have nothing to do with nervous system disorders. Migraine headaches, for example, are often treated with drugs that cause the autonomic nervous system to send out signals constricting the dilated blood vessels that cause the migraine.

AUTONOMIC NERVOUS SYSTEM

The autonomic, or involuntary, nervous system governs the actions of the muscles of the organs and glands. Such vital functions as heart beat and digestion continue without conscious direction, whether we are awake or asleep.

The autonomic nervous system is divided into two parts: the sympathetic and parasympathetic nervous systems. The effects of one generally balance those of the other; the sympathetic has an excitatory effect, while the parasympathetic, by contrast, has an opposite effect.

Although the functional pace of most organs results from the interplay between the two systems, the muscles in the blood vessel walls respond only to the signals of the sympathetic nervous system. Whether a vessel is dilated or constricted is determined by the relative stimulation of two sets of receptor sites: alpha sites and beta sites.

Blood vessels in the skin These are constricted by stimulation of alpha receptors by the sympathetic; the parasympathetic has no effect on them.

The heart The rate and strength of the heart are increased by the sympathetic and reduced by the parasympathetic.

The pupils These are dilated by the sympathetic and constricted by the parasympathetic.

The airways The bronchial muscles are relaxed and widened by the sympathetic and contracted and narrowed by the parasympathetic.

Intestines The activity of the intestinal wall muscles is reduced by the sympathetic and increased by the parasympathetic.

NEUROTRANSMITTERS

The sympathetic nervous system relies on epinephrine (adrenaline) and norepinephrine (noradrenaline), products of the adrenal glands and neurons that act as both hormones and neurotransmitters. The parasympathetic nervous system depends on the neurotransmitter acetylcholine to transmit signals from cell to cell.

DRUGS THAT ACT ON THE SYMPATHETIC NERVOUS SYSTEM

The drugs that stimulate the sympathetic nervous system are called adrenergics (or sympathomimetics). They either promote the release of epinephrine (adrenaline) and norepinephrine (noradrenaline) or mimic their effects. Drugs that interfere with the action of the sympathetic nervous system are called sympatholytics. Alpha blockers act on alpha receptors; beta blockers act on beta receptors (see also Beta blockers, p.28)

DRUGS THAT ACT ON THE PARA-SYMPATHETIC NERVOUS SYSTEM

Drugs that stimulate the parasympathetic nervous system are called cholinergics (or

parasympathomimetics); drugs that oppose its action are called anticholinergics. Many prescribed drugs have anticholinergic properties.

MAJOR DRUG GROUPS

◆ Analgesics
◆ Sleeping drugs
◆ Anti-anxiety drugs
◆ Antidepressant drugs
◆ Antipsychotic drugs
◆ Antimanic drugs
◆ Anticonvulsant drugs
◆ Drugs for parkinsonism
◆ Drugs for dementia
◆ Nervous system stimulants
◆ Drugs for migraine
◆ Anti-emetics

Analgesics

Analgesics (painkillers) are drugs that relieve pain. Since pain is not a disease but a symptom, long-term relief depends on treatment of the underlying cause. The pain of toothache, for example, can be relieved by drugs but can be cured only by appropriate dental treatment. If the underlying disorder cannot be cured (e.g., some rheumatic conditions) long-term analgesic treatment may be necessary.

Damage to body tissues as a result of disease or injury is detected by nerve endings that transmit signals to the brain. Interpretation of these sensations can be affected by an individual's psychological state, so that pain is worsened by anxiety and fear, for example. Often, a reassuring explanation of the cause of discomfort can make pain easier to bear and may even relieve it. Anti-anxiety drugs (see p.13) are helpful when pain is accompanied by anxiety, and some are also used to reduce painful muscle spasms. Antidepressant drugs (see p.14) block the transmission of impulses signalling pain and are particularly useful for nerve pains (neuralgia), which do not always respond to analgesics.

TYPES OF ANALGESIC

Analgesics are divided into the opioids (with similar properties to drugs derived from opium, such as morphine) and non-opioids. Non-opioids consist of all other analgesics, including paracetamol, nefopam, and also the non-steroidal anti-inflammatory drugs (NSAIDs), the most well known of which is aspirin. In most circumstances, the non-opioids are less powerful as painkillers than the opioids. Local anaesthetics (see facing page) are also used to relieve pain.

Opioid drugs and paracetamol act directly on the brain and spinal cord to alter the perception of pain. Opioids act like the endorphins, hormones naturally produced in the brain that stop the cell-to-cell transmission of pain sensation. NSAIDs prevent stimulation of nerve endings at the site of the pain.

When pain is treated under medical supervision, it is common to start with an NSAID or paracetamol; if neither provides adequate relief, they may be combined. A mild opioid (e.g., codeine) may also be used. If the less powerful drugs are ineffective, a strong opioid such as morphine may be given. As there is now a wide variety of oral analgesic formulations, injections are seldom necessary to control even the most severe pain.

When treating pain with over-the-counter preparations (e.g., taking aspirin for a headache), you should seek medical advice if the pain persists for longer than 48 hours, recurs, or is worse or different from previous pain.

NON-OPIOID ANALGESICS

Paracetamol This analgesic is believed to act by reducing the production of chemicals called prostaglandins in the brain. It does not affect prostaglandin production in the rest of the body, so it does not reduce inflammation, although it can reduce fever. Paracetamol can be used for aches and pains, such as headache and joint pain. It is given as liquid to treat pain and reduce fever in children.

As well as being the most widely used analgesic, it is one of the safest when taken correctly. It does not usually irritate the stomach, and allergic reactions are rare. However, an overdose can cause severe and possibly fatal liver or kidney damage. The toxic potential of paracetamol may be increased in heavy drinkers.

Non-steroidal anti-inflammatory drugs (NSAIDs):
Aspirin Used for many years to relieve pain and reduce fever, aspirin also reduces inflammation by blocking the production of prosta-

glandins, which contribute to the swelling and pain in inflamed tissue. It is useful for headaches, toothache, mild rheumatic pain, sore throat, and the discomfort of feverish illnesses. Given regularly, it can also relieve the pain and inflammation of chronic rheumatoid arthritis (see Antirheumatic drugs, p.50).

Aspirin is often combined with other substances in a variety of medicines (see Cold cures, p.26). It is also used in the treatment of some blood disorders, since it helps to prevent abnormal clotting (see Drugs that affect blood clotting, p.36). For this reason, it is sometimes unsuitable for people whose blood does not clot normally.

Aspirin in the form of soluble tablets, dissolved in water before being taken, is absorbed into the bloodstream more quickly, thereby relieving pain faster than tablets. Soluble aspirin is not, however, less irritating to the stomach lining. Aspirin is available in many forms, all of which have a similar effect but, because the amount of aspirin in a tablet of each type varies, it is important to read the packet for the correct dosage. It is not recommended for children aged under 12 years because its use has been linked to Reye's syndrome, a rare but potentially fatal liver and brain disorder.

Other NSAIDs These drugs can relieve both pain and inflammation. NSAIDs are related to aspirin and also work by blocking the production of prostaglandins. They are most commonly used to treat muscle and joint pain and may also be prescribed for menstrual pain. For further information on these drugs, see p.48.

COMBINED ANALGESICS

Mild opioids, such as codeine, are often found in combination preparations with non-opioids, such as NSAIDs or paracetamol. The prefix "co-" is used to denote a drug combination. These mixtures may combine the advantages of analgesics that act through two different pathways. Another advantage of combining analgesics is that the reductions in dose of the components may reduce the side effects of the preparation. Combinations can be helpful in reducing the number of tablets taken during long-term treatment.

OPIOID ANALGESICS

These drugs are related to opium, an extract of poppy seeds. They act directly on several sites in the central nervous system involved in pain perception and block the transmission of pain signals. Because they act directly on the parts of the brain where pain is perceived, opioids are the strongest analgesics and are therefore used to treat the pain arising from surgery, serious injury, and cancer. These drugs are particularly valuable for relieving severe pain during terminal illnesses. In addition, their ability to produce a state of relaxation and euphoria is often of help in relieving the stress that accompanies severe pain. Morphine is the best known opioid analgesic. Others include diamorphine (heroin) and pethidine. The use of these powerful opioids is strictly controlled because the euphoria produced can lead to abuse and addiction. When these opioids are given under medical supervision to treat severe pain, the risk of addiction is negligible.

Opioid analgesics may prevent clear thought and cloud consciousness. Other possible adverse effects include nausea, vomiting, constipation, drowsiness, and depressed breathing. Taken in overdose, these drugs may induce a deep coma and lead to fatal breathing difficulties.

In addition to the powerful opioids, some less powerful drugs in this group, such as dihydrocodeine, dextropropoxyphene, and codeine, are used to relieve mild to moderate pain. Their normally unwanted side effects of depressing respiration and causing constipation make them useful as cough suppressants (p.25) and antidiarrhoeal drugs (p.42).

LOCAL ANAESTHETICS

These drugs are used to prevent pain, usually in minor surgical procedures (for example, dental treatment and stitching cuts). They can also be injected into the space around the spinal cord to numb the lower half of the body. This use is called spinal or epidural anaesthesia and can be used for some major operations in people who are not fit for a general anaesthetic. Local anaesthetics are also used for childbirth.

Local anaesthetics block the passage of nerve impulses at the site of administration,

deadening all feeling conveyed by the nerves they come into contact with. They do not interfere with consciousness, however. Local anaesthetics are usually given by injection but can also be applied to the skin, mouth, and other areas lined with mucous membrane (such as the vagina), or the eye to relieve pain. Some local anaesthetics are formulated for injection together with epinephrine (adrenaline). Epinephrine constricts the blood vessels and prevents the local anaesthetic from being removed. This action prolongs the anaesthetic's effect.

Local anaesthetic creams are often used to numb the skin before injections in children and those people with a fear of needles.

COMMON DRUGS

Opioids Co-codamol, Co-codaprin, Codeine*, Co-dydramol, Co-proxamol*, Morphine*, Dipipanone, Fentanyl, Meptazinol, Methadone*, Morphine*, Pentazocine, Pethidine, Phenazocine, Tramadol*

NSAIDs (see p.48) Aspirin*, Diclofenac*, Etodolac, Fenbufen, Fenoprofen, Ibuprofen*, Indomethacin, Ketoprofen*, Ketorolac, Mefenamic acid*, Naproxen*, Piroxicam*

Other non-opioids Nefopam, Paracetamol*
* See part 2

Sleeping drugs

Difficulty in getting to sleep or staying asleep (insomnia) has many causes. Most people suffer from sleepless nights from time to time, usually as a result of a temporary worry or discomfort from a minor illness. Persistent sleeplessness can be caused by psychological problems, including anxiety or depression, or the pain and discomfort of a physical disorder.

WHY THEY ARE USED

For occasional sleeplessness, simple, common remedies, such as a warm bath or a hot milk drink before bedtime, promote relaxation and are usually the best treatment. Sleeping drugs (also known as hypnotics) are normally prescribed only when self-help remedies have failed and lack of sleep is beginning to affect your general health. They are used to re-establish the habit of sleeping and should be used in the smallest dose and for the shortest possible time (not more than three weeks). It is best not to use them every night (see Risks and special precautions, right). Do not use alcohol to help you sleep; it can cause disturbed sleep and insomnia. Long-term treatment of sleeplessness depends on resolving the underlying cause.

TYPES OF SLEEPING DRUG

Benzodiazepines are the most commonly used class of sleeping drugs because they have comparatively few adverse effects and are relatively safe in overdose. They are also used to treat anxiety (see p.13).

Barbiturates are now rarely used because of the risks of abuse, dependence, and toxicity in overdose. There is also a risk of prolonged sedation ("hangover").

Chloral derivatives are sometimes prescribed for the elderly. These drugs may irritate the stomach, causing nausea and vomiting.

Zopiclone and zolpidem are non-benzodiazepine sleeping drugs that work in a similar way to benzodiazepines. They are not intended for long-term use, and withdrawal symptoms have been reported.

Antihistamines are widely used to treat allergic symptoms (see p.56). Because they also cause drowsiness, they are sometimes used to promote sleep in children and the elderly.

Antidepressant drugs may be used to promote sleep in depressed people (see p.14), as well as being effective in treating underlying depressive illness.

HOW THEY WORK

Most sleeping drugs promote sleep by depressing brain function. They interfere with chemical activity in the brain and nervous system by reducing communication between nerve cells. This leads to reduced brain activity, allowing you to fall asleep more easily, but the nature of the sleep is affected by the drug. The benzodiazepines are the main class of sleeping drug.

HOW THEY AFFECT YOU

A sleeping drug rapidly produces drowsiness and slowed reactions. Some people find that that the drug makes them appear drunk, with slurred speech, especially if they delay going to bed after taking their dose. Most people find that they usually fall asleep within an hour of taking the drug.

Because drug-induced sleep is not the same as normal sleep, many people find they do not feel as well rested by it as by a night of natural sleep. This is the result of suppressed brain activity. Sleeping drugs also suppress the sleep during which dreams occur, and both dream sleep and non-dream sleep are essential components of a good night's sleep.

Some people experience a variety of "hangover" effects the following day. Some benzodiazepines may produce minor side effects such as daytime drowsiness, dizziness, and unsteadiness that can impair the ability to drive or operate machinery. Elderly people are especially likely to become confused; for them, selection of an appropriate drug is particularly important.

RISKS AND SPECIAL PRECAUTIONS

Sleeping drugs become less effective after the first few nights, and it may be tempting to increase the dose. Apart from the antihistamines, most sleeping drugs can produce psychological and physical dependence when they are taken regularly for more than a few weeks, especially if larger-than-normal doses are taken.

When sleeping drugs are suddenly withdrawn, anxiety, convulsions, and hallucinations sometimes occur. Nightmares and vivid dreams may be a problem because the time spent in dream sleep increases. Sleeplessness will recur and may lead to a temptation to use sleeping drugs again. Anyone who wishes to stop taking sleeping drugs, particularly after prolonged use, should seek his or her doctor's advice to prevent these withdrawal symptoms from occurring.

COMMON DRUGS

Benzodiazepines Loprazolam, Lormetazepam, Nitrazepam, Temazepam*
Barbiturate Amobarbital
Chloral derivatives Chloral betaine, Chloral hydrate
Other non-benzodiazepine sleeping drugs Chlormethiazole, Diphenhydramine, Zolpidem, Zopiclone*
* **See part 2**

Anti-anxiety drugs

A certain amount of stress can be beneficial, providing a stimulus to action. But too much will often result in anxiety, which might be described as fear or apprehension not caused by any real danger.

Clinically, anxiety arises when the balance of certain chemicals in the brain is disturbed. The feelings of fear or apprehension increase brain activity, stimulating the sympathetic nervous system (see Autonomic nervous system, p.8), and often trigger physical symptoms (e.g., breathlessness, shaking, palpitations, digestive distress, and headaches).

WHY THEY ARE USED

Anti-anxiety drugs (also known as anxiolytics or minor tranquillizers) are prescribed to alleviate persistent feelings of tension and nervousness caused by stress or other psychological problems. But these drugs cannot resolve the causes. Tackling the underlying problem through counselling and perhaps psychotherapy offer the best hope of a long-term solution. Anti-anxiety drugs are also used in hospitals to calm and relax people who are undergoing uncomfortable medical procedures.

There are two main classes of drugs for relieving anxiety: benzodiazepines and beta blockers. Benzodiazepines, which are the most widely used, are given as regular treatment for short periods to promote relaxation. Most benzodiazepines have a strong sedative effect, and they help to relieve the insomnia that accompanies anxiety (see also Sleeping drugs, p.11).

Beta blockers are mainly used to reduce the physical symptoms of anxiety, such as shaking and palpitations. These drugs are commonly prescribed for people who feel excessively anxious in certain situations, such as interviews or public appearances.

When anxiety occurs in a person with depression, the anxiety can be treated with an antidepressant drug (see p.14).

HOW THEY WORK

Benzodiazepines and related drugs depress activity in the part of the brain that controls emotion by promoting the action of the neurotransmitter gamma-aminobutyric acid (GABA) which binds to neurons, blocking transmission of electrical impulses and thus reducing communication between brain cells. Benzodiazepines increase the inhibitory effect of GABA on brain cells, preventing the excessive brain activity that causes anxiety.

Buspirone is different from other anti-anxiety drugs; it binds mainly to serotonin (another neurotransmitter) receptors, and it does not cause drowsiness. Its effect is not felt for at least two weeks after treatment has begun.

Beta blockers block the action of a chemical transmitter called norepinephrine (noradrenaline) in the body, reducing the physical symptoms of anxiety. These symptoms are produced by an increase in the activity of the sympathetic nervous system. Sympathetic nerve endings release norepinephrine, which stimulates the heart, digestive system, and other organs. For more information on beta blockers, see p.28.

HOW THEY AFFECT YOU

Benzodiazepines and related drugs reduce feelings of restlessness and agitation, slow mental activity, and often produce drowsiness. They are said to reduce motivation and, if they are taken in large doses, may lead to apathy. They also have a relaxing effect on the muscles, and some benzodiazepines are used specifically for that purpose (see Muscle relaxants, p.52).

Minor adverse effects of these drugs include dizziness and forgetfulness. People who need to drive or operate potentially dangerous machinery should be aware that their reactions may be slowed. Because the brain soon becomes tolerant to their effects, benzodiazepines are usually effective for only a few weeks at a time.

Beta blockers reduce the physical symptoms of anxiety. This in turn may promote greater mental calmness. Because they do not cause drowsiness, they are safer for people who need to drive.

RISKS AND SPECIAL PRECAUTIONS

The benzodiazepines are safe for most people and are not likely to be fatal in overdose. The main risk is psychological and physical dependence, especially for people who take them regularly or when larger-than-average doses have been used. For this reason, they are usually given for courses of two weeks or less. If they have been used for a longer period, they should be withdrawn gradually under medical supervision. If they are stopped suddenly, withdrawal symptoms, such as excessive anxiety, nightmares, and restlessness, may occur.

Benzodiazepines have been abused for their sedative effect, and are therefore prescribed with caution for people with a history of drug or alcohol abuse.

COMMON DRUGS

Benzodiazepines Chlordiazepoxide*, Diazepam*, Lorazepam, Oxazepam
Beta blockers Atenolol*, Oxprenolol, Propranolol*
Other non-benzodiazepines Buspirone, Promazine*
* See part 2

Antidepressant drugs

Occasional sadness or loss of heart are normal and usually pass quickly. But more severe depression, accompanied by despair, lethargy, loss of sex drive, and often poor appetite, may call for medical attention. Such depression can arise from life stresses such as the death of someone close, an illness, or sometimes from no apparent cause.

Three main types of antidepressant are used to treat depression: tricyclic antidepressants (TCAs), selective serotonin re-uptake inhibitors (SSRIs), and monoamine oxidase inhibitors (MAOIs). Treatment usually begins with either a TCA or an SSRI. Both groups of drugs are equally effective.

WHY THEY ARE USED

Minor depression does not usually require drug treatment, and support and help in coming to terms with the cause of the depression is often all that is needed. Moderate or severe depression usually requires drug treatment, which is effective in most cases. Antidepressants may have to be taken for many months. Treatment should not be stopped too soon because symptoms are likely to reappear. When treatment with some types

of antidepressant is stopped, the dose should be reduced gradually over several weeks because withdrawal symptoms may occur if they are stopped suddenly.

TYPES OF ANTIDEPRESSANT

TCAs Some TCAs (e.g., amitriptyline) cause drowsiness, which is useful for sleep problems in depression. TCAs also cause anticholinergic effects (see Drugs that act on the parasympathetic nervous system, p.9), including blurred vision, dry mouth, and urinary difficulties.

SSRIs These drugs generally have fewer side effects than TCAs. The main unwanted effects are nausea and vomiting. Anxiety, headache, and restlessness may also occur.

MAOIs These are especially effective in people who are anxious as well as depressed, or who suffer from phobias.

Lithium Salts of this metallic element are used to treat manic depression (see Antimanic drugs, p.16). They are sometimes used with an antidepressant drug for resistant depression.

Other antidepressants These include venlafaxine, nefazodone, maprotiline, mianserin, and trazodone.

HOW THEY WORK

Normally, the brain cells release sufficient quantities of certain chemicals (known as neurotransmitters) in the brain to stimulate neighbouring cells. The neurotransmitters are constantly reabsorbed into the brain cells where they are broken down by an enzyme called monoamine oxidase.

Depression is thought to be caused by a reduction in the level of neurotransmitters being released. Antidepressants bring these levels back to normal.

TCAs and venlafaxine work by blocking the reabsorption of the neurotransmitters serotonin and norepinephrine (noradrenaline), thereby increasing the level neurotransmitters in the brain.

SSRIs act by blocking the reabsorption of only one neurotransmitter, serotonin.

MAOIs act by preventing the breakdown of neurotransmitters – mainly serotonin and norepinephrine (noradrenaline) – by blocking the action of monoamine oxidase, which breaks them down.

HOW THEY AFFECT YOU

The antidepressant effect of these drugs starts after 10 to 14 days' treatment and it may be six to eight weeks before the full effect is seen. However, side effects may happen at once. Tolerance to these side effects usually occurs and treatment should be continued.

RISKS AND SPECIAL PRECAUTIONS

Overdose can be dangerous: TCAs can produce coma, fits, and disturbed heart rhythm, which may be fatal; MAOIs can also cause muscle spasms and even death. Both are prescribed with caution for people with heart problems or epilepsy.

MAOIs taken with certain drugs or foods rich in tyramine (e.g., cheese, meat, yeast extracts, and red wine) can produce a dramatic rise in blood pressure, with headache or vomiting. People taking MAOIs are given a card that lists prohibited drugs and foods. Apart from moclobemide, MAOIs are used much less frequently today because of this adverse interaction, and SSRIs or TCAs are prescribed in preference to them.

COMMON DRUGS

TCAs Amitriptyline*, Amoxapine, Clomipramine*, Dosulepin*, Doxepin, Imipramine*, Lofepramine*, Nortriptyline, Protriptyline, Trimipramine
SSRIs Citalopram*, Fluoxetine*, Fluvoxamine, Paroxetine*, Sertraline
MAOIs Isocarboxazid, Moclobemide, Phenelzine
Other drugs Flupentixol*, Maprotiline, Mianserin, Mirtazepine, Nefazodone, Reboxetine, Trazodone*, Venlafaxine*, Viloxazine
* **See Part 2**

Antipsychotic drugs

Psychosis is a term used to describe mental disorders that prevent the sufferer from thinking clearly, acting rationally, and recognizing reality. These disorders include schizophrenia, manic depression, and paranoia. Their precise causes are unknown, but several factors, including stress, heredity, and brain injury, may be involved. Temporary psychosis can also arise as a result of alcohol withdrawal or the abuse of mind-altering drugs. A variety

of drugs is used to treat psychotic disorders (see Common drugs, p.16), most of which have similar actions and effects. One exception, lithium, is particularly useful for manic depression (see Antimanic drugs, p.16).

WHY THEY ARE USED

A person with a psychotic illness may recover spontaneously, so a drug will not always be prescribed. Long-term treatment is started only when normal life is seriously disrupted. Antipsychotic drugs (also called major tranquillizers or neuroleptics) do not cure the disorder, but they do help to control symptoms.

By controlling the symptoms of psychosis, antipsychotic drugs enable most sufferers to live in the community and only be admitted to hospital for acute episodes.

The drug given to a particular individual depends on the nature of his or her illness and the expected adverse effects of that drug. Drugs differ in the amount of sedation produced; the need for sedation also influences the choice of drug.

Antipsychotics may also be given to calm or sedate a highly agitated or aggressive person, whatever the cause. Some antipsychotics also have a powerful action against nausea and vomiting (see Anti-emetics, p.21) and are therefore sometimes used as premedication before surgery.

HOW THEY WORK

It is thought that some forms of mental illness are caused by increased communication between brain cells due to overactivity of dopamine, an excitatory chemical. This may disturb normal thought processes and produce abnormal behaviour. Dopamine combines with receptors on the brain cells. Antipsychotic drugs reduce the transmission of nerve signals by binding to these receptors, thereby making the brain cells less sensitive to dopamine. Some new antipsychotic drugs, such as clozapine (see p.182), risperidone (see p.358), and sertindole, also bind to receptors for the chemical serotonin.

HOW THEY AFFECT YOU

Because antipsychotics depress the action of dopamine, they can disturb its balance with acetylcholine, another chemical in the brain.

If an imbalance occurs, extrapyramidal side effects (EPSE) may appear. These include restlessness, movement disorders, and parkinsonism (see Drugs for parkinsonism, p.18). In these circumstances, a change to a different type of antipsychotic may be necessary. If this is not possible, an anticholinergic drug (see Drugs that act on the parasympathetic nervous system, p.9) may be prescribed.

Antipsychotics may block the action of norepinephrine (noradrenaline), another neurotransmitter in the brain. This lowers blood pressure, especially when you stand up, causing dizziness. It may also prevent ejaculation.

RISKS AND SPECIAL PRECAUTIONS

It is important to continue taking these drugs even if all symptoms have gone, because the symptoms are controlled only by taking the prescribed dose.

Because antipsychotic drugs can have permanent as well as temporary side effects, the minimum dosage is used. This is found by starting with a low dose and increasing it until the symptoms are controlled. Sudden withdrawal after more than a few weeks can cause nausea, sweating, headache, and restlessness. Therefore, when treatment needs to be stopped, the dose is reduced gradually.

A major long-term risk of antipsychotic drug treatment is a disorder known as tardive dyskinesia, which may develop after one to five years. It consists of repeated jerking movements of the mouth, tongue, and face, and sometimes the hands and feet. Tardive dyskinesia is less common during treatment with the new antipsychotic drugs than with phenothiazine and butyrophenone drugs.

HOW THEY ARE ADMINISTERED

Antipsychotics may be given by mouth as tablets, capsules, or syrup, or by injection. They can also be given in the form of a depot injection which releases the drug slowly over several weeks. This is helpful for people who might forget to take their drugs or who might take an overdose.

COMMON DRUGS

Phenothiazine antipsychotics Chlorpromazine*, Fluphenazine, Methotrimeprazine, Perphenazine, Pipotiazine, Thioridazine*, Trifluoperazine

Butyrophenone antipsychotics
Benperidol, Droperidol, Haloperidol*
Other antipsychotics Amisulpride/sulpiride*
Clozapine*, Flupentixol*, Olanzapine*, Oxypertine, Pericyazine, Pimozide, Quetiapine*, Risperidone*, Zotepine, Zuclopenthixol
* See part 2

Antimanic drugs

Changes in mood are normal, but when a person's mood swings become grossly exaggerated, with peaks of elation or mania alternating with troughs of depression, it becomes an illness known as manic depression. It is usually treated with salts of lithium (p.278), a drug that reduces the intensity of the mania, lifts the depression, and lessens the frequency of mood swings. Because it can take three weeks for lithium salts to work, an antipsychotic may be prescribed with lithium at first to give immediate relief of symptoms.

Lithium can be toxic if levels of the drug in the blood rise too high. Regular checks on the blood concentration of lithium should therefore be carried out during treatment. Symptoms of lithium poisoning include blurred vision, twitching, vomiting, and diarrhoea.

COMMON DRUGS

Carbamazepine*, Lithium*
* See part 2

Anticonvulsant drugs

Electrical signals from nerve cells in the brain are normally finely coordinated to produce smooth movements of arms and legs, but these signals can become irregular and chaotic and trigger the disorderly muscular activity and mental changes characteristic of a fit (also called a seizure or convulsion). The most common cause of recurrent fits is the disorder known as epilepsy, often as a result of brain disease or injury. In epileptics, fits may be triggered by outside stimuli, such as flashing lights. They can also result from toxic effects of certain drugs and, in young children, a high temperature (febrile convulsions).

Anticonvulsants are used both to reduce the risk of an epileptic fit and to stop one that is in progress.

WHY THEY ARE USED

Isolated convulsions seldom require drug treatment, but anticonvulsants are usually given to prevent or reduce the frequency of epileptic fits. Anticonvulsants permit people with epilepsy to lead a normal life, and they reduce the possibility of brain damage, which can result from recurrent fits.

Most people with epilepsy need to take anticonvulsants on a regular basis to prevent fits. Usually a single drug is used, and treatment may need to be lifelong.

If one drug is not effective, then a different anticonvulsant will be tried. Occasionally, it is necessary to take a combination of drugs. Even when receiving treatment, a person can suffer fits. A prolonged fit can be halted by injection of diazepam or a similar drug.

The selection of anticonvulsant drug depends on the type of epilepsy, but the age and particular response of the individual to drug treatment are also important.

Generalized (grand mal) seizures This type of fit is characterized by a warning sensation, such as flashing lights or a sound, which is followed by a sudden loss of consciousness during which convulsions occur, and the sufferer may lose bowel or bladder control, bite the tongue, or foam at the mouth. The fit usually lasts for a few minutes only but can occasionally last longer. Prolonged attacks that last for over 20 minutes are called status epilepticus and can be fatal without emergency treatment.

The principal drugs used to prevent generalized seizures are phenytoin, sodium valproate, and carbamazepine. Doctors try to avoid prescribing phenytoin for young children because of its unpleasant side effects, which include overgrowth of the gums, acne, and increased body hair. These effects are less prominent in adults. If the patient is still having convulsions when medical help arrives, a benzodiazepine drug such as diazepam is given by injection or enema.

Absence (petit mal) seizures This form of epilepsy most commonly affects children. The fits consist of a momentary loss of consciousness, during which the child may stare off into space. Convulsions do not occur. Sodium valproate, ethosuximide, and, less commonly, clonazepam are used for the prevention of this type of fit.

Partial seizures There are a number of different variations of this form of epilepsy. Most cause a sudden severe disturbance of the senses and/or muscle spasm without loss of consciousness. Phenytoin and carbamazepine are the medicines most commonly prescribed to prevent partial seizures.

HOW THEY WORK

Brain cells bring about body movement by electrical activity that passes through the nerves to the muscles. In an epileptic fit, excessive electrical activity starts in one part of the brain and spreads to other parts, causing uncontrolled stimulation of brain cells. Most of the anticonvulsants have an inhibitory effect on brain cells and damp down electrical activity, preventing the excessive build-up that causes epileptic fits.

HOW THEY AFFECT YOU

Ideally, the only effect an anticonvulsant drug should have is to reduce the frequency of, or prevent, epileptic fits. Unfortunately, no drug prevents fits without potentially affecting normal brain function, leading to poor memory, inability to concentrate, lack of coordination, and lethargy. It is important, therefore, to find a dosage sufficient to prevent fits without causing any unacceptable side effects. The dose has to be carefully tailored to the individual. It is usual to start with a low dose of a selected drug and to increase it gradually until a balance is achieved between the effective control of fits and the occurrence of side effects. Many of these side effects wear off after the first few weeks of treatment.

Blood tests are used to monitor the levels of some anticonvulsant drugs in the body as an aid to dose adjustment. It may be several months before the correct dose is found.

RISKS AND SPECIAL PRECAUTIONS

Each anticonvulsant drug has its own specific adverse effects and risks. In addition, most of these drugs affect the ability of the liver to break down other drugs and may therefore influence the action of other drugs you are taking. Doctors try to prescribe no more than the minimum number of anticonvulsants needed to control the person's fits in order to reduce the risk of such interactions.

Most anticonvulsants have risks for a developing baby – if you are hoping to become pregnant, it is important to discuss the risks, and whether your medication should be changed, with your doctor. People taking anticonvulsants need to be careful to take their medicine regularly as prescribed. If the anticonvulsant levels in the body are allowed to fall suddenly, fits are very likely to occur. The dose should not be reduced or the treatment stopped, except on the advice of a doctor.

If, for any reason, anticonvulsant drug treatment needs to be stopped, the dose should be reduced gradually. People on anticonvulsant therapy are advised to carry an identification tag giving full details of their condition and treatment.

COMMON DRUGS
Carbamazepine*, Clobazam, Clomethiazole, Clonazepam*, Diazepam*, Ethosuximide*, Gabapentin, Lamotrigine*, Lorazepam, Phenobarbital*, Phenytoin*, Piracetam, Primidone*, Sodium valproate*, Tiagabine, Topiramate, Vigabatrin
* See part 2

Drugs for Parkinsonism

Parkinsonism is a general term that is used to describe shaking of the head and limbs, muscular stiffness, an expressionless face, and inability to control or initiate movement. It is caused by an imbalance of chemicals in the brain in which the effect of acetylcholine is increased by a reduction in the action of dopamine.

Parkinsonism has a variety of causes, but the most common is Parkinson's disease, in which there is degeneration of the dopamine-producing cells in the brain. Other causes include side effects of certain drugs, notably antipsychotics (see p.15), and narrowing of blood vessels in the brain.

WHY THEY ARE USED
Drugs can relieve the symptoms of parkinsonism, but unfortunately the degeneration of brain cells in Parkinson's disease cannot be halted, although drugs can minimize symptoms for many years.

HOW THEY WORK
Drugs treat parkinsonism by restoring the balance between dopamine and acetylcholine. There are two main groups: those that reduce the effect of acetylcholine (anticholinergics) and those that boost the effect of dopamine.

Anticholinergics combine with receptors on brain cells, preventing acetylcholine from binding to them. This action reduces acetylcholine's relative overactivity and restores the balance with dopamine.

Dopamine cannot pass from the blood to the brain and cannot therefore be given to boost its levels in the brain. Levodopa (L-dopa), the chemical from which it is naturally produced in the brain, is combined with carbidopa or benserazide to prevent it from being converted to dopamine before it reaches the brain. Amantadine (also used as an antiviral, see p.67) boosts levels of dopamine in the brain by stimulating its release. The action of dopamine can also be boosted by other drugs, including bromocriptine, lisuride, or apomorphine (injection only), which mimic the action of dopamine.

CHOICE OF DRUG
Anticholinergics are often effective in the early stages of Parkinson's disease and are used to treat parkinsonism due to antipsychotic drugs, which have dopamine-blocking properties. L-dopa is usually given when the disease impairs walking. Its effectiveness usually wanes after two to five years, in which case other dopamine-boosting drugs may also be prescribed.

COMMON DRUGS
Anticholinergic drugs Benzhexol, Benztropine, Biperiden, Orphenadrine*, Procyclidine*
Dopamine-boosting drugs Amantadine*, Apomorphine, Bromocriptine*, Cabergoline, Levodopa*, Lisuride, Pergolide, Pramipexole, Ropinirole, Selegiline
* See part 2

Drugs for Dementia

Dementia is a progressive decline in mental function that is severe enough to affect normal social or occupational activities. It usually develops gradually and may be a feature of a number of disorders, including poor circulation in the brain, multiple sclerosis, and Alzheimer's disease. A great deal of research is in progress on the cause of Alzheimer's disease, which is the single most common cause of dementia.

WHY THEY ARE USED
Drugs called acetylcholinesterase inhibitors have been found to lessen the symptoms of dementia in Alzheimer's disease, but they do not prevent its long-term progression.

HOW THEY WORK
In healthy people, acetylcholinesterase (an enzyme in the brain) breaks down the neurotransmitter acetylcholine, balancing its levels and limiting its effects. In Alzheimer's disease, there is a deficiency of acetylcholine. Acetylcholinesterase inhibitors block the action of acetylcholinesterase, raising the levels of acetylcholine in the brain, thereby increasing alertness and slowing the rate of deterioration.

HOW THEY AFFECT YOU
Following assessment of mental function by a specialist, drug treatment is started at a low dose and increased gradually to minimize side effects. Any improvements should begin to appear in about 3 weeks. Assessment is repeated after 3 months to see if the treatment has been beneficial. About half of those people treated show some improvement.

RISKS AND SPECIAL PRECAUTIONS
It is important to continue taking these drugs because there is a gradual loss of improvement after they are stopped. Side effects include urinary difficulties, nausea, vomiting, and diarrhoea.

COMMON DRUGS
Acetylcholinesterase inhibitors Donepezil*, Rivastigmine*
* See part 2

Nervous system stimulants

A person's state of mental alertness varies throughout the day and is under the control of chemicals in the brain. Some of these chemicals are depressant, causing drowsiness, and others are stimulant, which heightens awareness.

Increased activity of the depressant chemicals is thought to be responsible for a condition called narcolepsy, which is a tendency to fall asleep during the day for no obvious reason. In this case, nervous system stimulants are given to increase wakefulness. These drugs include the amphetamines (usually dexamfetamine), the related drug methylphenidate, and modafinil. Apart from their use in treating narcolepsy, amphetamines are no longer used because of the risk of dependence. The most common home remedy for increasing alertness is caffeine, a mild stimulant present in coffee, tea, and cola.

WHY THEY ARE USED
In adults who suffer from narcolepsy, some of these drugs prevent excessive drowsiness during the day. Stimulants do not cure narcolepsy and, since the disorder lasts throughout the sufferer's lifetime, may have to be taken indefinitely. Methylphenidate is also occasionally given to children suffering from attention deficit disorder. Stimulants have also been used as part of the treatment for obesity because reduced appetite is a side effect of amphetamines. Phentermine is a drug related to amfetamine but with a more modest stimulant action. It is used (for a maximum of 3 months) to promote weight loss in severe cases of obesity.

Caffeine is added to some analgesics to counteract the effects of caffeine withdrawal which can cause headaches, but no clear medical justification exists for this.

Respiratory stimulants such as doxapram are related to caffeine and are used to improve breathing. They act on the the respiratory centre – the part of the brain that controls breathing. They are sometimes used in hospitals to help people who have difficulty in breathing, mainly very young babies and adults with severe lung disease.

Apart from their use in narcolepsy, nervous system stimulants are not useful in the long term because the brain soon develops tolerance to them.

HOW THEY WORK

The level of wakefulness is controlled by a part of the brain stem called the reticular activating system (RAS). Activity in this area depends on the balance between chemicals, some of which are excitatory (including norepinephrine (noradrenaline) and some of which are inhibitory, such as gamma aminobutyric acid (GABA). Stimulants promote release of noradrenaline increasing activity in the RAS and other parts of the brain, thereby raising alertness.

HOW THEY AFFECT YOU

In adults, the central nervous system stimulants taken in the prescribed dose for narcolepsy increase wakefulness, thereby allowing normal concentration and thought processes to occur. They may also reduce appetite and cause tremors. In hyperactive children, they reduce the general level of activity to a more normal level and increase the attention span.

RISKS AND SPECIAL PRECAUTIONS

Some people, especially the elderly or those with previous psychiatric problems, are particularly sensitive to stimulants and may experience adverse effects, even when the drugs are given in comparatively low doses. They need to be used with caution in children because, taken for prolonged periods, they can retard growth. An excess of these drugs given to a child may depress the nervous system, producing drowsiness or even loss of consciousness. Palpitations may also occur.

These drugs reduce the level of natural stimulants in the brain, so after regular use for a few weeks a person may become physically dependent on them for normal function. If they are abruptly withdrawn, the excess of natural inhibitory chemicals in the brain depresses central nervous system activity, producing withdrawal symptoms. These may include lethargy, depression, increased appetite, and difficulty staying awake.

Stimulants can produce overactivity in the brain if they are used inappropriately or in excess, resulting in extreme restlessness, sleeplessness, nervousness, or anxiety. These drugs also stimulate the sympathetic branch of the autonomic nervous system (see p.9), causing shaking, sweating, and palpitations. More serious risks of exceeding the prescribed dose are fits and a major disturbance in mental functioning that may result in delusions and hallucinations. Because these drugs have been abused, amphetamines and methylphenidate are classified as controlled drugs.

COMMON DRUGS

Respiratory stimulants Doxapram, Theophylline/aminophylline*
Other drugs Caffeine, Methylphenidate, Modafinil
* **See part 2**

Drugs used for Migraine

Migraine is a term applied to recurrent severe headaches affecting only one side of the head and caused by changes in the blood vessels around the brain and scalp. They may be accompanied by nausea and vomiting and preceded by warning signs, usually an impression of flashing lights or numbness and tingling in the arms. Occasionally, speech may be impaired, or the attack may be disabling. The cause of migraine is unknown, but an attack may be triggered by a blow to the head, physical exertion, certain foods and drugs, or emotional factors such as excitement, tension, or shock. A family history of migraine also increases the chance of an individual suffering from it.

WHY THEY ARE USED

Drugs are used either to relieve symptoms of migraine or to prevent attacks. Different drugs are used in each approach, but none cures the underlying disorder. However, a susceptibility to migraine headaches can clear up spontaneously and, if you are taking drugs regularly, your doctor may recommend that you stop them after a few months to see if this has happened.

In most people, migraine headaches can be relieved by a mild analgesic (painkiller), for example, paracetamol or aspirin, or a stronger one like codeine (see Analgesics, p.9). If nausea and vomiting accompany the migraine, tablets may not be absorbed sufficiently from the gut. Absorption can be increased if drugs are taken as soluble tablets in water or with an anti-emetic.

Some drugs used to relieve attacks can be given by injection, inhaler, nasal spray, or suppository. Preparations that contain caffeine should be avoided since headaches may be caused by excessive use or on stopping treatment. Ergotamine or 5HT$_1$ agonist drugs (such as sumatriptan) are used if analgesics are not effective.

The factors that trigger an individual's attacks should be identified, in order for them to be avoided. Anti-anxiety drugs are not usually prescribed if stress is a precipitating factor because of the potential for dependence. If the attacks occur more often than once a month, drugs to prevent migraine may be taken every day. Drugs used to prevent migraine are propranolol (a beta blocker, see p.345) or pizotifen (an antihistamine, see p.334, and serotonin blocker). Other drugs that have been used include amitriptyline (an antidepressant, see p.134), clonidine, methysergide (which is given under hospital supervision), cyproheptadine, nifedipine (see p.315), and verapamil (see p.396).

HOW THEY WORK

A migraine attack begins when blood vessels surrounding the brain constrict (become narrower), producing the typical migraine warning signs. The constriction is thought to be caused by certain chemicals found in food or produced by the body. The neurotransmitter serotonin causes large blood vessels in the brain to constrict. Pizotifen and propranolol block the effect of chemicals on blood vessels and thereby prevent attacks.

The next stage of a migraine attack occurs when blood vessels in the scalp and around the eyes dilate (widen). As a result, chemicals called prostaglandins are released, producing pain. Aspirin and paracetamol relieve this pain by blocking prostaglandins. Codeine acts directly on the brain, altering pain

perception (see Analgesics, p.9). Ergotamine and 5HT$_1$ agonists relieve pain by narrowing dilated blood vessels in the scalp.

HOW THEY AFFECT YOU

Each drug has its own adverse effects. 5HT$_1$ agonists may cause drowsiness and chest tightness. Ergotamine may cause drowsiness, tingling sensations in the skin (paraesthesia), cramps, and weakness in the legs; and vomiting may be made worse. Pizotifen may cause drowsiness and weight gain. Clonidine may disturb sleep. For the effects of propranolol, see p.345, and for analgesics, see p.9.

RISKS AND SPECIAL PRECAUTIONS

5HT$_1$ agonists should not usually be used by people with high blood pressure, angina, or coronary heart disease. Ergotamine can damage blood vessels by prolonged overconstriction, so it should be used with caution by those with poor circulation. Excessive use of 5HT$_1$ agonists can lead to dependence and many adverse effects, including headache. You should not take more than your doctor advises in any one week.

HOW THEY ARE ADMINISTERED

These drugs are usually taken by mouth as tablets or capsules. Sumatriptan can also be taken as an injection or a nasal spray. Ergotamine can be taken by aerosol inhalation, as suppositories, or as tablets that dissolve under the tongue.

COMMON DRUGS

Drugs to prevent migraine Amitriptyline*,
Clonidine, Cyproheptadine, Methysergide,
Nifedipine*, Pizotifen*, Propranolol*, Verapamil*
5HT$_1$ agonists Naratriptan, Rizatriptan,
Sumatriptan*, Zolmitriptan
Other drugs to relieve migraine Aspirin*,
Codeine*, Dihydroergotamine, Ergotamine*,
Isometheptene, Paracetamol*, Tolfenamic acid
* **See part 2**

Anti-emetics

Drugs used to treat or prevent vomiting or the feeling of sickness (nausea) are known as anti-emetics. Vomiting is a reflex action for getting rid of harmful substances, but it may also be a symptom of disease. Vomiting and nausea are often caused by travel sickness, a digestive tract infection, pregnancy, or vertigo (a balance disorder involving the inner ear that causes a sensation of things turning around). They can also occur as a side effect of some drugs, especially those that are used in cancer treatment, radiation therapy, or general anaesthesia.

Commonly used anti-emetics include metoclopramide, domperidone, cyclizine, haloperidol, ondansetron, granisetron, prochlorperazine, and promethazine; the antihistamine cinnarizine is also commonly used. The phenothiazine and butyrophenone drug groups are also used as antihistamines (see p.56) and to treat some types of mental illness (see Antipsychotic drugs, p.15).

WHY THEY ARE USED

Doctors usually diagnose the cause of vomiting before prescribing an anti-emetic because vomiting may be due to an infection of the digestive tract or some other condition of the abdomen that might require treatment such as surgery. Treating only the vomiting and nausea might delay diagnosis, correct treatment, and recovery.

Anti-emetics may be taken to prevent travel sickness (using one of the antihistamines), vomiting resulting from anticancer (see p.94) and other drug treatments (using metoclopramide, haloperidol, domperidone, ondansetron, and prochlorperazine, for example). The anti-emetic prochlorperazine, betahistine, or an anti-anxiety drug (see p.13) are usually used to treat Ménière's disease, a disorder in which excess fluid builds up in the inner ear, causing vertigo, noises in the ear, and gradual deafness; a diuretic (see p.30) may also be given to reduce the excess fluid in the ear. Anti-emetics are also used to help the nausea in vertigo and are occasionally also used to relieve cases of severe vomiting occurring during pregnancy. You should not take an anti-emetic during pregnancy except on medical advice.

No anti-emetic drug should be taken for longer than a couple of days without consulting your doctor.

HOW THEY WORK

Nausea and vomiting occur when the vomiting centre in the brain is stimulated by signals from three places in the body: the digestive tract, the part of the inner ear controlling balance, and the brain itself through thoughts and emotions and via its chemoreceptor trigger zone, which responds to harmful substances in the blood. Anti-emetic drugs may act at one or more of these places. Some help the stomach to empty its contents into the intestine. A combination may be used that works at different sites and has an additive effect.

HOW THEY AFFECT YOU

As well as treating vomiting and nausea, many anti-emetic drugs may make you feel drowsy. However, to help prevent travel sickness on long journeys, a sedating antihistamine may be an advantage.

Some anti-emetics (in particular, antihistamines and phenothiazines) can block the parasympathetic nervous system (see Autonomic nervous system, p.8), causing a dry mouth, blurred vision, or difficulty in passing urine. The phenothiazines may also lower blood pressure, leading to dizziness or fainting.

RISKS AND SPECIAL PRECAUTIONS

Because some antihistamines can make you drowsy, it may be advisable not to drive while taking them. Phenothiazines, butyrophenones, and metoclopramide can produce uncontrolled movements of the face and tongue, so they are used with caution in people with parkinsonism.

COMMON DRUGS

Antihistamines Cinnarizine*, Cyclizine, Dimenhydrinate, Meclozine, Promethazine*

Phenothiazines Chlorpromazine*, Perphenazine, Prochlorperazine*

5HT$_3$ antagonists Granisetron, Ondansetron* Tropisetron

Butyrophenones Haloperidol*

Other drugs Betahistine*, Domperidone*, Hyoscine hydrobromide*, Metoclopramide*, Nabilone

* **See part 2**

RESPIRATORY SYSTEM

The respiratory system consists of the lungs and the air passages leading to them. Through the process of inhaling and exhaling air (breathing), the body obtains the oxygen necessary for survival, and expels carbon dioxide, the waste product of the basic human biological process.

Air enters the trachea (windpipe), which branches into two main bronchi, one for each lung. Within the lungs, the air passes into bronchioles, smaller tubes whose muscular walls may contract or dilate in response to drugs and nerve signals. The bronchioles open out into tiny, blood-vessel lined air sacs (alveoli) which allow oxygen to pass into the bloodstream and carbon dioxide to pass from the bloodstream for expiration.

WHAT CAN GO WRONG

Difficulty in breathing may be due to narrowing of the air passages from spasm, as in asthma and bronchitis, or swelling of the linings of the air passages, as in bronchiolitis and bronchitis. Breathing difficulties may also be due to infection of the lung tissue, as in pneumonia and bronchitis, or damage to the alveoli from smoking or inhaled dusts or moulds, which cause emphysema, pneumoconiosis and farmer's lung. Smoking and air pollution can affect the respiratory system as irritants and toxins, leading to diseases such as lung cancer and bronchitis.

Sometimes difficulty in breathing may be due to congestion of the lungs from heart disease, an inhaled object such as a peanut, or infection or inflammation of the throat. Symptoms of breathing difficulties often include a cough and a tight feeling in the chest.

WHY DRUGS ARE USED

Drugs with a variety of actions are used to clear the air passages, soothe inflammation, and reduce the production of mucus. Some can be bought without a prescription as single- or combined-ingredient preparations, often with an analgesic (see p.9).

Decongestants (p.24) reduce the swelling inside the nose, thereby making it possible to breathe more freely. If the cause of the congestion is an allergic response, an antihistamine (p.56) is often recommended to relieve symptoms or to prevent attacks. Infections of the respiratory tract are usually treated with antibiotics (p.60).

Bronchodilators (see below) are drugs that widen the bronchi. Used to relieve or prevent asthma attacks, this group includes drugs that relax the muscles around the airways, and corticosteroids (p.78) that reduce both inflammation and the narrowing of airways. Other drugs, such as sodium cromoglycate, may be used for treating allergies and preventing asthma attacks but they are not effective once an asthma attack has begun.

A variety of drugs are used to relieve a cough, depending on the type of cough involved. Some drugs make it easier to eliminate phlegm; others suppress the cough by inhibiting the cough reflex.

MAJOR DRUG GROUPS

◆ Bronchodilators
◆ Decongestants
◆ Drugs to treat coughs
◆ See also sections on Allergy (p.56) and Infections (p.59)

Bronchodilators

Air entering the lungs passes through narrow tubes called bronchioles. In bronchitis and asthma, the bronchioles become narrower, either as a result of contraction of the muscles in their walls, or as a result of mucus congestion. This narrowing of the bronchioles obstructs the flow of air into and out of the lungs and causes breathlessness.

Bronchodilators are prescribed to widen the bronchioles and improve breathing. There are three main groups of bronchodilator: sympathomimetics, anticholinergics, and xanthine drugs, which are related to caffeine.

Inhaling a bronchodilator drug directly into the lungs is the best way of getting benefit without excessive side effects. Devices for delivering the drug into the airways are described on page 24.

Inhalers or puffers release a small dose when they are pressed, but they require some skill to use effectively. A large hollow plastic "spacer" can help you to inhale your drug more easily.

Insufflation cartridges deliver larger amounts of drug than inhalers, and, as well as being almost as effective, are easier to use because the drug is taken in as you breathe normally.

Nebulizers pump compressed air through a solution of drug to produce a fine mist which is inhaled through a face mask. They deliver large doses of the drug to the lungs, rapidly improving breathing.

WHY THEY ARE USED

Bronchodilators help to dilate the bronchioles of people suffering from asthma and bronchitis. However, they are of little benefit to those people suffering from severe chronic bronchitis.

Bronchodilators can either be taken when they are needed, in order to relieve an attack of breathlessness that is in progress, or on a regular basis to prevent such attacks from occurring. Some people find it helpful to take an extra dose of their bronchodilator immediately before undertaking any activity that is likely to provoke an attack of breathlessness. A patient who requires treatment with a sympathomimetic inhaler more than once daily should see his or her doctor about preventative treatment with an inhaled corticosteroid. Sympathomimetic drugs are mainly used for the rapid relief of breathlessness; anticholinergic and xanthine drugs are used long term.

HOW THEY WORK

Bronchodilator drugs act by relaxing the muscles surrounding the bronchioles. Sympathomimetic and anticholinergic drugs achieve this by interfering with nerve signals that are passed to the muscles through the autonomic nervous system (see p.8). Xanthine drugs are thought to relax the muscle in the bronchioles by having a direct effect on the muscle fibres, but their precise action is not known.

Bronchodilator drugs usually improve breathing within a few minutes of administration. Corticosteroids usually start to increase the sufferer's capacity for exercise within a few days, and most people find that the frequency of their attacks of breathlessness is reduced.

Because sympathomimetics stimulate a branch of the autonomic nervous system that controls heart rate, they may sometimes cause palpitations and trembling. Typical side effects of anticholinergics include dry mouth, blurred vision, constipation, and difficulty in passing urine. Xanthine drugs may cause headaches and nausea, but these effects can usually be controlled by regulating the dosage.

RISKS AND SPECIAL PRECAUTIONS

Since most bronchodilators are not taken by mouth, but via inhalers (see left), they do not commonly cause serious side effects. However, because of their possible effect on the heart rate, xanthine and sympathomimetic drugs need to be prescribed with caution to people with heart problems, high blood pressure, or an overactive thyroid gland. The anticholinergic drugs may not be suitable for people with urinary retention or those who have a tendency to glaucoma.

COMMON DRUGS

Sympathomimetics Bambuterol, Eformoterol, Ephedrine*, Epinephrine*, Fenoterol, Reproterol, Salbutamol*, Salmeterol*, Terbutaline*, Tulobuterol
Anticholinergics Ipratropium bromide*, Oxitropium
Xanthines Theophylline/aminophylline*
Corticosteroids Beclometasone*, Budesonide*, Fluticasone*, Prednisolone*
Other drugs Antihistamines (see p.56), Ketotifen, Nedocromil, Sodium cromoglicate*
* See Part 2

Decongestants

The usual cause of a blocked nose is swelling of the delicate mucous membrane that lines the nasal passages, and excessive production of mucus as a result of inflammation. This swelling and inflammation may be caused by an infection, such as a common cold, or to an allergy to, for example, pollen – a condition known as allergic rhinitis or hay fever. Congestion can also occur in the sinuses (the air spaces in the skull), resulting in sinusitis. Decongestants are drugs that reduce the swelling of the mucous membrane and suppress the production of mucus, helping to clear blocked nasal passages and sinuses. Antihistamines (see p.56) counter the allergic response in allergy-related conditions. If the symptoms are persistent, either topical corticosteroids (see p.116) or sodium cromoglycate (p.366) may be preferred.

WHY THEY ARE USED

Most common colds and blocked noses do not need to be treated with decongestants. Simple home remedies such as steam inhalation, possibly with the addition of an aromatic oil such as menthol or eucalyptus, are often effective. Decongestants are used when such measures are ineffective or when there is a particular risk from untreated congestion – for example, in people who suffer from recurrent middle-ear or sinus infections.

Decongestants are available in the form of drops or sprays applied directly into the nose (topical decongestants), or they can be taken by mouth. Small quantities of decongestant drugs are added to many over-the-counter cold remedies (see Cold cures p.26).

HOW THEY WORK

When the mucous membrane lining the nose is irritated by infection or allergy, the blood vessels supplying the membrane become enlarged. This leads to fluid accumulation in the surrounding tissue and encourages the production of larger-than-normal amounts of mucus.

Most decongestants belong to the sympathomimetic group of drugs that stimulate the sympathetic branch of the autonomic nervous system (see p.9). One effect of this action is to constrict the blood vessels, thereby reducing swelling of the lining of the nose and sinuses.

HOW THEY AFFECT YOU

When applied topically in the form of drops or sprays, these drugs start to relieve congestion within a few minutes. Decongestants by mouth take a little longer to act, but their effect may also last longer. Used in moderation, topical decongestants have few adverse

effects, because they are not absorbed by the body in large amounts.

Used for too long or in excess, topical decongestants can, after giving initial relief, do more harm than good, causing a "rebound congestion". This can happen when decongestant nose drops and sprays are withdrawn or overused. The result is a sudden increase in congestion due to widening of the blood vessels in the nasal lining because blood vessels are no longer constricted by the decongestant. Rebound congestion can be prevented by taking the minimum effective dose and by using decongestant preparations only when absolutely necessary. Decongestants taken by mouth do not cause rebound congestion but are more likely to cause other side effects; they have been linked with strokes.

COMMON DRUGS

Used topically Ephedrine*, Ipratropium bromide*, Xylometazoline, Oxymetazoline, Phenylephrine
Taken by mouth Ephedrine*, Phenylephrine, Phenylpropanolamine*, Pseudoephedrine
* See Part 2

Drugs to treat coughs

Coughing is a natural response to irritation of the lungs and air passages that is designed to expel harmful substances from the respiratory tract. Common causes of coughing include infection of the respiratory tract (e.g., bronchitis or pneumonia), inflammation of the airways caused by asthma, or exposure to certain irritant substances such as smoke or chemical fumes. Depending on their cause, coughs may be productive – that is, phlegm-producing – or dry.

In most cases coughing is a helpful reaction that assists the body in ridding itself of excess phlegm and substances that irritate the respiratory system; suppressing a cough may delay recovery. However, repeated bouts of coughing can be distressing and may increase irritation. In such cases, medication to ease the cough may be recommended.

There are two main groups of cough remedies, according to whether the cough is productive or dry.

PRODUCTIVE COUGHS

Mucolytics and expectorants are sometimes recommended for productive coughs when simple home remedies such as steam inhalation have failed to "loosen" the cough and make it easier to cough up phlegm. Mucolytics alter the consistency of the phlegm, making it less sticky and easier to cough up. These drugs are often given by inhalation. However, there is little evidence that they are effective. Dornase alfa may be given to people who suffer from cystic fibrosis; the drug, which is inhaled via a nebulizer, is an enzyme that improves lung function by thinning the mucus. Expectorant drugs, such as ammonium chloride, are taken by mouth to loosen a cough. There is some evidence that guaifenesin is effective. Expectorants are included in many over-the-counter cough remedies.

DRY COUGHS

In dry coughs there is no advantage to be gained from promoting the expulsion of phlegm. Drugs used for dry coughs are given to suppress the coughing mechanism by calming the part of the brain that governs the coughing reflex. Antihistamines are often given for mild coughs, particularly in children. A demulcent, such as a simple linctus, can be used to soothe a dry, irritating cough. For persistent coughs, mild opioid drugs such as codeine may be prescribed (see also Analgesics, p.9). All cough suppressants have a generally sedating effect on the brain and nervous system and commonly cause drowsiness and other side effects.

SELECTING A COUGH MEDICATION

There is a bewildering variety of over-the-counter medications available for treating coughs. Most consist of a syrupy base to which active ingredients and flavourings are added. Many contain a number of different active ingredients, sometimes with contradictory effects: it is not uncommon to find an expectorant (for a productive cough) and a cough suppressant (for a dry cough) included in the same preparation.

Cough medicines, although soothing, are not often beneficial and can be harmful. For example, using a cough suppressant for the relief of a productive cough may prevent you from getting rid of excess infected phlegm and may delay your recovery. It is best to choose a preparation with a single active ingredient that is appropriate for your type of cough. Diabetics may need to select a sugar-free product. If you are in any doubt about which medication to select, ask your doctor or pharmacist for advice. Because there is a danger that use of over-the-counter cough remedies to alleviate symptoms may delay the diagnosis of a more serious underlying disorder, it is important that you seek medical advice for any cough that persists for longer than a few days or if a cough is accompanied by additional symptoms such as fever or blood in the phlegm.

COLD CURES

Many preparations are available over the counter to treat different symptoms of the common cold. The main ingredient in most of these preparations is a mild analgesic, such as aspirin or paracetamol, accompanied by a decongestant (p.24), an antihistamine (p.56), and sometimes caffeine. In some cases, the dose of each added ingredient is too low to provide any benefit. There is no evidence to suggest that vitamin C (see p.88) speeds recovery, but zinc supplements (see p.91) may be effective in shortening the duration of the cold, however.

While some people find these drugs help to relieve symptoms, over-the-counter cold cures do not alter the course of the illness. Most doctors recommend using a product with a single analgesic as the best way of alleviating symptoms. Other decongestants or antihistamines may be taken if needed. These medicines are not harmless, and care should be taken to to avoid overdose if different brands are used.

COMMON DRUGS

Expectorants Ammonium chloride, Guaifenesin
Mucolytics Carbocysteine, Dornase alfa, Mecysteine
Steam inhalation Eucalyptus, Menthol
Opioid cough suppressants Codeine*, Dextromethorphan, Pholcodine
Non-opioid cough suppressants Antihistamines (see p.56)
* **See Part 2**

HEART AND CIRCULATION

The blood transports oxygen, nutrients, and heat, contains chemical messages in the form of drugs and hormones, and carries away waste products for excretion by the kidneys. It is pumped by the heart through the lungs, and then in a separate circuit to the rest of the body, including the brain, digestive organs, muscles, kidneys, and skin.

The heart is a pump with four chambers – two atria and two ventricles. The atrium and ventricle on the left side pump oxygenated blood to the body, while those on the right pump deoxygenated blood to the lungs. Backflow of blood is stopped by one-way valves at the chamber exits. Arteries carry blood away from the heart. Their muscle walls are elastic, contracting and dilating in response to nerve signals. Veins carry blood back to the heart. Their walls are thinner and less elastic than those of arteries.

WHAT CAN GO WRONG

The efficiency of the circulation may be impaired by weakening of the heart's pumping action (heart failure), too fast a heart rate (tachycardia), or irregularity of the heart rate (arrhythmia). In addition, the blood vessels may be narrowed and clogged by fatty deposits (atherosclerosis). This may reduce blood supply to the brain, extremities (peripheral vascular disease), or heart muscle (coronary heart disease), causing angina. These last disorders can be complicated by the formation of clots that may block a blood vessel. A clot in the arteries supplying the heart muscle is known as coronary thrombosis; a clot in an artery inside the brain (cerebral thrombosis) is the most frequent cause of stroke.

One common circulatory disorder is abnormally high blood pressure (hypertension), in which the pressure of circulating blood on the blood vessel walls is increased for reasons not yet fully understood. One factor may be loss of elasticity of the vessel walls (arteriosclerosis). Several other conditions, such as migraine and Raynaud's disease, are caused by temporary alterations to blood vessel size.

WHY DRUGS ARE USED

Because people suffering from heart disease often have more than one problem, several drugs may be prescribed at once. Many act directly on the heart to alter the rate and rhythm of the heart beat. These drugs are known as anti-arrhythmics and include beta blockers and digoxin.

Other drugs affect the diameter of the blood vessels by either dilating them (vasodilators) to improve the blood flow and reduce blood pressure, or by constricting them (vasoconstrictors).

Drugs may also reduce blood volume and fat levels, and alter its clotting ability. Diuretics (used in the treatment of hypertension and heart failure) increase the body's excretion of water. Lipid-lowering drugs reduce the levels of cholesterol in the blood, thereby minimizing the risk of atherosclerosis. Drugs to reduce blood clotting are administered if there is a risk of abnormal blood clots forming in the heart, veins, or arteries. Drugs that increase clotting are given when the body's natural clotting mechanism is defective.

MAJOR DRUG GROUPS

◆ Digitalis drugs
◆ Beta blockers
◆ Vasodilators
◆ Diuretics
◆ Anti-arrhythmics
◆ Anti-angina drugs
◆ Antihypertensive drugs
◆ Lipid-lowering drugs
◆ Drugs that affect blood clotting

Digitalis drugs

Digitalis is the collective term for the naturally occurring substances (also called cardiac glycosides) found in the leaves of plants of the foxglove family and used to treat certain heart disorders. The principal drugs in this group are digoxin and digitoxin. Digoxin is more commonly used because it is shorter acting and dosage is easier to adjust (see also Risks and special precautions, p.28).

WHY THEY ARE USED

Digitalis drugs do not cure heart disease, but they improve the heart's pumping action and thereby relieve many of the symptoms that result from poor heart function. They are useful for treating conditions in which the heart beats irregularly or too rapidly (notably in atrial fibrillation, see Anti-arrhythmics, p.32), when it pumps too weakly (in congestive heart failure) or the heart muscle is damaged and weakened following a heart attack.

Digitalis drugs can be used for a short period when the heart is working poorly but have to be taken indefinitely in many cases. Their effect does not diminish with time. In heart failure, these drugs are often given together with a diuretic drug (see p.30).

HOW THEY WORK

The normal heart beat results from electrical impulses generated in nerve tissue within the heart. These cause the heart muscle to contract and pump blood. By reducing the flow of electrical impulses in the heart, digitalis makes the heart beat more slowly.

The force with which the heart muscle contracts depends on chemical changes in the heart muscle. By promoting these chemical changes, digitalis increases the force of muscle contraction each time the heart is stimulated. This compensates for the loss of power that occurs when some of the muscle is damaged following a heart attack. The stronger heart beat increases blood flow to the kidneys. This increases urine production and helps to remove the excess fluid that often accumulates as a result of heart failure.

HOW THEY AFFECT YOU

Digitalis relieves the symptoms of heart failure – fatigue, breathlessness, and swelling of the legs – and increases your capacity for exercise. The frequency with which you need to pass urine is also increased initially.

RISKS AND SPECIAL PRECAUTIONS

Digitalis drugs can be toxic and, if blood levels of the drugs rise too high, they may produce symptoms of digitalis poisoning. These include loss of appetite, nausea, vomiting, diarrhoea, confusion, and visual disturbance. If such symptoms occur, it is important that you to report them to your doctor promptly.

Digoxin is normally removed from the body by the kidneys; if kidney function is impaired, the drug is more likely to accumulate in the body and cause toxic effects. Digitoxin, which is broken down in the liver, is sometimes preferred in such cases. If liver function is severely impaired, digitoxin can accumulate after repeated dosage.

Both digoxin and digitoxin are more toxic when blood potassium levels are low. Potassium deficiency is commonly caused by diuretics. Therefore, people taking diuretics at the same time as digitalis drugs need to have the effects of both drugs, and their blood potassium levels, carefully monitored. They may be required to take potassium supplements.

COMMON DRUGS

Digitoxin, Digoxin*
* **See part 2**

Beta blockers

Beta blockers are drugs that interrupt the transmission of stimuli through the beta receptors of the body. Since the actions they block originate in the adrenal glands (and elsewhere), they are also sometimes called beta adrenergic blocking agents. There are two types of beta receptor in the body: beta 1 and beta 2. Beta 1 receptors are located mainly in the heart muscle; beta 2 receptors are found both in the airways and blood vessels. Cardioselective drugs act mainly on beta 1 receptors; non-cardioselective drugs act on both types of receptor. Used mainly in heart disorders, these drugs are occasionally prescribed for other conditions.

WHY THEY ARE USED

Beta blockers are used for treating angina (see p.33), hypertension (see p.34), and irregular heart rhythms (see p.32). They are usually given after a heart attack to reduce the likelihood of abnormal heart rhythms or further damage to the heart muscle. Beta blockers are also prescribed to improve heart function in heart muscle disorders (which are called cardiomyopathies).

Beta blockers may also be given to prevent migraine headaches (see p.20); and they are sometimes prescribed to reduce the physical symptoms of anxiety (see p.13). These drugs may be given to control symptoms of an overactive thyroid gland. A beta blocker is sometimes given in the form of eye drops to lower the fluid pressure inside the eye that occurs in glaucoma (see p.110).

HOW THEY WORK

By occupying the beta receptors in different parts of the body, beta blockers nullify the stimulating action of norepinephrine (noradrenaline), the main "fight or flight" hormone. Blocking the transmission of signals through beta receptors produces a wide variety of benefits and side effects depending on the disease being treated.

Heart Slowing of the heart rate and reduction of the force of the heart beat reduces the workload of the heart, helping to prevent angina and abnormal heart rhythms. This action may worsen heart failure, however.

Lungs Constriction of the airways may provoke breathlessness in asthmatics or those people with chronic bronchitis.

Brain Dilation of the blood vessels that surround the brain is inhibited, thereby preventing migraine.

Blood vessels Constriction of the blood vessels may cause coldness of the hands and feet.

Blood pressure The blood pressure is lowered because the rate and force at which the heart pumps blood into the circulatory system is reduced.

Eye Beta blocker eye drops reduce fluid production, thereby lowering pressure inside the eye.

Muscles Muscle tremor as a result of anxiety or overactivity of the thyroid gland is reduced.

HOW THEY AFFECT YOU

Beta blockers are taken to treat angina. They reduce the frequency and severity of attacks. As part of the treatment for hypertension, they help to lower the blood pressure and thus reduce the risks that are associated with this condition. Beta blockers help to prevent severe attacks of arrhythmia, in which the heart beat is wild and uncontrolled.

Because beta blockers affect many parts of the body, they often produce minor side effects. By reducing the heart rate and air flow to the lungs, they may reduce the capacity for strenuous exercise. This is unlikely to be noticed by somebody whose physical activity was previously limited by heart problems, however. Many people taking these drugs experience cold hands and feet as a result of a reduction in the blood supply to the limbs. Reduced circulation can, rarely, lead to temporary impotence during treatment.

RISKS AND SPECIAL PRECAUTIONS

The main risk of beta blockers is that of provoking breathing difficulties as a result of their blocking effect on beta receptors in the lungs. Cardioselective beta blockers act mainly on the heart and are thought to be less likely than non-cardioselective ones to cause such problems. But all beta blockers are prescribed with caution to people with asthma, bronchitis, or other forms of respiratory disease.

Beta blockers are not commonly prescribed to people who have poor circulation in the limbs because they reduce blood flow and may aggravate such conditions. Though helpful in small doses, large doses are not normally given to people who are subject to heart failure because they may further reduce the force of the heart beat. Diabetics needing to take beta blockers should be aware that they may notice a change in the warning signs of low blood sugar; in particular, they may find that symptoms such as palpitations and tremor are suppressed.

Beta blockers should not be stopped suddenly after prolonged use; this may provoke a sudden and severe recurrence of symptoms of the original disorder, even a heart attack. The blood pressure may also rise markedly. When treatment with beta blockers needs to be stopped, it should be withdrawn gradually under medical supervision.

COMMON DRUGS

Cardioselective Atenolol*, Betaxolol, Bisoprolol, Celiprolol, Metoprolol*

Non-cardioselective Acebutolol, Carvedilol, Labetalol, Nadolol, Pindolol, Propranolol*, Sotalol*, Timolol*

* **See part 2**

Vasodilators

Vasodilators are drugs that widen blood vessels. Their most obvious use is to reverse narrowing of blood vessels when this leads to reduced blood flow and, consequently, a lower oxygen supply to parts of the body. Vasodilators are often used to treat high blood pressure (hypertension) and angina because a widening of the body's blood vessels reduces the heart's workload.

WHY THEY ARE USED

Vasodilators improve blood flow and thus the oxygen supply to areas of the body where they are most needed. In angina, dilation of the blood vessels throughout the body reduces the force with which the heart needs to pump and thereby eases its workload (see also Anti-angina drugs, p.33). This may also be helpful in treating congestive heart failure when other treatments are not effective.

Because blood pressure is partly dependent on the diameter of blood vessels, vasodilators are often helpful in treating hypertension (see p.34).

In peripheral vascular disease, narrowed blood vessels in the legs cannot supply sufficient blood to the extremities, often leading to pain in the legs during exercise. Unfortunately, because the vessels are narrowed by atherosclerosis, vasodilators have little effect.

Vasodilators have also been used to treat senile dementia, in the hope of increasing the oxygen supply to the brain, but the benefits of this treatment have not yet been proved.

HOW THEY WORK

Vasodilators widen blood vessels by relaxing the muscles surrounding them. They achieve this either by directly affecting the action of the muscles (nitrates, calcium channel blockers, and hydralazine) or by interfering with the nerve signals that govern contraction of the blood vessels (alpha blockers). ACE (angiotensin-converting enzyme) inhibitors are powerful vasodilators that block the action of an enzyme in the bloodstream that is responsible for converting a chemical called angiotensin I into angiotensin II. Angiotensin II encourages constriction of the blood vessels; its absence permits them to dilate.

HOW THEY AFFECT YOU

As well as relieving the symptoms of the disorders for which they are taken, vasodilators can have many minor side effects related to their action on the circulation. Flushing and headaches are common at the start of treatment; and dizziness and fainting may also occur as a result of lowered blood pressure. Dilation of blood vessels can also cause a build-up of fluid, leading to swelling, particularly of the ankles.

RISKS AND SPECIAL PRECAUTIONS

The major risk is that blood pressure may fall too low, and this can lead to dizziness on standing because the blood vessels cannot contract to prevent pooling of the blood in the legs. Therefore vasodilators are prescribed with caution for people with unstable blood pressure. It is also advisable to sit or lie down after taking the first dose of a vasodilator.

COMMON DRUGS

ACE inhibitors Captopril*, Cilazapril, Enalapril*, Fosinopril*, Lisinopril*, Moexipril, Perindopril, Quinapril, Ramipril*, Trandolapril
Potassium channel activators Nicorandil*
Alpha blockers Doxazosin*, Indoramin, Prazosin*, Terazosin
Calcium channel blockers Amlodipine*, Diltiazem*, Felodipine, Isradipine, Lacidipine, Lercanidipine, Nicardipine, Nifedipine*, Verapamil*
Angiotensin II blockers Candesartan, Irbesartan*, Losartan*, Valsartan
Nitrates Glyceryl trinitrate*, Isosorbide dinitrate/mononitrate*
Other drugs Hydralazine, Minoxidil*
* See part 2

Diuretics

Diuretic drugs help to turn excess body water into urine. As the urine is expelled, two disorders are relieved: oedema is relieved as the tissues become less water-swollen, and the heart action improves because it has to pump a smaller volume of blood. There are several classes of diuretic, each of which has different uses, modes of action, and effects. But all diuretics act on the kidneys, the organs that govern the body's water content.

WHY THEY ARE USED

Diuretics are most commonly used in the treatment of high blood pressure (hypertension). By removing a larger amount of water than usual from the bloodstream, the kidneys reduce the total volume of blood circulating. It is thought that this drop in volume causes a reduction of the pressure within the blood vessels (see Antihypertensive drugs, p.34).

Diuretics are also widely used to treat heart failure (in which the heart's pumping mechanism has become weak). In the treatment of this disorder, they remove fluid that has accumulated in the tissues and lungs. The resulting drop in blood volume reduces the work of the heart.

Other conditions for which diuretics are often prescribed include nephrotic syndrome (a kidney disorder that causes oedema), liver cirrhosis (in which fluid may accumulate in the abdominal cavity), and premenstrual syndrome (when hormonal activity can lead to fluid retention and bloating).

Less commonly, diuretics are used to treat glaucoma (see p.110) and Ménière's disease. (See also Anti-emetics, p.22).

TYPES OF DIURETIC

Thiazides The most commonly prescribed diuretics, thiazides are often given with potassium supplements, or in conjunction with a potassium-sparing diuretic (see below), because they may lead to potassium deficiency.

Loop diuretics These fast-acting, powerful drugs increase urine output for a few hours and are therefore sometimes used in emergencies. They can cause excessive potassium loss, which may need to be countered as for thiazides.

Potassium-sparing diuretics These mild diuretics are usually used in conjunction with a thiazide or a loop diuretic to prevent excessive loss of potassium.

Osmotic diuretics Prescribed only rarely, osmotics are used to maintain the flow of urine through the kidneys after surgery or injury, and to reduce pressure rapidly in the brain or the eye.

Acetazolamide This mild diuretic is used principally in the treatment of glaucoma (see p.110).

HOW THEY WORK

The normal filtration process of the kidneys removes water, salts (mainly potassium and sodium), and waste products from the bloodstream. Most of the salts and water are subsequently returned to the bloodstream, but some are expelled from the body along with the waste products in the urine. Diuretics interfere with this process by reducing the amount of sodium and water taken back into the bloodstream, thereby increasing the volume of urine produced. Modifying the filtration process in this way means that the water content of the blood is reduced; less water in the blood causes excess water present in the tissues to be drawn out and eliminated in urine.

HOW THEY AFFECT YOU

All diuretics increase the frequency with which you need to pass urine, most noticeably at the start of treatment. People who have had oedema may notice reduction in swelling, particularly of the ankles; and those with heart failure may find that breathlessness is relieved.

RISKS AND SPECIAL PRECAUTIONS

Diuretics can cause blood chemical imbalances, of which hypokalaemia (a fall in potassium levels) is the most common. Hypokalaemia can cause confusion and weakness and can trigger abnormal heart rhythms (especially in people taking digitalis drugs). Potassium supplements or a potassium-sparing diuretic usually corrects the imbalance. A potassium rich diet (containing plenty of fresh fruits and vegetables) may be helpful.

Some diuretics may raise blood levels of uric acid, increasing the risk of gout. They may also raise blood sugar levels, causing problems for diabetics. The thiazides can cause impotence.

COMMON DRUGS

Loop diuretics Bumetanide*, Ethacrynic acid, Furosemide*, Torasemide

Potassium-sparing diuretics Amiloride*, Spironolactone*, Triamterene*

Thiazides Bendroflumethiazide*, Chlorothiazide, Chlortalidone, Cyclopenthiazide*, Hydrochlorothiazide*, Hydroflumethiazide, Indapamide*, Mefruside, Metolazone, Polythiazide, Xipamide

* **See part 2**

Anti-arrhythmics

The heart contains two upper and two lower chambers, which are known as the atria and ventricles (see p.27). The pumping actions of these two sets of chambers are normally coordinated by electrical impulses that originate in the heart's pacemaker and then travel along conducting pathways so that the heart beats with a regular rhythm. If this coordination breaks down, the heart will beat abnormally, either irregularly or faster or slower than usual. The general term for abnormal heart rhythm is arrhythmia.

Arrhythmias may occur as a result of a birth defect, coronary heart disease, or other less common heart disorders. A variety of more general conditions, including an overactive thyroid gland, and certain drugs, such as caffeine and anticholinergic drugs, can also disturb heart rhythm.

Arrhythmias can be divided into two groups: tachycardias (such as atrial fibrillation), in which the heart rate is faster than normal; and bradycardias (such as heart block), in which the rate is slower.

Atrial fibrillation In this common type of arrhythmia, the atria contract irregularly at such a high rate that the ventricles cannot keep pace. The condition is treated with digoxin, sometimes in combination with other drugs.

Ventricular tachycardia This condition arises from abnormal electrical activity in the ventricles that causes the ventricles to contract rapidly. Regular treatment with quinidine, disopyramide, or procainamide is usually given. Amiodarone may be used if these drugs are not effective.

Supraventricular tachycardia This condition occurs when extra electrical impulses arise in the pacemaker or atria. These extra impulses stimulate the ventricles into contracting rapidly. Attacks may disappear on their own without treatment, but drugs such as adenosine, digoxin, verapamil, or propranolol may be given.

Heart block When impulses are not conducted from the atria to the ventricles, the ventricles start to beat at a slower rate. Some cases of heart block do not require treatment. For more severe heart block accompanied by

dizziness and fainting, the fitting of an artificial pacemaker is usually necessary.

A wide range of drugs, including beta blockers, calcium channel blockers, and digitalis drugs, is used to regulate heart rhythm. Lignocaine, disopyramide, procainamide, and quinidine are also used.

WHY THEY ARE USED

Minor disturbances of heart rhythm are common and do not usually require drug treatment. However, if the heart's pumping action is seriously affected, the circulation of blood throughout the body may become inefficient, and drug treatment may be necessary.

Drugs may be taken to treat individual attacks of arrhythmia, or they may be taken on a regular basis to prevent or control abnormal heart rhythms. The particular drug prescribed depends on the type of arrhythmia to be treated but, because people differ in their response, it may be necessary to try several in order to find the most effective one. When the arrhythmia is sudden and severe, it may be necessary to inject a drug immediately to restore normal heart function.

HOW THEY WORK

The heart's pumping action is governed by electrical impulses under the control of the sympathetic nervous system (see Autonomic nervous system, p.8). These signals pass through the heart muscle, causing the two pairs of chambers – the atria and ventricles – to contract in turn.

All anti-arrhythmic drugs alter the conduction of electrical signals in the heart. However, each drug or drug group has a different effect on the sequence of events controlling the pumping action. Some block the transmission of signals to the heart (beta blockers); some affect the way in which signals are conducted within the heart (digitalis drugs); others affect the response of the heart muscle to the signals received (calcium channel blockers, disopyramide, procainamide, and quinidine).

HOW THEY AFFECT YOU

Anti-arrhythmics usually prevent the symptoms of arrhythmia and may restore a regular heart rhythm. Although they do not prevent all arrhythmias, they usually reduce the frequency and severity of any symptoms.

As well as suppressing arrhythmias, many of these drugs tend to depress normal heart function and may produce dizziness on standing, or increased breathlessness on exertion. Mild nausea and visual disturbance are also fairly frequent. Verapamil can cause constipation, especially when prescribed in high doses. Disopyramide may interfere with the parasympathetic nervous system (see Autonomic nervous system, p.8), resulting in a number of anticholinergic effects.

RISKS AND SPECIAL PRECAUTIONS

These drugs, in certain circumstances, may further disrupt heart rhythm and are used only when the likely benefit outweighs the risks.

Quinidine can be toxic if an overdose is taken, resulting in a syndrome called cinchonism, which includes disturbed hearing, giddiness, and impaired vision (even blindness). Because some people are particularly sensitive to this drug, a test dose is usually given before regular treatment is started.

Amiodarone may, over time, accumulate in the tissues and may lead to light-sensitive rashes, changes in thyroid function, and liver and lung problems.

COMMON DRUGS

Beta blockers (See p.28)
Calcium channel blockers Verapamil*
Digitalis drugs Digitoxin, Digoxin*,
Other drugs Adenosine, Amiodarone*, Bretylium, Disopyramide, Flecainide, Lignocaine, Mexiletine, Moracizine, Procainamide, Propafenone, Quinidine
* **See part 2**

Anti-angina drugs

Angina is chest pain that is produced when insufficient oxygen reaches the heart muscle. This is usually due to narrowing of the vessels (coronary arteries) that carry blood and oxygen to the heart muscle. In the most common type of angina (classic angina), the pain usually occurs during physical exertion or emotional stress. The pain may also occur at rest (variant angina). In classic angina, the narrowing of the coronary arteries results

from fat deposits (atheroma) on the artery walls. In the variant type, however, it is caused by contraction (spasm) of the muscle fibres in the artery walls. Pain not relieved by drugs may mean that a heart attack is imminent (unstable angina) and emergency treatment is needed.

Atheroma deposits build up more rapidly in the arteries of smokers and people who eat a high-fat diet. This is why, as a basic component of angina treatment, doctors recommend that smoking should be given up and the diet changed. Overweight people are also advised to lose weight in order to reduce the demands placed on the heart. While such changes in lifestyle often produce an improvement in symptoms, drug treatment to relieve angina is also frequently necessary.

The drugs used to treat angina include beta blockers, nitrates, calcium channel blockers, and potassium channel openers.

WHY THEY ARE USED

Frequent episodes of angina can be disabling and, if left untreated, can lead to increased risk of a heart attack. Drugs can both relieve angina attacks and reduce their frequency. People who suffer only occasional episodes are usually prescribed a rapid-acting drug to take at the first signs of an attack, or before an activity known to bring on an attack; glyceryl trinitrate is a rapid-acting drug that is usually prescribed for this purpose.

If the attacks become more frequent or more severe, regular preventative treatment may be advised. Beta blockers, calcium channel blockers, and long-acting nitrates are used as regular medication to prevent attacks. The introduction of adhesive patches to administer nitrates through the patient's skin has extended the duration of action of glyceryl trinitrate, making treatment easier.

Drugs can often control angina for many years, but they cannot cure the disorder. When severe angina cannot be controlled by drugs, then surgery to increase the blood flow to the heart may be recommended.

HOW THEY WORK

Nitrates and calcium channel blockers dilate blood vessels by relaxing the muscle layer in the blood vessel walls (see also Vasodilators, p.30). Blood is more easily pumped through the dilated vessels, reducing the strain on the heart.

Beta blockers protect the heart muscle from excessive stimulation by norepinephrine (noradrenaline) during exercise or stress by interrupting signal transmission in the heart. Decreased heart muscle stimulation means that less oxygen is required, reducing the risk of angina attacks. For further information on beta blockers, see p.28.

HOW THEY AFFECT YOU
Treatment with one or more of these medicines usually controls angina effectively. Drugs to prevent attacks allow sufferers to undertake more strenuous activities without provoking pain, and if an attack does occur, nitrates usually provide effective relief.

These drugs do not usually cause serious adverse effects, but they can produce a variety of minor symptoms. By dilating blood vessels throughout the body, the nitrates and calcium channel blockers can cause dizziness (especially on standing up) and may cause fainting. Other possible side effects are throbbing headaches at the start of treatment, flushing of the skin (especially of the face), and ankle swelling. Beta blockers often cause cold hands and feet, and they may sometimes produce tiredness and a feeling of heaviness in the legs.

COMMON DRUGS
Beta blockers (see p.28)
Calcium channel blockers Amlodipine*, Diltiazem*, Nicardipine, Nifedipine*
Nitrates Glyceryl trinitrate*, Isosorbide dinitrate/mononitrate*
Potassium channel opener Nicorandil*
Other drugs Aspirin*, Simvastatin* Heparin*
* **See part 2**

Antihypertensive drugs

Blood pressure is a measurement of the force exerted by the blood circulating in the arteries. Two readings are taken: one indicates force while the heart's ventricles are contracting (systolic pressure). This reading is a higher figure than the other one, which

measures the blood pressure during ventricle relaxation (diastolic pressure). Blood pressure varies among individuals, and in each person from moment to moment; it is lower at night, higher with stress or exercise, and normally increases with age. If a person's blood pressure is higher than normal on at least three separate occasions, a doctor may diagnose the condition as hypertension.

Blood pressure may be elevated as a result of an underlying disorder, which the doctor will try to identify. Usually, however, it is not possible to determine a cause. This condition is referred to as essential hypertension.

Although hypertension does not usually cause any symptoms, severely raised blood pressure may produce headaches, palpitations, and general feelings of ill-health. It is important to reduce high blood pressure because it can have serious consequences, including stroke, heart attack, heart failure, and kidney damage. Certain groups are at particular risk from high blood pressure. These risk groups include diabetics, smokers, people with pre-existing heart damage, and those whose blood contains a high level of fat. High blood pressure is more common in black people than whites, and in countries where the diet is high in salt. Processed foods are high in salt, and this contributes to high blood pressure.

A small reduction in blood pressure may be brought about by reducing weight, exercising regularly, and reducing the amount of salt in the diet. But for more severely raised blood pressure, one or more antihypertensives may be prescribed. Several classes of drugs have antihypertensive properties, including the centrally acting antihypertensives, diuretics (p.30), beta blockers (p.28), calcium channel blockers (p.33), ACE (angiotensin-converting enzyme) inhibitors (see Vasodilators, p.30), and alpha blockers.

WHY THEY ARE USED
Antihypertensive drugs are prescribed when diet, exercise, and other simple remedies have not reduced blood pressure adequately, and your doctor sees a risk of serious consequences if the condition is not treated. These drugs do not cure hypertension and usually have to be taken indefinitely. However, it is

sometimes possible to taper off drug treatment when blood pressure has been reduced to normal for a year or more.

HOW THEY WORK
Blood pressure depends, not only on the force with which the heart pumps blood, but also on the diameter of blood vessels and the volume of blood in circulation. It is increased either if the vessels are narrow or the volume of blood is high. Antihypertensive drugs lower blood pressure either by dilating the blood vessels or by reducing blood volume. Each type of antihypertensive acts in a different way to lower blood pressure.

Centrally acting drugs act on the mechanism in the brain that controls the diameter of the blood vessels.

Beta blockers reduce the force of the heart beat.

Diuretics act on the kidneys to reduce blood volume.

ACE inhibitors act on enzymes in the blood to dilate blood vessels.

Vasodilators and calcium channel blockers act on the arterial wall muscles to prevent constriction.

Alpha blockers block nerve signals that trigger constriction of blood vessels

CHOICE OF DRUG
Drug treatment depends on the severity of hypertension. At the start of treatment for mild or moderately high blood pressure, a single drug is used. A thiazide diuretic or beta blocker is often chosen initially, but it is also increasingly common to use a calcium channel blocker or ACE inhibitor. If a single drug does not reduce the blood pressure sufficiently, a diuretic in combination with one of the other drugs may be used. Some people who have moderate hypertension require a third drug, in which case a vasodilator, centrally acting antihypertensive, or alpha blocker, may also be prescribed.

Severe hypertension can usually be controlled using a combination of several drugs, which may need to be given in high doses. Your doctor may need to try a number of drugs before finding a combination that controls your blood pressure without causing unacceptable side effects.

HOW THEY AFFECT YOU
Treatment with antihypertensive drugs relieves symptoms such as headache and palpitations. However, since most people with hypertension have few, if any, symptoms, side effects may be more noticeable than any immediate beneficial effect. Some antihypertensive drugs may cause dizziness and fainting at the start of treatment because they can sometimes cause and excessive fall in blood pressure. It may take a while for your doctor to determine a dosage that avoids such effects. For detailed information on adverse effects of drugs used to treat hypertension, see the individual drug profiles in part 2.

RISKS AND SPECIAL PRECAUTIONS
Since your doctor needs to know exactly how treatment with a particular drug affects your hypertension – the benefits as well as the side effects – it is important for you to keep using the medication as prescribed, even though you may feel the problem is under control. Sudden withdrawal of some antihypertensive drugs may cause a potentially dangerous rebound increase in blood pressure. To stop treatment, the dose needs to be reduced gradually under medical supervision.

COMMON DRUGS
ACE inhibitors (see Vasodilators, p.30)
Beta blockers (see p.28)
Calcium channel blockers (see Anti-angina drugs, p.33)
Centrally acting antihypertensives Clonidine, Methyldopa*, Moxonidine*
Diuretics (see p.30)
Alpha blockers Doxazosin*, Prazosin, Terazosin
* **See part 2**

Lipid-lowering drugs

The blood contains several types of fats, or lipids. These are necessary for normal body function but can be damaging if they are present in excess, particularly cholesterol. The main risk is atherosclerosis, in which fatty deposits called atheroma build up in the arteries, restricting and disrupting the flow of blood. This can increase the likelihood of the formation of abnormal blood clots, leading to potentially fatal disorders such as stroke and heart attack.

For most people, reducing their fat intake lowers the risk of atherosclerosis. However, those with an inherited tendency to high levels of fat in the blood (hyperlipidaemia) may also be prescribed lipid-lowering drugs.

WHY THEY ARE USED

Lipid-lowering drugs are usually prescribed only when dietary measures have failed to control hyperlipidaemia. The drugs may be given at an earlier stage to individuals at increased risk of atherosclerosis – such as diabetics and people already suffering from circulatory disorders. They are also given to people who have had a heart attack to help prevent further attacks. The drugs may remove existing atheroma in the blood vessels and prevent accumulation of new deposits.

For maximum benefit, these drugs are used in conjunction with a low-fat diet and a reduction in other risk factors such as obesity and smoking. The choice of drug depends on the type of lipid causing problems, so a full medical history, examination, and laboratory analysis of blood samples are needed before drug treatment is prescribed.

HOW THEY WORK

Cholesterol and triglycerides are two of the major fats in the blood. One or both may be raised, influencing the choice of lipid-lowering drug. Bile salts contain a large amount of cholesterol and are normally released into the bowel to aid digestion before being reabsorbed into the blood. Drugs that bind to bile salts reduce cholesterol levels by blocking their reabsorption, allowing them to be lost from the body.

Other drugs act on the liver by altering the way in which the liver converts fatty acids in the blood into different types of lipids. Fibrates and nicotinic acid and its derivatives can reduce the level of both cholesterol and triglycerides in the blood. Statins and probucol lower blood cholesterol. Fish oil preparations reduce blood triglycerides, but they may raise cholesterol levels.

Lipid-lowering drugs do not correct the underlying cause of raised levels of fat in the blood, so it is usually necessary to continue with diet and drug treatment indefinitely. Stopping treatment usually leads to a return of high blood lipid levels.

HOW THEY AFFECT YOU

Because hyperlipidaemia and atherosclerosis are usually symptomless, you are unlikely to notice any short-term benefits from these drugs. Rather, the aim of treatment is to reduce long-term complications. There may be minor side effects from some of these drugs.

By increasing the amount of bile in the digestive tract, several drugs can cause gastrointestinal disturbances such as nausea and constipation or diarrhoea, especially at the start of treatment. The statin drugs appear to be well tolerated and are widely used to lower cholesterol levels when diet alone does not have sufficient effect.

RISKS AND SPECIAL PRECAUTIONS

Drugs that bind to bile salts can limit the absorption of some fat-soluble vitamins, and vitamin supplements may therefore be needed. The fibrates can increase susceptibility to gallstones and can occasionally upset the balance of fats in the blood. Statins are used with caution in people with reduced kidney or liver function, and monitoring of blood samples is often advised.

COMMON DRUGS

Fibrates Bezafibrate*, Ciprofibrate, Fenofibrate, Gemfibrozil
Statins Atorvastatin*, Fluvastatin, Pravastatin*, Simvastatin*
Drugs that bind to bile salts Colestyramine*, Colestipol, Ispaghula
Nicotinic acid and derivatives Acipimox, Nicotinic acid
Other drugs acting on the liver Omega-3 marine triglycerides
* **See part 2**

Drugs that affect blood clotting

When bleeding occurs from injury or surgery, the body normally acts swiftly to stem the flow by sealing the breaks in the blood vessels.

This occurs in two stages: when cells called platelets accumulate as a plug at the opening in the blood vessel wall, then when these platelets produce chemicals that activate clotting factors in the blood to form a protein called fibrin. Vitamin K plays an important role in this process. An enzyme in the blood called plasmin ensures that clots are broken down when the injury has been repaired.

Some disorders interfere with this process, either preventing clot formation or creating clots uncontrollably. If the blood does not clot, there is a danger of excessive blood loss. Inappropriate development of clots may block the supply of blood to a vital organ.

DRUGS USED TO PROMOTE BLOOD CLOTTING

Fibrin formation depends on the presence in the blood of several clotting-factor proteins. When Factor VIII is absent or at low levels, an inherited disease called haemophilia exists; the symptoms almost always appear only in males. Factor IX deficiency causes the bleeding condition called Christmas disease, named after the person in whom it was first identified. Lack of these clotting factors can lead to uncontrolled bleeding or excessive bruising following even minor injuries.

Regular drug treatment for haemophilia is not normally required. But if severe bleeding or bruising occurs, a concentrated form of the missing factor, extracted from normal blood, may be injected to promote clotting and thereby halt bleeding. Injections may need to be repeated for several days after injury.

It is sometimes useful to promote blood clotting in non-haemophiliacs when bleeding is difficult to stop (for example, after surgery). In such cases, blood clots are sometimes stabilized by reducing the action of plasmin with an antifibrinolytic (or haemostatic) drug like tranexamic acid; this is also occasionally given to haemophiliacs before minor surgery such as tooth extraction.

A tendency to bleed may also occur with deficiency of vitamin K, which is required for the production of several blood clotting factors. It is absorbed from the intestine in fats, but some diseases of the small intestine or pancreas cause fat to be poorly absorbed. As a result, the level of vitamin K in the circulation is low, causing impaired blood clotting. A similar problem sometimes occurs in newborn babies due to absence of vitamin K. Injections of phytomenadione, a vitamin K preparation, are used to restore levels to normal.

DRUGS USED TO PREVENT ABNORMAL BLOOD CLOTTING

Blood clots normally form only as a response to injury. In some people, however, there is a tendency for clots to form in the blood vessels without apparent cause. Damage to blood vessels that occurs as a result of the presence of fatty deposits (atheroma) inside them increases the risk of the formation of this type of abnormal clot (a thrombus). In addition, a portion of a blood clot (an embolus) formed in response to injury or surgery may sometimes break off and be removed in the bloodstream. The likelihood of this happening is increased by long periods of little or no activity. When an abnormal clot forms, there is a risk that it may become lodged in a blood vessel and block the blood supply to a vital organ such as the brain or heart.

Three main types of drugs are used to prevent and disperse clots: antiplatelet drugs, anticoagulants, and thrombolytics.

ANTIPLATELET DRUGS

Taken regularly by people with a tendency to form clots in the fast-flowing blood of the heart and arteries, these drugs are also given to prevent clots from forming after heart surgery. They reduce the tendency of platelets to stick together when the blood flow is disrupted.

The most widely used antiplatelet drug is aspirin (see also Analgesics, p.9), which has an antiplatelet action even when given in much lower doses than would be needed to reduce pain. In these low doses, adverse effects that may occur when aspirin is given in pain-relieving doses are unlikely. Other antiplatelet drugs are clopidogrel and dipyridamole.

ANTICOAGULANTS

Anticoagulant drugs help to maintain normal blood flow in people at risk from clot formation. They can either prevent the formation of blood clots in the veins or stabilize an existing clot so that it does not break away and become a circulation-stopping embolism. All anticoagulant drugs reduce the activity of certain blood clotting factors, although the mode of action of each drug differs. These medicines do not dissolve the clots that have already formed, however; these clots are treated with thrombolytic drugs (see right).

Anticoagulants fall into two groups: those that are given by intravenous injection and act immediately, and those that are given by mouth and take effect after a few days.

INTRAVENOUS ANTICOAGULANTS

Heparin is the most widely used drug of this type, and it is used mainly in hospital before or after surgery. It is also given during kidney dialysis to prevent clots from forming in the dialysis equipment. Because heparin cannot be taken by mouth, it is less suitable for long-term treatment in the home.

Heparin is sometimes given before starting regular treatment with one of the oral anticoagulants.

Versions of heparin such as certoparin, dalteparin, enoxaparin, and tinzaparin, are called low molecular weight heparins (LMWH). They are as effective as ordinary heparin, and their effects last longer.

ORAL ANTICOAGULANTS

Warfarin is the most widely used oral anticoagulant. These drugs are mainly prescribed to prevent the formation of clots in veins and the chambers of the heart; they are less likely to prevent blood clots from forming in arteries. Oral anticoagulants may be given following injury or surgery (in particular, heart valve replacement) when there is a high risk of embolism. They are also given long term as a preventative treatment to people at risk from strokes. A common problem experienced with these drugs is that overdosage may lead to bleeding from the nose or gums or in the urinary tract. For this reason, the dosage needs to be carefully calculated; regular blood tests are performed to ensure that the clotting mechanism is correctly adjusted.

The action of oral anticoagulants may be affected by many other drugs. It may therefore be necessary to alter the dosage of anticoagulant when other drugs also need to be given. People who are taking oral anticoagulants should carry a warning list of the drugs that they should avoid. In particular, none of the anticoagulants should be taken together with aspirin except under the direction of a doctor.

THROMBOLYTICS

Also known as fibrinolytics, thrombolytics are used to dissolve clots that have already formed. They are usually administered intravenously in hospital to clear a blocked blood vessel (e.g., in coronary thrombosis). The sooner they are given after symptoms have started, the more likely they are to reduce the size and severity of a heart attack. Thrombolytics may be given either intravenously or directly into the blocked blood vessel.

The main thrombolytic drugs are streptokinase, anistreplase, and alteplase. These drugs act by increasing the blood level of plasmin, the enzyme that breaks up the strands of fibrin that bind the clot together, allowing the clot to disperse and restoring the blood flow to normal. When given promptly, alteplase appears to be tolerated better than streptokinase and anistreplase.

The most common problems with use of these drugs are an increased susceptibility to bleeding and bruising, and allergic reactions to streptokinase and anistreplase, which often take the form of rashes, breathing difficulties, or general discomfort. Once streptokinase has been administered, patients are given a card indicating this, because further treatment with the same drug is generally not advised for several months.

COMMON DRUGS

Blood clotting factors Clopidogrel*, Factor VIIa, Factor VIII, Factor IX

Antifibrinolytic or haemostatic drugs Aprotinin, Etamsylate, Tranexamic acid, Vitamin K, Phytomenadione

Antiplatelet drugs Aspirin*, Dipyridamole*

Heparin-like anticoagulants Certoparin, Dalteparin, Danaparoid, Enoxaparin, Heparin*, Tinzaparin

Thrombolytic drugs Alteplase, Anistreplase, Reteplase, Streptokinase*, Urokinase

Oral anti-coagulants, Nicoumalone, Warfarin*

* **See part 2**

GASTROINTESTINAL TRACT

The gastrointestinal tract, also known as the digestive or alimentary tract, is the pathway through which food passes as it is processed to enable the nutrients it contains to be absorbed for use by the body. It consists of the mouth, oesophagus, stomach, duodenum, small intestine, large intestine (including the colon and rectum), and anus. A number of other organs are also involved in the digestion of food: the salivary glands in the mouth, the liver, pancreas, and gallbladder, which, together with the gastrointestinal tract, form the digestive system.

The digestive system breaks down the large, complex chemicals – proteins, fats, and carbohydrates, which are present in the food we eat – into simpler molecules that can be used by the body (see also Nutrition, p.88).

The stomach holds food and passes it into the intestine. The lining of the stomach releases gastric juice that partly digests food. The stomach wall continuously produces thick mucus that forms a protective coating.

The duodenum is the tube that connects the stomach to the intestine. Its lining may be damaged by excess acid produced by the stomach.

The pancreas produces enzymes that digest proteins, fats, and carbohydrates into simpler substances; pancreatic juices neutralize acidity of the stomach contents.

The gallbladder stores bile, which is produced by the liver, and releases it into the duodenum. Bile assists the digestion of fats by reducing them to smaller units that are more easily acted upon by digestive enzymes.

The small intestine is a long tube in which food is broken down by digestive juices from the gallbladder and pancreas. The mucous lining of the small intestine consists of tiny, finger-like projections called villi that provide a large surface area through which the products of digestion are absorbed into the bloodstream.

The large intestine receives both undigested food and indigestible material from the small intestine. Water and mineral salts pass through the lining into the bloodstream. When a sufficient mass of undigested or indigestible material, together with some of the body's waste products, has accumulated it is expelled from the body as faeces.

MOVEMENT OF FOOD THROUGH THE GASTROINTESTINAL TRACT

Food is propelled through the gastrointestinal tract by rhythmic waves of muscular contraction called peristalsis.

Muscle contraction in the gastrointestinal tract is controlled by the autonomic nervous system (p.8) and is therefore easily disrupted by drugs that either stimulate or inhibit the activity of the autonomic nervous system. Excessive peristaltic action may cause diarrhoea, and constipation may result from slowed peristalsis.

WHAT CAN GO WRONG

Inflammation of the lining of the stomach or intestine (gastroenteritis) is usually due to infection or parasitic infestation. Damage may also be done by inappropriate production of digestive juices, leading to minor complaints like acidity and more serious disorders like peptic ulcers. The intestinal lining can be damaged by abnormal functioning of the immune system (inflammatory bowel disease). The rectum and anus can become painful and irritated by damage to the lining, tears in the skin at the opening of the anus (anal fissure), or enlarged veins (haemorrhoids, or piles).

Constipation, diarrhoea, and irritable bowel syndrome are the most frequently experienced gastrointestinal complaints, and they usually occur when something disrupts the normal muscle contractions that propel food residue through the bowel.

WHY DRUGS ARE USED

Many drugs for gastrointestinal disorders are taken by mouth and act directly on the digestive tract without first entering the bloodstream. Such drugs include certain antibiotics and other drugs for treating infestations. Some antacids for peptic ulcers and excess stomach acidity, and the bulk-forming agents for constipation and diarrhoea, also pass through the system unabsorbed.

However, for many disorders, drugs with a systemic effect are required, including anti-ulcer drugs, opioid antidiarrhoeal drugs, and some of the drugs for inflammatory bowel disease.

MAJOR DRUG GROUPS

◆ Antacids
◆ Anti-ulcer drugs
◆ Antidiarrhoeal drugs (including drugs for irritable bowel syndrome)
◆ Laxatives
◆ Drugs for inflammatory bowel disease
◆ Drugs for rectal and anal disorders
◆ Drug treatment for gallstones

Antacids

Digestive juices in the stomach contain acid and enzymes that break down food before it passes into the intestine. The wall of the stomach is normally protected from the action of digestive acid by a layer of mucus that is constantly secreted by the stomach lining. Problems arise when the stomach lining is damaged or too much acid is produced and eats away at the mucous layer.

Excess acid that leads to discomfort, commonly referred to as indigestion, may result from anxiety, overeating or eating certain foods, coffee, alcohol, or smoking. Some drugs, most notably aspirin and nonsteroidal anti-inflammatory drugs, can irritate the stomach lining and even cause ulcers.

Antacids neutralize acid, thereby relieving pain. They are simple chemical compounds that are mildly alkaline and some also act as chemical buffers. Their chalky taste is often disguised with flavourings.

WHY THEY ARE USED

Antacids may be needed when simple remedies (a change in diet or a glass of milk) fail to relieve indigestion. They are especially useful one to three hours after meals to neutralize the effects of excess acid after meals.

Doctors prescribe antacids to relieve dyspepsia or heartburn (pain in the chest or upper abdomen caused or aggravated by acid) in disorders such as inflammation or ulceration of the oesophagus, stomach lining, and

duodenum. Antacids usually relieve the pain of ulcers in the oesophagus, stomach, or duodenum within a few minutes. Regular treatment with antacids reduces the acidity of the stomach, thereby encouraging the healing of any ulcers that may have formed.

TYPES OF ANTACID

Aluminium compounds These drugs have a prolonged action and are widely used, especially for the treatment of indigestion and dyspepsia. They may cause constipation, but this is often countered by combining this type of antacid with one containing magnesium. Aluminium compounds can interfere with the absorption of phosphate from the diet, causing muscle weakness and bone damage if taken in high doses over a long period.

Magnesium compounds Like the aluminium compounds, these have a prolonged action. In large doses magnesium compounds can cause diarrhoea, and in people who have impaired kidney function, a high blood magnesium level may build up, causing weakness, lethargy, and drowsiness.

Sodium bicarbonate This antacid, the only sodium compound used as an antacid, acts quickly, but its effect soon passes. It reacts with stomach acids to produce gas, which may cause bloating and belching. Sodium bicarbonate is not advised for people with heart or kidney disease, because the excess sodium can lead to accumulation of water (oedema) in the legs and lungs and may raise blood pressure.

Combined preparations Antacids may be combined with other substances called alginates and antifoaming agents. Alginates are intended to float on the contents of the stomach and produce a neutralizing layer to subdue acid that can otherwise rise into the oesophagus, causing heartburn.

Antifoaming agents (usually dimeticone) are used to relieve flatulence. In some preparations, a local anaesthetic is combined with the antacid to relieve discomfort in oesophagitis. The value of these additives is dubious.

HOW THEY WORK

By neutralizing stomach acid, antacids prevent inflammation, relieve pain, and allow the mucous layer and lining to mend. When used in the treatment of ulcers, they prevent acid from attacking damaged stomach lining and so allow the ulcer to heal.

HOW THEY AFFECT YOU

If antacids are taken according to the instructions, they are usually effective in relieving abdominal discomfort caused by acid. The speed of action, dependent on the ability to neutralize acid, varies. Their duration of action also varies; the short-acting drugs may have to be taken quite frequently.

Most antacids have few serious side effects when used only occasionally, but some may cause diarrhoea, and others may cause constipation (see Types of antacid, facing page).

RISKS AND SPECIAL PRECAUTIONS

Antacids should not be taken to prevent abdominal pain on a regular basis except under medical supervision, because they may suppress the symptoms of stomach cancer. Your doctor is likely to want to arrange tests such as endoscopy or barium X-rays before prescribing long-term treatment.

All antacids can interfere with the absorption of other drugs. Therefore, if you are taking a prescription medicine, you should check with your doctor before taking an antacid.

COMMON DRUGS

Antacids Aluminium hydroxide*, Calcium carbonate, Hydrotalcite, Magnesium hydroxide*, Sodium bicarbonate*
Antifoaming agent Dimeticone
* See Part 2

Anti-ulcer drugs

Normally, the linings of the oesophagus, stomach, and duodenum are protected from the irritant action of stomach acids or bile by a thin covering layer of mucus. If this is damaged, or if large amounts of stomach acid are formed, the underlying tissue may become eroded, causing a peptic ulcer (break in the gut lining) that may, if small enough, heal spontaneously. An established ulcer can lead to abdominal pain, vomiting, and changes in appetite. The most common type of ulcer occurs in the duodenum, just beyond the stomach. The exact cause of peptic ulcers is not understood, but a number of risk factors have been identified, including heavy smoking, the regular use of aspirin or similar drugs, and family history. An organism found in almost all patients who have peptic ulcers, *Helicobacter pylori*, is now believed to be the main causative agent.

Symptoms of ulcers may be relieved by an antacid (see facing page), but healing is slow. The usual treatment is with an anti-ulcer drug, such as an H_2 blocker, a proton pump inhibitor, bismuth, or sucralfate, often combined with antibiotics to eradicate *Helicobacter pylori* infection, which seems to cause many ulcers.

WHY THEY ARE USED

Anti-ulcer drugs are used to relieve symptoms and heal the ulcer. Untreated ulcers may erode blood vessel walls or perforate the stomach or duodenum.

Until recently, drugs could heal ulcers but not cure them. However, the eradication of *Helicobacter pylori* by a proton pump inhibitor, or ranitidine bismuth citrate combined with two antibiotics (triple therapy), may provide a cure in one to two weeks. Surgery is reserved for complications such as obstruction, perforation, haemorrhage, and when there is a possibility of cancer.

HOW THEY WORK

Drugs protect ulcers from the action of stomach acid, allowing the tissue to heal. H_2 blockers, misoprostol, and proton pump inhibitors reduce the amount of acid released; bismuth and sucralfate form a protective coating over the ulcer. Bismuth also has an antibacterial effect. It is combined with an H_2 blocker in ranitidine bismuth citrate.

HOW THEY AFFECT YOU

These drugs begin to reduce pain in a few hours and usually allow the ulcer to heal in four to eight weeks. They produce few side effects, although H_2 blockers can cause confusion in the elderly. Bismuth and sucralfate may cause constipation; misoprostol, diarrhoea; and proton pump inhibitors, either constipation or diarrhoea. Triple therapy is given for one or two weeks. If *Helicobacter pylori* is eradicated, maintenance therapy should not be necessary. Sucralfate is usually prescribed for up to 12 weeks, and bismuth and misoprostol for four to six weeks. As they may mask symptoms of stomach cancer, H_2 blockers and proton pump inhibitors are normally prescribed for older patients only when tests have ruled out this disorder.

COMMON DRUGS

Proton pump inhibitors Lansoprazole, Omeprazole*, Pantoprazole, Rabeprazole

H_2 blockers Cimetidine*, Famotidine, Nizatidine, Ranitidine*

Other drugs Antacids (see p.40), Antibiotics (see p.60), Bismuth, Carbenoxolone, Misoprostol*, Ranitidine bismuth citrate, Sucralfate*

* **See Part 2**

Antidiarrhoeal drugs

Diarrhoea is an increase in the fluidity and frequency of bowel movements. In some cases, diarrhoea protects the body from harmful substances in the intestine by hastening their removal. The most common causes of diarrhoea are travellers' diarrhoea, viral infection, food poisoning, and parasites. Diarrhoea also occurs as a symptom of other illnesses. It can be a side effect of some drugs and may follow radiation therapy for cancer. It may also be caused by anxiety.

Most attacks of diarrhoea usually clear up quickly without medical attention. The best treatment is to abstain from food and to drink plenty of clear fluids. Rehydration solutions containing sugar as well as potassium and sodium salts are widely recommended for preventing dehydration and chemical imbalances, particularly in children. You should consult your doctor if: the condition does not improve within 48 hours; the diarrhoea contains blood; severe abdominal pain and vomiting are present; you have just returned from a foreign country; or if the diarrhoea occurs in a small child or an elderly person.

Severe diarrhoea can impair the absorption of drugs; anyone taking prescribed drugs should seek advice from a doctor or pharmacist. Women taking oral contraceptives may require additional contraception (see p.101).

The main types of drug used to relieve non-specific diarrhoea are opioids and bulk-forming and adsorbent agents. Antispasmodic drugs may also be used to relieve accompanying pain (see Drugs for irritable bowel syndrome, facing page).

WHY THEY ARE USED

An antidiarrhoeal drug may be prescribed to provide relief when simple remedies are not effective, and after ruling out the more severe types of infectious diarrhoea.

Opioids are the most effective antidiarrhoeals. They are used when the diarrhoea is severe and debilitating. The bulking and adsorbent agents have a milder effect and are often used when it is necessary to regulate bowel action over a prolonged period (e.g., in people with colostomies or ileostomies).

HOW THEY WORK

Opioids decrease the muscles' propulsive activity so that faecal matter passes more slowly through the bowel. This allows more time for water to be absorbed from the food residue and therefore reduces the fluidity as well as the frequency of bowel movements.

Bulk-forming agents and adsorbents absorb water and irritants present in the bowel, thereby producing larger and firmer stools at less frequent intervals.

HOW THEY AFFECT YOU

Antidiarrhoeals reduce the urge to move the bowels. Opioids and antispasmodics may relieve abdominal pain. All antidiarrhoeals may cause constipation if used in excess.

RISKS AND SPECIAL PRECAUTIONS

Used in relatively low doses for limited periods, the opioid drugs are unlikely to produce adverse effects. They should be used with caution when diarrhoea is caused by an infection, however, since they may slow the elimination of microorganisms from the intestine. All antidiarrhoeals should be taken with plenty of water, and if the diarrhoea is prolonged or the patient is a child, an oral rehydration solution should be taken. Bulk- forming agents should not be taken together with opioid or antispasmodic drugs, because a bulky mass could form and obstruct the bowel.

COMMON DRUGS
Antispasmodics Atropine*, Dicycloverine*, Hyoscine*
Opioids Codeine*, Diphenoxylate*, Loperamide*
Bulk-forming agents and adsorbents Ispaghula, Kaolin, Methylcellulose*
Oral rehydration solutions
* See Part 2

Drugs for irritable bowel syndrome

Irritable bowel syndrome is a common, often stress-related, condition in which the normal coordinated waves of muscular contraction responsible for moving the bowel contents smoothly through the intestines become strong and irregular, often causing pain, and associated with diarrhoea or constipation.

Symptoms are often relieved by adjusting the amount of fibre in the diet, but medication may also be needed. Bulk-forming agents may be given to regulate consistency of the bowel contents. If pain is severe, an antispasmodic drug may be given. These anticholinergics (see Drugs that act on the parasympathetic nervous system, p.9) reduce the transmission of nerve signals to the bowel wall, preventing spasm. Tricyclic antidepressants are sometimes used because their anticholinergic action has a calming effect on the bowel.

COMMON DRUGS
Antispasmodics Dicycloverine*, Mebeverine*
Opioids Loperamide*
Other drugs Peppermint oil

Laxatives

When your bowels do not move as frequently as usual and the faeces are hard and difficult to pass, you are suffering from constipation. The most common cause is lack of sufficient fibre in your diet; fibre supplies the bulk that makes the faeces soft and easy to pass. The simplest remedy is more fluid and a diet that contains plenty of foods that are high in fibre, but laxative drugs may also be used.

Ignoring the urge to open the bowels can also cause constipation because the faeces become hard and dry, difficult to pass, and too small to stimulate the muscles that propel them through the intestine.

Certain drugs may be constipating (e.g., opioid analgesics, tricyclic antidepressants, and antacids containing aluminium). Painful conditions of the anus (e.g., diseases such as hypothyroidism (underactive thyroid gland) and fissures) can also lead to constipation.

The onset of constipation in a middle-aged or elderly person may be an early symptom of bowel cancer. Consult your doctor about any persistent change in bowel habit.

TYPES OF LAXATIVE
Bulk-forming agents These are relatively slow acting but are less likely than other laxatives to interfere with normal bowel action. If constipation is accompanied by abdominal pain, only take these after consulting your doctor because of the risk of intestinal obstruction.
Stimulant (contact) laxatives These laxatives are for occasional use when other treatments have failed or when rapid onset of action is needed. They should not normally be used for longer than a week at a time, because they can cause abdominal cramps and diarrhoea.
Softening agents These are often used (especially after surgery when straining must be avoided, or if there are haemorrhoids) when hard faeces cause pain as the bowels are opened. Liquid paraffin was once used to relieve faecal impaction (blockage of the bowel by faeces) but, because of its side effects, has largely been replaced by sodium docusate.
Osmotic laxatives Salts such as Epsom salts (magnesium sulphate) may be used to evacuate the bowel before surgery or investigative procedures. They are not normally used for long-term relief of constipation because they can cause chemical imbalances in the blood.
Lactulose is an alternative to bulk-forming laxatives for long-term treatment of chronic constipation. It may cause stomach cramps and flatulence but is usually well tolerated.

WHY THEY ARE USED
Because prolonged use of laxatives is harmful, they should be used only for very short periods. Laxatives may prevent pain and

straining in people with haemorrhoids (p.45) or hernias. Doctors may prescribe them for the same reason after childbirth or abdominal surgery. They are also used to clear the bowel before investigative procedures such as colonoscopy. They may be prescribed for elderly or bedridden patients because lack of exercise can often lead to constipation.

HOW THEY WORK

Laxatives act on the large intestine. They work by increasing the speed with which faecal matter passes through the bowel or by increasing its bulk and/or water content.

Stimulants cause the bowel muscles to contract, increasing the speed at which faecal matter goes through the intestine. Bulk-forming laxatives absorb water in the bowel, thereby increasing the volume of faeces, making them softer and easier to pass. Lactulose also causes fluid to accumulate in the intestine. Osmotic laxatives act by keeping water in the bowel, and thereby make the bowel movements softer. This also increases the bulk of the faeces and enables them to be passed more easily. Lubricant liquid paraffin preparations make bowel movements softer and easier to pass without increasing their bulk. Prolonged use can interfere with the absorption of some essential vitamins.

RISKS AND SPECIAL PRECAUTIONS

Laxatives can cause diarrhoea if taken in overdose, and constipation if overused. The most serious risk of prolonged use of most laxatives is developing dependence on them for normal bowel action. Therefore, laxative use should be discontinued as soon as normal bowel movements are re-established. Children should not be given laxatives except in special circumstances on the advice of a doctor.

COMMON DRUGS

Stimulant laxatives Bisacodyl, Co-danthramer, Co-danthrusate, Docusate, Senna
Bulk-forming agents Ispaghula, Methylcellulose*, Sodium alginate
Softening agents Liquid paraffin, Sodium docusate,
Osmotic laxatives Lactulose*, Magnesium citrate, Magnesium hydroxide*, Magnesium sulphate, Sodium acid phosphate
* **See Part 2**

Drugs for inflammatory bowel disease

Inflammatory bowel disease is the term used for disorders in which inflammation of the intestinal wall causes symptoms ranging from minor and infrequent attacks of diarrhoea to episodes of life-threatening illness. There may be recurrent attacks of abdominal pain, general feelings of ill-health, and, frequently, diarrhoea with blood and mucus in the faeces. Loss of appetite and poor absorption of food may often result in weight loss.

There are two main types of inflammatory bowel disease: Crohn's disease and ulcerative colitis. In Crohn's disease (also called regional enteritis), any part of the digestive tract may become inflamed, although the small intestine is the most commonly affected site. In ulcerative colitis, it is the large intestine (colon) that becomes inflamed and ulcerated, often producing bloodstained diarrhoea.

The exact cause of these disorders is unknown, but dietary, infectious, genetic, and stress-related factors may all be important.

Establishing a proper diet and less stressful lifestyle may help to alleviate these conditions. Bed rest during attacks is also advisable. However, these simple measures alone do not usually relieve or prevent attacks, and drug treatment is often necessary.

Three types of drug are used to treat inflammatory bowel disease: corticosteroids (p.78), immunosuppressants (p.96), and aminosalicylate anti-inflammatory drugs such as sulfasalazine. Nutritional supplements (used especially for Crohn's disease) and antidiarrhoeal drugs (p.42) may also be used. Surgery to remove damaged areas of the intestine may be needed in severe cases. Newer drugs are currently being developed; one new drug, infliximab, offers hope of controlling Crohn's disease.

WHY THEY ARE USED

Drugs cannot cure inflammatory bowel disease, but treatment is needed, not only to control symptoms, but also to prevent complications, especially severe anaemia and perforation of the intestinal wall. Aminosalicylates are used to treat acute attacks of ulcerative colitis and Crohn's disease, and they may be continued as maintenance therapy. People who have severe bowel inflammation are usually prescribed a course of corticosteroids, particularly during a sudden flare-up. Once the disease is under control, an immunosuppressant drug may be prescribed to prevent a relapse.

HOW THEY WORK

Corticosteroids and sulfasalazine damp down the inflammatory process, allowing the damaged tissue to recover. They act in different ways to prevent migration of white blood cells into the bowel wall, which may be partly responsible for the inflammation of the bowel.

HOW THEY AFFECT YOU

Taken to treat attacks, these drugs relieve symptoms within a few days, and general health improves gradually over a period of a few weeks. Aminosalicylates usually provide long-term relief from the symptoms of inflammatory bowel disease.

Treatment with an immunosuppressant drug may take several months before improvement of the condition occurs; and regular blood tests to monitor possible drug side effects are often required.

RISKS AND SPECIAL PRECAUTIONS

Immunosuppressants and corticosteroids can cause serious adverse effects and are only used when potential benefits outweigh the risks.

The side effects of corticosteroids can be reduced by the use of budesonide in a new, topical preparation which releases the drug at the site of inflammation.

It is important to continue taking these drugs as instructed because stopping them abruptly may cause a sudden flare-up of the disorder. Doctors usually supervise a gradual reduction in dosage when such drugs are stopped, even when they are given as a short course for an attack. Antidiarrhoeal drugs should not be taken on a routine basis because they may mask signs of deterioration or cause sudden bowel dilation or rupture.

HOW THEY ARE ADMINISTERED

Antidiarrhoeals are usually taken in the form of tablets, although mild ulcerative colitis in

the last part of the large intestine may be treated with suppositories or an enema containing a corticosteroid or aminosalicylate.

COMMON DRUGS

Corticosteroids Budesonide*, Hydrocortisone*, Prednisolone*
Immunosuppressants Azathioprine*, Mercaptopurine*, Methotrexate*
Aminosalicylates Balsalazide, Mesalazine*, Olsalazine, Sulfasalazine*
* **See Part 2**

Drugs for rectal and anal disorders

The most common disorder of the rectum (the last part of the large intestine) and anus (the opening from the rectum) is haemorrhoids, or piles. They occur when haemorrhoidal veins are swollen or irritated, often as a result of prolonged local pressure such as that caused by pregnancy or a job requiring long hours of sitting. Haemorrhoids may cause irritation and pain, especially on opening the bowels, and are aggravated by constipation and straining. In some cases haemorrhoids may bleed, and occasionally clots form in the swollen veins, leading to severe pain, a condition called thrombosed haemorrhoids.

Other common disorders include pruritus ani (itching around the anus) and anal fissure (painful cracks in the anus). Anal disorders of all kinds occur less often in people who have soft, bulky stools.

A number of both over-the-counter and prescription-only preparations are available for the relief of such disorders.

WHY THEY ARE USED

Preparations for relief of haemorrhoids and anal discomfort fall into two main groups: creams or suppositories that act locally to relieve inflammation and irritation; and measures that relieve constipation, which contributes to the formation of, and discomfort from, haemorrhoids and anal fissure.

The first group often contain a soothing agent with antiseptic, astringent, or vasoconstrictor properties. Such ingredients include zinc oxide, bismuth, hamamelis (witch hazel), and ephedrine. Some products also include a mild local anaesthetic (see p.11) such as lignocaine. In some cases a doctor may prescribe an ointment containing a corticosteroid to relieve inflammation around the anus (see Topical corticosteroids, p.116).

People who suffer from haemorrhoids or anal fissure are generally advised to include in their diets plenty of fluids and fibre-rich foods, such as fresh fruits, vegetables, and whole grain products, both to prevent constipation and to ease bowel movements. A mild bulk-forming or softening laxative may also be prescribed (see p.43).

Neither of these treatments can shrink large haemorrhoids, although they may provide relief while anal fissures heal naturally. Severe, persistently painful haemorrhoids that continue to be troublesome in spite of these measures may need to be removed surgically or, more commonly, by banding. This is a procedure in which a small rubber band is applied tightly to a haemorrhoid, thereby blocking off its blood supply; the haemorrhoid will eventually wither away.

HOW THEY AFFECT YOU

These treatments usually relieve discomfort, especially during bowel movement. Most people experience no adverse effects, but preparations containing local anaesthetics may cause irritation or even a rash in the anal area. It is rare for ingredients in locally acting preparations to be absorbed into the body in sufficient quantities to cause generalized side effects.

The main risk is that self-treatment of haemorrhoids may delay diagnosis of bowel cancer. It is therefore always wise to consult your doctor if symptoms of haemorrhoids are present, especially if you have noticed bleeding from the rectum or a change in bowel habits.

COMMON DRUGS

Soothing and astringent agents Aluminium acetate, Bismuth, Peru balsam, Zinc oxide
Vasoconstrictors Ephedrine*
Topical corticosteroids Hydrocortisone*
Local anaesthetics (see p.11)
Laxatives (see p.43)
* **See Part 2**

Drug treatment for gallstones

The formation of gallstones is the most common disorder of the gallbladder, which stores and concentrates bile, a digestive juice produced by the liver. During digestion, bile passes from the gallbladder via the bile duct into the small intestine, where it assists in the digestion of fats. Bile is composed of several ingredients, including bile acids, bile salts, and bile pigments. It also has a significant amount of cholesterol, which is dissolved in bile acid. If the amount of cholesterol in the bile increases, or if the amount of bile acid is reduced, a proportion of the cholesterol cannot remain dissolved, and under certain circumstances this excess accumulates in the gallbladder as gallstones.

Gallstones may be present in the gallbladder for years without causing symptoms. Sometimes they may cause the gallbladder to become infected and inflamed. They may also lodge in the bile duct, causing pain and blocking the flow of bile. Bile may then spill over into the blood and be apparent as jaundice.

Drug treatment with chenodeoxycholic acid and ursodeoxycholic acid is only effective against stones made principally of cholesterol (some contain other substances), and even these take many months to dissolve. Therefore, surgery and ultrasound have become widely used, as techniques have improved. Surgery and ultrasound treatments are always used to remove stones blocking the bile duct.

WHY THEY ARE USED

Even if you have not experienced any symptoms, once gallstones have been diagnosed your doctor may advise treatment because of the risk of blockage of the bile duct. Drug treatment is usually preferred to surgery for small cholesterol stones when there is a possibility that surgery may be risky.

HOW THEY WORK

Chenodeoxycholic acid is a substance that is naturally present in bile. It acts on chemical processes in the liver to regulate the amount of cholesterol in the blood by controlling the amount that passes into the bile. Once the cholesterol level in the bile is reduced, the bile acids can start dissolving the stones in the gallbladder. To achieve maximum effect, chenodeoxycholic acid treatment usually needs to be accompanied by adherence to a low-cholesterol, high-fibre diet.

HOW THEY AFFECT YOU

Drug treatment may often take years to dissolve gallstones completely. You will not, therefore, feel any immediate benefit from the drugs, but you may have some minor side effects, the most usual of which is diarrhoea. If this occurs, your doctor may adjust the dosage. The effect of drug treatment on the gallstones is usually monitored at regular intervals by means of ultrasound or X-ray examinations.

Even after successful treatment with drugs, gallstones often recur when the drug is stopped. In some cases drug treatment and dietary restrictions may be continued even after the gallstones have dissolved, to prevent a recurrence.

Although these drugs reduce cholesterol in the gallbladder, they increase the level of cholesterol in the blood because they reduce its excretion in the bile. Doctors therefore prescribe them with caution to people who have atherosclerosis (fatty deposits in the blood vessels). These drugs are not usually given to people who have liver disorders because they can interfere with normal liver function. Surgical or ultrasound treatment is used for those with liver problems.

AGENTS USED IN THE TREATMENT OF DISORDERS OF THE PANCREAS

The pancreas releases certain enzymes into the small intestine that are necessary for digestion of a range of foods. If the release of pancreatic enzymes is impaired (by chronic pancreatitis or cystic fibrosis, for example), enzyme replacement therapy may be necessary. Replacement of enzymes does not cure the underlying disorder, but it restores normal digestion. Pancreatic enzymes should be taken just before or with meals, and usually take effect immediately. Your doctor will probably advise you to eat a diet that is high in protein and carbohydrates and low in fat.

Pancreatin, the generic name for those preparations containing pancreatic enzymes, is extracted from pig pancreas. Treatment must be continued indefinitely as long as the pancreatic disorder persists.

COMMON DRUGS

Drugs for gallstones Chenodeoxycholic acid, Ursodeoxycholic acid

Pancreatic enzymes Amylase, Lipase, Pancreatin, Protease

MUSCLES, BONES, AND JOINTS

The basic architecture of the human body relies on 206 bones, over 600 muscles, and a complex assortment of other tissues that enable the body to move with remarkable efficiency.

Tendons attach the muscles that control body movement to the bones.

Muscles work bones that act as levers: when the muscle contracts, movement occurs at the joint.

Ligaments are bands of tough fibrous tissue that hold joints together.

Cartilage covers each bone end, reducing friction between the ends of two bones.

WHAT CAN GO WRONG

Although tough, these structures often suffer damage. Muscles, tendons, and ligaments can be strained or torn by violent movement, which may cause inflammation, making the affected tissue swollen and painful. Joints, especially those that bear the body's weight – hips, knees, ankles, and vertebrae – are prone to wear and tear. The cartilage covering the bone ends may tear, causing pain and inflammation. Joint damage also occurs in rheumatoid arthritis, which is thought to be a form of autoimmune disorder. Gout, in which uric acid crystals form in some joints, may also cause inflammation, a condition known as gouty arthritis.

Another problem affecting the muscles and joints includes nerve injury or degeneration, which alters nerve control over muscle contraction. Myasthenia gravis, in which transmission of signals between nerves and muscles is reduced, affects muscle strength as a result. Bones may also be weakened by vitamin, mineral, or hormone deficiencies.

WHY DRUGS ARE USED

A simple analgesic drug or one that has an anti-inflammatory effect will provide pain relief in most of the conditions described above. For severe inflammation, a doctor may inject a drug with a more powerful anti-inflammatory effect, such as a corticosteroid, into the affected site. In cases of severe progressive rheumatoid arthritis,

antirheumatic drugs may halt the disease's progression and relieve symptoms.

Drugs that help to eliminate excess uric acid from the body are often prescribed to treat gout. Muscle relaxants that inhibit transmission of nerve signals to the muscles are used to treat muscle spasm. Drugs that increase nervous stimulation of the muscle are prescribed for myasthenia gravis. Bone disorders in which the mineral content of the bone is reduced are treated with supplements of minerals, vitamins, and hormones.

MAJOR DRUG GROUPS

◆ Non-steroidal anti-inflammatory drugs
◆ Antirheumatic drugs
◆ Corticosteroids for rheumatic disorders
◆ Drugs for gout
◆ Muscle-relaxants
◆ Drugs used for myasthenia gravis
◆ Drugs for bone disorders

Non-steroidal anti-inflammatory drugs

Drugs in this group are used to relieve the pain, stiffness, and inflammation of painful conditions affecting the muscles, bones, and joints. For this reason, they are effective in rheumatoid arthritis. They are less effective in osteoarthritis, however, because there is usually pain, due to worn joints, without inflammation. NSAIDs are called "non-steroidal" to distinguish them from corticosteroid drugs (see p.78), which also relieve inflammation.

There are many NSAIDs currently available, and others are being investigated in the hope of finding new compounds with fewer side effects.

WHY THEY ARE USED

NSAIDs are widely prescribed for the treatment of osteoarthritis, rheumatoid arthritis, and other rheumatic conditions. They do not alter the progress of these diseases but reduce inflammation and thus relieve pain and swelling of joints.

The response to the various drugs in this group varies between individuals and the first drug chosen may not be effective. It is sometimes necessary for the doctor to prescribe a number of different NSAIDs before he or she finds the one that best suits a particular individual.

Because NSAIDs do not change the progress of the disease, additional treatment may be required, particularly for rheumatoid arthritis (see p.50).

NSAIDs are also commonly prescribed for back pain, headaches, gout (p.51), menstrual pain (p.100), mild pain following surgery, and pain from soft tissue injuries such as sprains and strains (see also Analgesics, p.9).

HOW THEY WORK
Prostaglandins are chemicals released by the body at the site of injury. They are responsible for producing inflammation and pain following tissue damage and in immune reactions. NSAIDs block the production of prostaglandins and thus reduce pain and inflammation.

HOW THEY AFFECT YOU
NSAIDs are usually effective in reducing joint pain and swelling. They are rapidly absorbed from the digestive system, and most start to relieve pain within an hour. When they are used regularly, NSAIDs reduce pain, inflammation, and stiffness and may restore or improve the function of a joint if this has been impaired.

Most NSAIDs are short acting and need to be taken a few times a day in order to provide optimal relief from pain. Some of them need to be taken only twice daily. Others, such as piroxicam, are very slowly eliminated from the body and are effective when taken once a day.

RISKS AND SPECIAL PRECAUTIONS
With a few exceptions, most NSAIDs are free from serious adverse effects, although nausea, indigestion, and altered bowel action are common. The main risk from NSAIDs, however, is that they can occasionally cause bleeding in the stomach or duodenum. They should therefore be avoided by people who have suffered from peptic ulcers.

Most NSAIDs are not recommended during pregnancy or for breast-feeding mothers. Caution is also advised for those people with kidney or liver abnormalities or with a history of hypersensitivity to other drugs.

NSAIDs may impair blood clotting and are, therefore, prescribed with caution to people with bleeding disorders or who are taking drugs that reduce blood clotting.

MISOPROSTOL
An NSAID causes the side effect of bleeding when its antiprostaglandin action occurs where it is not wanted, such as in the digestive tract. To protect against this side effect, a prostaglandin-like drug called misoprostol is sometimes prescribed with the NSAID. Preparations are now available that incorporate both misoprostol and an NSAID. Misoprostol is also used to help heal peptic ulcers (see p.41). As an alternative to giving drugs such as misoprostol, NSAIDs are being developed that work selectively by preventing prostaglandin production in the joints but not in the digestive tract.

COX-2 INHIBITORS
NSAIDs block the action of the enzyme cyclo-oxygenase (COX), which is involved in the manufacture of prostaglandins at different sites in the body. Research has shown that they block two types of COX (COX-1 and COX-2) and that blocking COX-1 leads to the stomach irritation of NSAIDs, while blocking COX-2 leads to the anti-inflammatory effect. As a result, a new class of NSAIDs, COX-2 inhibitors, has been developed, to block COX-2 but not COX-1. Thus, the benefits of NSAIDs can be obtained without increased risk of stomach pain, peptic ulcers, or intestinal bleeding. COX-2 inhibitors include etodolac, rofecoxib, and celecoxib.

COMMON DRUGS
Aceclofenac, Acemetacin, Aspirin*, Azapropazone, Benorylate, Benzydamine, Celecoxib, Diclofenac*, Diflunisal, Etodolac, Felbinac*, Fenbufen, Fenoprofen, Flurbiprofen, Ibuprofen*, Indomethacin, Ketoprofen*, Mefenamic acid*, Meloxicam*, Nabumetone, Naproxen*, Phenylbutazone, Piroxicam*, rofecoxib, Sulindac, Tenoxicam, Tiaprofenic acid
* **See Part 2**

Antirheumatic drugs

These drugs are used in the treatment of various rheumatic disorders, the most crippling and deforming of which is rheumatoid arthritis, an autoimmune disease in which the body's mechanism for fighting infection contributes to the damage of its own joint tissue. The disease causes pain, stiffness, and swelling of the joints that can, over many months, lead to deformity. Flare-ups of rheumatoid arthritis also cause a general feeling of being unwell, fatigue, and loss of appetite.

Treatments for rheumatoid arthritis include drugs, rest, physiotherapy, changes in diet, and immobilization of joints. The disorder cannot yet be cured, but in many cases it does not progress far enough to cause permanent disability. It sometimes subsides spontaneously for prolonged periods.

WHY THEY ARE USED

The aim of drug treatment is to relieve the symptoms of pain and stiffness, maintain mobility, and prevent deformity. There are two main forms of drug treatment for rheumatoid arthritis: the first alleviates symptoms, and the second modifies, halts, or slows the underlying disease process. Drugs in the first category include aspirin (see p.138) and the other NSAIDs (see Non-steroidal anti-inflammatory drugs, p.48). These drugs are usually prescribed as a first treatment.

However, if the rheumatoid arthritis is severe, or the initial drug treatment has proved ineffective, the second category of drugs may be given. These drugs may prevent any further joint damage and disability. They are not prescribed routinely because they have potentially severe adverse effects and because the disease may stop spontaneously.

Corticosteroids (p.78) are sometimes used in the long-term treatment of rheumatoid arthritis, but high doses are only used for limited periods of time because the risks from adverse effects outweigh the benefits.

TYPES OF ANTIRHEUMATIC DRUG

Chloroquine Originally developed to treat malaria (see p.73), chloroquine and related drugs are less effective than penicillamine or gold. Prolonged use may cause eye damage, but only if too high a dose is used.

Immunosuppressants These are prescribed if other drugs do not provide relief and if the rheumatoid arthritis is severe and disabling. Regular observation and blood tests must be carried out because immunosuppressants can cause severe complications.

Sulfasalazine Used mainly for ulcerative colitis (p.44), sulfasalazine was originally introduced to treat rheumatoid arthritis and is effective in some cases.

Gold-based drugs These are effective and may be given orally or by injection for many years. Side effects can include a rash and digestive disturbances. Gold may sometimes damage the kidneys, which recover once treatment is stopped; regular urine tests are usually carried out, however. Gold can also suppress blood cell production in bone marrow. Therefore, periodic blood tests are also carried out.

Penicillamine This drug may be used when rheumatoid arthritis is worsening, or when gold cannot be given. Improvement in symptoms may take 3 to 6 months. It has similar side effects to gold, and periodic blood and urine tests are usually performed.

HOW THEY WORK

It is not known precisely how most antirheumatic drugs stop or slow the disease process. Some may reduce the body's immune response, which is thought to be partly responsible for the disease (see also Immunosuppressant drugs, p.96). When they are effective, antirheumatic drugs prevent damage to the cartilage and bone, thereby reducing progressive deformity and disability. The effectiveness of each drug varies depending on the individual response.

HOW THEY AFFECT YOU

These drugs are generally slow acting; it may be weeks or even months before benefit is felt. Therefore, aspirin or other NSAID treatment is usually continued until remission occurs. Prolonged treatment with antirheumatic drugs can cause a marked improvement in symptoms. Arthritic pain is relieved, joint mobility increased, and general symptoms of ill health fade. Side effects (which vary between individual drugs) may be noticed before any beneficial effect, so patience is required. Severe adverse effects may necessitate abandoning the treatment.

COMMON DRUGS
Immunosuppressants Azathioprine*, Cyclophosphamide*, Ciclosporin*, Methotrexate*
NSAIDs (see p.48)
Gold-based drugs Auranofin, Sodium aurothiomalate
Other drugs Chloroquine*, Hydroxychloroquine, Penicillamine, Sulfasalazine*
* **See Part 2**

Corticosteroids for rheumatic disorders

The adrenal glands, which lie on the top of the kidneys, produce a number of important hormones. Among these are the corticosteroids, so named because they are made in the outer part (cortex) of the glands. The corticosteroids play an important role, influencing the immune system and regulating the carbohydrate and mineral metabolism of the body. A number of drugs that mimic the natural corticosteroids have been developed.

These drugs have many uses and are discussed in detail under Corticosteroids (p.78). This section concentrates on those corticosteroids injected into an affected site to treat joint disorders.

WHY THEY ARE USED
Corticosteroids given by injection are particularly useful for treating joint disorders – notably rheumatoid arthritis and osteoarthritis – when one or only a few joints are involved, and when pain and inflammation have not been relieved by other drugs. In such cases, it is possible to relieve symptoms by injecting each of the affected joints individually. Corticosteroids may also be injected to relieve pain and inflammation caused by strained or contracted muscles, ligaments, and/or tendons – for example, in frozen shoulder or tennis elbow. They may also be used to treat bursitis, tendinitis, or swelling

that is compressing a nerve. Corticosteroid injections are sometimes used in order to relieve pain and stiffness sufficiently for physiotherapy to be carried out.

HOW THEY WORK
Corticosteroids have two important actions that are believed to account for their effectiveness: they block the production of prostaglandins – chemicals responsible for triggering inflammation and pain – and they depress the accumulation and activity of the white blood cells that cause the inflammation. Injection concentrates the corticosteroids, and their effects, at the site of the problem, thereby giving the maximum benefit where it is most needed.

HOW THEY AFFECT YOU
Corticosteroids usually produce dramatic relief of symptoms when the drug is injected into a joint. Often a single injection is sufficient to relieve pain and swelling, and to improve mobility. When used to treat muscle or tendon pain, they may not always be effective because it is difficult to position the needle so that the drug reaches the right spot. In some cases, repeated injections are necessary.

Because these drugs are concentrated in the affected area, rather than being dispersed in significant amounts in the body, the generalized adverse effects that sometimes occur when corticosteroids are taken by mouth are unlikely. Minor effects, such as loss of skin pigment at the injection site, are uncommon. Occasionally, a temporary increase in pain (steroid flare) may occur. In such cases, rest, local application of ice, and analgesic medication may relieve the condition. Sterile injection technique is critically important.

COMMON DRUGS
Dexamethasone*, Hydrocortisone*, Prednisolone*, Triamcinolone, Methylprednisolone
* **See Part 2**

Drugs for gout

Gout is a disorder that arises when the blood contains increased levels of uric acid, which is a by-product of normal body metabolism.

When its concentration in the blood is excessive, uric acid crystals may form in various parts of the body, especially in the joints of the foot (most often the big toe), the knee, and the hand, causing intense pain and inflammation known as gouty arthritis. Crystals may form as white masses, known as tophi, in soft tissue, and in the kidneys as stones. Attacks of gouty arthritis can recur, and may lead to damaged joints and deformity. Kidney stones can cause kidney damage.

Excess uric acid can be due either to increased production or decreased elimination by the kidneys, which remove it from the body. Gout tends to run in families and is far more common in men than women. The risk of attack is increased by high alcohol intake, the consumption of certain foods (red meat, sardines, anchovies, and offal), and obesity. An attack may be triggered by drugs such as thiazide diuretics (see p.30) or anticancer drugs (see p.94), or excessive drinking. Changes in diet and reduced alcohol intake may be an important part of treatment.

Drugs to treat acute attacks of gouty arthritis include NSAIDs (see Non-steroidal anti-inflammatory drugs, p.48), and colchicine. Other drugs, which lower blood levels of uric acid, are for the long-term prevention of gout. These include the uricosuric drugs probenecid and sulfinpyrazone (both of which are now rarely used) and allopurinol. Aspirin is not prescribed for pain relief because it slows the excretion of uric acid.

WHY THEY ARE USED

Drugs may be prescribed either to treat an attack of gout or to prevent recurrent attacks that could lead to deformity of the affected joints and to kidney damage. The NSAIDs and colchicine are both used to treat an attack of gout and should be taken as soon as it begins. Because colchicine is relatively specific in relieving the pain and inflammation arising from gout, doctors sometimes administer it in order to confirm their diagnosis of the condition before prescribing an NSAID.

If symptoms recur, your doctor may advise long-term treatment with either allopurinol or a uricosuric drug. One of these drugs usually has to be taken indefinitely. Because these drugs can trigger acute attacks of gout

at the beginning of treatment, they are only given once the attack has settled. NSAIDs are widely used to treat acute attacks.

HOW THEY WORK

Allopurinol lowers the level of uric acid in the blood by reducing the activity of xanthine oxidase, an enzyme involved in the production of uric acid in the body. Both sulfinpyrazone and probenecid increase the rate at which uric acid is excreted by the kidneys. The process by which colchicine reduces inflammation and relieves pain is not understood. The actions of NSAIDs are described on p.48.

HOW THEY AFFECT YOU

Drugs used in long-term gout treatment are usually successful in preventing attacks and joint deformity, but response may be slow.

Colchicine can disturb the digestive system, causing abdominal pain and diarrhoea, which your doctor can control by prescribing other drugs.

RISKS AND SPECIAL PRECAUTIONS

Because they increase the output of uric acid through the kidneys, uricosuric drugs can cause uric acid crystals to form in the kidneys. They are not, therefore, usually prescribed for those people who already have kidney problems. In such cases, allopurinol is preferred. It is always important to drink plenty of fluids while taking drugs for gout in order to prevent kidney crystals from forming. Blood tests to monitor levels of uric acid may be required until its concentration in the blood has been successfully reduced.

COMMON DRUGS

Drugs to treat attacks Colchicine*, NSAIDs (but not aspirin, see p.48)
Drugs to prevent attacks Allopurinol*, Probenecid, Sulfinpyrazone
* See Part 2

Muscle relaxants

Several drugs are available to treat muscle spasm – the involuntary, painful contraction of a muscle or a group of muscles that can stiffen an arm or leg, or make it nearly impossible to straighten your back. There are various causes. It can follow an injury, or come on without warning. It may also be brought on by a disorder like osteoarthritis, the pain in the affected joint triggering abnormal tension in a nearby muscle.

Spasticity is another form of muscle tightness seen in some neurological disorders, such as multiple sclerosis, stroke, or cerebral palsy. Spasticity can sometimes be helped by physiotherapy but in severe cases drugs may be used to relieve symptoms.

WHY THEY ARE USED
Muscle spasm resulting from direct injury is usually treated with an NSAID (see Nonsteroidal anti-inflammatory drugs, p.48) or an analgesic. However, if the spasm is severe, a muscle relaxant may also be tried for a short period.

In spasticity, the legs may become so stiff and uncontrollable that walking unaided is impossible. In such cases, a drug may be used to relax the muscles. Relaxation of the muscles often permits physiotherapy to be given for longer-term relief from spasms.

The muscle relaxant, botulinum toxin, may be injected locally to relieve muscle spasm in small groups of accessible muscles, such as those around the eye or in the neck.

HOW THEY WORK
Muscle-relaxant drugs work in one of several ways. The centrally acting drugs damp down the passage of the nerve signals from the brain and spinal cord that cause muscles to contract, thus reducing excessive stimulation of muscles as well as unwanted muscular contraction. Tizanidine stimulates the alpha receptors in the blood vessels. Dantrolene reduces the sensitivity of the muscles to nerve signals. When injected locally, botulinum toxin prevents the transmission of impulses between nerves and muscles.

HOW THEY AFFECT YOU
Drugs taken regularly for a spastic disorder of the central nervous system usually reduce stiffness and improve mobility. They may restore the use of the arms and legs when this has been impaired by muscle spasm.

Unfortunately, most centrally acting drugs can have a generally depressant effect on nervous activity and produce drowsiness, particularly at the beginning of treatment. Too high a dosage can excessively reduce the muscles' ability to contract and can therefore cause weakness. For this reason, the dosage needs to be carefully adjusted to find a level that controls symptoms while maintaining sufficient muscle strength.

RISKS AND SPECIAL PRECAUTIONS
The main long-term risk associated with centrally acting muscle relaxants is that the body becomes dependent. If the drugs are withdrawn suddenly, the stiffness may become worse than before drug treatment.

Rarely, dantrolene can cause serious liver damage, especially when given in high doses. Anyone taking this drug should have his or her blood tested regularly to assess liver function.

Unless used very cautiously, botulinum toxin can paralyse unaffected muscles, and might interfere with functions such as speech and swallowing.

COMMON DRUGS
Centrally acting drugs Baclofen*, Carisoprodol, Cyclobenzaprine, Diazepam*, Methocarbamol, Orphenadrine*
Other drugs Botulinum toxin, Dantrolene, Quinine*, Tizanidine
* **See Part 2**

Drugs used for myasthenia gravis

Myasthenia gravis occurs when the immune system (see p.93) becomes defective and produces antibodies that disrupt the signals being transmitted between the nervous system and muscles that are under voluntary control. As a result, the body's muscular response is progressively weakened. The first muscles to be affected are those controlling the eyes, eyelids, face, pharynx, and larynx, with muscles in the arms and legs becoming involved as the disease progresses. Typical symptoms that result include drooping eyelids, double vision, and a weak voice, which worsens during the day. The disease is often linked to a disorder of the thymus gland, which is the source of the destructive antibodies concerned. Located in the upper part of the chest, this gland is thought to be partly responsible for the abnormal antibody activity in this disease.

Various methods can be used in the treatment of myasthenia gravis, including removal of the thymus gland (thymectomy) or temporarily clearing the blood of antibodies using a procedure known as plasmapheresis. Drugs that improve muscle function, principally neostigmine and pyridostigmine, may be prescribed. They may be used either alone or together with other drugs that depress the immune system – usually azathioprine (see Immunosuppressant drugs, p.96) or corticosteroids (see p.78).

WHY THEY ARE USED

Drugs that improve the muscle response to nerve impulses have several uses. One such drug, edrophonium, acts very quickly and, once administered, brings about a dramatic improvement in the symptoms. This effect is used to confirm the diagnosis of myasthenia gravis. However, because of its short duration of action, edrophonium is not used for long-term treatment. Pyridostigmine and neostigmine are preferred for long-term treatment, especially when surgery to remove the thymus gland is not feasible or does not provide adequate relief.

These drugs may be given following surgery to counteract the effects of a muscle-relaxant drug given prior to certain surgical procedures.

HOW THEY WORK

Normal muscle action occurs when a nerve impulse triggers a nerve ending to release a neurotransmitter, which combines with a specialized receptor on the muscle cells and causes contraction of the muscles. In myasthenia gravis, the body's immune system destroys many of these receptors, so that the muscles are less responsive to nervous stimulation. Drugs used to treat the disorder increase the amount of neurotransmitter at the nerve ending by blocking the action of

an enzyme that normally breaks it down. Increased levels of the neurotransmitter permit the remaining receptors to function more efficiently.

HOW THEY AFFECT YOU

These drugs usually restore the muscle function to a normal or near-normal level, particularly when the myasthenia gravis takes a mild form. Unfortunately, the drugs can produce unwanted muscular activity by enhancing the transmission of nerve impulses elsewhere in the body.

Common side effects include vomiting, nausea, diarrhoea, and muscle cramps in the arms, legs, and abdomen.

RISKS AND SPECIAL PRECAUTIONS

Muscle weakness can suddenly worsen even when it is being treated with drugs. Should this occur, it is important not to take larger doses of the drug in an attempt to relieve the symptoms, since excessive levels can interfere with the transmission of nerve impulses to muscles, causing further weakness. The administration of other drugs, including some antibiotics, can also markedly increase the symptoms of myasthenia gravis. If your symptoms suddenly become worse, you should consult your doctor.

COMMON DRUGS

Azathioprine*, Edrophonium, Distigmine, Neostigmine, Pyridostigmine*, Corticosteroids (see p.78)
* **See Part 2**

Drugs for bone disorders

Bone is a living structure. Its hard, mineral quality is created by the action of the bone cells. These cells continuously deposit and remove phosphorus and calcium, which are stored in a honeycombed protein framework called the matrix. Because the rates of deposit and removal (the bone metabolism) are about equal in adults, the bone mass remains fairly constant.

Removal and renewal is regulated by hormones and influenced by a number of factors, notably the level of calcium in the blood, which depends on the intake of calcium and vitamin D from the diet, the actions of various hormones, plus everyday movement and weight-bearing stress. When normal bone metabolism is altered, various bone disorders result.

OSTEOPOROSIS

In osteoporosis, the strength and density of bone are reduced. Such wasting occurs when the rate of removal of mineralized bone exceeds the rate of deposit. In most people, bone density decreases very gradually from the age of 30. But bone loss can dramatically increase when a person is immobilized for a period, and this is an important cause of osteoporosis in elderly people. Hormone deficiency is another important cause, commonly occurring in women with lowered oestrogen levels after the menopause or removal of the ovaries. Osteoporosis is therefore much more common with increasing age in women than in men. It also occurs in disorders in which there is excess production of adrenal or thyroid hormones, and it is a major adverse effect of long-term treatment with corticosteroid drugs.

People with osteoporosis often have no symptoms, but, if the vertebrae become so weakened that they are unable to bear the body's weight, they may collapse spontaneously or after a minor accident. Subsequently, the individual suffers from back pain, reduced height, and a round-shouldered appearance. Osteoporosis also makes a fracture of a wrist, thigh, or hip bone more likely.

Most doctors stress the need to prevent osteoporosis by ensuring adequate intake of protein and calcium, giving up smoking, and taking regular exercise throughout adult life. Oestrogen supplements during and after the menopause may be used to prevent osteoporosis in older women. (See Hormone replacement therapy, p.87.)

The condition of bones damaged by osteoporosis cannot usually be improved, but drug treatment can help prevent further deterioration and help fractures to heal. For people whose diet is deficient in calcium or vitamin D, supplements may be prescribed. However, these are of limited value and are often less useful than drugs that inhibit the removal of calcium from the bones. In the past, the hormone calcitonin was used, but it has now been largely superseded by drugs such as etidronate and alendronate. These drugs, known as bisphosphonates, bind very tightly to bone matrix, preventing its removal by bone cells. They reduce the incidence of vertebral fractures, but there is less evidence of their effectiveness in reducing hip fractures.

OSTEOMALACIA AND RICKETS

In osteomalacia (called rickets when it affects children), lack of vitamin D leads to loss of calcium, resulting in softening of the bones. Sufferers experience pain, tenderness, and reduced muscle strength, and there is a risk of fracture and bone deformity. In children, growth is retarded.

Osteomalacia is most commonly caused by a lack of vitamin D. This can result from an inadequate diet, inability to absorb the vitamin, or insufficient exposure of the skin to sunlight (the action of the sun on the skin produces vitamin D inside the body). People at special risk include those whose absorption of vitamin D is impaired by an intestinal disorder, like Crohn's disease or coeliac disease. People with dark skins living in Northern Europe are also susceptible. Chronic kidney disease is an important cause of rickets in children and of osteomalacia in adults, since healthy kidneys play an essential role in the body's metabolism of vitamin D.

Long-term relief depends on treating the underlying disorder where possible. In rare cases, treatment may be lifelong.

VITAMIN D

A number of substances that are related to vitamin D may be used in the treatment of bone disorders. These include alfacalcidol, calcitriol, and ergocalciferol. The drug prescribed depends on the underlying problem. (See also page 87.)

COMMON DRUGS

Alendronate, Alfacalcidol, Calcitonin, Calcitriol, Calcium carbonate, Conjugated estrogens*, Ergocalciferol, Etidronate*, Fluoride, Salcatonin (calcitonin (salmon)), Vitamin D

* **See Part 2**

ALLERGY

Allergy, which is a hypersensitivity to certain substances, is a reaction of the body's immune system. Through a variety of mechanisms (see Malignant and immune disease, p.93), the immune system protects the body by eliminating foreign substances that it does not recognize, such as microorganisms (bacteria or viruses).

One way in which the immune system acts is through the production of antibodies. When the body encounters a particular foreign substance (or allergen) for the first time, one type of white blood cell, the lymphocytes, produces antibodies that attach themselves to another type of white blood cell, the mast cells. If the same substance is encountered again, the allergen binds to the antibodies on the mast cells, causing the release of chemicals known as mediators.

The most important mediator is histamine. Released in response to injury or the presence of allergens, it acts on H_1 receptors in the skin, blood vessels, nasal passages, and airways, and on H_2 receptors in the stomach lining. This can produce a rash, swelling, narrowing of the airways, and a drop in blood pressure. Despite being important in protecting the body against infection, these effects may be triggered inappropriately in an allergic reaction. (see also Antihistamines, right, and Anti-ulcer drugs, p.41).

WHAT CAN GO WRONG

One of the most common allergic disorders, hay fever, is caused by an allergic reaction to inhaled grass pollen leading to allergic rhinitis – swelling and irritation of the nasal passages and watering of the nose and eyes. Other substances, such as house-dust mites, animal fur, and feathers, may cause a similar reaction in susceptible people.

Asthma may result from the action of leukotrienes rather than histamine. Other allergic conditions include urticaria (hives) or other rashes (sometimes in response to a drug), and some forms of eczema and dermatitis. Anaphylaxis is a serious systemic allergic reaction that occurs when an allergen reaches the tissues. (See also Epinephrine, p.219.)

WHY DRUGS ARE USED

Antihistamines and drugs that inhibit mast cell activity are used to prevent and treat allergic reactions. Other drugs minimize allergic symptoms, such as decongestants (p.24) to clear the nose in allergic rhinitis, bronchodilators (p.23) to widen the airways of people with asthma, and corticosteroids applied to skin affected by eczema (p.116).

MAJOR DRUG GROUPS

◆ Antihistamines
◆ Corticosteroids (see p.78)

Antihistamines

Antihistamines are the most widely used drugs in the treatment of allergic reactions of all kinds. They can be subdivided according to their chemical structure; each subgroup has slightly different actions and characteristics. (see table, p.58). Their main action is to counter the effects of histamine, one of the chemicals released in the body when there is an allergic reaction (see Allergy, left).

Histamine is also involved in other body functions, including blood-vessel dilation and constriction, contraction of muscles in the respiratory and gastrointestinal tracts, and the release of digestive juices. The antihistamines described here are also known as H_1 blockers because they only block the action of histamine on certain receptors, called H_1 receptors. Another group of antihistamines, called H_2 blockers, is used in the treatment of peptic ulcers (see Anti-ulcer drugs, p.41).

Some antihistamines have a significant anticholinergic action (see Drugs that act on the parasympathetic nervous system, p.9). This is used to advantage in a variety of conditions, but it also accounts for certain undesired side effects.

WHY THEY ARE USED

Antihistamines relieve allergy-related symptoms when it is not possible to prevent exposure to the substance that has provoked the reaction. They are most commonly used in the prevention of allergic rhinitis (hay fever), in which histamine released in response to an allergen, such as pollen, house dust, or animal fur, acts on histamine receptors and produces dilation of the blood vessels supplying the lining of the nose, leading to swelling and increased mucus production. There is also irritation that causes sneezing, and often redness and watering of the eyes. The drugs are more effective when taken before an attack starts; if taken after the start of an attack, beneficial effects may be delayed.

Antihistamines are not usually effective in asthma caused by similar allergens because the symptoms of this allergic disorder are not solely caused by the action of histamine, but are likely to be the result of more complex mechanisms. Antihistamines are usually the first drugs to be tried in the treatment of allergic disorders but alternatives can be prescribed (see Other allergy treatments, p.58).

Antihistamines are also prescribed for the itching, swelling, and redness of allergic reactions involving the skin (e.g., urticaria (hives) and dermatitis) and the irritation of chickenpox. Allergic reactions to insect stings may also be reduced by these drugs . In such cases the drug may be taken by mouth or applied topically. Applied as drops, antihistamines can reduce inflammation and irritation of the eyes and eyelids in allergic conjunctivitis.

An antihistamine is often included in cough and cold preparations (see p.26), when the anticholinergic effect of drying mucus secretions and their sedative effect on the coughing mechanism may be helpful.

Because most antihistamines have a depressant effect on the brain, they are sometimes used to promote sleep, especially when it is disturbed by itching (see also Sleeping drugs, p.11). Antihistamines' depressant effect on the brain also extends to the centres that control nausea and vomiting. The drugs are therefore often effective in preventing and controlling these symptoms (see Anti-emetics, p.21).

Occasionally, antihistamines are used to treat fever, rash, and breathing difficulties that may occur in adverse reactions to blood transfusions and allergic reactions to drugs. Promethazine and trimeprazine are also used as premedication and to dry secretions during surgery, particularly in children.

HOW THEY WORK

Antihistamines block the action of histamine on H_1 receptors, which are found in various body tissues, particularly the small blood vessels in the skin, nose, and eyes. This helps prevent the dilation of the vessels, caused by the release of histamine in allergic reactions, thus reducing the redness, watering, and swelling typical of many types of allergy. Also, the drugs' anticholinergic action contributes to this effect by reducing the secretions from tear glands and nasal passages.

Antihistamines pass from the blood into the brain, where they produce general sedation and depression of various brain functions, including the vomiting and coughing mechanisms.

HOW THEY AFFECT YOU

Some antihistamines can cause a degree of drowsiness and may adversely affect coordination, leading to clumsiness. However, there are a number of newer drugs which have little or no sedative effect (see table, p.58).

Anticholinergic side effects, including dry mouth, blurred vision, and difficulty passing urine, are common. Most diminish with continued use and can often be helped by adjusting the dose or changing to a different drug.

RISKS AND SPECIAL PRECAUTIONS

It may be advisable to avoid driving or operating machinery while taking antihistamines, particularly those that are more likely to cause drowsiness (see table, p.58). The sedative effects of alcohol, sleeping drugs, opioid analgesics, and anti-anxiety drugs will add to those of antihistamines.

In high doses, or in children, some antihistamines can cause excitement, agitation, and, in extreme cases, hallucinations and convulsions. Abnormal heart rhythms have occurred after high doses or when drugs that interact with them (e.g., antifungals and antibiotics) have been taken at the same time. Heart-rhythm problems may also affect people with liver disease, electrolyte disturbances, or abnormal heart activity. People with these conditions, or glaucoma or prostate trouble, should seek medical advice before taking antihistamines because the various actions of these drugs may make such conditions worse.

COMMON DRUGS

Non-sedating Acrivastine, Cetirizine*, Fexofenadine, Loratadine*, Mizolastine

Sedating Azatadine, Brompheniramine, Chlorphenamine, Clemastine, Dimenhydrinate, Diphenhydramine, Diphenylpyraline, Doxylamine, Promethazine*, Trimeprazine, Triprolidine

* **See Part 2**

OTHER ALLERGY TREATMENTS

Sodium cromoglicate This drug (p.366) prevents the release of histamine from mast cells (see p.56) in response to exposure to an allergen, thus preventing the physical symptoms of allergies. It is commonly given by inhaler for the prevention of allergy-induced rhinitis (hay fever) or asthma attacks and by drops for the treatment of allergic eye disorders.

Leukotriene antagonists Like histamine, leukotrienes are substances that occur naturally in the body and seem to play an important part in asthma. Drugs such as zileuton, montelukast (p.308), and zafirlukast (leukotriene antagonists) have been developed to prevent asthma attacks, but they are not bronchodilators and will not relieve an existing attack.

Corticosteroids These drugs for allergic rhinitis and asthma are usually given by inhaler, providing a high dose to the affected area. The dose to the rest of the body is very low, reducing the risk of long-term adverse effects.

Desensitization This may be tried in conditions such as allergic rhinitis due to pollen sensitivity and insect venom hypersensitivity, when avoidance, antihistamines, and other treatments have not been effective and tests have shown one or two specific allergens be responsible. Desensitization often provides incomplete relief and can be time consuming.

Treatment involves a series of injections containing increasing doses of an extract of the allergen. It is not understood how this prevents allergic reactions, but controlled exposure may trigger the immune system into producing increasing levels of antibodies so that the body no longer responds dramatically when the allergen is encountered naturally.

Desensitization must be carried out under medical supervision because it can provoke a severe allergic response. It is important to remain near emergency medical facilities for at least one hour after each injection.

COMPARISON OF ANTIHISTAMINES

The table below indicates the main uses of some common antihistamines and lists their relative strength of anticholinergic action, sedative effects, and duration of action.

KEY
● Drug used ■ Strong ◨ Medium □ Minimal
▲ Long (over 12 hours) ▲ Medium (6–12 hours)
△ Short (4–6 hours)

DRUGS	COMMON USES — Allergic rhinitis	Skin allergy	Sedation	Premedication	Nausea/vomiting	Cough/cold remedies	ACTIONS AND EFFECTS — Sedation/drowsiness	Anticholinergic action	DURATION OF ACTION
Alimemazine	●	●	●				■	□	▲
Azatadine	●	●					◨	◨	▲
Brompheniramine	●	●				●	◨	□	△
Cetirizine	●	●					□	□	▲
Chlorphenamine	●	●	●				◨	◨	△
Dimenhydrinate				●			◨	◨	△
Diphenhydramine			●		●	●	◨	◨	△
Diphenylpyraline	●	●				●	■	◨	▲
Fexofenadine	●	●					□	□	▲
Hydroxyzine		●	●				◨	◨	△
Loratadine	●	●					□	□	▲
Promethazine	●	●	●	●		●	■	◨	▲
Triprolidine	●	●				●	◨	□	▲

INFECTIONS AND INFESTATIONS

The human body provides a suitable environment for the growth of many types of microorganisms, including bacteria, viruses, fungi, yeasts, and protozoa. It may also become the host for animal parasites such as insects, worms, and flukes.

Microorganisms (microbes) exist all around us and can be transmitted from person to person in many ways: direct contact, inhalation of infected air, and consumption of contaminated food or water. Not all microorganisms cause disease; many types of bacteria exist on the skin surface or in the bowel without causing ill effects, while others cannot live either in or on the body.

Normally the immune system protects the body from infection. Invading microbes are killed before they can multiply in sufficient numbers to cause serious disease. (See also Malignant and immune disease, p.93.)

TYPES OF INFECTING ORGANISM

A typical bacterium consists of a single cell that has a protective wall. Some bacteria are aerobic – that is, they require oxygen – and therefore are more likely to infect surface areas such as the skin or respiratory tract. Others are anaerobic and multiply in oxygen-free surroundings such as the bowel or deep puncture wounds. Bacteria can cause symptoms of disease in two principal ways: first, by releasing toxins that harm body cells; second, by provoking an inflammatory response in the infected tissues.

Viruses are smaller than bacteria and consist simply of a core of genetic material surrounded by a protein coat. A virus can multiply only in a living cell by using the host tissue's replicating material.

Protozoa are single-celled parasites and are slightly bigger than bacteria. Many protozoa live in the human intestine and are harmless. However, some types cause malaria, sleeping sickness, and dysentery.

INFESTATIONS

Invasion by parasites that live on the body (such as lice) or in the body (such as tapeworms) is known as infestation. Since the body lacks strong natural defences against infestation, antiparasitic treatment is necessary. Infestation is often associated with tropical climates and poor standards of hygiene.

WHAT CAN GO WRONG

Infectious diseases occur when the body is invaded by microbes. This may be caused by the body having little or no natural immunity to the invading organism, or the number of invading microbes being too great for the body's immune system to overcome. Serious infections can occur when the immune system does not function properly, as in the malnourished or the elderly, or when a disease that weakens or destroys the immune system, as occurs in AIDS (acquired immune deficiency syndrome).

Infections (such as childhood infectious diseases or those with flu-like symptoms) can cause generalized illness, or they may affect a specific part of the body (as in wound infections). Some parts are more susceptible to infection than others – respiratory tract infections are relatively common, whereas bone and muscle infections are rare.

Some symptoms are the result of damage to body tissues by the infection, or by toxins released by the microbes. In other cases, they result from the body's defence mechanisms.

Most bacterial and viral infections cause fever; and bacterial infections may also cause pus formation and inflammation in the affected area.

WHY DRUGS ARE USED

Treatment of an infection is necessary only when the type or severity of symptoms shows that the immune system has not overcome the infection.

Bacterial infection can be treated with antibiotic or antibacterial drugs. Some of these drugs kill the infecting bacteria; others simply prevent them from multiplying.

Unnecessary use of antibiotics may result in the development of resistant bacteria.

Some antibiotics can be used to treat a broad range of infections, while others are effective against particular types of bacteria or in a certain part of the body. Antibiotics are most commonly given by mouth, or by injection in severe infections, but they may be applied topically for a local action.

Antiviral drugs are used for severe viral infections that threaten body organs or survival. Antivirals may be used in topical preparations, given by mouth, or administered in hospital by injection.

Other drugs used to fight infection include antiprotozoal drugs for protozoal infections such as malaria; antifungal drugs for infection by fungi and yeasts, including *Candida* (thrush); and anthelmintics to eradicate worm and fluke infestations. Infestation by skin parasites is usually treated with the topical application of insecticides (see p.118.)

MAJOR DRUG GROUPS
◆ Antibiotics and antibacterial drugs (including drugs for meningitis, drug treatment for Hansen's disease, and antituberculous drugs)
◆ Antiviral drugs
◆ Vaccines and immunizations
◆ Antiprotozoal drugs (including antimalarial drugs)
◆ Antifungal drugs
◆ Anthelmintic drugs

Antibiotics

One in six prescriptions that British doctors write every year is for antibiotics. These drugs are usually safe and effective in the treatment of bacterial disorders ranging from minor infections, like conjunctivitis, to life-threatening diseases like pneumonia, meningitis, and septicaemia. They are similar in function to the antibacterial drugs (see p.64), but the early antibiotics all had a natural origin in moulds and fungi, although most are now synthesized.

Since 1941, when the first antibiotic, penicillin, was introduced, many different classes have been developed. Each one has a different chemical composition and is effective against a particular range of bacteria. None is effective against viral infections (see Antiviral drugs, p.67).

Some of the antibiotics have a broad spectrum of activity against a wide variety of bacteria. Others are used in the treatment of infection by only a few specific organisms. For a description of each common class of antibiotic, see Classes of antibiotics p.62.

WHY THEY ARE USED
We are surrounded by bacteria – in the air we breathe, on the mucous membranes of our mouth and nose, on our skin, and in our intestines – but we are protected, most of the time, by our immunological defences. When these break down, or when bacteria already present migrate to a vulnerable new site, or when harmful bacteria not usually present invade the body, infectious disease sets in.

The bacteria multiply uncontrollably, destroying tissue, releasing toxins, and, in some cases, threatening to spread via the bloodstream to such vital organs as the heart, brain, lungs, and kidneys. The symptoms of infectious disease vary widely, depending on the site of the infection and type of bacteria.

Confronted with a sick person and suspecting a bacterial infection, the doctor should identify the organism causing the disease before prescribing any drug. However, tests to analyse blood, sputum, urine, stool, or pus usually take 24 hours or more. In the meantime, especially if the person is in discomfort or pain, the doctor usually makes a preliminary drug choice, something of an educated guess as to the causative organism. In starting this "empirical" treatment, as it is called, the doctor is guided by the site of the infection, the nature and severity of the symptoms, the likely source of infection, and the prevalence of any similar illnesses in the community at that time.

In such circumstances, pending laboratory identification of the trouble-making bacteria, the doctor may initially prescribe a broad-spectrum antibiotic, which is effective against a wide variety of bacteria. As soon as tests provide more exact information, the doctor may switch the person to the recommended antibiotic treatment for the identified bacteria. In some cases, more than one antibiotic is prescribed, to be sure of eliminating all strains of bacteria.

In most cases, antibiotics can be given by mouth. However, in serious infections when high blood levels of the drug are needed

USES OF ANTIBIOTICS

The table below shows common drugs in each class of antibiotic that are used to treat infections in different parts of the body; it is not intended for use as a guide to prescribing. For comparison, some antibacterial drugs (p.64) are included under 'Other drugs'.

ANTIBIOTIC	Ear, nose, throat, and mouth	Respiratory tract	Skin and soft tissue	Gastrointestinal tract	Eye	Kidney and urinary tract	Brain and nervous system	Heart	Bones and joints	Genital tract
Penicillins										
Amoxicillin	●	●	●			●		●	●	●
Ampicillin	●	●	●			●	●		●	●
Benzylpenicillin	●	●	●			●	●	●	●	●
Co-amoxiclav	●	●	●			●		●		
Flucloxacillin	●		●					●	●	
Phenoxymethylpenicillin	●	●	●							
Cephalosporins										
Cefaclor	●	●				●				
Cefalexin		●	●			●				
Cefotaxime		●					●			
Cefoxitin		●	●			●				●
Macrolides										
Azithromycin	●	●	●							●
Erythromycin	●	●	●	●	●				●	●
Tetracyclines										
Doxycycline	●	●				●				●
Oxytetracycline	●	●								
Tetracycline	●	●			●	●				●
Aminoglycosides										
Amikacin		●	●	●		●	●		●	
Gentamicin		●	●	●	●	●	●	●	●	
Neomycin			●	●						
Netilmicin		●	●	●		●	●		●	
Streptomycin		●						●		
Tobramycin		●	●	●		●	●		●	
Sulphonamides										
Co-trimoxazole		●				●				
Sulphafurazole	●	●				●				
Other drugs										
Chloramphenicol	●	●		●	●	●				
Ciprofloxacin		●		●		●				
Clindamycin		●	●	●					●	
Colistin		●				●				
Dapsone			●							
Fusidic acid			●						●	
Metronidazole	●		●	●			●	●	●	●
Nalidixic acid						●				
Nitrofurantoin						●				
Teicoplanin			●						●	●
Trimethoprim	●					●				
Vancomycin				●				●		

rapidly, or when a type of antibiotic is needed that cannot be given by mouth, the drug may be given by injection. Antibiotics are also included in topical preparations for localized skin, eye, and ear infections (see also Anti-infective skin preparations, p.116, and Drugs for ear disorders, p.113).

HOW THEY WORK

Depending on the type of drug and the dosage, antibiotics are either bactericidal, killing organisms directly, or bacteriostatic, halting the multiplication of bacteria and enabling the body's natural defences to overcome the remaining infection.

Penicillins and cephalosporins are bactericidal, destroying bacteria by preventing them from making normal cell walls; most other antibiotics act inside the bacteria by interfering with the chemical activities essential to their life cycle.

CLASSES OF ANTIBIOTIC

Penicillins The first antibiotic drugs to be developed, penicillins are still widely used to treat many common infections. Some are not effective when they are taken by mouth and therefore have to be given by injection in hospital. Unfortunately, certain strains of bacteria are resistant to penicillin treatment, and other drugs may have to be substituted. Penicillins often cause allergic reactions.

Cephalosporins These broad-spectrum antibiotics, similar to the penicillins, are often used when penicillin treatment has proved ineffective. Some can be given by mouth, but others are only given by injection. About 10 per cent of people who are allergic to penicillins are also allergic to cephalosporins. Some cephalosporins can occasionally damage the kidneys, particularly if used with aminoglycosides. Another serious, although rare, adverse effect of a few cephalosporins is that they occasionally interfere with normal blood clotting, leading to abnormally heavy bleeding, especially in the elderly.

Macrolides Erythromycin is the most common drug in this group. It is a broad-spectrum antibiotic that is often prescribed as an alternative to penicillins or cephalosporins. Erythromycin is also effective against certain diseases, such as Legionnaires' disease (a rare type of pneumonia), that cannot be treated with other antibiotics. The main risk with erythromycin is that it can occasionally impair liver function.

Tetracyclines These have a broader spectrum of activity than other classes of antibiotic. However, increasing bacterial resistance (see Antibiotic resistance, facing page) has limited their use, but they are still widely prescribed. As well as being used for the treatment of infections, tetracyclines are also used in the long-term treatment of acne, although this application is probably not related to their antibacterial action. A major drawback to the use of tetracycline antibiotics in pregnant women and young children is that they are deposited in developing bones and teeth.

With the exception of doxycycline, drugs from this group are poorly absorbed through the intestines, and when given by mouth they have to be administered in high doses in order to reach effective levels in the blood. Such high doses increase the likelihood of diarrhoea as a side effect. The absorption of tetracyclines can be further reduced by interaction with calcium and other minerals. Drugs from this group should not therefore be taken with iron tablets or milk products. Tetracyclines deteriorate and may become poisonous with time, so leftover tablets or capsules should always be discarded.

Aminoglycosides These potent drugs are effective against a wide range of bacteria. They are not as widely used as some other antibiotics, however, since they have to be given by injection and have potentially serious side effects. Their use is therefore limited to hospital treatment of serious infections. They are often given with other antibiotics. Possible adverse effects include a severe skin rash and damage to the kidneys and nerves in the ear.

Lincosamides The lincosamide clindamycin is not commonly used as it is more likely to cause serious disruption of bacterial activity in the bowel than other antibiotics. It is mainly reserved for the treatment of bone, joint, abdominal, and pelvic infections that do not respond well to the safer antibiotics. Clindamycin is also used topically for acne and vaginal infections.

Quinolones These drugs, often called antibacterials, are derived from chemicals rather than living organisms. Quinolones have a wide spectrum of activity. They are used in the treatment of urinary infections and are widely effective in acute diarrhoeal diseases, including that caused by salmonella, as well as in the treatment of enteric fever.

The absorption of quinolones is reduced by antacids containing magnesium and aluminium. They are well tolerated but should be avoided by epileptics, as they may rarely cause convulsions, and by children, as studies have shown that they may cause arthritis.

HOW THEY AFFECT YOU

Antibiotics stop most common types of infection within days. Because they do not relieve symptoms directly, your doctor may advise additional medication, such as analgesics (see p.9), to relieve pain and fever until the antibiotics take effect.

It is important to complete the course of medication as prescribed by your doctor, even if all your symptoms have disappeared. Failure to do this can lead to a resurgence of the infection in an antibiotic-resistant form (see Antibiotic resistance, below).

Most antibiotics used in the home do not cause adverse effects if taken in the recommended dosage. In people who do experience them, nausea and diarrhoea are common. (See also individual drug profiles in Part 2.) Some people may be sensitive to certain types of antibiotics, which can result in a variety of serious adverse effects.

ANTIBIOTIC RESISTANCE

The increasing use of antibiotics in the treatment of infection has led to resistance in certain types of bacteria to the effects of particular antibiotics. This resistance to the drug usually occurs when bacteria develop mechanisms of growth and reproduction that are not disrupted by the effects of the antibiotics. In other cases, bacteria produce enzymes that neutralize the antibiotics.

Antibiotic resistance may develop in a person during prolonged treatment when a drug has failed to eliminate the infection quickly. The resistant strain of bacteria is able to multiply, thereby prolonging the illness. It may also infect other people and result in the spread of resistant infection.

One particularly important example is methicillin-resistant staphylococcus aureus, which resists most antibiotics but can be treated with other drugs such as teicoplanin and vancomycin.

Doctors try to prevent the development of antibiotic resistance by selecting the drug most likely to eliminate the bacteria present in each individual case as quickly and as thoroughly as possible. Failure to complete a course of antibiotics that has been prescribed by your doctor increases the likelihood that the infection will recur in a resistant form.

RISKS AND SPECIAL PRECAUTIONS

Most antibiotics used for short periods outside a hospital setting are safe for most people. The most common risk, especially with cephalosporins and penicillins, is a severe allergic reaction to the drug that can cause a rash and sometimes swelling of the face and throat. If this happens, you should stop the drug and seek immediate medical advice. If you have had a previous allergic reaction to an antibiotic, all other drugs in that class and related classes should be avoided. It is therefore important to inform your doctor if you have previously suffered an adverse reaction to treatment with an antibiotic (with the exception of minor bowel disturbances).

Another risk of antibiotic treatment, especially if it is prolonged, is that the balance among microorganisms normally inhabiting the body may be disturbed. In particular, antibiotics may destroy the bacteria that normally limit the growth of *candida*, a yeast that is often present in small amounts in the body. This can lead to overgrowth of *Candida* (thrush) in the mouth, vagina, or bowel, and an antifungal drug (p.74) may be needed.

A rarer, but more serious, result of disruption of normal bacterial activity in the body is a disorder known as pseudomembranous colitis, in which bacteria that are resistant to the antibiotic multiply in the bowel, causing violent, bloody diarrhoea. This potentially fatal disorder can occur with any antibiotic, but is most common with the lincosamides.

COMMON DRUGS

Aminoglycosides Amikacin, Gentamicin*, Neomycin, Netilmicin, Streptomycin, Tobramycin

Cephalosporins Cefadroxil, Cefaclor, Cefalexin*, Cefamandole, Cefazolin, Cefixime, Cefodizime, Cefoxitin, Cefpodoxime, Cefradine, Ceftazidime
Lincosamides Clindamycin
Macrolides Azithromycin, Clarithromycin, Erythromycin*
Penicillins Amoxicillin*, Ampicillin, Azlocillin, Aztreonam, Benzylpenicillin, Co-amoxiclav, Co-fluampicil, Flucloxacillin, Imipenem, Phenoxymethylpenicillin*
Tetracyclines Doxycycline*, Oxytetracycline, Tetracycline*
Other drugs Chloramphenicol*, Colistin, Fusidic acid, Metronidazole*, Rifampicin*, Spectinomycin, Teicoplanin, Trimethoprim*, Vancomycin
∗ See Part 2

Drugs for meningitis

Meningitis is inflammation of the meninges (the membranes surrounding the brain and spinal cord) and is caused by both bacteria and viruses. Bacterial meningitis can kill previously well individuals within hours.

If bacterial meningitis is suspected, intramuscular or intravenous antibiotics are needed immediately and admission to hospital is arranged.

In cases of bacterial meningitis caused by *Haemophilus influenzae* or *Neisseria meningitidis*, contacts are advised to have a preventative course of antibiotics, usually rifampicin.

Antibacterial drugs

This broad classification of drugs comprises agents similar to the antibiotics (p.60) in function but dissimilar in origin. The original antibiotics were derived from living organisms such as moulds and fungi. Antibacterials were developed from chemicals. The sulphonamides were the first drugs to be given for the treatment of bacterial infections and were the mainstay of the treatment of infection before penicillin (the first antibiotic) became generally available. Increasing bacterial resistance and the development of more effective and less toxic antibiotics have reduced the use of sulphonamides.

WHY THEY ARE USED

Sulphonamides have a number of uses. Because certain strains of bacteria have developed a resistance to the actions of sulphonamides (see Antibiotic resistance, p.63), the sulphonamides have, in many cases, been superseded by antibiotics that are more effective and safer. However, there are still many circumstances in which doctors prescribe the sulphonamides.

Because sulphonamides reach high concentrations in the urine, they are especially useful for treating many urinary tract infections. They are often used for chlamydial pneumonia and some middle-ear infections. Trimethoprim is used for chest and urinary tract infections. The drug used to be combined with sulfamethoxazole as co-trimoxazole, but because of the side effects of sulfamethoxazole, trimethoprim on its own is now usually preferred.

Not all antibacterials are sulphonamides. Antibacterials used in the treatment of tuberculosis are discussed on the facing page. Others, sometimes classified as antimicrobials, include metronidazole, which is prescribed to treat a variety of genital infections and for some serious infections of the abdomen, pelvic region, heart, and central nervous system. Other antibacterials are used to treat urinary infections. These include nitrofurantoin and drugs in the quinolone group such as nalidixic acid (see Classes of antibiotic, p.62), which is used as a urinary tract antiseptic and to cure or prevent recurrent infections. Two more potent relatives of nalidixic acid are norfloxacin and ciprofloxacin. Norfloxacin is used to treat urinary tract infections, and ciprofloxacin is prescribed for many serious bacterial infections.

HOW THEY WORK

Most antibacterials function by preventing the growth and multiplication of bacteria. Folic acid, a chemical necessary for their growth, is produced within bacterial cells by an enzyme that acts on a chemical called para-aminobenzoic acid. Sulphonamides interfere with the release of the enzyme. This prevents folic acid from being formed. The bacterium is therefore unable to function properly and dies.

HOW THEY AFFECT YOU

Antibacterials usually take several days to eliminate bacteria. During this time your doctor may recommend additional medication to alleviate pain and fever. Possible side effects of sulphonamides include loss of appetite, nausea, a rash, and drowsiness.

RISKS AND SPECIAL PRECAUTIONS

Like antibiotics, most antibacterials can cause allergic reactions in susceptible people. Possible symptoms that should always be brought to your doctor's attention include rashes and fever. If such symptoms occur, a change to another drug is likely to be necessary. Treatment with sulphonamides carries a number of serious but rare risks. Some drugs in this group can cause crystals to form in the kidneys, a risk that can be reduced by drinking adequate amounts of fluid during prolonged treatment. Because sulphonamides may also occasionally damage the liver, they are not usually prescribed for people with impaired liver function. There is also a slight risk of damage to bone marrow, lowering the production of white blood cells and increasing the chances of infection. Doctors therefore try to avoid prescribing sulphonamides for prolonged periods. Liver function and blood composition are often monitored during unavoidable long-term treatment.

COMMON DRUGS

Quinolones Cinoxacin, Ciprofloxacin*, Grepafloxacin, Levofloxacin*, Nalidixic acid, Norfloxacin, Ofloxacin
Sulphonamides Co-trimoxazole*, Sulfadiazine, Sulfadimidine
Urinary antiseptic Nitrofurantoin
Other drugs Clofazimine, Dapsone, Metronidazole*, Tinidazole, Trimethoprim*
* See Part 2

Drug treatment for Hansen's disease

Hansen's disease, more commonly known as leprosy, is a bacterial infection caused by *Mycobacterium leprae*. It is rare in the United

Kingdom, but relatively common in parts of Africa, Asia, and Latin America.

The disease progresses slowly, first affecting the peripheral nerves and causing loss of sensation in the hands and feet. This leads to frequent unnoticed injuries and consequent scarring. Later, the nerves of the face may also be affected.

Treatment uses three drugs together to prevent the development of resistance. Usually, dapsone, rifampicin, and clofazimine will be given for at least 2 years. If one of these cannot be used, then a second line drug (ofloxacin, minocycline, or clarithromycin) might be substituted. Complications during treatment may require use of prednisolone, aspirin, chloroquine, or even thalidomide.

Antituberculous drugs

Tuberculosis is a contagious bacterial disease that is acquired, often in childhood, by inhaling the tuberculosis bacilli present in the spray caused by a sneeze or cough from someone who is actively infected. It may also be acquired from infected cow's milk. The disease usually starts in a lung and takes one of two forms: either primary infection or reactivated infection.

In 90 to 95 per cent of those people with a primary infection, the body's immune system suppresses the infection, but it does not kill the bacilli. They remain alive but dormant and may cause the reactivated form of tuberculosis. After the tuberculosis bacilli are reactivated, they may spread throughout the body via the lymphatic system and the bloodstream.

The first symptoms of the primary infection may include a cough, fever, tiredness, night sweats, and loss of weight. Tuberculosis is confirmed through clinical investigations, which may include a chest X-ray, isolation of the bacilli from the person's sputum, and a positive reaction – localized inflammation – to the Mantoux test, an injection of tuberculin (a protein extracted from tuberculosis bacilli) into the skin.

The gradual emergence in adults of the destructive and progressive form of tuberculosis is caused by the reactivated infection.

It occurs in 5 to 10 per cent of those who have had a previous primary infection. Another form, reinfection tuberculosis, occurs when someone with the dormant, primary form is reinfected. This type of tuberculosis is clinically identical to the reactivated form. Reactivation is more likely in those people whose immune system is suppressed, such as the elderly, those on corticosteroids or other immunosuppressant drugs, and those who have AIDS. Reactivation tuberculosis may be difficult to identify because the symptoms may start in any part of the body seeded with the bacilli. It is most often first seen in the upper lobes of the lung, and it is frequently diagnosed after a chest X-ray. The early symptoms may be identical to those of primary infection: a cough, tiredness, night sweats, fever, and loss of weight.

If left untreated, tuberculosis continues to destroy tissue, spreading throughout the body and eventually causing death. It was one of the most common causes of death in the United Kingdom until the 1940s and the disease is on the increase again. Vulnerable groups are people with suppressed immune systems and the homeless.

WHY THEY ARE USED

A person diagnosed as having tuberculosis is likely to be treated with three or four antituberculous drugs. This helps to overcome the risk of drug-resistant strains of the bacilli emerging (see Antibiotic resistance, p.63).

The standard drug combination for the treatment of tuberculosis consists of four drugs, usually including rifampicin, isoniazid, pyrazinamide, and ethambutol. Other drugs may be substituted if the initial treatment fails or if drug sensitivity tests indicate that the bacilli are resistant to these drugs.

The standard duration of treatment for a newly diagnosed tuberculosis infection is a six-month regimen as follows: isoniazid, rifampicin, pyrazinamide and ethambutol daily for two months, followed by isoniazid and rifampicin for four months. The duration of treatment can be extended from nine months to up to two years in people at particular risk, such as those whose immune system has been suppressed. Ethambutol can sometimes be omitted if resistance is unlikely.

Corticosteroids may be added to the treatment, if the immune system is not suppressed, to reduce the amount of tissue damage; and pyridoxine (see Vitamins, p.88) is also often prescribed to protect the nerves from damage by isoniazid.

Both the number of drugs required and the long duration of treatment may make treatment difficult, particularly for those who are homeless. To help with this problem, supervised administration of treatment is available when required, both in the community and in hospital.

Tuberculosis infection in patients with HIV infection or AIDS is treated with the standard antituberculous drug regimen; but lifelong preventative treatment with isoniazid may be necessary.

HOW THEY WORK

Antituberculous drugs act in the same way as antibiotics, either by killing bacilli or preventing them from multiplying. (See also antibiotics, p.60.)

HOW THEY AFFECT YOU

Although the drugs start to combat the disease within days, the benefits of drug treatment are not usually noticeable for a few weeks. As the infection is eradicated, the body repairs the damage caused by the disease. Symptoms such as fever and coughing gradually subside, and the appetite and general health improve.

RISKS AND SPECIAL PRECAUTIONS

Antituberculous drugs may cause adverse effects (nausea, vomiting, and abdominal pain), and they occasionally lead to serious allergic reactions. When this happens, another drug is substituted.

Rifampicin and isoniazid may affect liver function; isoniazid may adversely affect the nerves as well. Ethambutol can cause changes in colour vision. Dosage is carefully monitored, especially in children, the elderly, and those with reduced kidney function.

TUBERCULOSIS PREVENTION

A vaccine prepared from an artificially weakened strain of cattle tuberculosis bacteria can provide immunity from tuberculosis by provoking the development of natural resistance to the disease (see Vaccines and immunization, p.68). The BCG (Bacille Calmette-Guérin) vaccine is a form of tuberculosis bacillus that provokes the body's immune response but does not cause the illness because it does not invade tissues. The vaccine is usually given to children between the ages of 10 and 14 years who are shown to have no natural immunity when given a skin test. BCG vaccination may be given to newborn babies if, for example, someone in the family has tuberculosis.

The vaccine is usually injected into the upper arm. A small pustule usually appears 6–12 weeks later, by which time the person can be considered immune.

COMMON DRUGS

Capreomycin, Cycloserine, Ethambutol*, Isoniazid*, Pyrazinamide, Rifampicin*, Rifabutin, Streptomycin
* See Part 2

Antiviral drugs

Viruses are simpler and smaller organisms than bacteria and are less able to sustain themselves. These organisms can survive and multiply only by penetrating body cells. In order to reproduce, a virus requires a living cell. The invaded cell eventually dies and the new viruses are released, spreading and infecting other cells. Because viruses perform few functions independently, medicines that disrupt or halt their life cycle without harming human cells have been difficult to develop.

There are many different types of virus, and viral infections cause illnesses with various symptoms and degrees of severity. Common viral illnesses include colds, influenza and flu-like illnesses, cold sores, and childhood diseases such as chickenpox and mumps. Throat infections, pneumonia, acute bronchitis, gastroenteritis, and meningitis are often, but not always, caused by a virus.

Fortunately, the body's natural defences are usually strong enough to overcome infections such as these, with drugs given to ease pain and lower fever. However, the more serious viral diseases, such as pneumonia and meningitis, need close medical supervision.

Another difficulty with viral infections is the speed with which the virus multiplies. By the time symptoms appear, the viruses are so numerous that antiviral drugs have little effect. Antiviral agents must be given early in the course of the infection; they may also be used as a prophylactic (preventative). Some viral infections can be prevented by vaccination (see p.68).

WHY THEY ARE USED

The main area where antiviral drugs are helpful is in the treatment of various conditions caused by the herpes virus: cold sores, encephalitis, genital herpes, chickenpox, and shingles.

Some drugs are applied topically to treat cold sores, herpes eye infections, and genital herpes. They can reduce the severity and duration of an outbreak but do not eliminate the infection permanently. Other antiviral drugs are given by mouth or, under exceptional circumstances, by injection to prevent chickenpox or severe, recurrent attacks of the herpes virus infections in those who are already weakened by other conditions.

Antiviral agents are also given to prevent influenza A, as is amantadine, a drug for parkinsonism that also has antiviral properties.

The interferons are proteins produced by the body and involved in the immune response and cell function. Interferon alpha and beta have recently been shown to be effective in reducing disease activity in people infected with hepatitis B and hepatitis C. Further research into the antiviral activity of these agents is under way, including their use in the treatment of central nervous system conditions, such as multiple sclerosis.

AIDS (acquired immune deficiency syndrome) is caused by infection with the human immunodeficiency virus (HIV), which reduces the body's resistance to infection by other viruses, bacteria, and protozoa, and to some types of cancer. Drug treatment for AIDS is discussed more fully on p.97.

HOW THEY WORK

Some antiviral drugs, such as idoxuridine, act by altering the cell's genetic material (DNA) so that the virus cannot use it to multiply. Other drugs stop multiplication of viruses by blocking enzyme activity within the host cell. Halting multiplication prevents the virus from spreading to uninfected cells and improves symptoms rapidly. However, in herpes infections, it does not eradicate the virus from the body. Infection may therefore flare up on another occasion.

Amantadine has a different action: it stops the virus from entering cells. It is therefore most effective when given prophylactically, before the infection has spread widely.

HOW THEY AFFECT YOU

Topical antiviral drugs usually start to act at once. Providing that the treatment is applied early enough, an outbreak of herpes can be cut short. Symptoms usually clear up within two to four days. Antiviral ointments may cause irritation and redness. Antiviral drugs given by mouth or injection can occasionally cause nausea and dizziness.

RISKS AND SPECIAL PRECAUTIONS

Because some of these drugs may affect the kidneys adversely, they are prescribed with caution for people with reduced kidney function. Some antiviral drugs can adversely affect the activity of normal body cells, particularly those in the bone marrow. Idoxuridine is, for this reason, available only for topical application.

COMMON DRUGS

Aciclovir*, Amantadine* Cidofovir, Famciclovir, Foscarnet, Ganciclovir, Idoxuridine, Inosine pranobex, Interferon*, Penciclovir, Tribavirin, Valaciclovir, Zanamivir*, See also Drugs for HIV, p.97

* **See Part 2**

Vaccines and immunization

Many infectious diseases, including most of the common viral infections, occur only once during a person's lifetime. The reason is that the antibodies produced in response to the disease remain afterwards, prepared to repel any future invasion as soon as the first infectious germs appear. The duration of such immunity varies, but it can last a lifetime.

Protection against many infections can now be provided artificially by the use of vaccines derived from altered forms of the infecting organism. These vaccines stimulate the immune system in the same way as a genuine infection, and provide lasting, active immunity. Because each type of microbe stimulates the production of a specific antibody, a different vaccine must be given for each disease.

Another type of immunization, called passive immunization, relies on giving antibodies (see Immune globulins, p.70).

WHY THEY ARE USED

Some infectious diseases cannot be treated effectively or are potentially so serious that prevention is the best treatment. Routine immunization not only protects the individual but may gradually eradicate the disease completely, as has been achieved with smallpox.

Newborn babies receive antibodies for many diseases from their mothers, but this protection lasts only for about three months. Most children between the ages of 2 months and 15 years are routinely vaccinated against common childhood infectious diseases. In addition, travellers to many underdeveloped countries, especially those in the tropics, are often advised to be vaccinated against the diseases common in those regions.

Effective lifelong immunization can sometimes be achieved by a single dose of the vaccine. However, in many cases, reinforcing doses, commonly called booster shots, are needed later to maintain reliable immunity.

Vaccines do not provide immediate protection against infection and it may be up to four weeks before full immunity is able to develop. When immediate protection from infectious disease is needed – for example, following exposure to infection – it may be necessary to establish passive immunity with immune globulins (see p.70).

HOW THEY WORK

Vaccines provoke the immune system into creating antibodies that help the body to resist specific infectious diseases. Many vaccines (known as live vaccines) are made from artificially weakened forms of the disease-causing germ. But even these weakened

COMMON VACCINATIONS

Most vaccinations are given during infancy and childhood as part of a routine immunization schedule, and most are given by injection. Those people at particular risk through their work or travel can have additional immunization in adulthood.

DISEASE	AGE AT WHICH VACCINATION IS GIVEN
Diphtheria	2 months, 3 months, 4 months, 3–5 years. Booster on leaving school.
Tetanus	2 months, 3 months, 4 months, 3–5 years. Boosters on leaving school and every 10 years thereafter.
Pertussis (whooping cough)	2 months, 3 months, 4 months.
Polio	2 months, 3 months, 4 months, 3–5 years. Boosters on leaving school.
Haemophilus influenzae type b (Hib)	2 months, 3 months, 4 months.
Rubella (German measles)	12–15 months and 3–5 years.
Measles	12–15 months and 3–5 years.
Mumps	12–15 months and 3–5 years.
Tuberculosis (BCG) (Bacille Calmette-Guérin)	6 weeks or 10–14 years.
Influenza	People of any age who are at risk of serious illness or death if they develop influenza.
Hepatitis A	Single dose for people of any age who are at risk. Booster 6–12 months after initial shot. Boosters every 10 years if needed.
Hepatitis B	3 inoculations at any age, with the second and third shots 1 and 6 months after the first. Booster after 5 years if needed.
Pneumococcal pneumonia	Single dose for people of any age who are at risk.
Meningococcal meningitis	Single dose for people of any age who are at risk.

germs are effective in stimulating sufficient growth of antibodies. Other vaccines rely either on inactive (or killed) disease-causing germs, or inactive derivatives of these germs, but their effect on the immune system remains the same. Effective antibodies are created, thereby establishing active immunity.

HOW THEY AFFECT YOU

The degree of protection varies among different vaccines. Some provide reliable life-long immunity; others may not give full protection against a disease, or the effects may last for as little as six months. Influenza vaccines usually protect only against the variety of virus causing the latest outbreak of flu. New varieties appear during most years.

Any vaccine may cause side effects but they are usually mild and soon disappear. The most common reactions are a red, slightly raised, tender area at the site of injection and a slight fever or a flu-like illness lasting for one or two days.

RISKS AND SPECIAL PRECAUTIONS

Serious reactions are rare and, for most children, the risk is far outweighed by the protection given. Children who have had fits may be advised against vaccinations for pertussis (whooping cough) or measles. Children who have any infection more severe than a common cold will not be given any routine vaccination until they have recovered.

Live vaccines should not be given during pregnancy because they can affect the developing baby, nor should they be given to people whose immune systems are weakened by disease or drug treatment. It is also advisable for those taking high doses of corticosteroids (p.78) to delay their vaccinations until the end of drug treatment.

The risk of high fever following the DPT (combined diphtheria, pertussis, and tetanus) vaccine can be reduced by giving paracetamol at the time of vaccination. The pertussis vaccine may rarely cause a mild fit, which is brief, usually associated with fever, and stops without treatment. Children who have experienced such fits recover completely without neurological or developmental problems.

IMMUNE GLOBULINS

Antibodies, which can result from exposure to snake and insect venom as well as infectious disease, are found in the serum of the blood (the part remaining after the red cells and clotting agents are removed). The concentrated serum of people who have survived diseases or poisonous bites is called immune globulin, and, given by injection, it creates passive immunity. Immune globulin from blood donated by a wide cross-section of donors is likely to contain antibodies to most common diseases. Specific immune globulins against rare diseases or toxins are derived from the blood of selected donors likely to have high levels of antibodies to that disease. These are called hyperimmune globulins. Some immune globulins are extracted from horse blood following repeated doses of the toxin.

Because immune globulins do not stimulate the body to produce its own antibodies, their effect is not long-lasting and diminishes progressively over three or four weeks. Continued protection requires repeated injections of immune globulins.

Adverse effects from immune globulins are uncommon. Some people are sensitive to horse globulins, and about a week after the injection they may experience a reaction known as serum sickness, with fever, a rash, joint swelling, and pain. This usually ends in a few days but should be reported to your doctor before any further immunization.

TRAVEL VACCINATIONS

These are not normally necessary for travel to Western Europe, North America, Australia, or New Zealand (although you should make sure that your tetanus and poliomyelitis boosters are up to date). Consult your doctor if you are visiting other destinations. Check that children travelling with you have had the full set of routine childhood vaccinations as well as any that are necessary for the areas in which you will be travelling.

If you are visiting an area where there is yellow fever, an International Certificate of Vaccination will be needed. You may also need this certificate in the future. Many countries that you might want to visit require an International Certificate of Vaccination if you have already been to a country where yellow fever is present.

You are at risk of other infectious diseases in many parts of the world, and appropriate vaccinations are a wise precaution. For example, there is a zone called the "Meningitis Belt" that runs across northern India, Nepal, Bhutan, and Pakistan, and continues across Africa from the Sahara down to Kenya. Anyone intending to visit this zone should have meningococcal vaccine A and C. Visitors to Saudi Arabia at certain times of the year may also be required to have had the meningitis group A and C vaccine.

You may need extra vaccinations if you are backpacking or planning to stay for a long time. For example, hepatitis A vaccine would be sensible for anyone travelling to a developing country, but a long-stay traveller should consider having the hepatitis B vaccine and BCG (tuberculosis) as well. Anyone travelling into remote areas is recommended to have rabies vaccination.

All immunization should be completed well before departure as the vaccinations do not give instant protection (BCG needs 3 months), and some (for example, typhoid) need more than one dose to be effective.

The Department of Health booklet called "Health Advice for Travellers Anywhere in the World" (available with the E111 form from some travel agents and post offices) and The Hospital for Tropical Diseases Travel Clinic Healthline, provide information on requirements for vaccination.

TRAVEL IMMUNIZATION

The immunizations needed before travelling depend on the part of the world you intend to visit, but some diseases can be contracted almost anywhere. Make sure that you have been immunized against tetanus and polio and have had boosters if necessary. Ask your doctor or pharmacist for the most up-to-date information on vaccination for specific areas.

DISEASE	NUMBER OF DOSES	WHEN EFFECTIVE	PERIOD OF PROTECTION	WHO SHOULD BE IMMUNIZED
Diphtheria	1 injection	Immediately	10 years	People travelling to the countries of the former USSR and expatriates living in developing countries.
Hepatitis A	1 injection (gamma globulin)	Immediately	3–6 months	People travelling to Mediterranean or developing countries on a single occasion.
	2 injections (active vaccine)	2–4 weeks after 1st dose	10 years	Frequent travellers to Mediterranean or developing countries.
Hepatitis B	3 injections over 6 months, at least 4 weeks apart	Immediately after 2nd dose	3–5 years	People travelling to countries in which hepatitis B is prevalent; those who might need medical or dental treatment while travelling in a developing country; and people likely to have unprotected sex.
Japanese B encephalitis	2–3 injections 1–2 weeks apart	10–14 days after last dose	About 2 years	People staying for an extended period in rural areas of the Indian subcontinent, China, Southeast Asia, and the Far East.
Meningitis A and C	1 injection	After 15 days	3–5 years	People travelling to Saudi Arabia and remote areas of sub-Saharan Africa, Nepal, and Brazil; immunization certificate needed if travelling to Mecca.
Rabies	3 injections. 1 week between 1st and 2nd doses, 3 weeks between 2nd and 3rd doses	Immediately after 3rd dose	2–3 years	People travelling to areas where rabies is endemic and who are at high risk (e.g., veterinary surgeons, people working with animals, and those travelling into remote country).
Typhoid	1 or 2 injections or 3 oral doses	10 days after last dose or injection	3 years	People travelling to areas with poor sanitation.
Yellow fever	1 injection	After 10 days	10 years	People travelling to parts of South America and Africa.

Antiprotozoal drugs

Protozoa are single-celled organisms that are present in soil and water. They may be transmitted to or between humans through contaminated food or water, sexual contact, or insect bites. There are many different types of protozoal infection, each one causing a different disease depending on the organism that is involved.

Many types of protozoa infect the bowel, causing diarrhoea and generalized symptoms of ill-health. Others may infect the genital tract or skin. Some protozoa may penetrate vital organs such as the lungs, brain, and liver. Prompt diagnosis and treatment are important in order to limit the spread of the infection within the body and, in some cases, prevent it from spreading to other people. Increased attention to hygiene is an important factor in controlling the spread of the disease.

A variety of medicines is used in the treatment of these diseases. Some, such as metronidazole and tetracycline, are also commonly used for their antibacterial action. Others, such as pentamidine, are rarely used except in treating specific protozoal infections.

HOW THEY AFFECT YOU

Protozoa are often difficult to eradicate from the body. Drug treatment may therefore need to be continued for several months in order to eliminate the infecting organisms completely and thus prevent recurrence of the disease. In addition, unpleasant side effects such as nausea, diarrhoea, and abdominal cramps are often unavoidable because of the limited choice of drugs and the need to maintain dosage levels that will effectively cure the disease. For detailed information on the risks and adverse effects of individual antiprotozoal drugs, consult the appropriate drug profile in Part 2.

TYPES OF PROTOZOAL DISEASE

Amoebiasis (*Entamoeba histolytica*), or amoebic dysentery, is an infection of the bowel (and sometimes the liver and other organs) usually transmitted in contaminated food or water. Its major symptom is violent, sometimes bloody, diarrhoea. Treatment is with diloxanide, metronidazole, or tinidazole.

Balantidiasis (*Balantidium coli*) is an infection of the bowel, specifically the colon, usually transmitted through contact with infected pigs. Possible symptoms include diarrhoea and abdominal pain. Treatment is with tetracycline, metronidazole, or diodohydroxyquinoline

Cryptosporidiosis (*Cryptosporidium*) affects the bowel (and occasionally the respiratory tract and bile ducts). It is spread through contaminated food or water or by contact with animals or other humans. Symptoms include diarrhoea and abdominal pain. There are no specific drugs to treat it, but paromomycin, azithromycin, or eflornithine may be effective.

Giardiasis (*Giardia lamblia*), or lambliasis, affects the bowel and is usually transmitted in contaminated food or water; but it may also be spread by some types of sexual contact. Its

major symptoms are generalized ill-health, diarrhoea, flatulence, and abdominal pain. Treatment is with mepacrine, metronidazole, or tinidazole.

Leishmaniasis (*Leishmania*) is a mainly tropical and subtropical disease caused by organisms spread through sandfly bites. It affects the mucous membranes of the mouth, nose, and throat and may, in its severe form, invade organs such as the liver. Treatment is with paromomycin, sodium stibogluconate, pentamidine, or amphotericin.

Pneumocystis pneumonia (*Pneumocystis carinii*) is a potentially fatal lung infection usually affecting, only those people with reduced resistance to infection, such as AIDS sufferers. Symptoms include cough, breathlessness, fever, and chest pain. Treatment is with drugs such as atovaquone, co-trimoxazole, pentamidine, and trimetrexate.

Toxoplasmosis (*Toxoplasma gondii*) is usually spread via cat faeces or by eating undercooked meat. Although usually symptomless, toxoplasmosis may cause generalized ill-health, mild fever, and eye inflammation. Treatment is necessary only if the eyes are involved or the patient is immunosuppressed (such as in AIDS). It may also pass from mother to baby during pregnancy, leading to severe disease in the fetus. Treatment usually consists of pyrimethamine with sulfadiazine, azithromycin, clarithromycin, or clindamycin, or, during pregnancy, spiramycin.

Trichomoniasis (*Trichomonas vaginalis*) most often affects the vagina, causing irritation and an offensive discharge. In men, it may occur in the urethra. It is usually sexually transmitted. Treatment is with metronidazole or tinidazole.

Trypanosomiasis (*Trypanosoma*), or African trypanosomiasis (sleeping sickness), is spread by the tsetse fly and causes fever, swollen glands, and drowsiness. South American trypanosomiasis (Chagas' disease) is spread by assassin bugs and causes inflammation, enlargement of internal organs, and infection of the brain. Sleeping sickness is treated with pentamidine, suramin, eflornithine, or melarsoprol. Chagas' disease is treated with primaquine or nifurtimox.

Trichomoniasis, toxoplasmosis, cryptosporidium, giardiasis, and pneumocystis pneumonia are probably the most common protozoal infections seen in the United Kingdom. The rarer infections are usually contracted as a result of exposure to infection in another part of the world.

Antimalarial drugs

Malaria is one of the main killing diseases in the tropics and is most likely to affect people who live in or travel to such places.

The disease is caused by protozoa (see p.71) whose life cycle is far from simple. The malaria parasite, which is called *Plasmodium*, lives in and depends on the female *Anopheles* mosquito during one part of its life cycle. It lives in and depends on human beings during other parts of its life cycle.

Transferred to humans in the saliva of the female mosquito as she penetrates ("bites") the skin, the malaria parasite enters the bloodstream and settles in the liver, where it multiplies asexually.

Following its stay in the liver, the parasite (or plasmodium) enters another phase of its life cycle, circulating in the bloodstream, penetrating and destroying red blood cells, and reproducing again. If the plasmodia then transfer back to a female *Anopheles* mosquito via another "bite", they breed sexually, and are again ready to start a human infection.

Following the emergence of plasmodia from the liver, the symptoms of malaria occur: episodes of high fever and profuse sweating alternate with equally agonizing episodes of shivering and chills. One of the four strains of malaria (*Plasmodium falciparum*) can produce a single severe attack that can be fatal unless treated. The others cause recurrent attacks, sometimes extending over many years.

A number of drugs are available for preventing malaria, the choice depending on the region in which the disease can be contracted and the resistance to the commonly used drugs. In most malarial areas, *Plasmodium falciparum* is resistant to chloroquine. In all regions, three drugs are commonly used: quinine, mefloquine, and Malarone.

CHOICE OF DRUGS

The parts of the world in which malaria is prevalent, and travel to which may make antimalarial drug treatment advisable, can be divided into six zones. Due to drug resistance, specific antimalarials are recommended for each zone.

Zone 1 North Africa and the Middle East Chloroquine, plus proguanil in areas of chloroquine resistance

Zone 2 Sub-Saharan Africa Mefloquine, or chloroquine with proguanil

Zone 3 South Asia Mefloquine, or chloroquine with proguanil

Zone 4 Southeast Asia Mefloquine in high-risk areas, or chloroquine with proguanil; doxycycline in mefloquine-resistant areas

Zone 5 Oceania Mefloquine, or doxycycline

Zone 6 Latin America Central America: chloroquine or proguanil. South America: mefloquine in high-risk areas, or chloroquine with proguanil

As prevalent strains of malaria change very rapidly, you must always seek specific medical advice before travelling to any of these areas.

WHY THEY ARE USED

The medical response to malaria takes three forms: prevention, treatment of attacks, and the complete eradication of the plasmodia (radical cure).

For someone planning a trip to an area where malaria is prevalent, drugs are given that destroy the parasites in the liver. Dosing begins one week (2–3 weeks for mefloquine) before the traveller arrives in the malarial area and should continue for four to six weeks after return from the area.

Drugs such as mefloquine and Fansidar can produce a radical cure but chloroquine does not. So, after chloroquine treatment of non-falciparum malaria, a 14- to 21-day course of primaquine is administered. Although it is highly effective in destroying plasmodia in the liver, the drug is weak against the plasmodia circulating in the bloodstream. Primaquine is recommended only after a person leaves the malarial area because of the high risk of reinfection.

HOW THEY WORK

Taken to prevent the disease, the drugs kill the plasmodia in the liver, preventing them from multiplying. Once plasmodia have multiplied in the liver, the same drugs may be used in higher doses to kill those that re-enter the bloodstream. If these drugs are not effective, primaquine may be used to destroy any plasmodia still present in the liver.

HOW THEY AFFECT YOU

The low doses of antimalarial drugs taken to prevent the disease rarely produce noticeable effects. Drugs taken for an attack usually begin to relieve symptoms within a few hours. Most of them can cause nausea, vomiting, and diarrhoea. Quinine can cause disturbances in vision and hearing. Mefloquine can cause sleep disturbance, dizziness, and difficulties in coordination.

RISKS AND SPECIAL PRECAUTIONS

When drugs are given to prevent or cure malaria, the full course of treatment must be taken. No drugs give long-term protection; a new course of treatment is needed for each journey.

Most of these drugs do not produce severe adverse effects, but primaquine can cause the blood disorder haemolytic anaemia, particularly in people with glucose-6-phosphate dehydrogenase (G6PD) deficiency. Blood tests are taken before treatment to identify susceptible individuals. Halofantrine can have an adverse effect on heart rhythm. Mefloquine is not prescribed for those who have had psychological disorders or convulsions.

OTHER PROTECTIVE MEASURES

Because *Plasmodium* strains continually develop resistance to the available drugs, prevention using drugs is not absolutely reliable. Protection from mosquito bites is of the highest priority. Such protection includes the use of insect repellents, such as DEET, and mosquito nets impregnated with permethrin insecticide, as well as covering any areas of exposed skin after dark.

COMMON DRUGS

Artemether, Chloroquine*, Doxycycline*, Halofantrine, Mefloquine*, Primaquine, Proguanil*, Proguanil/atovaquone ("Malarone")*, Pyrimethamine/dapsone ("Malaprim")*, Pyrimethamine/sulphadoxine ("Fansidar"), Quinine*
* **See Part 2**

Antifungal drugs

We are continually exposed to fungi – in the air we breathe, the food we eat, and the water we drink. Fortunately, most of them cannot live in the body, and few are harmful. But some can grow in the mouth, skin, hair, or nails, causing irritating or unsightly changes, and a few can cause serious and possibly fatal disease. The most common fungal infections are caused by the tinea group. These include tinea pedis (athlete's foot), tinea corporis (ringworm), tinea cruris (groin ringworm), and tinea capitis (scalp ringworm). Caused by a variety of organisms, they are spread by direct or indirect contact with infected humans or animals. Infection is encouraged by warm, moist conditions.

Problems may also result from the proliferation of a fungus that is normally present in the body; the most common example is excessive growth of *Candida*, a yeast that causes thrush infection of the mouth, vagina, and bowel. It can also infect other organs if it spreads through the body via the bloodstream. Overgrowth of *Candida* may occur in people taking antibiotics (p.60) or oral contraceptives (p.101), pregnant women, or those with diabetes or immune system disorders such as AIDS.

Superficial fungal infections – those that attack only the outer layer of the skin and mucous membranes – are relatively common and, although irritating, do not usually present a threat to general health. Internal fungal infections – for example, of the lungs, heart, or other organs – are rare but may be serious and prolonged.

Because antibiotics and other antibacterial drugs have no effect on fungi and yeasts, it is necessary to use a different type of drug. Drugs for fungal infections are either applied topically to treat minor infections of the skin, nails, and mucous membranes, or they are given by mouth or injection to eliminate serious fungal infections of the internal organs and nails.

WHY THEY ARE USED

Drug treatment is necessary for most fungal infections since they rarely improve alone. Measures such as careful washing and drying

CHOICE OF ANTIFUNGAL DRUG

The table below shows the range of uses for some of the more common antifungal drugs. The particular drug chosen in each case depends on the precise nature and site of the infection. The usual route of administration for each drug is also indicated.

DRUG	INFECTION	Oesophageal thrush	Cryptococcal meningitis	Skin ringworm	Scalp ringworm	Nail infection	Mouth thrush	Vaginal thrush	Candida of the skin	Systemic candida	ADMINISTRATION	Topical	Injection	Oral
Amphotericin		●	●				●		●	●		▲	▲	
Clotrimazole				●	●		●	●	●			▲		
Fluconazole		●	●					●		●			▲	▲
Flucytosine		●	●							●			▲	▲
Griseofulvin				●	●	●								▲
Ketoconazole				●	●			●	●	●		▲		▲
Miconazole							●	●	●			▲		▲
Nystatin							●	●	●			▲		▲
Terbinafine				●	●	●								▲

of affected areas may help, but they are not a substitute for antifungal drugs. The use of over-the-counter preparations to increase the acidity of the vagina is not usually effective except when it is accompanied by drug treatment.

Fungal infections of the skin and scalp are usually treated with a cream or shampoo. Drugs for vaginal thrush are most commonly applied in the form of vaginal pessaries or cream applied with a special applicator. For very severe or persistent vaginal infections, fluconazole or itraconazole may be given as a short course by mouth. Mouth infections are usually eliminated by lozenges dissolved in the mouth or an antifungal solution or gel applied to the affected areas. When Candida infects the bowel, an antifungal drug that is not absorbed into the bloodstream, such as nystatin, is given in the form of tablets. For severe or persistent infections of the nails, either griseofulvin or terbinafine are given by mouth and are continued until the infected nails have grown out.

In the rare cases of fungal infections affecting internal organs, such as the blood, the heart, or the brain, potent drugs such as fluconazole and itraconazole are given by mouth, or amphotericin and flucytosine are given by injection. These drugs pass into the bloodstream to fight the fungi.

HOW THEY WORK

Most antifungals alter the permeability of the fungal cell's walls. Chemicals needed for cell life leak out and the fungal cell dies.

HOW THEY AFFECT YOU

The speed with which antifungal drugs provide benefit varies with the type of infection. Most fungal or yeast infections of the skin, mouth, and vagina improve within a week. The condition of nails affected by fungal infections improves only when new nail growth occurs, which takes months. Systemic infections of the internal organs can take weeks to cure.

Antifungal drugs applied topically rarely cause side effects, although they may irritate the skin. However, treatment by mouth or injection for systemic and nail infections may produce more serious side effects. Amphotericin, injected in cases of life-threatening, systemic infections, can cause potentially dangerous effects, including kidney damage.

COMMON DRUGS

Amorolfine, Amphotericin*, Benzoyl peroxide*, Co-trimazole*, Econazole, Fenticonazole, Fluconazole*, Griseofulvin, Isoconazole, Itraconazole, lucytosine, Ketoconazole*, Miconazole*, Nystatin*, Sulconazole, Terbinafine*, Tioconazole

* See Part 2

Anthelmintic drugs

Anthelmintics are drugs that are used to eliminate the many types of worm (helminths) that can enter the body and live there as parasites, producing a general weakness in some cases and serious harm in others. The body may be host to many different worms (see Types of infestation, below). Most species spend part of their life cycle in another animal, and the infestation is often passed on to humans in food contaminated with the eggs or larvae. In some cases, such as hookworm, larvae enter the body through the skin. Larvae or adults may attach themselves to the intestinal wall and feed on the bowel contents; others feed off the intestinal blood supply, causing anaemia. Worms can also infest the bloodstream or lodge in the muscles or internal organs.

Many people have worms at some time during their life, especially during childhood. Most infestations can be effectively eliminated with anthelmintic drugs.

WHY THEY ARE USED

Most worms common in the United Kingdom cause only mild symptoms and usually do not pose a serious threat to general health. Anthelmintic drugs are usually necessary, however, because the body's natural defences against infection are not effective against most worm infestations. Certain types of infestation must always be treated since they can cause serious complications. In some cases, such as threadworm infestation, doctors may recommend anthelmintic treatment for the whole family to prevent reinfection. If worms have invaded tissues and formed cysts, they may have to be removed surgically. Laxatives are given with some anthelmintics to hasten expulsion of worms from the bowel. Other drugs may be prescribed to ease symptoms or to compensate for any blood loss or nutritional deficiency.

TYPES OF INFESTATION

Threadworm (*enterobiasis*) The most common worm infection in the UK, especially among young children. It lives in the intestine but travels to the anus at night to lay eggs, causing itching; scratching leaves eggs on the fingers, usually under the fingernails. Sucking the fingers or eating food with unwashed hands often transfers these eggs to the mouth. Keeping the nails short and good hygiene, including washing the hands after using the toilet and before each meal, and an early morning bath to remove the eggs, are important in eradication of the infection.
Drugs Mebendazole, piperazine.
All members of the household should be treated simultaneously.

Common roundworm (*ascariasis*) The most common worm infection worldwide. It is transmitted to humans in contaminated raw food or in soil. The worms are large, and they infect the intestine, which can be blocked by dense clusters of them.
Drugs Levamisole, mebendazole, piperazine

Tropical threadworm (*strongyloidiasis*) Occurs in the tropics and southern Europe. The larvae from contaminated soil penetrate the skin, pass into the lungs, and are swallowed into the gut.
Drugs Albendazole, thiabendazole, ivermectin

Whipworm (*trichuriasis*) Mainly occurs in tropical areas as a result of eating contaminated raw vegetables. The worms infest the intestines.
Drug Mebendazole

Hookworm (*uncinariasis*) Mainly found in tropical areas. The worm larvae penetrate the skin and pass via the lymphatic system and bloodstream to the lungs. They then travel up the airways, are swallowed, and attach themselves to the intestinal wall, where they feed off the intestinal blood supply.
Drug Mebendazole

Pork roundworm (*trichinosis*) Transmitted in infected undercooked pork. Initially, the worms lodge in the intestines, but larvae may invade muscle to form cysts that are often resistant to drug treatment and may require surgery.
Drugs Mebendazole, thiabendazole

Toxocariasis (*visceral larva migrans*) Usually occurs as a result of eating soil or eating with fingers contaminated with dog or cat faeces. The eggs hatch in the intestine and may travel to the lungs, liver, kidney, brain, and eyes. Treatment is not always effective.
Drugs Mebendazole, thiabendazole, diethylcarbamazine

Creeping eruption (*cutaneous larva migrans*) Mainly occurs in tropical areas and coastal areas of the southeastern US as a result of skin contact with larvae from cat and dog faeces. Infestation is usually confined to the skin.
Drugs Thiabendazole, ivermectin, albendazole

Filariasis (including *onchocerciasis* and *loiasis*) Occurs in tropical areas only. It may affect the lymphatic system, blood, eyes, and skin. Infection by this group of worms is spread by bites of insects that are carriers of worm larvae or eggs.
Drugs Diethylcarbamazine, ivermectin

Flukes Sheep liver fluke (*fascioliasis*) is indigenous to the UK. Infestation usually results from eating watercress grown in contaminated water. It mainly affects the liver and biliary tract. Other flukes only found abroad may infect the lungs, intestines, or blood.
Drug Praziquantel

Tapeworms (including beef, pork, fish, and dwarf tapeworms) Depending on the type, it may be carried by cattle, pigs, or fish and transmitted to humans in undercooked meat. Most types affect the intestines. Larvae of the pork tapeworm may form cysts in muscle and other tissues.
Drugs Niclosamide, praziquantel

Hydatid disease (*echinococciasis*) The eggs are transmitted in dog faeces, and the larvae may form cysts over many years, commonly in the liver. Surgery is the usual treatment for cysts.
Drug Albendazole

Bilharzia (*schistosomiasis*) Occurs in polluted water in tropical areas. The larvae may be swallowed or penetrate the skin. Once inside the body, they migrate to the liver; adult worms live in the bladder.
Drug Praziquantel

HOW THEY WORK

The anthelmintic drugs act in several ways. Many of them kill or paralyse the worms, which pass out of the body in the faeces. Others, which act systemically, are used to treat infection in the tissues.

Many anthelmintics are specific for particular worms, and the doctor must identify the worm before selecting the most appropriate treatment (see Types of infestation, facing page). Most of the common intestinal infestations are easily treated, often with only one or two doses of the drug. However, tissue infections may require more prolonged treatment.

HOW THEY AFFECT YOU

Once the drug has eliminated the worms, symptoms caused by infestation rapidly disappear. Taken as a single dose or a short course, anthelmintics do not usually produce side effects. However, treatment can disturb the digestive system, causing abdominal pain, nausea, and vomiting.

COMMON DRUGS

Albendazole, Diethylcarbamazine, Ivermectin, Levamisole, Mebendazole, Niclosamide, Piperazine, Praziquantel, Thiabendazole

* **See Part 2**

HORMONES AND ENDOCRINE SYSTEM

The endocrine system is a collection of endocrine glands located throughout the body that produce hormones and release them into the bloodstream.

The pituitary gland produces hormones that regulate growth, sexual and reproductive development, and also stimulate other endocrine glands (see p.83). Each endocrine gland produces one or more hormones, each of which governs a particular body function, including growth and repair of tissues, sexual development and reproductive function, and the body's response to stress.

The thyroid gland regulates metabolism. Hyperthyroidism or hypothyroidism may occur if the thyroid does not function well (see p.82).

The adrenal glands produce hormones that regulate the body's mineral and water content and reduce inflammation (see Corticosteroids, right).

The pancreas produces insulin to regulate blood glucose levels, and glucagon, which helps the liver and muscles to store glucose (see p.80).

The kidneys produce a hormone, erythropoietin, needed for red blood cell production. Patients with kidney failure lack this hormone and become anaemic; they may be given epoetin (p.220), a version of the hormone.

The ovaries (in women) secrete oestrogen and progesterone, responsible for female sexual and physical development (see p.86).

The testes (in men) produce testosterone, which controls the development of male sexual and physical characteristics (see p.85).

Most hormones are released continuously from birth, but the amount produced fluctuates with the body's needs. Others are produced mainly at certain times – for example, growth hormone is released mainly during childhood and adolescence. Sex hormones are produced by the testes and ovaries from puberty onwards (see p.99).

Many endocrine glands release their hormones in response to triggering hormones produced by the pituitary gland. The pituitary releases a variety of pituitary hormones, each of which, in turn, stimulates the appropriate endocrine gland to produce its hormone.

A "feedback" system usually regulates blood hormone levels; if the blood level rises too high, the pituitary responds by reducing the amount of stimulating hormone produced, thereby allowing the blood hormone level to return to normal.

WHAT CAN GO WRONG

Endocrine disorders, usually resulting in too much or too little of a particular hormone, have a variety of causes. Some are congenital in origin; others may be caused by autoimmune disease (including some forms of diabetes mellitus), malignant or benign tumours, injury, or certain drugs.

WHY DRUGS ARE USED

Natural hormone preparations or their synthetic versions are often prescribed to treat deficiency. Sometimes, drugs are given to stimulate increased hormone production in the endocrine gland, such as oral antidiabetic drugs, which act on the insulin-producing cells of the pancreas. When too much hormone is produced, drug treatment may be able to reduce the activity of the gland.

Hormones or related drugs are also used to treat certain other conditions. Corticosteroids related to adrenal hormones are prescribed to relieve inflammation and to suppress immune system activity (see p.96). Several types of cancer (see p.94) are treated with sex hormones. Female sex hormones are used as contraceptives (see p.101) and to treat menstrual disorders (see p.100).

MAJOR DRUG GROUPS

◆ Corticosteroids
◆ Drugs used in diabetes
◆ Drugs for thyroid disorders
◆ Drugs for pituitary disorders
◆ Male sex hormones
◆ Female sex hormones

Corticosteroids

Corticosteroid drugs, often referred to simply as steroids, are derived from, or are synthetic variants of, the natural corticosteroid hormones formed in the outer part (cortex) of the adrenal glands, situated on top of each kidney. Release of these hormones is governed by the pituitary gland (see p.83).

Corticosteroids may have either mainly glucocorticoid or mineralocorticoid effects. Glucocorticoid effects include the maintenance of normal levels of sugar in the blood and the promotion of recovery from injury and stress. The main mineralocorticoid effects are the regulation of the balance of mineral salts and the water content of the body. When present in large amounts, corticosteroids reduce inflammation and suppress allergic reactions and immune system activity. They are distinct from another group of steroid hormones, the anabolic steroids (see p.86).

Although corticosteroids have broadly similar actions, they vary in their relative strength and duration of action. Their mineralocorticoid effects also vary in strength.

WHY THEY ARE USED

Corticosteroid drugs are used primarily for their effect in controlling inflammation, whatever its cause. Topical preparations containing corticosteroids are often used for the treatment of many inflammatory skin disorders (see p.116). These drugs may also be injected directly into a joint or around a tendon to relieve inflammation caused by injury or disease (see p.51). However, when local administration of the drug is either not possible or not effective, corticosteroids may be given systemically, either by mouth or by intravenous injection.

Corticosteroids are commonly part of the treatment of many disorders in which inflammation is thought to be due to excessive or inappropriate activity of the immune system. These disorders include inflammatory bowel disease (p.44), rheumatoid arthritis (p.50), glomerulonephritis (a kidney disease), and some rare connective tissue disorders, such as systemic lupus erythematosus. In these conditions corticosteroids relieve symptoms and may also temporarily halt the disease.

Corticosteroids may be given regularly, by mouth or inhaler, to treat asthma but are not effective for the relief of asthma attacks that are in progress (see Bronchodilators, p.23).

An important use of oral corticosteroids is to replace the natural hormones that are deficient when adrenal gland function is reduced, as in Addison's disease. In these cases, the drugs most closely resembling the actions of the natural hormones are selected and a combination of these may be used.

Some cancers of the lymphatic system (lymphomas) and blood (leukaemias) may also respond to corticosteroid treatment. These drugs are also widely used to prevent or treat rejection of organ transplants, usually in conjunction with other drugs, such as azathioprine (see Immunosuppressants, p.96).

HOW THEY WORK

Given in high doses, corticosteroids reduce inflammation by blocking the action of chemicals called prostaglandins that are responsible for triggering the inflammatory response. These drugs also temporarily depress the immune system by reducing the activity of certain types of white blood cell.

HOW THEY AFFECT YOU

Corticosteroids often dramatically improve symptoms. Given systemically, they may also act on the brain to produce a heightened sense of well-being and, in some people, a sense of euphoria.

Troublesome day-to-day side effects are rare. Long-term corticosteroid treatment, however, carries a number of serious risks for the patient.

RISKS AND SPECIAL PRECAUTIONS

In the treatment of Addison's disease, corticosteroids can be considered as "hormone replacement therapy", with the drugs replacing the natural hormone hydrocortisone. Because replacement doses are given, the adverse effects of high-dose corticosteroids do not occur.

Drugs with strong mineralocorticoid effects, such as fludrocortisone, may cause water retention, swelling (especially of the ankles), and an increase in blood pressure. Because corticosteroids reduce the effect of insulin, they may create problems in diabetics, and may even give rise to diabetes in susceptible individuals. They can also cause peptic ulcers.

Because corticosteroids suppress the immune system, they increase susceptibility to infection. They also suppress symptoms of infectious disease. People taking corticosteroids should avoid exposure to chickenpox or shingles, but if they catch either disease, aciclovir tablets may be prescribed.

With long-term use, corticosteroids may cause a variety of adverse effects such as mood changes, acne, a moon-shaped face, increased blood pressure and fluid retention, peptic ulcers, reduced effect of insulin, a fat pad on the top of the back, muscle weakness and wasting, osteoporosis, cataracts, thin skin, and easy bruising. Doctors try to avoid prescribing corticosteroids to children in the long term because it may retard growth.

Long-term use of corticosteroids suppresses production of the body's own corticosteroid hormones. Therefore, treatment lasting longer than a few weeks should be withdrawn gradually to give the body time to adjust. Stopping abruptly may lead to sudden collapse due to lack of the hormones.

People taking corticosteroids by mouth for longer than one month are advised to carry a warning card. If someone taking steroids long term has an accident or serious illness, his or her defences against shock may need to be quickly strengthened with extra hydrocortisone, administered intravenously.

COMMON DRUGS

Alclometasone, Beclometasone*, Betamethasone*, Budesonide*, Clobetasol*, Clobetasone, Desoximetasone, Dexamethasone*, Diflucortolone, Fludrocortisone, Flunisolide, Flumetasone, Fluocinonide, Fluocinolone, Fluocortolone, Fluticasone*, Flurandrenolone, Halcinonide, Hydrocortisone*, Methylprednisolone, Mometasone*, Prednisolone*, Triamcinolone

* **See Part 2**

Drugs used in diabetes

The body obtains most of its energy from glucose, a simple form of sugar made in the intestine from the breakdown of starch and other sugars. Insulin, one of the hormones produced in the pancreas, enables body tissues to take up glucose from the blood either to use for energy or to store. In diabetes mellitus (or sugar diabetes) insulin production is defective. This results in reduced uptake of glucose by the tissues, and therefore the glucose level in the blood rises abnormally. This is known medically as hyperglycaemia.

There are two main types of diabetes mellitus. Insulin-dependent (Type 1) diabetes usually affects young people; 50 per cent of cases occur at around puberty. The insulin-secreting cells in the pancreas are gradually destroyed. An autoimmune condition (where the body recognizes its pancreas as "foreign" and tries to eliminate it) or a childhood viral infection is the most likely cause. Despite slow insulin production, the condition often appears suddenly, brought on by periods of stress (e.g., infection or puberty) when the body's insulin requirements are high. Symptoms of Type 1 diabetes include extreme thirst, increased urination, lethargy, and weight loss. Left untreated, this type of diabetes is fatal.

In Type 1 diabetes, insulin treatment is the only treatment option. It has to be continued for the rest of the patient's life. Several types of insulin are available, which are broadly classified by their duration of action (short-, medium-, and long-acting).

Non-insulin-dependent diabetes mellitus (NIDDM), also called Type 2 or maturity-onset diabetes, appears at an older age (usually over 40) and tends to come on much more gradually – there may be a delay in its diagnosis for several years because of the gradual onset of symptoms. In this type of diabetes, insulin is present, but the cells of the body are often resistant to the effects of insulin and have a reduced glucose uptake despite the presence of insulin. This results in hyperglycaemia. Obesity is the most common cause of Type 2 diabetes.

In both types of diabetes, an alteration in diet is vital. A healthy diet consisting of a low-fat, high-fibre, low simple sugar (cakes, sweets) and high complex sugar (pasta, rice, potatoes) intake is advised.

In Type 2 diabetes, a reduction in weight alone may be sufficient to lower the body's energy requirements and restore blood glucose to normal levels. If an alteration in diet fails, oral antidiabetic drugs, such as metformin, acarbose, or sulphonylureas, are prescribed. Insulin may need to be given to people with Type 2 diabetes if the above treatments fail, or in pregnancy, during severe illness, and before the patient undergoes any surgery requiring a general anaesthetic.

IMPORTANCE OF TREATING DIABETES

If diabetes is left untreated, the continuous high blood glucose levels damage various parts of the body. The major problems are caused by the build-up of atherosclerosis in arteries, which narrows the vessels, reducing blood flow. This can result in heart attacks, blindness, kidney failure, reduced circulation in the legs, and even gangrene. With treatment, the risk of these conditions is greatly reduced. Careful control of diabetes in young people, during puberty and afterwards, is of great importance in reducing possible long-term complications. Good diabetic control before conception reduces the chance of miscarriage or abnormalities in the baby.

HOW ANTIDIABETIC DRUGS WORK

Most drugs for diabetes promote the uptake of glucose into body tissues and help to prevent an excessive rise in the level of glucose in the blood. Insulin treatment directly replaces the natural hormone that is deficient in diabetes mellitus. Human and pork insulins are the most widely available. When transferring between animal and human insulin, alteration of the dose may be required.

Unfortunately, insulin cannot be given by mouth because it is broken down in the digestive tract before it reaches the blood-stream. Regular injections are therefore necessary (see Administration of insulin, below).

Sulphonylurea oral antidiabetics encourage the pancreas to produce insulin. They are therefore effective only when some insulin-secreting cells remain active. This is why they are ineffective in the treatment of Type 1 diabetes. Metformin alters the way in which the body metabolizes sugar. Acarbose slows digestion of starch, thereby slowing the increase in blood glucose that occurs after a meal.

ADMINISTRATION OF INSULIN

The body normally produces a background level of insulin, with additional insulin being produced as required in response to meals.

The insulin delivery systems currently available cannot mimic this precisely. In young people with Type 1 diabetes, short-acting insulin is usually given before meals, and medium-acting either before the evening meal or at bedtime. Insulin pen injectors are especially useful for daytime administration because they are discreet and easy to carry and use. In patients with Type 2 diabetes who require insulin, a mixture of short- and medium-acting insulin may be given twice a day. Special pumps that deliver continuous subcutaneous insulin seem to have no advantage over multiple subcutaneous injections. Some new types of insulins called "insulin analogues" (e.g. Insulin lispro) act very rapidly and may be better at mimicking the insulin-producing behaviour of the normal pancreas.

INSULIN TREATMENT AND YOU

The insulin requirements in diabetes vary greatly between individuals and also depend on physical activity and calorie intake. Hence, insulin regimens are tailored to each person's particular needs, and the diabetic is encouraged to take an active role in his or her own management.

A regular record of home blood glucose monitoring should be kept. This is the basis on which insulin doses are adjusted, preferably by diabetics themselves. They need to check either their blood or urine glucose level, although blood tests give the most accurate results. Testing kits are available that consist of a programmable meter that reads the glucose levels in blood samples applied to a special card testing strip.

A person with diabetes should learn to recognize the warning signs of hypoglycaemia. A hypoglycaemic event may be induced by giving insulin under medical supervision. The symptoms of sweating, faintness, or palpitations are produced but disappear with the administration of glucose, so a diabetic should always carry glucose tablets or sweets. Recurrent "hypos" at specific times of the day or night may require a reduction of insulin dose. Rarely, undetected low glucose levels may lead to coma. The injection of glucagon (a substance that raises blood glucose) rapidly reverses this. A relative may be instructed how to perform this procedure.

Insulin requirements are increased during illness and pregnancy. During an illness, the urine should be checked for ketones, which are produced when there is insufficient insulin to permit the normal uptake of glucose by the tissues. If high ketone levels occur in a diabetic's urine during an illness, urgent medical advice should be sought. The combination of high blood glucose, high urinary ketones, and vomiting is a diabetic emergency and the person should attend an Accident and Emergency department immediately.

Exercise increases the body's need for glucose, so extra calories should be taken prior to exertion. The effects of vigorous exercise on blood glucose levels may last up to 18 hours, and the subsequent (post-exercise) doses of insulin may need to be reduced by 10–25 per cent to avoid hypoglycaemia (low blood glucose).

It is advisable for diabetics to carry a card or bracelet detailing their treatment. This may be useful in an emergency.

ANTIDIABETIC DRUGS AND YOU

Oral antidiabetics relieve symptoms of diabetes by returning the blood glucose to normal. A normal, healthy, active lifestyle should be encouraged. However, the sulphonylureas may lower the blood glucose too much. Hypoglycaemia can be avoided by starting treatment with low doses and ensuring a regular food intake. Rarely, these drugs cause a decrease in the blood cell count, a rash, or intestinal or liver disturbances. Interactions may occur with other drugs, so your doctor should be informed of your treatment before prescribing any medicines for you.

Unlike the sulphonylureas, metformin does not cause hypoglycaemia. Its most common side effects are nausea, weight loss, abdominal distension, and diarrhoea. It should not be used in people with liver, kidney, or heart problems. Acarbose does not cause hypoglycaemia if used on its own. The tablets must either be chewed with the first mouthful of food at mealtimes or swallowed whole with a little liquid immediately before food.

COMMON DRUGS

Sulphonylurea drugs Chlorpropamide, Glibenclamide*, Gliclazide*, Glimepiride, Gliquidone,

Glipizide, Tolbutamide*, Tolazamide
Other drugs Acarbose , Glucagon, Guar gum, Insulin*, Insulin lispro, Metformin*, Repaglinide*
* **See Part 2**

Drugs for thyroid disorders

The thyroid gland produces the hormone thyroxine, which regulates the body's metabolism. During childhood, thyroxine is essential for normal physical and mental development. Calcitonin, also produced by the thyroid, regulates calcium metabolism and is used as a drug for certain bone disorders (p.54).

HYPERTHYROIDISM

In this condition (often called thyrotoxicosis), the thyroid is overactive and produces too much thyroxine. Women are more commonly affected than men. Symptoms include anxiety, palpitations, weight loss, increased appetite, heat intolerance, diarrhoea, and menstrual disturbances. Graves' disease, the most common form of hyperthyroidism, is an autoimmune disease in which the body produces antibodies that stimulate the thyroid to produce excess thyroxine. Patients with Graves' disease may develop exophthalmos (protuberant eyes) or pretibial myxoedema (a swelling involving the skin over the shins).

Hyperthyroidism can be caused by a benign single tumour of the thyroid. It can also be caused by a pre-existing multinodular goitre (see below). Rarely, an overactive thyroid may follow a viral infection, a condition called thyroiditis. Inflammation of the gland leads to the release of stored thyroxine. **Goitre** is a swelling of the thyroid gland that may occur only temporarily, during puberty or pregnancy, or may be due to abnormal growth of thyroid tissue that requires surgical removal. Goitre may also, rarely, be brought about by iodine deficiency, which can be prevented or treated with iodine supplements.

MANAGEMENT OF HYPERTHYROIDISM

There are three possible treatments: antithyroid drugs, radio-iodine, and surgery. The most commonly used antithyroid drug is carbimazole. This drug inhibits the formation of thyroid hormones and reduces their levels to normal over a period of about 4–8 weeks. In the early stage of treatment a beta blocker (p.28) may be prescribed to control symptoms. This should be stopped once thyroid function returns to normal. Long-term carbimazole is usually given for 18 months to prevent relapse. A "block and replace" regimen may also be used. In this treatment, the thyroid gland is blocked by high doses of carbimazole and thyroxine is added when the level of thyroid hormone in the blood falls below normal.

Carbimazole may produce minor side effects such as nausea, vomiting, rashes, or headaches. Rarely, the drug may reduce the white blood cell count. Propylthiouracil may be used as an alternative antithyroid drug.

Radio-iodine (radioactive iodine) is often chosen as first-line therapy, especially in the elderly, usually after giving a course of carbimazole until up to a week before treatment. It is the second choice if hyperthyroidism recurs following use of carbimazole. It acts by destroying thyroid tissue. Hypothyroidism occurs in up to 80 per cent of people within 20 years after treatment. Long-term studies show radio-iodine to be safe, but its use should be avoided during pregnancy.

Surgery is a third-line therapy. Its use may be favoured for patients with a large goitre, particularly if it causes difficulty in swallowing or breathing. Exophthalmos may require corticosteroids (p.78) as it does not respond to other treatments.

HYPOTHYROIDISM

This is a condition resulting from too little thyroxine. Sometimes it may be caused by an autoimmune disorder, in which the body's immune system attacks the thyroid gland. Other cases may follow treatment for hyperthyroidism. In newborn babies, hypothyroidism may be the result of an inborn enzyme disorder. In the past, it also arose from a deficiency of iodine in the diet.

The symptoms of adult hypothyroidism develop slowly and include weight gain, mental slowness, dry skin, hair loss, increased sensitivity to cold, and heavy menstrual periods. In babies, low levels of thyroxine cause permanent mental and physical retardation. For this reason, babies are tested for hypothyroidism within a week of birth.

MANAGEMENT OF HYPOTHYROIDISM

Lifelong oral treatment with synthetic thyroid hormones (thyroxine (levothyroxine) or liothyronine) is the only option. Blood tests are performed regularly to monitor treatment and permit dosage adjustments. In the elderly and people with heart disease, thyroxine is introduced gradually to prevent heart strain.

In severely ill patients, thyroid hormone may be given by injection. This method of administration may also be used to treat newborn infants with low levels of thyroxine.

Symptoms of thyrotoxicosis may appear if excess thyroxine replacement is given. Otherwise, no adverse events occur since treatment is adjusted to replace the natural hormone that the body should produce itself.

COMMON DRUGS

Drugs for hypothyroidism Liothyronine, Thyroxine (levothyroxine)*

Drugs for hyperthyroidism Carbimazole*, Iodine, Nadolol, Propranolol*, Propylthiouracil,* Radio-iodine

* **See Part 2**

Drugs for pituitary disorders

The pituitary gland, which lies at the base of the brain, produces a number of hormones that regulate physical growth, metabolism, sexual development, and reproductive function. Many of these hormones act indirectly by stimulating other glands, such as the thyroid, adrenal glands, ovaries, and testes, to release their own hormones.

Thyroid-stimulating hormone stimulates production and release of thyroid hormones.

Prolactin stimulates glands in the breast to produce milk in women and helps sperm production in men.

Corticotrophin (ACTH) controls production and release of adrenal corticosteroid hormones.

Gonadotrophins follicle-stimulating hormone (FSH) and luteinizing hormone (LH) act on the sex glands to stimulate egg production and release, and sperm production. They also control the output of the sex hormones oestrogen, progesterone, and testosterone.

Growth hormone promotes normal growth and development.

Melanocyte-stimulating hormone controls skin pigmentation.

Antidiuretic hormone (ADH or vasopressin) regulates the output of water in the urine.

An excess or a lack of one of the pituitary hormones may produce serious effects, the nature of which depends on the hormone involved. Abnormal levels of a particular hormone may be caused by a pituitary tumour, which may be treated with surgery, radiotherapy, or drugs. In other cases, drugs may be used to correct the hormonal imbalance.

The more common pituitary disorders that can be treated with drugs are those involving growth hormone, antidiuretic hormone, prolactin, adrenal hormones, and the gonadotrophins. The first three are discussed below. For information on the use of drugs to treat infertility arising from inadequate levels of gonadotrophins, see p.105. Lack of corticotrophin, leading to inadequate production of adrenal hormones, is usually treated with corticosteroids (see p.78).

DRUGS FOR GROWTH HORMONE DISORDERS

Growth hormone (somatotropin) is the principal hormone required for normal growth in childhood and adolescence. Lack of growth hormone impairs normal physical growth. Doctors administer hormone treatment only after tests have proven that a lack of this hormone is the cause of the disorder. If treatment is started at an early age, regular injections of somatropin, a synthetic form of natural growth hormone administered until the end of adolescence, usually allow normal growth and development to take place.

Less often, the pituitary produces excess growth hormone. In children this can result in pituitary gigantism; in adults, it can produce a disorder known as acromegaly. This disorder, which is usually the result of a pituitary tumour, is characterized by thickening of the skull, face, hands, and feet, and enlargement of some internal organs.

The pituitary tumour may either be surgically removed or destroyed by radiotherapy. In the frail or elderly, drugs such a bromocriptine and octreotide are used to reduce growth hormone levels. Octreotide is also used as an adjunctive treatment before surgery and in those with increased growth hormone levels occurring after surgery. People who have undergone surgery and/or radiotherapy may require long-term replacement with other hormones (such as sex hormones, thyroid hormone, or corticosteroids).

DRUGS FOR DIABETES INSIPIDUS

Antidiuretic hormone (also known as ADH or vasopressin) acts on the kidneys, controlling the amount of water retained in the body and returned to the blood. A lack of ADH is usually caused by damage to the pituitary, and this in turn causes diabetes insipidus. In this rare condition, the kidneys cannot retain water and large quantities pass into the urine. The chief symptoms of diabetes insipidus are constant thirst and the production of large volumes of urine.

Diabetes insipidus is treated with ADH or a related synthetic drug, desmopressin. These replace naturally produced ADH and may be given by injection or in the form of a nasal spray. Chlorpropamide may be used to treat mild cases; it works by increasing ADH release from the pituitary and by sensitizing the kidneys to the effect of ADH.

Alternatively, a thiazide diuretic (such as chlortalidone) may be prescribed for mild cases (see Diuretics, p.30). The usual effect of such drugs is to increase urine production, but in diabetes insipidus they have the opposite effect, reducing water loss from the body.

DRUGS TO REDUCE PROLACTIN LEVELS

Prolactin, also called lactogenic hormone, is produced in both men and women. In women, prolactin controls the secretion of breast milk following childbirth. The function of this hormone in men is not understood, although it appears to be necessary for normal sperm production.

The disorders associated with prolactin are all concerned with overproduction. High levels of prolactin in women can cause lactation that is unassociated with pregnancy and birth (galactorrhoea), lack of menstruation (amenorrhoea), and infertility. If excessive amounts of prolactin are produced in men, the result may be galactorrhoea, impotence, or infertility.

Some drugs, notably methyldopa, oestrogen, and the phenothiazine antipsychotics, can raise the prolactin level in the blood. More often, however, the increased prolactin results from a pituitary tumour and is usually treated with bromocriptine or cabergoline. These drugs inhibit prolactin production.

COMMON DRUGS

Drugs for growth hormone disorders
Bromocriptine*, Lanreotide, Octreotide, Somatropin
Drugs for diabetes insipidus Carbamazepine*,
Chlorpropamide, Chlortalidone, Desmopressin*,
Vasopressin (ADH)
Drugs to reduce prolactin levels Bromocriptine*,
Cabergoline, Quinagolide
* **See Part 2**

Male sex hormones

Male sex hormones, or androgens, are responsible for the development of male sexual characteristics. The principal androgen is testosterone, which in men is produced by the testes from puberty onwards. Women produce testosterone in small amounts in the adrenal glands, but its exact function in the female body is not known.

Testosterone has two major effects: an androgenic effect and an anabolic effect. Its androgenic effect is to stimulate the appearance of the secondary sexual characteristics at puberty, such as the growth of body hair, deepening of the voice, and an increase in genital size. Its anabolic effects are to increase muscle bulk and accelerate growth rate.

There are a number of synthetically produced derivatives of testosterone that produce varying degrees of the androgenic and anabolic effect mentioned above. Derivatives that have a mainly anabolic effect are known as anabolic steroids (see p.86).

Testosterone and its derivatives have been used under medical supervision in both men and women to treat a number of conditions.

WHY THEY ARE USED

Male sex hormones are mainly given to men to promote the development of male sexual characteristics when hormone production is deficient. This may be the result of an abnormality of the testes or of inadequate production of the pituitary hormones that stimulate the testes to release testosterone.

A course of treatment with male sex hormones is sometimes prescribed for adolescent boys in whom the onset of puberty is delayed by pituitary problems. The treatment may also help to stimulate development of secondary male sexual characteristics and to increase sex drive (libido) in adult men who are producing inadequate testosterone levels. However, this type of hormone treatment has been found to reduce the production of sperm. (For information on the drug treatment of male infertility, see p.105.)

Androgens may also be prescribed for women to treat certain types of cancer of the breast and uterus (see Anticancer drugs, p.94). Testosterone can be given by injection, capsules, patches, or pellets that are surgically inserted.

HOW THEY WORK

Taken in low doses as part of replacement therapy when natural production is low, male sex hormones act in the same way as the natural hormones. In adolescents suffering from delayed puberty, hormone treatment produces both androgenic and anabolic effects, initiating the development of secondary sexual characteristics over a few months; full sexual development usually takes place over three to four years. When sex hormones are given to adult men, the effects on physical appearance and libido may begin to be felt within a few weeks.

RISKS AND SPECIAL PRECAUTIONS

The main risks with these drugs occur when they are given to boys with delayed puberty and to women with breast cancer. Given to initiate the onset of puberty, they may stunt growth by prematurely sealing the growing ends of the long bones. Doctors normally try to avoid prescribing hormones in these circumstances until growth is complete. High doses given to women have various masculinizing effects, including increased facial and body hair, and a deeper voice. The drugs may also produce enlargement of the clitoris, changes in libido, and acne.

ANABOLIC STEROIDS

Anabolic steroids are synthetically produced variants that mimic the anabolic effects of the natural hormones. They increase muscle bulk and body growth.

Doctors occasionally prescribe anabolic steroids and a high-protein diet to promote recovery after serious illness or major surgery. The steroids may also help to increase the production of blood cells in some forms of anaemia and to reduce itching in chronic obstructive jaundice.

Anabolic steroids have been widely abused by athletes because these drugs speed up the recovery of muscles after a session of intense exercise. This enables the athlete to go through a more demanding daily exercise programme, which results in a significant improvement in muscle power. The use of anabolic steroids by athletes to improve their performance is condemned by doctors and athletic organizations because of the risks to health, particularly for women. The side effects range from acne and baldness to psychological changes, fluid retention, testicular atrophy and impotence (men), reduced fertility (women), hardening of the arteries, a long-term risk of liver disease, and certain forms of cancer.

COMMON DRUGS

Primarily androgenic Mesterolone, Testosterone*
Primarily anabolic Nandrolone, Oxymetholone, Stanozolol
Anti-androgens Cyproterone, Finasteride*
* **See Part 2**

Female sex hormones

There are two natural female sex hormones: oestrogen and progesterone which, in women, are secreted by the ovaries from puberty until the menopause. Each month, oestrogen and progesterone levels fluctuate, producing the menstrual cycle (see p.100). At the start of pregnancy, progesterone is made by the

corpus luteum (empty egg follicle); both hormones are made by the placenta thereafter. The adrenal gland also makes small amounts of oestrogen. Production of oestrogen and progesterone is regulated by the two gonadotrophin hormones (FSH and LH) produced by the pituitary gland (see p.83).

Oestrogen is responsible for development of female sexual characteristics, including breast development, growth of pubic hair, and widening of the pelvis. Progesterone prepares the lining of the uterus for implantation of a fertilized egg; it is also important for the maintenance of pregnancy.

Synthetic forms of these hormones are used medically to treat a number of conditions and are known as oestrogens and progestogens.

WHY THEY ARE USED

The best known use of oestrogens and progestogens is in oral contraceptives These drugs are discussed on p.101. Other uses include the treatment of menstrual disorders (p.100) and certain hormone-sensitive cancers (p.94). This page discusses the drug treatments that are used for natural hormone deficiency.

HORMONE DEFICIENCY

Deficiency of female sex hormones may occur as a result of deficiency of gonadotrophins caused by a pituitary disorder or by abnormal development of the ovaries (ovarian failure). This may lead to the absence of menstruation and lack of sexual development. If tests show a deficiency of gonadotrophins, preparations of these hormones may be prescribed (see p.105). These trigger the release of oestrogen and progesterone from the ovaries. If pituitary function is normal and ovarian failure is diagnosed as the cause of hormone deficiency, oestrogens and progestogens may be given as supplements. In this situation, these supplements ensure development of normal female sexual characteristics but cannot stimulate ovulation.

MENOPAUSE

A decline in levels of oestrogen and progesterone occurs naturally after the menopause, when the menstrual cycle ceases. The sudden reduction in levels of oestrogen often causes distressing symptoms and many doctors suggest that hormone supplements be used following the menopause (see Effects of hormone replacement therapy (HRT), right). HRT helps to reduce the symptoms of the menopause and to delay some of the long-term consequences of reduced oestrogen levels in old age, including osteoporosis (p.55) and atherosclerosis (the deposition of fat in the arteries). A balance between the benefits and risk for individual women must be considered, however, because there can be a slight increase in risk of breast cancer. When dryness of the vagina is a particular problem, a cream containing an oestrogen drug may be prescribed. For long-term treatment, it is used together with a progestogen unless the woman has had a hysterectomy, in which case the oestrogen alone is used. Some women with very severe symptoms respond poorly to oral drugs and may be helped by oestrogen implants. HRT may also be prescribed for women who have undergone premature menopause as a result of surgical removal of the ovaries or radiotherapy for ovarian cancer.

HOW THEY AFFECT YOU

Hormones given to treat ovarian failure or delayed puberty take three to six months to produce a noticeable effect on sexual development. Taken for menopausal symptoms, they can dramatically reduce the number of hot flushes within a week.

Both oestrogens and progestogens can cause fluid retention; and oestrogens may cause nausea, vomiting, breast tenderness, headache, dizziness, and depression. Progestogens may cause "breakthrough" bleeding between menstrual periods. In the comparatively low doses used to treat these disorders, side effects are unlikely.

RISKS AND SPECIAL PRECAUTIONS

The use of oestrogens and progestogens for the treatment of ovarian failure carries few risks for otherwise healthy young women. However, because oestrogens increase the risk of hypertension (high blood pressure) and thrombosis (abnormal blood clotting), there are risks associated with long-term treatment in older women. For this reason, they are prescribed with caution for women who have heart or circulatory disorders, or those who are overweight or smoke. Oestrogens may also trigger the onset of diabetes mellitus in susceptible people or may aggravate blood glucose control in diabetic women. Tibolone has both oestrogen and progestogen properties and can therefore be used on its own.

EFFECTS OF HORMONE REPLACEMENT THERAPY (HRT)

Besides alleviating the symptoms of the menopause, such as hot flushes and vaginal dryness, HRT has a beneficial effect on many parts of the body, including the cardiovascular system and the brain, and is important in preventing osteoporosis (p.55). Benefits must, however, be weighed against a slightly increased risk of breast cancer.

Brain The risk of stroke is reduced, and HRT may play a part in delaying or preventing Alzheimer's disease and Parkinsonism.

Heart HRT prevents the accumulation of fat deposits in the artery walls, reducing the risk of coronary artery disease.

Breasts There is a slightly increased risk of breast cancer with long-term use of HRT, especially in older women.

Bones HRT reduces the thinning of bone that occurs in osteoporosis and thus protects against fractures.

Reproductive organs Thinning of the vaginal tissues leading to painful intercourse can be prevented by HRT.

COMMON DRUGS

Oestrogens Conjugated estrogens*, Diethylstilbestrol*, Estradiol*, Estriol, Estrone, Estropipate, Mestranol, Tibolone*

Progestogens Dydrogesterone*, Hydroxyprogesterone, Levonorgestrel*, Medroxyprogesterone*, Norethisterone*, Norgestrel, Progesterone, Raloxifene*

* **See Part 2**

NUTRITION

Food provides energy (in the form of calories) and materials called nutrients needed for growth and renewal of tissues. Protein, carbohydrate, and fat are the major nutrient components of food.

Proteins are vital for tissue growth and repair. The moderate amounts required can be found in meat and dairy products, cereals, and pulses.

Carbohydrates are a major energy source, and are stored as fat when taken in excess. They can be found in cereals, sugar, and vegetables. Starchy foods are preferable to sugar.

Fats are a concentrated energy form needed only in small quantities. They are contained in animal products such as butter and in the oils of plants such as corn and nuts.

Vitamins and minerals are found only in small amounts in food but are very important for normal function of the body.

Fibre (non-starch polysaccharides) is the indigestible part of any plant product and is needed for a healthy digestive system. It contains no nutrients but adds bulk to faeces. It is found only in foods from plants.

During digestion, large molecules of food are broken down into smaller molecules, releasing nutrients that are absorbed into the bloodstream. Carbohydrate and fat are then metabolized by body cells to produce energy. They may also be incorporated with protein into the cell structure. Each metabolic process is promoted by a specific enzyme and often requires the presence of a particular vitamin or mineral.

WHY DRUGS ARE USED

Dietary deficiency of essential nutrients can lead to illness. In poorer countries where there is a shortage of food, marasmus (resulting from lack of food energy) and kwashiorkor (from lack of protein) are common. In the developed world, however, excessive food intake leading to obesity is more common. Nutritional deficiencies in developed countries result from poor food choices and usually stem from a lack of a specific vitamin or mineral, such as in iron-deficiency anaemia.

Some nutritional deficiencies may be caused by an inability of the body to absorb nutrients from food (malabsorption) or to utilize them once they have been absorbed. Malabsorption may be caused by lack of an enzyme or an abnormality of the digestive tract. Errors of metabolism are often inborn and are not yet fully understood. They may be caused by failure of the body to produce the chemicals that are required to process nutrients for use.

WHY SUPPLEMENTS ARE USED

Deficiencies such as kwashiorkor or marasmus are usually treated by dietary improvement and, in some cases, food supplements, rather than drugs. Vitamin and mineral deficiencies are usually treated with appropriate supplements. Malabsorption disorders may require changes in diet or long-term use of supplements. Metabolic errors are not easily treated with supplements or drugs, and a special diet may be the main treatment.

Obesity was formerly treated with appetite-suppressants related to amphetamines. The use of amphetamines is now discouraged, however, and the preferred treatment includes reduction of food intake, altered eating patterns, and increased exercise.

MAJOR DRUG GROUPS
◆ Vitamins
◆ Minerals

Vitamins

Vitamins are complex chemicals that are essential for a variety of body functions. With the exception of vitamin D, the body cannot manufacture these substances itself and therefore we need to include them in our diet. There are 13 major vitamins: A, C, D, E, K, and the B complex vitamins – thiamine (B_1), riboflavin (B_2), niacin (B_3), pantothenic acid (B_5), pyridoxine (B_6), and cobalamin (B_{12}) folic acid and biotin. Most vitamins are required in very small amounts and each vitamin is present in one or more foods (see Main food sources of vitamins, p.90). Vitamin D is also produced in the body when the skin is exposed to sunlight. Vitamins fall into two groups, depending on whether they dissolve in fat or water.

Water-soluble vitamins Vitamin C and the B vitamins dissolve in water. Most are stored in the body for only a short period and are rapidly excreted by the kidneys if taken in higher amounts than the body needs. Vitamin B_{12} is the exception; it is stored in the liver, which may hold up to six years' supply. For these reasons, foods containing water-soluble vitamins need to be eaten daily. These vitamins are easily lost in cooking, so uncooked foods containing them should be eaten regularly. An overdose does not usually cause toxic effects, but adverse reactions to large dosages of vitamin C and pyridoxine (vitamin B_6) have been reported.

Fat-soluble vitamins Vitamins A, D, E, and K are absorbed from the intestine into the bloodstream together with fat. Deficiency of these vitamins may occur as a result of any disorder that affects the absorption of fat (for example, coeliac disease). These vitamins are stored in the liver and reserves of some of them may last for several years. Taking an excess of a fat-soluble vitamin for a long period may cause it to build up to a harmful level in the body. Ensuring that foods rich in these vitamins are regularly included in the diet usually provides a sufficient supply without the risk of overdosage.

A number of vitamins, such as vitamins A, C, and E, have now been recognized as having strong antioxidant properties (neutralizing the effect of free radicals, which are believed to play a role in ageing and disease).

A balanced diet that includes a variety of different types of food is likely to contain adequate amounts of all the vitamins. Inadequate intake of any vitamin over an extended period can lead to symptoms of deficiency. The nature of these symptoms depends on the vitamin concerned.

A doctor may recommend supplements of one or more vitamins in a variety of circumstances: to prevent deficiency occurring in people who are considered at special risk, to treat symptoms of deficiency, and in the treatment of certain medical conditions.

WHY VITAMINS ARE USED

Preventing deficiency Most people in the UK obtain enough vitamins from their diet, and supplements are not usually necessary. People unsure if their diet is adequate are advised to look at the table on p.90 to check that vitamin-rich foods are eaten regularly. Vitamin intake can often be boosted simply by increasing the quantities of fresh food and raw fruit and vegetables in the diet. Certain groups of people are at increased risk of vitamin deficiency, however. These include people with increased need of certain vitamins that may not be met from dietary sources – in particular, pregnant or breast-feeding women and infants and young children. The elderly, who may not be eating a varied diet, may also be at risk. Strict vegetarians, vegans, and other people on restricted diets may not receive adequate amounts of all vitamins.

In addition, people who suffer from disorders in which absorption of nutrients from the bowel is impaired, or who need to take drugs that reduce the absorption of vitamins (for example, some types of lipid-lowering drugs), are usually given additional vitamins.

In these cases, the doctor is likely to advise supplements of one or more vitamins. Most preparations are available without a prescription, but it is important to seek specialist advice before starting a course of vitamin supplements, so that a proper assessment is made of your individual requirements.

Vitamin supplements should not be used as a tonic to improve well-being – they are ineffective for this purpose – nor should they be used as a substitute for a balanced diet.

Vitamin deficiency It is rare for a diet to totally lack a particular vitamin. But if intake of a vitamin is regularly lower than the body needs (see Vitamin requirements, p.90), the stores of vitamins may, over time, become depleted and symptoms of deficiency may begin to appear. In the UK, vitamin deficiency disorders are most common among vagrants and alcoholics and those on low incomes who fail to eat an adequate diet. Deficiencies of water-soluble vitamins are more likely since most of these are not stored in large quantities in the body.

Dosages of vitamins prescribed to treat deficiency are likely to be larger than those

MAIN FOOD SOURCES OF VITAMINS

The table below lists especially good sources of particular vitamins. A balanced diet helps to maintain adequate intake without the need for supplements. Processed and overcooked foods are likely to contain fewer vitamins than fresh, raw, or lightly cooked foods.

VITAMINS	Red meat	Poultry	Liver	Milk	Cheese	Butter/margarine	Eggs	Fish	Cereals and bread	Green vegetables	Root vegetables	Pulses/legumes	Nuts	Fruit
Biotin			•				•					•	•	
Folic acid			•				•			•				•
Niacin as nicotinic acid	•	•	•				•	•				•	•	
Pantothenic acid			•				•	•						
Pyridoxine	•	•	•				•	•	•					
Riboflavin			•	•	•		•		•			•	•	•
Thiamine	•		•					•				•	•	
Vitamin A			•	•	•	•	•			•	•			•
Vitamin B12	•		•	•	•		•	•						
Vitamin C										•	•			•
Vitamin D				•			•							
Vitamin E						•	•		•	•		•	•	
Vitamin K									•	•				

used to prevent it. Medical supervision is required when correcting vitamin deficiency.

Other medical uses of vitamins Various claims have been made for the value of vitamins in the treatment of other medical disorders. High doses of vitamin C have been said to be effective in preventing and treating the common cold. Such claims are not proved, but zinc may be helpful for this purpose. Supplements do not improve IQ in well-nourished children, but quite small dietary deficiencies can cause poor academic performance.

Certain vitamins also have recognized medical uses. Vitamin D has long been used to treat bone-wasting disorders (p.54). Niacin is sometimes used (in the form of nicotinic acid) as a lipid-lowering drug (p.35). Vitamin A derivatives (retinoids) are an established part of the treatment for severe acne (p.119). Many women suffering from premenstrual syndrome take pyridoxine (vitamin B_6) supplements to relieve their symptoms. See also Drugs for menstrual disorders, p.100.

VITAMIN REQUIREMENTS

Normal daily vitamin requirements are usually based on the Reference Nutrient Intake (RNI). Deficiency needs much higher doses, which should be determined by your doctor.

Biotin No RNI established; 10–200 micrograms is safe.

Folic acid (as folate): 50 micrograms (birth–1 year); 70 micrograms (1–3 years); 100 micrograms (4–6 years); 150 micrograms (7–10 years); 200 micrograms (11 years and over); 400 micrograms per day to prevent first occurrence of neural tube defects, then 5mg per day to prevent recurrence (pregnancy and breast-feeding).

Niacin 3mg (birth–3 months); 4mg (7–9 months); 5mg (10–12 months); 8mg (1–3 years); 11mg (4–6 years); 12mg (males 7–10 years and females 7–14 years); 15mg (males 11–14 years); 18mg (males 15–18 years); 14mg (females 15–18 years); 17mg (males 19–50 years); 13mg (females 19–50 years); 16mg (males 51 years and over); 12mg (females 51 years and over); no extra requirement (pregnancy); 2mg extra (breast-feeding).

Pantothenic acid No RNI established; adults require 3–7mg daily.

Pyridoxine 0.2mg (birth–6 months); 0.3mg (7–9 months); 0.4mg (10 months–1 year); 0.7mg (1–3 years); 0.9mg (4–6 years); 1mg (males 7–10 years and females 7–14 years); 1.2mg (males 11–14 years); 1.5mg (males 15–18 years); 1.2mg (females 15 and over); 1.4mg (males 19 and over).

Riboflavin 0.4mg (birth–1 year); 0.6mg (1–3 years); 0.8mg (4–6 years); 1mg (7–10 years); 1.2mg (males 11–14 years); 1.1mg (females 11 and over); 1.3mg (males 15 and over). Requirements rise by 0.3mg (pregnancy) and 0.5mg (breast-feeding).

Thiamine 0.2mg (birth–9 months); 0.3mg (10–12 months); 0.5mg (1–3 years); 0.7mg (males 4–10 years and females 4–14 years); 0.9mg (males 11–14 years); 1.1mg (males 15–18 years); 0.8mg (females 15 and over); 1mg (males 19–50 years); and 0.9mg (males 51 and over). 0.1mg extra (last three months of pregnancy); 0.2mg extra (breast-feeding).

Vitamin A 350 micrograms (up to 1 year); 400 micrograms (1–3 years); 500 micrograms (4–10 years); 600 micrograms (males 11–14 years, females 11 years and over); 700 micrograms (males 15 and over, and pregnant women); 950 micrograms (breast-feeding).

Vitamin B$_{12}$ Only minute quantities required. 0.3 micrograms (birth–6 months); 0.4 micrograms (7–12 months); 0.5 micrograms (1–3 years); 0.8 micrograms (4–6 years); 1 microgram (7–10 years); 1.2 micrograms (11–14 years); 1.5 micrograms (15 years and over); no extra requirements (pregnancy); 2 micrograms (breast-feeding).

Vitamin C 25mg (birth–1 year); 30mg (1–10 years); 35mg (11–14 years); 40mg (15 years and over); 50mg (pregnancy); 70mg (breast-feeding).

Vitamin D 8.5 micrograms (birth–6 months); 7 micrograms (7 months–3 years); 10 micrograms (over 65 years, pregnancy, and breast-feeding). Most people outside these groups do not require supplements.

Vitamin E No UK recommendations (requirement depends on intake of polyunsaturated fatty acid, which varies widely); 3–15mg (approx) recommended.

Vitamin K 10 micrograms (newborn); no RNI established (other age groups); no extra requirements (pregnancy and breast-feeding).

RISKS AND SPECIAL PRECAUTIONS

Vitamins are natural substances, and supplements can be taken without risk by most people. It is important not to exceed the recommended dosage, however, particularly in the case of fat-soluble vitamins, which may accumulate in the body. Dosage needs to be carefully calculated, taking into account the degree of deficiency, dietary intake, and duration of treatment. Overdosage has at best no therapeutic value and at worst may incur the risk of serious harmful effects. Multivitamin preparations containing a large number of different vitamins are widely available. Fortunately, the amounts of each vitamin in each tablet are not usually large and are not likely to be harmful unless the dose is greatly exceeded. Single vitamin supplements can be harmful because an excess of one vitamin may increase requirements for others; hence, they should be used only on medical advice.

Minerals

Minerals are elements – the simplest form of substance – many of which are essential in trace amounts for normal metabolic processes. A balanced diet usually contains all of the minerals that the body requires; mineral deficiency diseases, except iron-deficiency anaemia, are uncommon.

Dietary supplements are necessary only when a doctor has diagnosed a specific deficiency or as part of the prevention or treatment of a medical disorder. Doctors often prescribe minerals for people with intestinal diseases that reduce the absorption of minerals from the diet. Iron supplements are often advised for pregnant or breast-feeding women, and iron-rich foods are recommended for infants over six months.

Taking mineral supplements unless under medical direction is not advisable, exceeding the body's daily requirements is not beneficial, and large doses may be harmful.

MINERAL REQUIREMENTS

As with vitamins, normal daily mineral requirements are usually based on the Reference Nutrient Intake (RNI).

Calcium 525mg (birth–1 year); 350mg (1–3 years); 450mg (4–6 years); 550mg (7–10 years); 1,000mg (males 11–18 years); 800mg (females 11–18 years); 700mg (19 years and older). No extra requirement (pregnancy); 550mg extra (breast-feeding).

Chromium Only minute quantities needed. RNI not established; about 25 micrograms is safe.

MAIN FOOD SOURCES OF MINERALS

The table below indicates foods that are especially good sources of particular minerals. A balanced diet usually contains all the minerals required by the body, without the need for supplements. Some, known as trace elements, are required in only minute amounts.

MINERALS	Red meat	Poultry	Liver	Milk	Cheese	Butter/margarine	Eggs	Fish	Cereals and bread	Green vegetables	Root vegetables	Pulses/legumes	Nuts	Fruit
Calcium				●	●					●		●	●	
Chromium	●				●				●	●				
Copper	●	●	●				●	●	●			●	●	
Fluoride								●						
Iodine				●	●				●	●				
Iron	●	●	●				●	●	●	●				
Magnesium				●				●	●			●	●	
Phosphorus	●	●	●	●	●		●	●	●	●	●	●	●	●
Potassium								●	●	●	●			●
Selenium	●		●	●				●	●					
Sodium	●	●	●	●	●	●	●	●	●	●	●	●	●	●
Zinc	●				●			●	●			●		

Copper 0.2mg (birth–3 months); 0.3mg (4 months–1 year); 0.4mg (1–3 years); 0.6mg (4–6 years); 0.7mg (7–10 years); 0.8mg (11–14 years); 1.0mg (15–18 years); 1.2mg (19 years and over); no extra requirement (pregnancy); 0.3mg extra (breast-feeding).

Fluoride No RNI established; about 0.15mg (infants under 3 months) and 0.5mg (up to 2 years) is safe.

Iodine 50 micrograms (birth–3 months); 60 micrograms (4–12 months); 70 micrograms (1–3 years); 100 micrograms (4–6 years); 110 micrograms (7–10 years); 130 micrograms (11–14 years); 140 micrograms (15 years and over); slightly increased requirement (breast-feeding); one vitamin tablet with calcium and iodine recommended for nursing mothers.

Iron 1.7mg (birth–3 months); 4.3mg (4–6 months); 7.8mg (7–12 months); 6.9mg (1–3 years); 6.1mg (4–6 years); 8.7mg (7–10 years); 11.3mg (males 11–18 years); 14.8mg (females 11–50 years); 8.7mg (males 19 and over, and females 51 and over); requirements may be increased (pregnancy) and for 2 to 3 months after childbirth).

Magnesium 55mg (birth–3 months); 60mg (4–6 months); 75mg (7–9 months); 80mg (10–12 months); 85mg (1–3 years); 120mg (4–6 years); 200mg (7–10 years); 280mg (11–14 years); 300mg (males 15 and over, and females 15–18 years); 270mg (females 19 and over); no extra requirement (pregnancy); 50mg extra (breast-feeding).

Potassium 0.8g (birth–3 months); 0.85g (4–6 months); 0.7g (7–12 months); 0.8g (1–3 years); 1.1g (4–6 years); 2g (7–10 years); 3.1g (11–14 years); 3.5g (15 years and over).

Selenium 10 micrograms (birth–3 months); 13 micrograms (4–6 months); 10 micrograms (7–12 months); 15 micrograms (1–3 years); 20 micrograms (4–6 years); 30 micrograms (7–10 years); 45 micrograms (11–14 years); 70 micrograms (males 15–18 years); 60 micrograms (females 15 and over); 75 micrograms (males 19 and over); no extra requirement (pregnancy); 15 micrograms extra (breast-feeding).

Sodium 0.21g (birth–3 months); 0.28g (4–6 months); 0.32g (7–9 months); 0.35g (10–12 months); 0.5g (1–3 years); 0.7g (4–6 years); 1.2g (7–10 years); and 1.6g (11 years and over).

Zinc 4mg (birth–6 months); 5mg (7 months–3 years); 6.5mg (4–6 years); 7mg (7–10 years); 9mg (11–14 years); 9.5mg (males 15 years and over); and 7mg (females 15 years and over); no extra requirement (pregnancy); 13mg (first 4 months of breast-feeding and 9.5mg thereafter).

MALIGNANT AND IMMUNE DISEASE

New cells are continuously needed by the body to replace those that wear out and die naturally and to repair injured tissue. In normal circumstances the rate at which cells are created is carefully regulated. Sometimes, however, abnormal cells are formed that multiply uncontrollably. They may form lumps, warts, or nodules of abnormal tissue. These tumours are usually confined to one place and cause few problems; these are benign growths. In other types of tumour the cells may invade or destroy the structures around the tumour, and abnormal cells may spread to other parts of the body, forming satellite or metastatic tumours. These malignant growths are also called cancers.

Opposing the development of tumours is the body's immune system. This can recognize as foreign not only invading bacteria and viruses but also transplanted tissue and cells that have become cancerous. Interferons are natural proteins that limit viral infection by inhibiting viral replication within body cells. Some of these substances also assist in the destruction of cancer cells. The immune system relies on different types of white blood cell produced in the lymph glands and bone marrow.

Overactivity of the immune system also causes allergic reactions (see Allergy, p.56).

TYPES OF CANCER

Uncontrolled multiplication of cells leads to the formation of tumours that may be benign or malignant. Benign tumours do not spread to other tissues; malignant (cancerous) tumours do, however.

Carcinomas affect the skin and glandular tissue lining cells of internal organs.

Sarcomas affect muscles, bones, and fibrous tissues and lining cells of blood vessels.

Leukaemia affects white blood cells.

Lymphomas affect the lymph glands.

WHAT CAN GO WRONG

A single cause for cancer has not been identified, and an individual's risk of developing cancer may depend both upon genetic predisposition (some types of cancer run in families) and upon exposure to external risk factors, known as carcinogens. These include tobacco smoke, which increases the risk of lung cancer, and ultraviolet light, which makes skin cancer more likely in those who spend long periods in the sun. Long-term suppression of the immune system by disease (as in AIDS) or by drugs (e.g., those given to prevent rejection of transplanted organs) also increases the risk of developing not only infections but also certain cancers. This fact demonstrates the importance of the immune system in removing abnormal cells with the potential to cause a tumour.

Excessive activity of the immune system may also cause problems. It may respond excessively to an innocuous stimulus, as in hay fever, or may mount a reaction against normal tissues, leading to a variety of disorders known as autoimmune diseases. These include rheumatoid arthritis, certain inflammatory skin disorders (for example, systemic lupus erythematosus), pernicious anaemia, and some forms of hypothyroidism. Immune system activity can also be troublesome following an organ or tissue transplant, when it may lead to rejection of the foreign tissue. This shows the need for medication that can dampen the immune system and enable the body to accept the foreign tissue.

WHY DRUGS ARE USED

In cancer treatment, cytotoxic (cell-killing) drugs are used to eliminate abnormally dividing cells. This has the effect of slowing the growth rate of tumours and sometimes leading to their complete disappearance. Because these drugs act against all rapidly dividing cells, they also reduce the number of normal cells, including blood cells, being produced from the bone marrow. This can produce serious adverse effects, like anaemia and neutropenia in cancer patients, but it can be useful in limiting white cell activity in autoimmune disorders.

Other drugs that have immunosuppressant effects include corticosteroids and ciclosporin, which are used following transplant surgery. No drugs are yet available that directly stimulate the entire immune system. However, growth factors may be used to increase the number and activity of some white blood cells, and antibody infusions may help those people with deficient production or may be used against specific targets in organ transplantation and cancer.

MAJOR DRUG GROUPS

◆ Anticancer drugs
◆ Immunosuppressant drugs
◆ Drugs for AIDS and HIV

Anticancer drugs

Cancer is a general term that covers a wide range of disorders, ranging from the leukaemias (blood cancers) to solid tumours of the lung, breast, and other organs. In all cancers, a group of cells escape from the normal controls on cell growth, multiplication, and spread. As a result, the malignant (cancerous) cells begin to crowd out the normal cells and a tumour develops. Cancerous cells are frequently unable to perform their usual functions, and this may lead to progressively impaired function of the organ or area concerned. Cancers may develop from cells of the blood, skin, muscle, or any other tissue.

Malignant tumours spread into nearby structures, blocking blood vessels and compressing nerves and other structures. Fragments of the tumour may become detached and carried in the bloodstream to other parts of the body, where they form secondary growths (metastases).

Many different factors, or a combination of them, can provoke cancerous changes in cells. These include an individual's genetic background, immune system failure, and exposure to cancer-causing agents (carcinogens). Known carcinogens include strong sunlight, tobacco smoke, radiation, certain chemicals, viruses, and dietary factors.

Treating cancer is a complicated process that depends on the type of cancer, its stage of development, and the patient's condition and wishes. Any of the following treatments may be used alone or in combination with the others: surgical removal of the cancer,

radiation treatment, and chemotherapy (that is, the use of anticancer drugs).

Anticancer drugs that kill cancer cells are sometimes referred to as cytotoxic drugs. They fall into several classes, depending on their chemical composition and principal mode of action. Alkylating agents, antimetabolites, and cytotoxic antibiotics are among the most widely used classes. In addition to these drugs, sex hormones and related substances are also used to treat some types of cancer. Increasingly, attempts are being made to stimulate the body's own immune defences using drugs like interferon or interleukin and antibodies which recognise specific tumour types.

WHY THEY ARE USED

Cytotoxic drugs can cure rapidly growing cancers and are the treatment of choice for leukaemias, lymphomas, and certain cancers of the testis. They are less effective against slow-growing solid tumours, such as those of the breast and bowel, but they can relieve symptoms and prolong life (see Successful chemotherapy, facing page). Adjuvant (effect enhancing) chemotherapy is increasingly being used after surgery, especially for breast and bowel tumours, to prevent regrowth of the cancer from cells left behind after surgery.

Hormone treatment is offered in cases of hormone-sensitive cancer, including many breast, uterine, and prostatic cancers.

Since all anticancer drugs may produce severe adverse effects (see facing page), they are used only in cases where there is a reasonable chance of achieving a complete cure, significantly prolonging life, or relieving distressing symptoms. Their effectiveness varies a great deal, depending primarily on the type of cancer and the extent of its spread.

The choice of anticancer drug depends on the type of cancer and the condition of the person who is being treated. Often a combination of several drugs is used, either simultaneously or successively. Special regimes of different drugs used together and in succession have been devised to maximize their activity and minimize side effects.

Certain anticancer drugs are also used for their effect in suppressing immune system activity (see p.96).

HOW THEY WORK

All cytotoxic anticancer drugs kill cancer cells by preventing them from growing or dividing. Cells grow and divide in several stages. Most anticancer drugs act at one specific stage of cell growth or division. During treatment, several drugs may be given in sequence to eliminate abnormal cells at all stages of development.

Hormone treatments act by opposing the effects of the hormone that is encouraging growth of the cancer. For example, some breast cancers are stimulated by the female sex hormone oestrogen, whose action is opposed by the drug tamoxifen. Other cancers are damaged by high doses of a particular sex hormone. For example, medroxyprogesterone, a progestogen, often halts the spread of endometrial cancer.

Monoclonal antibodies, such as rituximab, bind to certain cells, marking them out for destruction. Interferon alfa and interleukin 2 are cytokines which stimulate the immune system to attack certain cancers by mechanisms that are not entirely understood.

HOW THEY AFFECT YOU

At the start of treatment, adverse effects of cytotoxic drugs are likely to be more noticeable than benefits. The most common side effect is nausea and vomiting, for which an anti-emetic drug (see p.21) will usually be prescribed. Effects on the blood are also common. Many anticancer drugs cause hair loss because of the effect of their activity on the hair follicle cells, but the hair usually starts to grow back after chemotherapy has been completed. Individual drugs may produce other side effects.

Anticancer drugs are, in most cases, administered in the highest doses that can be tolerated in order to kill as many cancer cells as quickly as possible.

The unpleasant side effects of intensive chemotherapy, combined with a delay of several weeks before any beneficial effects are seen, and the seriousness of the underlying disease, often lead to depression in those who are receiving anticancer drugs. Specialist counselling, support from family and friends, and, in some cases, treatment with antidepressant drugs, may be helpful.

SUCCESSFUL CHEMOTHERAPY

Not all cancers respond to treatment with anticancer drugs. Some cancers can be cured by drug treatment. In others, drug treatment can slow or temporarily halt the disease's progress. In certain cases, drug treatment has no beneficial effect, but other treatments, such as surgery, often produce significant benefits. The main cancers that fall into each of the three groups are described below.

Cancers that can often be cured by drugs

◆ Some cancers of the lymphatic system (including Hodgkin's disease)
◆ Acute leukaemias (forms of blood cancer)
◆ Choriocarcinoma (cancer of the placenta)
◆ Germ cell tumours (cancers affecting sperm and egg cells)
◆ Wilms' tumour (a rare form of kidney cancer that affects children)
◆ Cancer of the testis

Cancers in which drugs may produce worthwhile benefits

◆ Breast cancer
◆ Ovarian cancer
◆ Some leukaemias
◆ Multiple myeloma (a bone marrow cancer)
◆ Many types of lung cancer
◆ Head and neck cancers
◆ Cancer of the stomach
◆ Cancer of the prostate
◆ Some cancers of the lymphatic system
◆ Bladder cancer
◆ Cancer of the islet cells of the pancreas
◆ Endometrial cancer (cancer affecting the lining of the uterus)
◆ Cancer of the large intestine
◆ Cancer of the oesophagus

Cancers in which drugs are unlikely to be of benefit

◆ Thyroid cancer
◆ Brain cancer in adults
◆ Malignant melanoma (a form of skin cancer)
◆ Liver cancer
◆ Cancer of the pancreas
◆ Cancer of the cervix
◆ Kidney cell cancer

Successful drug treatment of cancer usually requires repeated courses of anticancer drugs because the treatment needs to be halted periodically to allow the blood-pro-ducing cells in the bone marrow to recover.

RISKS AND SPECIAL PRECAUTIONS

All cytotoxic anticancer drugs interfere with the activity of noncancerous cells and, for this reason, often produce serious adverse effects during long-term treatment. In par-ticular, these drugs often adversely affect rapidly dividing cells such as the blood-producing cells in the bone marrow. The numbers of red and white cells and the num-ber of platelets (particles in the blood re-sponsible for clotting) may all be reduced. In some cases, symptoms of anaemia (weakness and fatigue) and an increased risk of abnor-mal or excessive bleeding may develop as a result of treatment with anticancer drugs. Reduction in the number of white blood cells may result in an increased susceptibility to infection. A simple infection such as a sore throat may be a sign of depressed white cell production in a patient taking anticancer drugs, and it must be reported to the doctor without delay. In addition, wounds may take longer to heal, and susceptible people can develop gout as a result of increased uric acid production due to cells being broken down.

Because of these problems, anticancer chemotherapy is often given in hospital, where the adverse effects can be closely mon-itored. Several short courses of drug treat-ment are usually given, allowing the bone marrow time to recover in the period bet-ween courses (see Successful chemotherapy, p.95). Blood tests are performed regularly. When necessary, blood transfusions, anti-biotics, or other forms of treatment are used to overcome the adverse effects. When rele-vant, contraceptive advice is given early in treatment because most anticancer drugs can damage a developing baby.

In addition to these general effects, indi-vidual drugs may have adverse effects on particular organs. These are described under individual drug profiles in Part 2.

COMMON DRUGS

Alkylating agents Chlorambucil, Cyclophosphamide*, Melphalan
Antimetabolites Azathioprine*, Cytarabine,

Fluorouracil, Mercaptopurine*, Methotrexate*
Cytotoxic antibiotics Doxorubicin*, Epirubicin
Hormone treatments Anastrozole, Bicalutamide, Cyproterone acetate, Flutamide*, Formestane, Goserelin*, Letrozole, Leuprorelin, Medroxyprogesterone*, Megestrol*, Tamoxifen*
Cytokines Interferon alfa*, Interleukin 2
Taxanes Docetaxel, Paclitaxel
Other drugs Carboplatin, Cisplatin*, Etoposide, Irinotecan, Rituximab
* See Part 2

Immunosuppressant drugs

The body is protected against attack from bacteria, fungi, and viruses by the specialized cells and proteins in the blood and tissues that make up the immune system. They res-pond to foreign cells in a variety of ways: white blood cells known as lymphocytes res-pond to infection and foreign tissue, either by killing invading organisms directly or by producing special proteins (antibodies) to destroy them; B-lymphocytes produce anti-bodies to attack invading organisms, whereas T-lymphocytes attack invading cells directly; other blood cells help the action of the B- and T-cells. These mechanisms are also responsible for eliminating abnormal or unhealthy cells that could otherwise multiply and develop into a cancer.

In certain conditions it is medically neces-sary to dampen the immune system's activity. They include a number of autoimmune dis-orders (in which the immune system attacks normal body tissue), which may affect a single organ (e.g., the adrenal glands in Addison's disease or the thyroid gland in Hashimoto's disease), or they may result in widespread damage (e.g., in rheumatoid arthritis or sys-temic lupus erythematosus).

Immune system activity may also need to be reduced following an organ transplant, when the body's defences would otherwise attack and reject the transplanted tissue.

Several types of drug are used as immuno-suppressants.
Anticancer drugs (p.94) slow the production of all cells in the bone marrow.
Corticosteroids (p.78) reduce the activity of both B- and T-lymphocytes.

Ciclosporin p.170) inhibits the activity of T-lymphocytes only and not B-lymphocyte activity.

WHY THEY ARE USED

Immunosuppressants are given for autoimmune disorders such as rheumatoid arthritis when symptoms are severe and other treatments have not given adequate relief. Corticosteroids are usually prescribed initially; their anti-inflammatory effect and immunosuppressant action help to promote healing of tissue damaged by abnormal immune system activity. A drug such as methotrexate may be used in addition to corticosteroids, to reduce the activity of lymphocytes, if these do not produce sufficient improvement or their effect wanes (see also Antirheumatic drugs, p.50).

Immunosuppressant drugs are given before and after organ and other tissue transplants. Treatment may have to be continued indefinitely to prevent rejection. Several drugs and drug combinations are used, depending on the organ being transplanted and the underlying condition. However, ciclosporin, along with the related drug tacrolimus, is now the most widely used drug for preventing organ rejection. It is also increasingly used to treat autoimmune disorders. It is often used in combination with a corticosteroid or the more specific drug mycophenolate mofetil.

Monoclonal antibodies which attack those parts of the immune system responsible for organ rejection are also being introduced to aid transplantation.

HOW THEY WORK

Immunosuppressant drugs reduce the effectiveness of the immune system, either by depressing the production of lymphocytes or by altering their activity.

HOW THEY AFFECT YOU

When immunosuppressants are given to treat an autoimmune disorder, they reduce the severity of symptoms and may temporarily halt the progress of the disease. They cannot repair major tissue damage, however.

Immunosuppressants can produce a range of unwanted side effects; those of corticosteroids are described on p.79. Anticancer drugs prescribed as immunosuppressants are given in low doses that produce only mild side effects. They may cause nausea and vomiting, for which an anti-emetic (p.21) may be prescribed. Hair loss is rare and regrowth usually occurs when treatment is stopped. Ciclosporin may cause increased facial hair growth, swelling of the gums, and tingling in the hands.

RISKS AND SPECIAL PRECAUTIONS

All of these drugs may produce potentially serious adverse effects. By reducing the activity of the patient's immune system, immunosuppressant drugs can affect the body's ability to fight invading microorganisms, thereby increasing the risk of serious infections. Because lymphocyte activity is also important for preventing the multiplication of abnormal cells, there is an increased risk of certain types of cancer. A major drawback of anticancer drugs is that, in addition to their effect on the production of lymphocytes, they interfere with the growth and division of other blood cells in the bone marrow. Reduced production of red blood cells can cause anaemia; when the production of blood platelets is suppressed, blood clotting may be less efficient.

Although ciclosporin is more specific in its action than either corticosteroids or anticancer drugs, it can cause kidney damage and, in too high a dose, may affect the brain, causing hallucinations or fits. Ciclosporin also tends to raise blood pressure, and another drug may be required to counteract this effect (see Antihypertensive drugs, p.34).

COMMON DRUGS

Anticancer drugs Azathioprine*, Chlorambucil, Cyclophosphamide*, Methotrexate, Mycophenolate mofetil
Corticosteroids (see p.78)
Antibodies Anti-lymphocyte globulin, Basiliximab, Daclizumab
Other drugs Ciclosporin*, Tacrolimus
* **See Part 2**

Drugs for HIV and AIDS

The disease AIDS (acquired immune deficiency syndrome) is caused by infection with HIV (the human immunodeficiency virus).

HIV invades certain cells of the immune system, particularly white blood cells called T-helper lymphocytes, which normally activate other cells in the immune system to fight infection. Since HIV kills T-helper lymphocytes, the body cannot fight the virus or subsequent infections. Currently, it is not known whether all individuals who become infected with HIV will develop full-blown AIDS, which is defined by the occurrence of certain infections and/or cancers.

WHY THEY ARE USED
Drug treatments for HIV infection can be divided into treatment of the initial infection and of diseases associated with AIDS.

There are two groups of drugs which act directly against HIV. Both work by interfering with enzymes that are vital for virus replication. The first group, which inhibit an enzyme known as reverse transcriptase, are divided according to their chemical structure into nucleoside and non-nucleoside inhibitors. The second group interfere with an enzyme called protease.

These drugs are much more effective when used in combination. Treatment is now usually started with a combination of two nucleoside transcriptase inhibitors plus a non-nucleoside drug or a protease inhibitor. If this so-called "triple therapy" is started before damage to the immune system is too great, it can dramatically reduce the levels of HIV virus in the body and improve the outlook for HIV-infected patients. It is not a cure for the disease, however, and the blood and secretions of patients remain infectious.

The mainstay of drug treatment for AIDS-related diseases are the antimicrobial drugs for the bacterial, viral, fungal, and protozoal infections to which people with AIDS are susceptible. These drugs include the antituberculous drugs (p.65), co-trimoxazole for the treatment of pneumocystis carinii pneumonia (PCP), and ganciclovir for the treatment of CMV (cytomegalovirus) infection.

COMMON DRUGS
Nucleoside reverse transcriptase inhibitors
Didanosine*, Lamivudine*, Stavudine, Zalcitabine*, Zidovudine (AZT)*

Non-nucleoside transcriptase inhibitors Efavirenz, Nevirapine
Protease inhibitors Indinavir, Nelfinavir, Ritonavir, Saquinavir
* **See Part 2**

REPRODUCTIVE & URINARY TRACTS

The reproductive systems of men and women consist of those organs that produce and release sperm (male), or store and release eggs, and then nurture a fertilized egg until it develops into a baby (female).

The urinary system filters wastes and water from the blood, producing urine, which is then expelled from the body. The reproductive and urinary systems of men are partially linked, but those of women form two physically close but functionally separate systems.

The female reproductive organs comprise the ovaries, fallopian tubes, and uterus (womb). The uterus opens via the cervix (neck of the uterus) into the vagina. The principal male reproductive organs are the two sperm-producing glands, the testes (testicles), which lie within the scrotum, and the penis. Other structures of the male reproductive tract include the prostate gland and several tubular structures – the tightly coiled epididymides, the vas deferens, the seminal vesicles, and the urethra.

The urinary organs in both sexes comprise the kidneys, which filter the blood and excrete urine (see also Diuretics, p.30), the ureters down which urine passes, and the bladder, where urine is stored until it is released from the body via the urethra.

WHAT CAN GO WRONG

The reproductive and urinary tracts are both subject to infection. Such infections (apart from those transmitted by sexual activity) are relatively uncommon in men because the long male urethra prevents bacteria and other organisms passing easily to the bladder and upper urinary tract, and to the male sex organs. The shorter female urethra allows urinary tract infections, especially of the bladder (cystitis) and of the urethra (urethritis), to occur commonly. The female reproductive tract is also vulnerable to infection, which, in some cases, is sexually transmitted.

Reproductive function may also be disrupted by hormonal disturbances that lead to reduced fertility. Women may be troubled by symptoms arising from normal activity of the reproductive organs, including menstrual disorders as well as problems associated with childbirth.

The most common urinary problems, apart from infection, are those that are related to bladder function. Urine may be released involuntarily (incontinence), or it may be retained in the bladder. Such disorders are usually the result of damage occurring during childbirth. The filtering action of the kidneys may be affected by alteration of the composition of the blood or the hormones that regulate urine production, or by damage (from infection or inflammation) to the filtering units of the kidneys themselves.

WHY DRUGS ARE USED

Antibiotic drugs (p.60) are used to eliminate infections of both the urinary and reproductive tracts (including sexually transmitted infections). Certain infections of the vagina are caused by fungi or yeasts and require antifungal drugs (p.74).

Hormone drugs are used both to reduce fertility deliberately (oral contraceptives) and to increase fertility in certain conditions in which it has not been possible for a couple to conceive. Hormones may also be used to regulate menstruation when it is irregular or excessively painful or heavy. Analgesic drugs (p.9) are used to treat menstrual period pain and are also widely used for pain relief in labour. Other drugs used in labour include those that increase contraction of the muscles of the uterus and those that limit blood loss after the birth. Drugs may also be used to halt premature labour.

Drugs that alter the transmission of nerve signals to the bladder muscles have an important role in the treatment of urinary incontinence and retention. Drugs that increase the kidneys' filtering action are commonly used to reduce blood pressure and fluid retention (see Diuretics, p.30). Other drugs may alter the composition of the urine – for example, the uricosuric drugs that are used in the treatment of gout (p.51) increase the amount of uric acid.

THE MENSTRUAL CYCLE

A monthly cycle of hormone interactions allows an egg to be released and, if it is fertilized, creates the correct environment for it to implant in the uterus. Major changes occur in the body, the most obvious of which is monthly vaginal bleeding (menstruation). The menstrual cycle usually starts between the ages of 11 and 14 years and continues until the menopause, which occurs at around the age of 50. After the menopause, childbearing is no longer possible. The cycle is usually 28 days, but this varies with individuals.

Menstruation If no egg is fertilized, the endometrium is shed (days 1–5).

Fertile period Conception may take place in the two days after ovulation (days 14–16).

MAJOR DRUG GROUPS

◆ Drugs used to treat menstrual disorders
◆ Oral contraceptives
◆ Drugs for infertility
◆ Drugs used in labour
◆ Drugs used for urinary disorders

Drugs used to treat menstrual disorders

The menstrual cycle results from the actions of female sex hormones that cause ovulation (the release of an egg) and thickening of the endometrium (the lining of the uterus) each month in preparation for pregnancy. Unless the egg is fertilized, the endometrium will be shed about two weeks later during menstruation (see also The menstrual cycle, above).

The main problems associated with menstruation that may require medical treatment are excessive blood loss (menorrhagia), pain during menstruation (dysmenorrhoea), and distressing physical and psychological symptoms occurring prior to menstruation (premenstrual syndrome). The most common cause of absent periods (amenorrhoea), in women of childbearing age, is pregnancy.

The drugs most commonly used to treat the menstrual disorders described above include oestrogens, progestogens, danazol, and analgesics.

WHY THEY ARE USED

Drug treatment for menstrual disorders is undertaken only when the doctor has ruled out the possibility of an underlying gynaecological disorder, such as a pelvic infection or fibroids. In some cases, especially in women over the age of 35, a D and C (dilatation and curettage) may be recommended. When no underlying reason for the problem is found, drug treatment aimed primarily at the relief of symptoms is usually prescribed.

Dysmenorrhoea is painful menstrual periods. It is usually treated initially with a simple analgesic. NSAIDs (see Non-steroidal anti-inflammatory drugs, p.48) are often most effective because they counter the effects of prostaglandins, chemicals that are partly responsible for the painful cramps of the uterus that occur. Diclofenac and mefenamic acid are also used to reduce the excessive blood loss of menorrhagia (see below).

When these drugs are not sufficient to provide adequate pain relief, hormonal drug treatment may be recommended. If contraception is also required, treatment may involve an oral contraceptive pill containing both an oestrogen and a progestogen, or a progestogen alone. Non-contraceptive progestogen preparations may also be prescribed, however. These are usually taken for only a few days during each month.

Menorrhagia is excessive blood loss during menstruation that can sometimes be reduced by some NSAIDs. Tranexamic acid, an anti-fibrinolytic drug, is an effective treatment for menorrhagia. Alternatively, danazol, a drug that reduces production of the female sex hormone oestrogen, may be prescribed to reduce blood loss.

Premenstrual syndrome is a collection of psychological and physical symptoms that affect many women to some degree in the days before menstruation. Psychological symptoms include mood changes such as increased irritability, depression, and anxiety. Principal physical symptoms are bloating, headache, and breast tenderness. Because some doctors believe that premenstrual syndrome is the result of a drop in progesterone levels in the last half of the menstrual cycle, non-contraceptive supplements of this hormone may be given in the week or so before menstruation.

Oral contraceptives may be considered as an alternative. Other drugs sometimes used include pyridoxine (vitamin B$_6$), diuretics (p.30) if bloating due to fluid retention is a problem, and bromocriptine when breast tenderness is the major symptom. Antidepressants (p.14) may be prescribed in cases where severe premenstrual psychological disturbance is experienced.

Endometriosis is a condition in which fragments of endometrial tissue (uterine lining) occur outside the uterus in the pelvic cavity. It causes severe pain during menstruation, often causes pain during intercourse, and may sometimes lead to infertility. Drugs used for this disorder are similar to those prescribed for heavy periods (menorrhagia). In this case, however, the intention is to suppress endometrial development for an extended period so that the abnormal tissue eventually withers away. Progesterone supplements that suppress endometrial thickening may be prescribed throughout the menstrual cycle. Alternatively, danazol, which suppresses endometrial development by reducing oestrogen production, may be prescribed. Any drug treatment usually needs to be continued for a minimum of six months. When drug treatment is unsuccessful, surgical removal of the abnormal tissue is usually necessary.

HOW THEY WORK
Drugs used in menstrual disorders act in a variety of ways. Hormonal treatments are aimed at suppressing the pattern of hormonal changes that is causing troublesome symptoms. Contraceptive preparations override the woman's normal menstrual cycle. Ovulation does not occur, and the endometrium does not thicken normally. Bleeding that occurs at the end of a cycle is less likely to be abnormally heavy, to be accompanied by severe discomfort, or to be preceded by distressing symptoms. For further information on oral contraceptives, see right.

Non-contraceptive progestogen preparations taken in the days before menstruation do not suppress ovulation. Increased progesterone during this time reduces premenstrual symptoms and prevents excessive thickening of the endometrium.

Danazol, a potent drug, prevents the thickening of the endometrium, thereby correcting excessively heavy periods. Blood loss is reduced, and in some cases menstruation ceases altogether during treatment.

COMMON DRUGS
Oestrogens and progestogens (see p.86)
NSAID analgesics Aspirin*, Diclofenac*, Diflunisal, Flurbiprofen, Ibuprofen*, Ketoprofen*, Mefenamic acid*, Naproxen*
Diuretics (see p.30)
Other drugs Bromocriptine*, Buserelin, Danazol*, Gamolenic acid*, Gestrinone, Goserelin*, Leuprorelin, Nafarelin, Pyridoxine, Tranexamic Acid
* **See Part 2**

Oral contraceptives

There are many different methods of ensuring that conception and pregnancy do not follow sexual intercourse, but for most women the oral contraceptive is the most effective method.

The following list indicates the number of pregnancies occurring with each contraceptive method per 100 users each year. The wide variation with some methods takes into account pregnancies that occur through incorrect use:
◆ Combined and phased pills 2–3
◆ Progestogen-only pill 2.5–10
◆ IUD (Intrauterine device) 4–9
◆ Condom 3–4
◆ Diaphragm 10–20
◆ Rhythm 25–30
◆ Contraceptive sponge 9–27
◆ Vaginal spermicide alone 2–30
◆ Norethisterone implant Less than 1
◆ No contraception 80–85
◆ "Morning after" pill 20–25

Oral contraceptives have the added advantage of being convenient and unobtrusive during lovemaking. About 25 per cent of the women who seek contraceptive protection in Britain choose a form of oral contraceptive.

There are three main types: the combined pill, the progestogen-only pill, and the phased pill. All three types contain a progestogen (a synthetic form of the female sex hormone, progesterone). Both the combined and phased pills also contain a natural or synthetic oestrogen (see also Female sex hormones, p.86).

WHY THEY ARE USED

The combined pill The combined pill is the most widely prescribed form of oral contraceptive and has the lowest failure rate in terms of unwanted pregnancies. It is the type thought most suitable for young women who want to use a hormonal form of contraception. The combined pill is particularly suitable for those women who regularly experience exceptionally painful, heavy, or prolonged periods (see Drugs used to treat menstrual disorders, p.100).

There are many different products available containing a fixed dose of an oestrogen and a progestogen drug. They are generally divided into three groups according to their oestrogen content (see Hormone content of common oral contraceptives, below). Low-dose products are chosen when possible to minimize the risk of adverse effects.

Progestogen-only pill This pill is often recommended for women who react adversely to the oestrogen in the combined pill or for whom this pill is not considered suitable because of their age or medical history (see Risks and special precautions, facing page). It is also prescribed for women who are breast-feeding since it does not reduce milk production. The progestogen pill has a higher failure rate than the combined pill and must be taken at precisely the same time each day for maximum contraceptive effect.

Phased pills The newest form of oral contraceptive is a pack of pills divided into two or three groups or phases. Each phase contains a different proportion of an oestrogen and a progestogen. The aim is to provide a hormonal balance that closely resembles the fluctuations of a normal menstrual cycle. Phased pills provide effective protection for many women who suffer side effects from other available forms of oral contraceptive.

HOW THEY WORK

In a normal menstrual cycle, the ripening and release of an egg and preparation of the uterus for implantation of the fertilized egg are the result of a complex interplay between the natural female sex hormones, oestrogen and progesterone, and the pituitary hormones follicle-stimulating hormone (FSH) and luteinizing hormone (LH) (see also

HORMONE CONTENT OF COMMON ORAL CONTRACEPTIVES

The oestrogen-containing forms are classified according to oestrogen content as follows: Low: 20 micrograms; standard: 30–35 micrograms; high: 50 micrograms; phased pills: 30–40 micrograms; morning after pills: 100 micrograms dose.

TYPE OF PILL (oestrogen content)	BRAND NAMES
Combined (20 micrograms)	Loestrin 20, Mercilon
(30–35 micrograms)	Binovum, Brevinor, Cilest, Eugynon 30, Femodene, Femodene ED, Loestrin 30, Norimin, Marvelon, Microgynon 30, Microgynon 30 ED, Minulet, Ovran 30, Ovranette, Ovysmen
(50 micrograms)	Norinyl-1, Ovran
Phased (30–40 micrograms)	Logynon, Logynon ED, Synphase, Triadene, Tri-Minulet, Trinordiol, TriNovum
Progestogen-only (no oestrogen)	Femulen, Micronor, Microval, Neogest, Norgeston, Noriday
Post-coital (morning after) (50 micrograms x 2)	Schering PC4

p.86). The oestrogen and progestogens contained in oral contraceptives disrupt the normal menstrual cycle in such a way that conception is less likely.

With combined and phased pills, the increased levels of oestrogen and progesterone produce similar effects to the hormonal changes of pregnancy. The actions of the hormones inhibit the production of FSH and LH, preventing the egg from ripening in the ovary and from being released.

The progestogen-only pill has a slightly different effect. It does not always prevent the release of an egg; its main contraceptive action may be on the mucus that lines the cervix, which thickens so that sperm cannot cross it. This effect occurs to some extent with combined pills and phased pills.

HOW THEY AFFECT YOU

Each course of combined and phased pills lasts for 21 days, followed by a pill-free seven days, during which time menstruation occurs. Some brands contain seven additional inactive pills. With these, the new course directly follows the last so that the habit of taking the pill daily is not broken. Progestogen-only pills are taken for 28 days each month. Menstruation usually occurs during the last few days of the menstrual cycle.

Women taking oral contraceptives, especially drugs that contain oestrogen, usually find that their menstrual periods are lighter and relatively pain-free. Some women cease to menstruate altogether. This is not a cause for concern in itself, provided no pills have been missed, but it may make it difficult to determine if pregnancy has occurred. An apparently missed period probably indicates a light one, rather than pregnancy. However, if you have missed two consecutive periods and you feel that you may be pregnant, it is advisable to have a pregnancy test.

All forms of oral contraceptive may cause spotting of blood in mid-cycle ("breakthrough bleeding"), especially at first, but this can be a particular problem of the progestogen-only pill.

Oral contraceptives that contain oestrogen may produce any of a large number of mild side effects depending on the dose. Symptoms similar to those experienced early in pregnancy may occur, particularly in the first few months of pill use: some women complain of nausea and vomiting, weight gain, depression, altered libido, increased appetite, and cramps in the legs and abdomen. The pill may also affect the circulation, producing minor headaches and dizziness. All of these effects usually disappear within a few months, but if they persist, it may be advisable to change to a brand containing a lower dose of oestrogen or to some other contraceptive method.

RISKS AND SPECIAL PRECAUTIONS

All oral contraceptives need to be taken regularly for maximum protection against pregnancy. Contraceptive protection can be reduced by missing a pill. (see What to do if you miss a pill, p.104). It may also be reduced by vomiting or diarrhoea. If you have either of these symptoms, it is advisable to act as if you had missed your last pill. Many drugs may also affect the action of oral contraceptives; it is essential to tell your doctor that you taking are oral contraceptives before you take additional prescribed medications.

Oral contraceptives, particularly those containing an oestrogen, have been found to carry a number of risks (see Balancing the risks and benefits of oral contraceptives, p.104). One of the most serious potential adverse effects of oestrogen-containing pills is development of a thrombus (blood clot) in a vein or artery that may travel to the lungs or cause a stroke or heart attack. The risk of thrombus formation increases with age and other factors, notably obesity, high blood pressure, and smoking. Doctors assess these risk factors for each person when prescribing oral contraceptives. A woman aged over 35 may be advised against taking a combined pill, especially if she smokes or has an underlying medical condition such as diabetes mellitus. Concerns have been expressed about contraceptive pills containing the progestogens gestodene or desogestrel because several studies have found these preparations to carry a higher risk of thrombus formation than those containing other progestogens. The Committee on the Safety of Medicines has advised that these preparations should be used only by those women who are intolerant of other contraceptive pills and are aware of the higher risk. The drugs that contain desogestrel include Marvelon and Mercilon, while those that contain gestodene include Femodene, Femodene ED, Minulet, Triadene, and Tri-Minulet.

For some women, high blood pressure is a possible complication of oral contraceptives. All women prescribed oral contraceptives are advised to have their blood pressure measured before they start taking them, and every six months thereafter.

Some very rare liver cancers have occurred, and breast cancer may be slightly more common, but cancers of the ovaries and uterus are less common.

There is no evidence that oral contraceptives reduce a woman's fertility or damage the babies conceived after they are discontinued; but doctors recommend that you wait for at least one normal menstrual period before attempting to become pregnant.

BALANCING THE RISKS AND BENEFITS OF ORAL CONTRACEPTIVES

Oral contraceptives are safe for the vast majority of young women. However, every woman who is considering oral contraception should discuss with her doctor the risks and possible adverse effects of the drugs before deciding that a hormonal method is the most suitable in her case. A variety of factors must be taken into account, including the woman's age, her own medical history and that of her close relatives, and factors such as whether she is a smoker. The importance of such factors varies depending on the type of contraceptive. The main advantages and disadvantages of oestrogen-containing and progestogen-only pills are listed below.

Advantages of oestrogen-containing combined and phased pills Very reliable; convenient and unobtrusive; regularizes menstruation; reduced menstrual pain and blood loss; reduced risk of benign breast disease, endometriosis, ectopic pregnancy, ovarian cysts, pelvic infection, ovarian and endometrial cancer.

Advantages of progestogen-only pill Reasonably reliable; convenient and unobtrusive; suitable during breast-feeding; avoids any oestrogen-related side effects and risks; allows rapid return to fertility.

Side effects of oestrogen-containing combined and phased pills Weight gain; depression; breast swelling; reduced sex drive; headaches; increased vaginal discharge; nausea.

Side effects of progestogen-only pill Irregular menstruation.

Risks of oestrogen-containing combined and phased pills Thrombosis/embolism; heart disease high blood pressure; jaundice; cancer of the liver (rare); gallstones.

Risks of progestogen-only pill Ectopic pregnancy; ovarian cysts.

Factors that may prohibit use of oestrogen-containing combined and phased pills Previous thrombosis*; heart disease; high levels of lipid in blood; liver disease; blood disorders; high blood pressure; unexplained vaginal bleeding; migraine; otosclerosis; presence of several risk factors (see below).

Factors that may prohibit use of progestogen-only pill Previous ectopic pregnancy; heart or circulatory disease; unexplained vaginal bleeding.

Factors that increase risks of oestrogen-containing combined and phased pills Smoking*; obesity*; increasing age; diabetes mellitus; family history of heart or circulatory disease*; current treatment with other drugs.

Factors that increase risks of progestogen-only pill As for oestrogen-containing pills, but to a lesser degree.

* Products containing desogestrel or gestodene have a higher excess risk with these factors than other progestogens.

HOW TO MINIMIZE YOUR HEALTH RISKS WHILE TAKING THE PILL

◆ Give up smoking.
◆ Maintain a healthy weight and diet.
◆ Have regular blood pressure and blood lipid checks.
◆ Have regular cervical smear tests.
◆ Remind your doctor that you are taking oral contraceptives before taking other prescription drugs.
◆ Stop taking oestrogen-containing oral contraceptives four weeks before planned major surgery (use alternative contraception).

WHAT TO DO IF YOU MISS A PILL

Contraceptive protection may be reduced if blood levels of the hormones in the body fall as a result of missing a pill. It is particularly important to ensure that the progestogen-only pills are taken punctually. If you miss a pill, the action you should take depends on the degree of lateness and the type of pill being used (see below).

Combined and phased pills If you are 3–12 hours late, take the missed pill now; no additional precautions are necessary. If you are over 12 hours late, take the missed pill now and take the next pill on time (even if it is on the same day). If more than one pill has been missed, take the latest missed pill now and the next on time; take additional precautions for the next 7 days. If the 7 days extends into the pill-free (or inactive pill) period, start the next packet without a break (or without taking inactive pills).

Progestogen-only pills If you are 3–12 hours late, take the missed pill now; take additional precautions for the next 7 days. If you are over 12 hours late, take the missed pill now, and take the next on time; take additional precautions for the next 7 days.

POSTCOITAL CONTRACEPTION

Pregnancy following intercourse without contraception may be avoided by taking a short course of postcoital ("morning after") pills. These preparations usually contain either a progestogen alone or an oestrogen plus a progestogen. They are usually taken in two doses, 12 hours apart, within 72 hours of intercourse. They postpone ovulation and act on the lining of the uterus to prevent implantation of the egg. The high doses needed make them unsuitable for regular frequent use, however. This method has a higher failure rate than the usual oral contraceptives.

COMMON DRUGS

Progestogens Desogestrel, Gestodene, Levonorgestrel*, Norethisterone*, Norgestimate
Oestrogens Ethinylestradiol*, Mestranol
* See Part 2

Drugs for infertility

Conception and the establishment of pregnancy require a healthy reproductive system in both partners. The man must be able to produce sufficient numbers of healthy sperm; the woman must be able to produce a healthy egg that is able to pass freely down the fallopian tube to the uterus. The lining of the uterus must be in a condition that allows the implantation of the fertilized egg.

The cause of infertility may sometimes remain undiscovered, but in the majority of cases it is due to one of the following factors: intercourse taking place at the wrong time during the menstrual cycle; the man producing too few or unhealthy sperm; the woman either failing to ovulate (release an egg) or having blocked fallopian tubes perhaps as a result of previous pelvic infection. Alternatively, production of gonadotrophin hormones – follicle-stimulating hormone (FSH) and luteinizing hormone (LH) – needed for ovulation and implantation of the egg may be affected by illness or psychological stress.

If no simple explanation can be found, the man's semen will be analysed. If these tests show abnormally low sperm production, or if a large proportion of the sperm produced are unhealthy, drug treatment may be tried.

If no abnormality of sperm production is found, the woman will be given a thorough medical examination. Ovulation is monitored and blood tests may be performed to assess hormone levels. If ovulation does not occur, the woman may be offered drug treatment.

WHY THEY ARE USED

In men, low sperm production may be treated with gonadotrophins (FSH or HCG) or a pituitary-stimulating drug (for example, clomifene) and some problems may be controlled with corticosteroids.

In women, drugs are useful in helping to achieve pregnancy only when a hormone defect inhibiting ovulation has been diagnosed. Treatment may continue for months and does not always produce a pregnancy. Women in whom the pituitary gland produces some FSH and LH may be given courses of clomifene for several days during each month. Usually, up to three courses may be tried. An effective dose produces ovulation five to ten days after the last tablet is taken.

Clomifene may thicken cervical mucus, impeding the passage of sperm, but the advantage of achieving ovulation outweighs the risk of this side effect. If treatment with clomiphene fails to produce ovulation, or if a disorder of the pituitary gland prevents production of FSH and LH, treatment with FSH and human chorionic gonadotrophin (HCG) may be given. FSH is given during the second week of the menstrual cycle, followed by an injection of HCG.

HOW THEY WORK

Ovulation (release of an egg) and implantation are governed by hormones produced by the pituitary gland. FSH stimulates ripening of the egg follicle. LH triggers ovulation and ensures that progesterone is produced to prepare the uterus for the implantation of the egg. Drugs for female infertility boost the actions of these hormones.

Fertility drugs raise the chance of ovulation by boosting levels of LH and FSH. Clomifene stimulates the pituitary gland to increase its output of these hormones. Artificially produced FSH and HCG mimic the action of naturally produced FSH and LH respectively. Both treatments, when successful, stimulate ovulation and implantation of the fertilized egg.

HOW THEY AFFECT YOU

Clomifene may produce hot flushes, nausea, headaches, and, rarely, ovarian cysts and visual disturbance, while HCG can cause tiredness, headaches, and mood changes. FSH can cause the ovaries to enlarge, producing abdominal discomfort. These drugs increase the likelihood of multiple births, usually twins.

DRUGS FOR IMPOTENCE

Impotence is a common male disorder defined as inability to achieve or maintain an erection. The penis contains three cylinders of erectile tissue, the corpora cavernosa and corpus spongiosum. Normally, when a man is sexually aroused, the arteries in the penis relax and widen, allowing more blood than usual to flow into the organ, filling the corpora cavernosa and corpus spongiosum. As these tissues expand and harden, the veins that carry blood out of the penis are compressed, reducing outflow and resulting in an erection. In some forms of impotence, this does not happen. Drugs can be used to increase blood flow into the penis to produce an erection.

Sildenafil (p.363), taken by mouth, not only increases the blood flow into the penis but also prevents the muscle wall from relaxing, so the blood does not drain out of the blood vessels and the penis remains erect.

Alprostadil (p.128) is a prostaglandin drug that helps men achieve an erection by widening the blood vessels, but it must be injected directly into the penis, or applied into the urethra using a special pipette.

COMMON DRUGS

Chorionic gonadotrophin (HCG)*, Clomifene*, Follicle-stimulating hormone (FSH), Follitropin, Goserelin, Luteinizing hormone (LH), Menotrophin, Menopausal gonadotrophins, Tamoxifen*, Urofollitropin
Drugs for impotence Alprostadil*, Sildenafil*
* See Part 2

Drugs used in labour

Normal labour has three stages. In the first stage, the uterus begins to contract, initially irregularly and then gradually more regularly and powerfully, while the cervix dilates until it is fully stretched. During the second stage, powerful contractions of the uterus push the baby down the mother's birth canal and out of her body. The third stage involves the delivery of the placenta.

Drugs may be needed during one or more stages of labour for any of the following reasons: to induce or augment labour, delay premature labour (see Uterine muscle relaxants, facing page), and relieve pain. The administration of some drugs may be viewed as part of normal obstetric care; for example, ergometrine, a uterine stimulant, may be injected routinely before the third stage of labour. Other drugs are given only when the condition of the mother or baby requires intervention. The possible adverse effects of the drug on both mother and baby are always carefully balanced against the benefits.

DRUGS TO INDUCE OR AUGMENT LABOUR

Induction of labour may be advised when a doctor considers it risky for the health of the mother or baby for the pregnancy to continue (e.g., if natural labour does not occur within two weeks of the due date or when a woman has pre-eclampsia. Other common reasons for inducing labour include premature rupture of the membrane surrounding the baby (breaking of the waters), slow growth of the baby due to poor nourishment by the placenta, or death of the fetus in the uterus.

When it is necessary to induce labour, oxytocin, a uterine stimulant, may be administered intravenously. Alternatively, a prostaglandin pessary may be given to soften and dilate the cervix. If these methods are ineffective or cannot be used because of potential adverse effects (see Risks and special precautions, below), a caesarean delivery may have to be performed.

Oxytocin may also be used to strengthen the force of contractions in labour that has started spontaneously but has not continued normally.

A combination of oxytocin and another uterine stimulant, ergometrine, is given to most women as the baby is being born or immediately following birth to prevent excessive bleeding after the delivery of the placenta. This combination encourages the uterus to contract after delivery, which restricts the flow of blood.

RISKS AND SPECIAL PRECAUTIONS

When oxytocin is used to induce labour, the dosage is carefully monitored throughout to prevent the possibility of excessively violent contractions. It is administered to women who have had surgery of the uterus only with careful monitoring. The drug is not known to affect the baby adversely. Ergometrine is not given to women who have had high blood pressure during the course of pregnancy.

DRUGS USED FOR PAIN RELIEF

Opioid analgesics Pethidine, morphine, or other opioids may be given once active labour has been established (see Analgesics, p.9). Possible side effects for the mother include drowsiness, nausea, and vomiting. Opioid drugs may cause breathing difficulties for the newborn baby, but these problems can be reversed by the antidote naloxone, if necessary.

Epidural anaesthesia This provides pain relief during labour and birth by numbing the nerves leading to the uterus and pelvic area. It is often used during a planned caesarean delivery, thus enabling the mother to be fully conscious for the birth.

An epidural involves the injection of a local anaesthetic drug (see p.11) into the epidural space between the spinal cord and the vertebrae. An epidural may block the mother's urge to push during the second stage, and a forceps delivery may be necessary. Headaches may occasionally occur following epidural anaesthesia.

Oxygen and nitrous oxide These gases are combined to produce a mixture that reduces the pain caused by contractions. During the first and second stages of labour, gas is self-administered by inhalation through a mouthpiece or mask. If it is used over too long a period, it may produce nausea, confusion, and dehydration in the mother.

Local anaesthetics These drugs are injected inside the vagina or near the vaginal opening and are used to numb sensation during forceps delivery, before an episiotomy (an incision made to enlarge the vaginal opening), and when stitches are necessary. Side effects of these drugs are rare.

UTERINE MUSCLE RELAXANTS

When contractions of the uterus start before the 34th week of pregnancy, doctors usually advise bed rest and may also administer a drug that relaxes the muscles of the uterus and thus halts labour. Initially, the drug is given in hospital by injection, but it may be continued orally at home. These drugs work by stimulating the sympathetic nervous system (see Autonomic nervous system, p.8) and may cause palpitations and anxiety in the mother. They have not been shown to have adverse effects on the baby.

DRUGS USED TO TERMINATE PREGNANCY

Drugs may be used in a hospital or clinic to terminate pregnancy up to 20 weeks, or to empty the uterus after the death of the baby. Before the 14th week of pregnancy, a prostaglandin may be given as a vaginal pessary to dilate the cervix before removing the fetus under general anaesthetic.

After the 14th week, labour is induced by a prostaglandin drug in a vaginal pessary, injected into the uterus, or via a catheter placed through the cervix. These methods may be supplemented by oxytocin given by intravenous drip (see Drugs to induce or augment labour, p.106).

COMMON DRUGS

Prostaglandins Carboprost, Dinoprostone, Gemeprost
Pain relief Entonox® (oxygen and nitrous oxide)
Opioids Fentanyl, Morphine*, Pethidine
Uterine muscle relaxants Ritodrine, Salbutamol*, Terbutaline*
Uterine stimulants Ergometrine, Oxytocin
Local anaesthetics Bupivacaine, Lignocaine
Sex hormones Mifepristone
* See Part 2

Drug used for urinary disorders

Urine is produced by the kidneys and stored in the bladder. As the urine accumulates, the bladder walls stretch and pressure within the bladder increases. Eventually, the stretching stimulates nerve endings that produce the urge to urinate. The ring of muscle (sphincter) around the bladder neck normally keeps the bladder closed until it is consciously relaxed, allowing urine to pass out of the body via the urethra.

A number of disorders can affect the urinary tract. The most common of these disorders are infection in the bladder (cystitis) or the urethra (urethritis), and loss of reliable control over urination (urinary incontinence). A less common problem is inability to expel urine (urinary retention). Drugs used to treat these problems include antibiotics and antibacterial drugs, analgesics, drugs to increase the acidity of the urine, and drugs that act on nerve control over the muscles of the bladder and sphincter.

DRUGS FOR URINARY INFECTION

Almost all infections of the bladder are caused by bacteria. Symptoms include a continual urge to urinate, although often nothing is passed; pain on urinating; and lower abdominal pain.

Many antibiotic and antibacterial drugs are used to treat urinary tract infections. Among the most widely used – because of their effectiveness – are trimethoprim and amoxicillin (see Antibiotics, p.60, and Antibacterial drugs, p.64).

Measures are also sometimes taken to increase the acidity of the urine, thereby making it hostile to bacteria. Ascorbic acid (vitamin C) and acid fruit juices have this effect, although making the urine less acidic with potassium or sodium citrate during an attack of cystitis helps to relieve the discomfort. Symptoms are commonly relieved within a few hours of the start of treatment.

For maximum effect, all drug treatments prescribed for urinary tract infections need to be accompanied by increased fluid intake.

DRUGS FOR URINARY INCONTINENCE

Urinary incontinence can occur for a several reasons. A weak sphincter muscle allows the involuntary passage of urine when abdominal pressure is raised by coughing or physical exertion. This is known as stress incontinence and commonly affects women who have had children. Urgency – a sudden need to urinate – stems from oversensitivity of the bladder muscle; small quantities of urine stimulate the urge to urinate frequently.

Incontinence can also occur due to loss of nerve control in neurological disorders such as multiple sclerosis. In children, inability to control urination at night (nocturnal enuresis) is also a form of urinary incontinence.

Drug treatment is not necessary or appropriate for all forms of incontinence. In stress incontinence, exercises to strengthen the pelvic floor muscles or surgery to tighten stretched ligaments may be effective. In urgency, regular emptying of the bladder often avoids the need for medical intervention. Incontinence caused by loss of nerve control is unlikely to be helped by drug treatment. Frequency of urination in urgency may be reduced by anticholinergic (see Drugs that act on the parasympathetic nervous system, p.9) and antispasmodic drugs. These reduce nerve signals from the muscles in the bladder, allowing greater volumes of urine to accumulate without stimulating the urge to pass urine. Tricyclic antidepressants, such as imipramine, have a strong anticholinergic action and have been prescribed to treat nocturnal enuresis in children. However, many doctors believe the risk of overdosage is unacceptable. Desmopressin, a synthetic derivative of antidiuretic hormone (see p.83), is also used to treat nocturnal enuresis.

DRUGS FOR URINARY RETENTION

Urinary retention is the inability to empty the bladder. This usually results from failure of the bladder muscle to contract sufficiently to expel accumulated urine. Possible causes include an enlarged prostate gland or tumour, or a longstanding neurological disorder. Some drugs can cause urinary retention.

Most cases of urinary retention need to be relieved by inserting a tube (catheter) into the urethra. Surgery may be needed to prevent a recurrence of the problem. Drugs that relax the sphincter or stimulate bladder contraction are now rarely used in the treatment of urinary retention, but two types of drug are used in the long-term management of prostatic enlargement. Finasteride prevents production of male hormones that stimulate prostatic growth and alpha blockers, such as prazosin, indoramine, and terazosin, relax prostatic and urethral smooth muscle, thereby improving urine outflow. Long-term drug treatment can relieve symptoms and delay the need for surgery.

COMMON DRUGS

Antibiotics and antibacterials (see pp.60–65)
Anticholinergics Flavoxate, Imipramine*, Oxybutynin*, Propiverine, Tolterodine*
Parasympathomimetic Distigmine
Alpha blockers Alfuzosin, Doxazosin*, Indoramin*, Prazosin, Tamsulosin*, Terazosin
Other drugs Desmopressin*, Finasteride*, Potassium citrate, Vitamin C, Dimethyl sulphoxide
* **See Part 2**

EYES AND EARS

The eyes and ears are the two sense organs that provide us with the most information about the world around us. The eye is the organ of vision that converts light images into nerve signals, which are transmitted to the brain for interpretation. The ear not only provides the means by which sound is detected and communicated to the brain, but it also contains the organ of balance that tells the brain about the position and movement of the body. It is divided into three parts – outer, middle, and inner ear.

WHAT CAN GO WRONG

The most common eye and ear disorders are infection and inflammation (sometimes caused by allergy). Many parts of the eye may be affected, notably the conjunctiva (the membrane that covers the front of the eye and lines the eyelids) and the iris. The middle and outer ear are more commonly affected by infection than the inner ear.

The eye may also be damaged by glaucoma, a disorder in which pressure of fluid within the eye builds up and may eventually threaten vision. Eye problems such as retinopathy (disease of the retina) or cataracts (clouding of the lens) may occur as a result of diabetes or for other reasons, but both are now treatable. Disorders for which no drug treatment is appropriate are beyond the scope of this book.

Other disorders affecting the ear include build-up of wax (cerumen) in the outer ear canal and disturbances to the balance mechanism within the ear (vertigo and Ménière's disease, see Anti-emetics, p.21).

WHY DRUGS ARE USED

Doctors usually prescribe antibiotics (see p.60) to clear ear and eye infections. These may be given by mouth or topically. Topical eye and ear preparations may contain a corticosteroid (p.78) to reduce inflammation. When inflammation has been caused by allergy, antihistamines (p.56) may also be taken. Decongestant drugs (p.24) are often prescribed to help clear the eustachian tube in middle ear infections.

Various drugs are used to reduce fluid pressure in glaucoma. These include diuretics (p.30), beta blockers (p.28), and miotics to narrow the pupil. In other cases, the pupil may need to be widened by mydriatic drugs. (See also Drugs affecting the pupil, p.112.)

MAJOR DRUG GROUPS

◆ Drugs for glaucoma
◆ Drugs affecting the pupil
◆ Drugs for ear disorders

Drugs for Glaucoma

Glaucoma is the name given to a group of conditions in which the pressure in the eye builds up to an abnormally high level. This compresses the blood vessels that supply the nerve connecting the eye to the brain (optic nerve) and may result in irreversible nerve damage and permanent loss of vision.

In the most common type of glaucoma, chronic (open-angle), reduced fluid drainage from the eye causes pressure inside the eye to build up slowly. Progressive reduction in the peripheral field of vision may take months or years to be noticed. Acute (closed-angle) glaucoma occurs when drainage of fluid is suddenly blocked by the iris. Fluid pressure usually builds up quite suddenly, blurring vision in the affected eye. The eye becomes red and painful, and a headache and sometimes vomiting also occurs. The main attack is often preceded by milder warning attacks, such as seeing haloes around lights, in the previous weeks or months. Elderly, far-sighted people are particularly at risk of developing acute glaucoma. The angle may also narrow suddenly after injury or taking certain drugs such as anticholinergics (see Drugs that act on the parasympathetic nervous system, p.9). Closed-angle glaucoma may develop more slowly (chronic closed-angle glaucoma).

Drugs are used in the treatment of both types of glaucoma and include miotics (See Drugs affecting the pupil, p.112), beta blockers (p.28), and certain diuretics (carbonic anhydrase inhibitors and osmotics, p.30).

WHY THEY ARE USED

Chronic glaucoma In this form of glaucoma, drugs are used to reduce pressure inside the eye. These drugs will prevent further deterioration of vision but cannot restore damage that has already been sustained, and therefore these drugs may be required lifelong. In most patients, treatment is begun with eye drops containing a beta blocker to reduce the production of fluid inside the eye. Miotic eye drops to constrict the pupil and improve fluid drainage may be given. The prostaglandin, latanoprost, is also used to increase fluid outflow. If none of these drugs are effective, epinephrine, dipivefrine, or brimonidine may be tried to reduce secretion and help outflow. Sometimes a carbonic anhydrase inhibitor such as acetazolamide may be given by mouth to reduce fluid production. Laser treatment and surgery may also be used to improve fluid drainage from the eye.

Acute glaucoma In acute glaucoma immediate medical treatment is required in order to prevent total loss of vision. Drugs are used initially to bring down the pressure within the eye. Laser treatment or surgery is then carried out to prevent a recurrence of the problem so that long-term drug treatment is seldom required.

Acetazolamide is often the first drug to be administered when the condition is diagnosed. This drug may be injected for rapid effect and thereafter administered by mouth. Frequent applications of eye drops containing pilocarpine or another miotic drug are given. An osmotic diuretic such as mannitol may be administered. This drug draws fluid out of all body tissues, including the eye, and reduces pressure within the eye.

HOW THEY WORK

Drugs used to treat glaucoma act in various ways to reduce the pressure of fluid in the eye. Miotics improve drainage of fluid out of the eye. In chronic glaucoma, this is achieved by increasing the outflow of aqueous humour through the drainage channel called the trabecular meshwork. In acute glaucoma, the pupil-constricting effect of miotics pulls the iris away from the drainage channel, allowing the aqueous humour to flow out normally. Latanoprost acts by improving drainage

from the eye but has no miotic action. Beta blockers and carbonic anhydrase inhibitors act on the fluid-producing cells inside the eye to reduce the output of aqueous humour. Sympathomimetic drugs such as epinephrine (adrenaline), brimonidine, and apraclonidine are also thought to act partly in this way and partly by improving fluid drainage.

HOW THEY AFFECT YOU

Drugs for acute glaucoma relieve pain and other symptoms within a few hours of their being used. The benefits of treatment in chronic glaucoma, however, may not be immediately apparent since treatment is only able to halt a further deterioration of vision.

People receiving miotic eye drops are likely to notice darkening of vision and difficulty seeing in the dark. Increased shortsightedness may be noticeable. Some miotics also cause irritation and redness of the eyes.

Beta blocker eye drops have few day-to-day side effects but carry risks for a few people (see below). Acetazolamide usually causes an increase in frequency of urination and thirst. Nausea and general malaise are also common.

RISKS AND SPECIAL PRECAUTIONS

Miotics can cause alteration in vision. Beta blockers are absorbed into the body and can affect the lungs, heart, and circulation. As a result, a cardioselective beta blocker, such as betaxolol, may be prescribed with caution to people with asthma or certain circulatory disorders and, in some cases, such drugs are withheld altogether. The amount of the drug absorbed into the blood can be reduced by pressing on the the lacrimal (tear) duct in the corner of the eye and applying the number of eye drops prescribed by your doctor. Acetazolamide may cause troublesome adverse effects, including painful tingling of the hands and feet, the formation of kidney stones, and, rarely, kidney damage. People with existing kidney problems are not usually given this drug.

COMMON DRUGS

Miotics Carbachol, Physostigmine, Pilocarpine*
Carbonic anhydrase inhibitors Acetazolamide, Dorzolamide*
Other drugs Latanoprost

Beta blockers Betaxolol, Carteolol, Levobunolol, Metipranolol, Timolol*
Sympathomimetics Apraclonidine, Brimonidine, Dipivefrine, Epinephrine*, Guanethidine
* **See Part 2**

Drugs affecting the pupil

The pupil of the eye is the circular opening in the centre of the iris (the coloured part of the eye) through which light enters. It continually changes in size to adjust to variations in the intensity of light; in bright light it becomes quite small (constricts), but in dim light the pupil enlarges (dilates).

Eye drops containing drugs that act on the pupil are widely used by specialists. There are two categories: mydriatics, which dilate the pupil, and miotics, which constrict it.

WHY THEY ARE USED

Mydriatics are most often used to allow the doctor to view the inside of the eye – particularly the retina, the optic nerve head, and the blood vessels that supply the retina. Many of these drugs cause temporary paralysis of the eye's focusing mechanism, a state called cycloplegia. Cycloplegia is sometimes induced to help determine the presence of any focusing errors, especially in babies and young children. By producing cycloplegia, it is possible to determine the precise optical prescription required for a small child, especially in the case of a squint.

Dilation of the pupil is part of the treatment for uveitis, an inflammatory disease of the iris and focusing muscle. In uveitis, the inflamed iris may stick to the lens, severely damaging the eye. This complication can be prevented by early dilation of the pupil so that the iris is no longer in contact with the lens.

Constriction of the pupil with miotic drugs is often required in the treatment of glaucoma (see p.110). Miotics can also be used to restore the pupil to a normal size after dilation is induced by drugs.

HOW THEY WORK

The size of the pupil is controlled by two separate sets of muscles in the iris, the circular muscle and the radial muscle. The two sets of muscles are governed by separate branches of the autonomic nervous system (see p.8): the radial muscle is controlled by the sympathetic nervous system, and the circular muscle is controlled by the parasympathetic nervous system.

Individual mydriatic and miotic drugs affect different parts of the autonomic nervous system, and cause the pupil to dilate or contract, depending on the type of drug used.

HOW THEY AFFECT YOU

Mydriatic drugs – especially the long-acting types – impair the ability to focus the eye(s) for several hours after use. This interferes particularly with close activities such as reading. Bright light may cause discomfort. Miotics often interfere with night vision and may cause temporary short sight.

Normally, these eye drops produce few serious adverse effects. Sympathomimetic mydriatics may raise blood pressure and are used with caution in people with hypertension or heart disease. Miotics may irritate the eyes, but rarely cause generalized effects.

ARTIFICIAL TEAR PREPARATIONS

Tears are continually produced to keep the front of the eye covered with a thin moist film. This is essential for clear vision and for keeping the front of the eye free from dirt and other irritants. In some conditions, known collectively as dry eye syndromes (for example, Sjögren's syndrome), inadequate tear production may make the eyes feel dry and sore. Sore eyes can also occur in disorders where the eyelids do not close properly, causing the eye to become dry.

Why they are used Since prolonged deficiency of natural tears can damage the cornea, regular application of artificial tears in the form of eye drops is recommended for all of the conditions described above. Artificial tears may also be used to provide temporary relief from any feeling of discomfort and dryness in the eye caused by irritants, exposure to wind or sun, or following the initial wearing of contact lenses.

Although artificial tears are non-irritating, they often contain a preservative (e.g., thimerosal or benzalkonium chloride) that may cause irritation. This risk of irritation is increased for wearers of soft contact lenses, who should ask their optician for advice before using any type of eye drops.

COMMON DRUGS
Sympathomimetic mydriatics Epinephrine*, Phenylephrine
Miotics Carbachol, Pilocarpine*
Anticholinergic mydriatics Atropine*, Cyclopentolate, Homatropine, Physostigmine, Tropicamide
* See Part 2

Drugs for ear disorders

Inflammation and infection of the outer and middle ear are the most common ear disorders treated with drugs. Drug treatment for Ménière's disease, which affects the inner ear, is described under Anti-emetics, p.21.

The type of drug treatment given for ear inflammation depends on the cause of the trouble and the site affected.

INFLAMMATION OF THE OUTER EAR
Inflammation of the external ear canal (otitis externa) can be caused by eczema or a bacterial or fungal infection. The risk of inflammation is increased by swimming in dirty water, accumulation of wax in the ear, or scratching or poking too frequently at the ear.

Symptoms vary, but in many cases there is itching, pain (which may be severe if there is a boil in the ear canal), tenderness, and possibly some loss of hearing. If the ear is infected there will probably be a discharge.
Drug treatment A corticosteroid (see p.78) in the form of ear drops may be used to treat inflammation of the outer ear when there is no infection. Aluminium acetate solution, as drops or applied on a piece of gauze, may also be used. Relief is usually obtained within a day or two. Prolonged use of corticosteroids is not advisable because they may reduce the ear's resistance to infection.

If there is both inflammation and infection, your doctor may prescribe ear drops containing an antibiotic (see p.60) combined with a corticosteroid to relieve the inflammation. Usually, a combination of antibiotics is prescribed to make the treatment effective

against a wide range of bacteria. Commonly used antibiotics include framycetin, neomycin, and polymyxin B. These are not used if the eardrum is perforated and are not usually applied for long periods because they can irritate the skin lining the ear canal.

Sometimes an antibiotic given as drops is not effective, and another type of antibiotic may have to be taken by mouth also.

INFECTION OF THE MIDDLE EAR
Infection of the middle ear (otitis media) often causes severe pain and hearing loss. It is particularly common in young children in whom infecting organisms are able to spread easily into the middle ear from the nose or throat via the eustachian tube.

Viral infections of the middle ear usually cure themselves and are less serious than those caused by bacteria, which are treated with antibiotics given by mouth or injection. Bacterial infections often cause the eustachian tube to swell and become blocked. When a blockage occurs, pus builds up in the middle ear and puts pressure on the eardrum, which may perforate as a result.
Drug treatment Doctors usually prescribe a decongestant (see p.24) or antihistamine (see p.56) to reduce swelling in the eustachian tube, thus allowing the pus to drain out of the middle ear. Usually, an antibiotic is also given by mouth to clear the infection.

Although antibiotics are not effective against viral infections, it is often difficult to distinguish between a viral and a bacterial infection of the middle ear, so your doctor may prescribe an antibiotic as a precautionary measure. Paracetamol, an analgesic (see p.9), may be given to relieve pain.

COMMON DRUGS
Antibiotic and antibacterial ear drops
Chloramphenicol*, Clioquinol, Clotrimazole*, Framycetin, Gentamicin*, Neomycin
Decongestants Ephedrine*, Oxymetazoline, Xylometazoline
Corticosteroids Betamethasone*, Dexamethasone*, Flumethasone, Hydrocortisone*, Prednisolone*, Triamcinolone
Other drugs Aluminium acetate, Antihistamines (see p.56)
* See Part 2

SKIN

The skin waterproofs, cushions, and protects the body and is its largest organ. It provides a barrier against innumerable infections and infestations, helps the body to retain its vital fluids, plays a major role in temperature control, and houses the sensory nerves of touch.

The skin consists of two main layers: a thin, tough top layer, the epidermis, and a thicker layer, the dermis, beneath. The epidermis also has two layers: the skin surface, or stratum corneum (horny layer) consisting of dead cells, and below, a layer of active cells. The cells in the active layer divide and eventually die, maintaining the horny layer. Living cells produce keratin, which toughens the epidermis and is the basic substance of hair and nails. Some living cells in the epidermis produce melanin, a pigment released in increased amounts following exposure to sunlight.

The dermis contains different types of nerve ending for sensing pain, pressure, and temperature; sweat glands to cool the body; sebaceous glands to lubricate and waterproof the skin; and white blood cells to help keep the skin free of infection.

WHAT CAN GO WRONG

Most skin complaints are not serious but may be distressing if visible. They include infection, inflammation and irritation, infestation by skin parasites, and changes in skin structure and texture (e.g., psoriasis, eczema, and acne). Serious skin conditions include cancers such as malignant melanoma.

WHY DRUGS ARE USED

Skin problems often resolve without drug treatment. Preparations containing drugs are available over the counter, but their use is generally discouraged without medical supervision because they can aggravate some skin conditions if used inappropriately. Prescribed drugs, including antibiotics (p.60) for bacterial infections, antifungals (p.74) for fungal infections, agents for skin parasites (p.118), and topical corticosteroids (p.116) for inflammatory conditions are often highly effective, however. Specialized drugs are available for conditions like psoriasis and acne.

Although many drugs are topical, they must be used carefully because, like drugs taken orally, they can also cause adverse effects; and some can lead to allergy when they are used on the skin.

MAJOR DRUG GROUPS

◆ Antipruritics
◆ Topical corticosteroids
◆ Anti-infective skin preparations
◆ Drugs to treat skin parasites
◆ Drugs used to treat acne
◆ Drugs for psoriasis
◆ Treatments for eczema
◆ Drugs for dandruff
◆ Drugs for hair loss
◆ Sunscreens

Antipruritics

Itching (irritation of the skin that creates the urge to scratch), also called pruritus, most often occurs as a result of minor physical irritation or chemical changes in the skin due to disease, allergy, inflammation, or exposure to irritant substances. People have differing tolerance thresholds, which can be altered by stress and other psychological factors.

Itching is a common symptom of many skin disorders (e.g., eczema and psoriasis) and allergic conditions such as urticaria (hives). It is also sometimes caused by a localized fungal infection, parasitic infestation, or diseases such as chickenpox. Less commonly, itching may also occur as a symptom of diabetes mellitus, jaundice, and kidney failure.

Generalized itching is caused, in many cases, by dry skin. Itching in particular parts of the body is often due to a specific problem. For example, itching around the anus (pruritus ani) may result from haemorrhoids or worm infestation, while genital itching in women (pruritus vulvae) may be due to vaginal infection or diabetes or, in older women, it may be the result of a hormone deficiency.

Although scratching frequently provides temporary relief, it can often increase inflammation and make the condition worse.

Continued scratching of irritated skin may occasionally lead to a vicious cycle of scratching and itching that continues long after the original cause has been removed.

Many types of medication, including soothing topical preparations and drugs taken by mouth, relieve skin irritation. The main drugs in antipruritic products include local anaesthetics (p.11), topical corticosteroids (p.116), and antihistamines (p.56). Simple emollient or cooling creams or ointments such as emulsifying ointment contain no active ingredients and are often recommended.

WHY THEY ARE USED

For mild itching arising from sunburn, urticaria, or insect bites, a cooling lotion such as calamine, perhaps containing menthol, phenol, or camphor, may be the most appropriate treatment. Local anaesthetic creams can be helpful for small areas of irritation such as insect bites but are unsuitable for widespread itching. The itching caused by dry skin is often soothed by a simple emollient. Avoiding excessive use of soap and water and using moisturizing bath oils may also help.

Severe itching in eczema or other inflammatory skin conditions may be treated with a topical corticosteroid preparation. When the irritation prevents sleep, a doctor may prescribe an antihistamine to be taken at night to promote sleep as well as to relieve the itching (see also Sleeping drugs, p.11). Antihistamines are also often included in topical preparations for the relief of skin irritation, but their effectiveness when administered in this way is doubtful. For the treatment of pruritus ani, see Drugs for rectal and anal disorders (p.45). Post-menopausal pruritus vulvae may be helped by vaginal creams containing oestrogen (see Female sex hormones, p.86). Itching caused by an underlying illness cannot be helped by skin creams and requires treatment for the principal disorder.

HOW THEY WORK

Irritation of the skin causes the release of substances, such as histamine, that cause blood vessels to dilate and fluid to accumulate under the skin, which results in itching and inflammation. Antipruritic drugs act either by reducing inflammation, and therefore

irritation, or by numbing the nerve impulses that transmit sensation to the brain.

Corticosteroids applied to the skin reduce itching caused by allergy within a few days, but the cream's soothing effect may produce an immediate improvement. They pass into the underlying tissues and blood vessels and reduce the release of histamine, the chemical that causes itching and inflammation.

Antihistamines act within a few hours to reduce allergy-related skin inflammation. Applied to the skin, they pass into the underlying tissue and block the effects of histamine on the blood vessels beneath the skin. Taken by mouth, they also act on the brain to reduce the perception of irritation.

Local anaesthetics absorbed through the skin numb the transmission of signals from the nerves in the skin to the brain.

Soothing and emollient creams such as calamine lotion applied to the skin surface reduce inflammation and itching by cooling the skin. Emollient creams lubricate the skin surface and prevent dryness.

RISKS AND SPECIAL PRECAUTIONS

The main risk of any antipruritic (except simple emollient and soothing preparations) is skin irritation, and therefore aggravated itching, caused by prolonged or heavy use. Antihistamine and local anaesthetic creams are especially likely to cause a reaction and must be stopped if they do so. Antihistamines taken by mouth to relieve itching are likely to cause drowsiness. The special risks of topical corticosteroids are discussed on p.116.

Because itching can be a symptom of many underlying conditions, self-treatment should be continued for no longer than a week before seeking medical advice.

COMMON DRUGS

Antihistamines (see also p.56) Antazoline, Diphenhydramine , Mepyramine, Trimeprazine
Corticosteroids (see also p.78), Hydrocortisone*
Local anaesthetics Amethocaine, Benzocaine, Lignocaine
Emollient and cooling preparations Aqueous cream, Calamine lotion, Cold cream, Emulsifying ointment
Other drugs Colestyramine*, Crotamiton, Doxepin
* **See Part 2**

Topical corticosteroids

Corticosteroid drugs (often simply called steroids) are related to the hormones produced by the adrenal glands. For a full description of these drugs, see p.78. Topical preparations containing a corticosteroid are often used to treat skin conditions in which inflammation is a prominent symptom.

WHY THEY ARE USED

Corticosteroid creams and ointments are most commonly given to relieve itching and inflammation associated with skin diseases such as eczema and dermatitis. These preparations may also be prescribed for psoriasis (see p.120). Corticosteroids do not affect the underlying cause of skin irritation, and the condition is therefore likely to recur unless the substance (allergen or irritant) that has provoked the irritation is removed, or the underlying condition is treated.

A doctor might not prescribe a corticosteroid as the initial treatment, preferring to try a topical medicine that has fewer adverse effects (see Antipruritics, p.114).

In most cases, treatment is started with a preparation containing a low concentration of a mild corticosteroid drug. A stronger preparation may be prescribed subsequently if the first product is ineffective.

HOW THEY WORK

Irritation of the skin, caused by allergens or irritant factors, provokes white blood cells to release substances that dilate the blood vessels, making the skin hot, red, and swollen.

Applied to the skin surface, corticosteroids are absorbed into the underlying tissue. There they inhibit the action of the substances that cause inflammation, allowing the blood vessels to return to normal and reducing the swelling.

HOW THEY AFFECT YOU

Because corticosteroids prevent the release of chemicals that trigger inflammation, conditions treated with these drugs improve within a few days of starting the drug. Applied topically, corticosteroids rarely cause side effects, but the stronger drugs used in high concentrations have certain risks.

RISKS AND SPECIAL PRECAUTIONS

Prolonged use of potent corticosteroids in high concentrations usually leads to permanent skin changes, most commonly thinning of the skin, sometimes resulting in permanent stretch marks. Fine blood vessels under the skin may become prominent (a condition known as telangiectasia). Because the skin on the face and genital area is especially vulnerable to such damage, only weak corticosteroids may be prescribed for use on these parts of the body. Dark-skinned people sometimes suffer temporary reduction in pigmentation at the site of application.

When topical corticosteroids are used for a prolonged period, abrupt discontinuation can cause rebound erythroderma (a reddening of the skin). This may be avoided by gradual dosage reduction. Corticosteroids suppress the body's immune system (see p.96), increasing the risk of infection. For this reason, they are never used alone to treat skin inflammation caused by bacterial or fungal infection. However, they are sometimes included in a topical preparation also containing an antibiotic or antifungal agent (see Anti-infective skin preparations, below).

COMMON DRUGS

Very potent Clobetasol*, Halcinonide
Potent Beclometasone*, Betamethasone*, Desoxymetasone, Diflucortolone, Fluocinolone, Fluocinonide, Fluticasone*, Mometasone*, Triamcinolone
Moderate Alclometasone, Clobetasone, Fluocortolone, Flurandrenolone
Mild Hydrocortisone*
* See Part 2

Anti-infective skin preparations

The skin is the body's first line of defence against infection. Yet the skin can also become infected itself, especially if the outer layer (epidermis) is damaged by a burn, cut, scrape, insect bite, or an inflammatory skin condition such as eczema or dermatitis.

Several different types of organism may infect the skin, including bacteria, viruses, fungi, and yeasts. This section concentrates on topical drugs for bacterial skin infections and includes antiseptics, antibiotics, and other antibacterial agents. Infection by other organisms is covered elsewhere (see Antiviral drugs, p.67, Antifungal drugs, p.74, and Drugs used to treat skin parasites, p.118).

WHY THEY ARE USED
Bacterial infection of a skin wound can usually be prevented by thorough cleansing of the damaged area and the application of antiseptic creams or lotions. If infection does occur, the wound usually becomes inflamed and swollen, and pus may form. If you develop these signs, you should see your doctor. The usual treatment for a wound infection is an antibiotic taken orally, although often an antibiotic cream is also prescribed.

An antibiotic or antibacterial skin cream may also be used to prevent infection when your doctor considers this to be a particular risk (e.g., in the case of severe burns).

Other skin disorders in which topical antibiotic treatment may be prescribed include impetigo and infected eczema, skin ulcers, bedsores, and nappy rash.

Often, a preparation containing two or more antibiotics is used to ensure that all bacteria are eradicated. The antibiotics selected for inclusion in topical preparations are usually drugs that are poorly absorbed through the skin (e.g., the aminoglycosides). Thus the drug remains concentrated on the surface and in the skin's upper layers where it is intended to have its effect. However, if the infection is deep under the skin, or is causing fever and malaise, antibiotics may need to be given by mouth or injection.

RISKS AND SPECIAL PRECAUTIONS
Any topical antibiotic product can irritate the skin or cause an allergic reaction. Irritation is sometimes provoked by another ingredient of the preparation rather than the active drug (e.g., a preservative contained in the product). An allergic reaction causing swelling and reddening of the skin is more likely to be caused by the antibiotic itself. Any adverse reaction of this kind should be reported to your doctor, who may substitute another drug or a different preparation.

Always follow your doctor's instructions on how long the treatment with antibiotics should be continued. Stopping too soon may cause the infection to flare up again.

Never use a skin preparation that has been prescribed for someone else because it may aggravate your condition. Always throw away any unused medication.

BASES FOR SKIN PREPARATIONS
Drugs applied to the skin are usually in a preparation known as a base (or vehicle), such as a cream, lotion, ointment, or paste. Many bases are beneficial on their own.
Creams These have an emollient effect. They are usually composed of an oil-in-water emulsion and are used in the treatment of dry skin disorders, such as psoriasis and dry eczema. They may contain other ingredients, such as camphor or menthol.
Barrier preparations These may be creams or ointments. They protect the skin against water and irritating substances. They may be used in the treatment of nappy rash and to protect the skin around an open sore. They may contain powders and water-repellent substances, such as silicones.
Lotions These thin, semi-liquid preparations are often used to cool and soothe inflamed skin. They are most suitable for use on large, hairy areas. Preparations called shake lotions contain fine powder that remains on the skin surface when the liquid has evaporated. They are used to encourage scabs to form.
Ointments These are usually greasy and are suitable for treating wet (weeping) eczema.
Pastes These are ointments containing large amounts of finely powdered solids such as starch or zinc oxide. Pastes protect the skin and absorb unwanted moisture. They are used for skin conditions that affect clearly defined areas, such as psoriasis.
Collodions These are preparations that, when applied to damaged areas of the skin such as ulcers and minor wounds, dry to form a protective film. They are sometimes used to keep a dissolved drug in contact with the skin.

COMMON DRUGS
Antibiotics Bacitracin, Chlortetracycline, Colistin, Framycetin, Fusidic acid, Gramicidin, Mupirocin, Neomycin, Polymyxin B, Tetracycline*

Antiseptics and other antibacterials Cetrimide, Chlorhexidine, Hexachlorophene, Metronidazole*, Povidone iodine, Silver sulfadiazine, Triclosan
* See Part 2

Drugs to treat skin parasites

Mites and lice are the most common parasites that live on the skin. One common mite causes the skin disease scabies. The mite burrows into the skin and lays eggs, causing intense itching. Scratching the affected area results in bleeding and scab formation, as well as increasing the risk of infection.

There are three types of lice, each of which infests a different part of the human body: the head louse, the body (or clothes) louse, and the crab louse, which often infests the pubic areas but is also sometimes found on other hairy areas such as the eyebrows. All of these lice cause itching and lay eggs (nits) that look like white grains attached to hairs.

Both mites and lice are passed on by direct contact with an infected person (during sexual intercourse in the case of pubic lice) or, particularly in the case of body lice, by contact with infected bedding or clothing.

The drugs most often used to eliminate skin parasites are insecticides that kill both the adult insects and their eggs. The most effective drugs for scabies are malathion and permethrin; benzyl benzoate is occasionally used. For lice infestations, carbaryl, malathion, permethrin, and phenothrin are used.

WHY THEY ARE USED

Skin parasites do not represent a serious threat to health, but prompt treatment is needed since they can cause severe irritation and spread rapidly if untreated. Drugs are used to eradicate them from the body, but bedding and clothing should be disinfected to avoid the possibility of reinfestation.

ELIMINATING PARASITES FROM BEDDING AND CLOTHING

Most skin parasites may also infest bedding and clothing that has been next to an infected person's skin. To avoid reinfestation following treatment of the body, any insects and eggs lodged in the bedding or clothing must also be eradicated.

Washing Since all skin parasites are killed by heat, washing affected items of clothing and bedding in hot water and drying them in a hot dryer is an effective and convenient method of dealing with the problem.

Non-washable items Items that cannot be washed should be isolated in plastic bags. The insects and their eggs cannot survive long without their human hosts and die within days. The length of time they can survive, and therefore the period of isolation, varies depending on the type of parasite.

HOW THEY ARE USED

Lotions for the treatment of scabies are applied to the whole body – with the exception of the head and neck – after a bath or shower. Many people find lotions messy to use but should not wash them off for 12 hours (malathion) or 48 hours (benzyl benzoate), or they will not be effective. It is probably most convenient to apply malathion before going to bed. The lotion may then be washed off the following morning.

One or two treatments are normally sufficient to remove the scabies mites. However, the itch associated with scabies may persist after the mite has been removed, so a soothing cream or medication containing an antipruritic drug (see p.114) may be needed to ease it. People who have direct skin-to-skin contact with a sufferer from scabies, such as family members, classmates, and sexual partners, should also be treated with antiparasitic preparations at the same time.

Head and pubic lice infestations are usually treated by applying a preparation of one of the products and washing it off with water when and as instructed by the leaflet given with the preparation. If the skin has become infected as a result of scratching, a topical antibiotic (see Anti-infective skin preparations, p.116) may also be prescribed.

RISKS AND SPECIAL PRECAUTIONS

Lotions prescribed to control parasites can cause intense irritation and stinging if they are allowed to come into contact with the eyes, mouth, or other moist membranes.

Therefore, lotions and shampoos should be applied carefully, following the instructions of your doctor or the manufacturer.

Because antiparasitic drugs are topical, they do not usually have generalized effects. Nevertheless, it is important not to apply these preparations more often than directed.

COMMON DRUGS

Benzyl benzoate, Carbaryl*, Crotamiton, Malathion*, Permethrin*, Phenothrin

* See Part 2

Drugs used to treat acne

Acne, known medically as acne vulgaris, is a common condition caused by excess production of the skin's natural oil (sebum), leading to blockage of hair follicles. It chiefly affects adolescents but may occur at any age, due to certain drugs, exposure to industrial chemicals, oily cosmetics, or hot, humid conditions.

Acne primarily affects the face, neck, back, and chest. The main symptoms are blackheads, papules (inflamed spots), and pustules (raised pus-filled spots with a white centre). Mild acne may produce only blackheads and an occasional papule or pustule. Moderate cases are characterized by larger numbers of pustules and papules. In severe cases, painful, inflamed cysts also develop, causing permanent pitting and scarring.

Medication for acne can be divided into two groups: topical preparations applied directly to the skin and systemic treatments taken by mouth.

WHY THEY ARE USED

Mild acne usually does not need medical treatment. It can be controlled by regular washing and by moderate exposure to sunlight or ultraviolet light. Over-the-counter antibacterial soaps and lotions are limited in use and may cause irritation.

Acne that is severe enough to need medication is usually treated with a topical preparation containing benzoyl peroxide or salicylic acid. If this does not produce an improvement, an ointment containing tretinoin (a drug related to vitamin A), azelaic acid, or tetracycline (an antibiotic), may be prescribed.

If acne is severe or does not respond to topical treatments, a doctor may prescribe a course of antibiotics by mouth (usually tetracycline or minocycline). If these measures are unsuccessful, isotretinoin (a more powerful vitamin A-like drug), taken by mouth, may be prescribed.

Oestrogen drugs may have a beneficial effect on acne. A woman with acne who also needs contraception may be given an oestrogen-containing oral contraceptive (p.101). Alternatively, a preparation containing an oestrogen and cyproterone (a drug that opposes male sex hormones) may be prescribed.

HOW THEY WORK

Drugs used to treat acne act in different ways. Some have a keratolytic effect – that is, they loosen the dead cells on the skin surface. Others work by countering bacterial activity in the skin or reducing sebum production.

Topical preparations, such as benzoyl peroxide, salicylic acid, and tretinoin, have a keratolytic effect. Benzoyl peroxide also has an antibacterial effect. Topical or systemic tetracyclines reduce bacteria but may also have a direct anti-inflammatory effect on the skin. Isotretinoin reduces sebum production, soothes inflammation, and helps to unblock hair follicles.

HOW THEY AFFECT YOU

Keratolytic preparations often cause soreness of the skin, especially at the start of treatment. If this persists, a change to a milder preparation may be recommended. Day-to-day side effects are rare with antibiotics.

Treatment with isotretinoin often causes dry and scaly skin, particularly on the lips. The skin may become itchy and some hair loss may occur.

RISKS AND SPECIAL PRECAUTIONS

Antibiotics in skin ointments may, rarely, provoke an allergic reaction requiring discontinuation of treatment. The tetracyclines, which are some of the most commonly used antibiotics for acne, have the advantage of being effective both topically and systemically. They are not suitable for use by mouth in pregnancy, however, since they can affect the bones and teeth of the developing baby.

Isotretinoin sometimes increases blood lipid levels. More seriously, it is known to damage the developing baby if taken during pregnancy. Women need to ensure that they avoid conception during treatment.

COMMON DRUGS

Topical treatments Adapalene, Azelaic acid, Benzoyl peroxide*, Isotretinoin*, Nicotinamide (Niacin), Salicylic acid, Tretinoin

Oral and topical antibiotics Clindamycin, Erythromycin*, Minocycline*, Tetracycline*

Other oral drugs Cyproterone acetate, Isotretinoin*

* **See Part 2**

Drugs for psoriasis

The skin is constantly being renewed; as fast as dead cells in the outer layer (epidermis) are shed, they are replaced by cells from the base of the epidermis. Psoriasis occurs when production of new cells increases while shedding of old cells remains normal. As a result, the live skin cells accumulate and produce patches of inflamed, thickened skin covered by silvery scales. In some cases, the affected area is extensive and causes severe embarrassment and physical discomfort. Psoriasis may occasionally be accompanied by arthritis, in which the joints become swollen and painful.

The underlying cause of psoriasis is not known. The disorder usually first occurs between the ages of 10 and 30 and recurs throughout life. Outbreaks may be triggered by stress, skin damage, and physical illness. Psoriasis can also occur as a consequence of the withdrawal of corticosteroid drugs.

There is no complete cure for psoriasis; simple measures, including careful sunbathing or using an ultraviolet lamp, may help to clear mild cases. An emollient cream (see Antipruritics, p.114) often soothes the irritation. When such measures fail to provide adequate relief, additional drug therapy is needed.

WHY THEY ARE USED

Drugs are used to decrease the size of affected areas and reduce inflammation and scaling. Mild and moderate psoriasis are usually treated topically. Calcipotriol, applied as an ointment, is very effective for small areas of skin. Coal tar creams, pastes, or bath additives are also often helpful, but some people dislike the smell. Dithranol is also widely used. Applied to the affected areas, it is left for a few minutes or overnight (depending on the product), then washed off. Dithranol and coal tar can stain clothes and bed linen.

If these agents alone do not produce adequate benefit, ultraviolet light therapy in the form of regulated exposure to natural sunlight or ultraviolet lamps (UVB) may be advised. Salicylic acid may be applied to help remove thick scale and crusts, especially from the scalp.

Topical corticosteroids (see p.116) may be used in difficult cases that do not respond to those treatments. They are particularly useful for the skinfold areas and may be given to counter irritation caused by dithranol.

If psoriasis is very severe, and other treatments have not been effective, specialist treatment may include the use of more powerful drugs. These drugs include vitamin A derivatives (acitretin) taken by mouth in courses lasting approximately six months, and methotrexate, which is an anticancer drug.

PUVA

PUVA is the combined use of a psoralen drug (methoxsalen) and ultraviolet A light (UVA). The drug is applied topically or taken by mouth some hours before exposure to UVA, which enhances the effect of the drug on skin cells. The drug is activated by exposure of the skin to the ultraviolet light; it acts on the cell's genetic material (DNA) to regulate its rate of division.

This therapy is given two to three times a week and produces an improvement within about four to six weeks. Possible adverse effects include nausea, itching, and painful reddening of the normal areas of skin. More seriously, there is a risk of the skin ageing prematurely and a long-term risk of skin cancer, particularly in fair-skinned people. For these reasons, PUVA therapy is generally recommended only for severe psoriasis, when other treatments have failed.

HOW THEY WORK

Dithranol and methotrexate slow down the rapid rate of cell division that causes skin thickening. Acitretin also reduces production of keratin, the hard protein that forms in the outer layer of the skin. Salicylic acid and coal tar remove layers of dead skin cells. Corticosteroids reduce inflammation of the underlying skin.

HOW THEY AFFECT YOU
Appropriate treatment of psoriasis usually improves the appearance of the skin. However, since drugs cannot cure the underlying cause, psoriasis tends to recur, even following successful treatment of an outbreak.

Individual drugs may cause side effects. Topical preparations can cause stinging and inflammation, especially if they are applied to normal skin. Coal tar and methoxsalen increase the skin's sensitivity to sunlight; excessive sunbathing or overexposure to artificial ultraviolet light may damage skin and worsen the condition.

Acitretin and methotrexate can have several serious side effects, including gastro-intestinal upset, liver damage, and bone marrow damage (methotrexate). Both are unsuitable in pregnancy, and women are advised to avoid pregnancy for two years after completing treatment with acitretin. Topical corticosteroids may cause rebound worsening of psoriasis when they are stopped.

COMMON DRUGS
Acitretin, Calcipotriol*, Coal tar, Ciclosporin*, Dithranol, Methotrexate*, Methoxsalen, Salicylic acid, Tacalcitol, Tazarotene, Topical corticosteroids (see p.116)
* See Part 2

Treatments for eczema

Eczema, often called dermatitis, is a skin condition causing a dry, itchy rash that may be inflamed and blistered. It can be triggered by allergy but often occurs for no known reason. In the long term, eczema can thicken the skin as a result of persistent scratching.

The most common type, atopic eczema, may appear in infancy, but many children grow out of it. There is often a family history of eczema, asthma, or allergic rhinitis. Atopic eczema commonly appears over joints such as the fronts of the wrists and behind the knees.

Contact dermatitis, another common form of eczema, is caused by chemicals, detergents, or soap. It may only appear after repeated exposure to the substance, but strong acids or alkalis can cause a reaction within minutes. It can also result from irritation of the skin by traces of detergent on clothes and bedding.

Allergic contact dermatitis can appear days or even years after initial contact has been made with triggers such as nickel, rubber, elastic, or drugs (e.g., antibiotics, antihistamines, antiseptics, or local anaesthetics). Sunlight can also trigger contact dermatitis following use of aftershave or perfume.

In nummular eczema, circular dry, scaly, itchy, patches develop anywhere on the body, and bacteria are often found in these areas. The cause of nummular eczema is unknown.

Seborrhoeic dermatitis mainly affects the scalp and face (see Dandruff and hair loss p.122–123).

WHY THEY ARE USED
Emollients are used to soften and moisten the skin. Oral antihistamines (p.56) may be prescribed for a particularly itchy rash (topical antihistamines make the skin more sensitive and should not be used). Coal tar or ichthammol may be used for chronic atopic eczema, but topical corticosteroids (p.116) may be needed to help control a flare up. Rarely, severe cases that are resistant to other treatments may need treatment with the immunosuppressant drug (p.96) ciclosporin. Oral corticosteroids may be used to treat contact dermatitis. Nummular eczema usually requires corticosteroid treatment. If it is resistant, infection is likely, and antibiotics (p.60) may be prescribed.

HOW THEY WORK
Emollients make the skin less dry and itchy. They are available as ointments, creams, lotions, soap substitutes, or bath oils. The effect is not long-lasting, so they need to be applied frequently. Emollients do not usually contain an active drug.

Antihistamines block the action of histamine (a chemical that is present in all cells). Histamine dilates the blood vessels in the skin, causing redness and swelling of the surrounding tissue due to fluid leaking from the circulation. Antihistamines also prevent histamine from irritating the nerve fibres, which causes itching.

Topical corticosteroids are absorbed into the tissues to relieve itching and inflammation. The least potent one that is effective is given. Hydrocortisone 1 percent is often used in 1 to 2-week courses.

Oral or topical antibiotics destroy the bacteria sometimes present in broken, oozing, or blistered skin.

Ciclosporin blocks the action of white blood cells, which are involved in the immune response. The drug is given in short courses when the immune system responds inappropriately to an allergen.

RISKS AND SPECIAL PRECAUTIONS

All types of eczema can become infected, and antibiotics may be needed. Herpes virus may infect atopic eczema, so direct contact with people who have a herpes infection, such as a cold sore, should be avoided. Emollients are generally well tolerated, as are topical mild corticosteroids used in the short term. Ciclosporin, however, may produce some adverse effects.

PREVENTING ECZEMA

Trigger substances can be identified using patch testing (see below), and then avoided. PVC gloves should be worn to protect the hands from detergents; and cotton, rather than wool or synthetic, garments should be worn next to the skin. Cosmetic moisturizers should be avoided because they usually contain perfumes and other sensitizers.

PATCH TESTING

Low concentrations of suspected substances are applied to the skin of the back and are held in place with non-absorbent adhesive tape. This method allows a number of potential allergens (substances that can cause an allergic reaction) to be tested at the same time. After 48 hours, the adhesive tape is removed and the skin inspected for any redness, swelling, or blistering, which would indicate a positive reaction. The skin is checked after a further 24 and 48 hours, in case the reaction has taken longer to develop.

COMMON DRUGS

Emollient and cooling preparations Aqueous cream, Cold cream, Calamine lotion, Emulsifying ointment

Corticosteroids See also p.78, Hydrocortisone*

Antihistamines See also p.56, Antazoline, Chlorphenamine*, Diphenhydramine, Mepyramine, Trimeprazine

Other drugs Coal tar, Ichthammol, Ciclosporin*

* See Part 2

Drugs for dandruff

Dandruff is an irritating, but harmless, condition that involves an acceleration in the normal shedding of skin cells from the scalp. Extensive dandruff is considered to be a mild form of a type of dermatitis known as seborrhoeic dermatitis, which is caused by an overgrowth of a yeast organism that lives in the scalp. In severe cases, a rash and reddish yellow, scaly pimples appear along the hairline and on the face.

WHY THEY ARE USED

Frequent washing with a detergent shampoo usually keeps the scalp free of dandruff, but more persistent dandruff can be treated with shampoos medicated with zinc pyrithione or selenium sulphide, or with shampoos containing coal tar or salicylic acid. Severe cases of seborrhoeic dermatitis are best treated with shampoo containing the antifungal drug ketoconazole (p.267). Ointments containing coal tar and salicylic acid are also available. Corticosteroid gels and lotions may be needed to treat an itchy rash, especially in cases of severe seborrhoeic dermatitis or psoriasis on the scalp (p.120).

HOW THEY WORK

Coal tar and salicylic acid preparations reduce the overproduction of new skin cells and break down scales, which are then washed off during shampooing. Antifungals (p.74) reduce the overgrowth of yeast on the scalp by altering the permeability of the fungal cell walls. Corticosteroids (p.78) help to relieve an itchy rash by reducing inflammation of the underlying skin.

COMMON DRUGS
Antifungals Ketoconazole*, Zinc pyrithione
Other drugs Coal tar, Corticosteroids (see p.78), Salicylic acid, Selenium sulphide
* See Part 2

Drugs for hair loss

Hair loss (alopecia) is the result of greater-than-normal shedding of hairs or reduced hair production. Hair loss can be caused by a skin condition such as scalp ringworm or scalp psoriasis.

Other forms of hair loss are due to a disorder of the follicles themselves and may be a response to illness, malnutrition, or a reaction to some drugs, such as anticancer drugs or anticoagulants. The hair loss may be diffuse or in a pattern, as in male-pattern baldness which is caused by oversensitivity to testosterone.

WHY THEY ARE USED
If the hair loss is caused by a skin disorder such as scalp ringworm, an antifungal will be used to kill the fungal growth. If male-pattern baldness is a response to the male hormone, testosterone, finasteride may be used to reduce the hormone's effect. The anti-hypertensive drug minoxidil (p.305) can be applied to the scalp to promote hair growth.

HOW THEY WORK
Hair loss can be reversed when the underlying illness is treated, or drug treatment stops. Oral finasteride inhibits conversion of testosterone to its more active form and reduces sensitivity to androgens. The role of minoxidil in hair growth is not fully understood, but it is thought to stimulate follicles.

RISKS AND SPECIAL PRECAUTIONS
Finasteride can lead to loss of libido or impotence. Anyone with a history of heart disease or hypertension should consult their doctor before using minoxidil, because the drug can be absorbed through the skin.

COMMON DRUGS
Antifungals Griseofulvin, Itraconazole
Other drugs Finasteride*, Minoxidil*
* See Part 2

Sunscreens

Sunscreens and sunblocks are chemicals, usually formulated as creams or oils, that protect the skin from the damaging effects of ultraviolet radiation from the sun.

People vary in their sensitivity to sunlight. Fair-skinned people generally have the least tolerance and tend to burn easily when exposed to the sun, while those with darker, especially brown or black, skin can withstand exposure for longer periods. Fair skin unprotected by a sunscreen suffers damage as ultraviolet rays pass through to the layers beneath, causing pain and inflammation. Sunscreens act by blocking out some of these ultraviolet rays, while allowing a proportion of them to pass through the skin surface to the epidermis to stimulate the production of melanin, the pigment that gives the skin a tan and helps to protect it during further exposure to the sun.

In a few cases, the skin's sensitivity to sunlight is increased by a disease such as pellagra or herpes simplex infection. Some drugs, such as thiazide diuretics, phenothiazine antipsychotics, psoralens, sulphonamide antibacterials, tetracycline antibiotics, and nalidixic acid, can also increase the skin's sensitivity.

Apart from sunburn and premature skin ageing, the most serious effect from sunlight is skin cancer. Reducing the skin's exposure to sunlight can help to prevent skin cancers.

HOW THEY WORK
Sunlight consists of different wavelengths of radiation. Of these, ultraviolet (UV) radiation is particularly harmful to the skin. UV radiation ages the skin and causes burning. Excessive exposure to UV radiation also increases the risk of developing skin cancer. UV radiation is mainly composed of UVA and UVB rays, both of which age the skin. In addition, UVA rays cause tanning and UVB rays cause burning. Especially vulnerable are fair-skinned people and those being treated with immunosuppressant drugs.

Sunscreens absorb some of the UVB radiation, ensuring that less of it reaches the skin. They are graded using the Sun Protection Factor (SPF), which refers to the degree of protection given by a sunscreen against sunburn. SPF is a measure of the amount of

UVB radiation a sunscreen absorbs. The higher the number, the greater the protection. This number only describes the protection against UVB radiation. Some sunscreens, which contain chemicals such as zinc oxide and titanium dioxide, protect against UVA radiation as well; these are often called sunblocks. Some preparations carry a "star" classification for the UVA protection they give. The stars do not describe an absolute measure but indicate a ratio of UVA to UVB protection. Four stars means that the product gives balanced protection against both UVA and UVB. Ratings of 1, 2, or 3 stars mean that the sunscreen has more protection against UVB than UVA.

Sunscreens are particularly advisable for visitors to tropical, subtropical, and mountainous areas, and for those who wish to sunbathe, because they can prevent burning while allowing the skin to tan. Sunscreens must be applied before exposure to the sun. People with fair skin should use a sunscreen with a higher SPF than people with darker skin.

RISKS AND SPECIAL PRECAUTIONS

Sunscreens only form a physical barrier to the passage of UV radiation. They do not alter the skin to make it more resistant to sunlight. Sunscreen lotions must be applied frequently during exposure to the sun to maintain protection. People who are very fair skinned or are known to be very sensitive to sunlight should never expose their skin to direct sunlight, even if they are using a sunscreen, since not even sunscreens with high SPF values give complete protection.

Sunscreens can irritate the skin and some preparations may cause an allergic rash. People who are sensitive to some drugs, such as procaine and benzocaine, and some hair dyes, may develop a rash after applying a sunscreen containing aminobenzoic acid or a benzophenone derivative such as oxybenzone.

COMMON DRUGS

Ingredients in sunscreens and sunblocks

Aminobenzoic acid, Benzones, Dibenzoylmethanes, Ethylhexyl methoxycinnamate, Methylbenzylidene camphor, Mexenone, Oxybenzone, Padimate-O, Titanium dioxide, Zinc oxide

* **See Part 2**

PART 2

A–Z OF DRUGS

This part of the book contains 247 generic drugs, individually profiled, and written to a standard format to help you find specific information quickly and easily; cross-references to the relevant major drug groups are provided.

Aciclovir

Brand names Boots Avert, Herpetad, Soothelip, Virasorb, Virovir, Zovirax
Used in the following combined preparations
None

QUICK REFERENCE

Drug group Antiviral drug (p.67)
Overdose danger rating Low
Dependence rating Low
Prescription needed No (cold sore cream) Yes (other preparations)
Available as generic Yes

GENERAL INFORMATION

Aciclovir is an antiviral drug used in the treatment of herpes infections of all types. Most commonly given as a cream, aciclovir reduces the severity of outbreaks of cold sores and herpes. The drug's effectiveness is greatest if it is given when symptoms have just started. It may be given by mouth or injection for severe or recurrent genital herpes. Herpes zoster (shingles) infections are treated with tablets. Aciclovir is prescribed on a regular basis for people with reduced immunity and is administered as ointment for herpes infections affecting the eye.

The injected form is given with caution to those with impaired kidney function due to the risk of aciclovir accumulating in the body.

INFORMATION FOR USERS

Follow instructions on the label. Call your doctor if symptoms worsen.
How taken Tablets, liquid, injection, cream, eye ointment.
Frequency and timing of doses 2–5 x daily. Start as soon as possible.
Adult dosage range Tablets, liquid 1–4 daily (treatment); 800mg daily, occasionally 1.6g daily (prevention). Cream, eye ointment As directed.
Onset of effect Within 24 hours.
Duration of action Up to 8 hours.
Diet advice It is necessary to drink plenty of water when taking high doses by mouth or injection.
Storage Keep in a closed container in a cool, dry place out of reach of children. Protect from light.

Missed dose Tablets/liquid/cream, eye ointment Take as soon as you remember.
Stopping the drug Unless rash, confusion, or hallucinations occur, complete the full course as directed.
Exceeding the dose An occasional unintentional extra dose is unlikely to be a cause for concern. But if you notice any unusual symptoms, or if a large overdose has been taken, notify your doctor.

POSSIBLE ADVERSE EFFECTS

Serious adverse effects are rare. The cream may cause stinging or itching at the site of application. Rarely, a rash may develop. Taken by mouth, aciclovir can occasionally cause nausea, vomiting, headache, or dizziness. Confusion or hallucinations may occur rarely with injections; if these or rash occur, stop taking the drug and consult your doctor immediately.

INTERACTIONS (tablets/liquid only)

General note Any drug that affects the kidneys increases the risk of side effects with aciclovir.
Probenecid This drug may increase the level of aciclovir in the blood.
Mycophenolate mofetil Aciclovir may increase blood levels of this drug and vice versa.

SPECIAL PRECAUTIONS (tablets/liquid only)

Be sure to consult your doctor or pharmacist before taking this drug if:
◆ You have a long-term kidney problem.
◆ You have reduced immunity.
◆ You are taking other medications.
Pregnancy No known risk with topical preparations; oral and injectable forms are not usually prescribed, as effects on the developing baby are unknown. Discuss with your doctor.
Breast-feeding No evidence of risk with topical forms. The drug passes into the breast milk following injection or oral administration. Discuss with your doctor.
Infants and children Reduced dose necessary in young children.
Over 60 Reduced dose may be necessary.
Driving and hazardous work Avoid such activities until you know how aciclovir affects you because the drug may cause dizziness if it is taken by mouth.
Alcohol No known problems.

PROLONGED USE
Aciclovir is usually given as single courses of treatment and is not given long term, except to people with reduced immunity.

Allopurinol

Brand names Caplenal, Cosuric, Rimapurinol, Xanthomax, Zyloric
Used in the following combined preparations
None

QUICK REFERENCE
Drug group Drug for gout (p.51)
Overdose danger rating Medium
Dependence rating Low
Prescription needed Yes
Available as generic Yes

GENERAL INFORMATION
Allopurinol is prescribed as a long-term preventative of recurrent attacks of gout. It acts by reducing production of uric acid, which may form crystals in a joint, causing the inflammation characteristic of gout. The drug is also used to prevent high uric acid levels (hyperuricaemia) caused by other drugs, such as anticancer drugs.

Allopurinol is not effective for the pain of acute flare-ups, and attacks may increase initially; an anti-inflammatory is often also given.

Unlike the gout drugs that reduce uric acid levels by increasing the quantity excreted in the urine, allopurinol does not raise the risk of uric acid kidney stones, making it particularly suitable for people with poor kidney function or a tendency to form kidney stones.

INFORMATION FOR USERS
Your drug prescription is tailored for you. Do not alter dosage without checking with your doctor.
How taken Tablets.
Frequency and timing of doses Once daily after food.
Adult dosage range 100–300mg daily.
Onset of effect Within 24–48 hours. Full effect may not be felt for several weeks.
Duration of action Up to 30 hours. Some effect may last for 1–2 weeks after the drug has been stopped.

Diet advice A high fluid intake (2 litres daily) is recommended.
Storage Keep in a closed container in a cool, dry place out of reach of children.
Missed dose If your next dose is not due for another 12 hours or more, take a dose as soon as you remember and take the next one as usual. Otherwise, skip the missed dose and take your next dose on schedule.
Stopping the drug Unless rash, sore throat, fever, or shivering occur, do not stop taking the drug without consulting your doctor; symptoms may recur.
Exceeding the dose An occasional unintentional extra dose is unlikely to cause problems. Large overdoses may cause nausea, vomiting, abdominal pain, diarrhoea, and dizziness. Notify your doctor.

POSSIBLE ADVERSE EFFECTS
Adverse effects of allopurinol are uncommon. The most serious are an allergic rash, sore throat, fever, or shivering, which may require treatment to be substituted. Stop taking the drug and consult your doctor. Nausea can be avoided by taking allopurinol after food.

INTERACTIONS
Mercaptopurine and azathioprine Allopurinol blocks the breakdown of these drugs, requiring a reduction in their dosage.
Aspirin Large doses of this drug may reduce the effects of allopurinol.
Anticoagulant drugs Allopurinol may increase the effects of these drugs.
Chlorpropamide The hypoglycaemic effects of this drug may be increased with allopurinol.
Ciclosporin Allopurinol may increase the effects of this drug.
ACE inhibitors Allopurinol may increase the effects of these drugs.

SPECIAL PRECAUTIONS
Be sure to tell your doctor if:
◆ You have long-term liver or kidney problems.
◆ You have had a previous sensitivity reaction to allopurinol.
◆ You have a current attack of gout.
◆ You are taking other medications.
Pregnancy Safety in pregnancy not established. Discuss with your doctor.

Breast-feeding The drug passes into the breast milk and may affect the baby. Discuss with your doctor.

Infants and children Reduced dose necessary.

Over 60 Reduced dose may be necessary.

Driving and hazardous work No problems expected.

Alcohol Keep consumption low. Large amounts of alcohol may worsen gout.

PROLONGED USE

Apart from an increased risk of gout in the first weeks or months, no problems expected.

Monitoring Periodic checks on uric acid levels in the blood are usually performed until the levels are stable/controlled.

Alprostadil

Brand names Caverject, MUSE, Prostin VR, Viridal
Used in the following combined preparations
None

QUICK REFERENCE

Drug group Prostaglandin and drug for impotence (p.105)
Overdose danger rating Medium
Dependence rating Low
Prescription needed Yes
Available as generic No

GENERAL INFORMATION

Alprostadil is a member of a group of drugs known as the prostaglandins and is used to treat patent ductus arteriosus, a congenital heart disorder in newborn babies. It works by keeping the ductus blood vessel (which would normally have shut off at birth) open until it can be closed permanently by surgery.

Alprostadil is also used to help men who are impotent to achieve an erection. It is either injected directly into the penis or applied as a gel into the urethra.

The drug is usually only administered to babies in hospital. Side effects such as heart, circulatory, and respiratory problems are common, and there is a risk of unusual bone growth, particularly with long-term use. The most common side effect in men is pain in the penis.

INFORMATION FOR USERS

Your drug prescription is tailored for you. Do not alter dosage without checking with your doctor.

How taken Injection, gel.

Frequency and timing of doses Up to 3 x per week. Not more than one dose in any 24 hour period.

Dosage range 2.5 micrograms (starting dose), individually adjusted by your doctor to produce an erection lasting not more than 1 hour.

Onset of effect Within a few minutes.

Duration of action Erection should not last more than 1 hour.

Diet advice None.

Storage Store in a refrigerator, out of reach of children. Do not freeze.

Missed dose Take the next dose when needed. Use no more than one dose in any 24-hour period and no more than 3 doses per week.

Stopping the drug The drug can be safely stopped as soon as you no longer need it.

Exceeding the dose An occasional unintentional extra dose is unlikely to be a cause for concern. But if you notice any unusual symptoms or if a large overdose has been taken, notify your doctor.

POSSIBLE ADVERSE EFFECTS

Breathing difficulties are a side effect of the drug in newborn babies. In men, pain or bruising may occur at the injections site, and there is a risk of prolonged erection. Report any erection lasting more than 4 hours to your doctor and stop taking the drug immediately.

INTERACTIONS

None.

SPECIAL PRECAUTIONS

Be sure to tell your doctor if:
◆ You are taking other medications for impotence.

Pregnancy Not prescribed.

Breast-feeding Not prescribed.

Infants and children Other than for new born babies, not prescribed.

Over 60 Doses are adjusted individually.

Driving and hazardous work No special problems.

Alcohol Excessive use of alcohol with alprostadil can contribute to erectile problems.

PROLONGED USE

Prolonged use of alprostadil in the newborn may cause abnormal bone development and weakening of some blood vessel walls. Prolonged use by injection for impotence may lead to development of scarring of the penis. **Monitoring** Regular examinations for penile scarring are required.

Aluminium Hydroxide

Brand names Alu-Cap, Aludrox
Used in the following combined preparations
Asilone, Co-magaldrox, Gaviscon, Maalox, Mucaine, Mucogel, Topal, and others

QUICK REFERENCE

Drug group Antacid (p.40)
Overdose danger rating Low
Dependence rating Low
Prescription needed No
Available as generic Yes

GENERAL INFORMATION

Aluminium hydroxide is the ingredient basic to many over-the-counter remedies for indigestion and heartburn. The drug is constipating (it is sometimes used to treat diarrhoea), so it is usually combined with a magnesium-containing antacid with a balancing laxative effect. The combination is sometimes referred to by the generic name of co-magaldrox.

The drug's action makes it useful in preventing pain in stomach and duodenal ulcers or reflux oesophagitis. It can also promote the healing of ulcers.

In the intestine aluminium hydroxide binds with, and thereby reduces absorption of, phosphate. This makes it helpful in treating high blood phosphate (hyperphosphataemia), which occurs in some people with impaired kidney function. Prolonged heavy use can lead to phosphate deficiency and consequent weakening of the bones.

Some preparations include large amounts of sodium and should be used with caution by those people on low-sodium diets; special preparations that are low in sodium are available in these circumstances. Aluminium hydroxide may be more effective as an antacid in liquid form than as tablets.

INFORMATION FOR USERS

Follow instructions on the label. Call your doctor if symptoms worsen.

How taken Tablets, capsules, liquid (gel suspension). The tablets should be well chewed.

Frequency and timing of doses *As antacid* 4–6 x daily as needed, or 1 hour before and after meals. *Peptic ulcer* 6–7 x daily. *Hyperphosphataemia* 3–4 x daily with meals. *Diarrhoea* 2–6 x daily.

Dosage range *Adults* Up to 70ml daily (liquid), 2–10g daily (tablets or capsules). *Children over 6 years* Reduced dose according to age and weight.

Onset of effect Within 15 minutes.

Duration of action 2–4 hours.

Diet advice For hyperphosphataemia, a low-phosphate diet may be advised in addition to treatment with aluminium hydroxide.

Storage Keep in a closed container in a cool, dry place out of reach of children.

Missed dose Do not take the missed dose. Take your next dose as usual.

Stopping the drug Can be safely stopped as soon as you no longer need it (for indigestion). When taken as ulcer treatment, or for hyperphosphataemia resulting from kidney failure, do not stop taking the drug without consulting your doctor.

Exceeding the dose An occasional unintentional extra dose is unlikely to be a cause for concern. But if you notice any unusual symptoms, or if a large overdose has been taken, notify your doctor.

POSSIBLE ADVERSE EFFECTS

Constipation is a common adverse effect of aluminium hydroxide; nausea and vomiting may occur due to the granular, powdery nature of the drug. Bone pain occurs only when large doses of the drug have been taken regularly for months or years.

INTERACTIONS

General note Aluminium hydroxide may interfere with the absorption or excretion of many drugs, including oral anticoagulants, digoxin, many antibiotics, penicillamine, corticosteroids, antipsychotics, and phenytoin.

Enteric-coated tablets Aluminium hydroxide may lead to break-up of the enteric coating (e.g., bisacodyl, or enteric-coated pred-nisolone) before tablets leave the stomach, causing stomach irritation.

SPECIAL PRECAUTIONS
Be sure to consult your doctor or pharmacist before taking this drug if:
◆ You have a long-term kidney problem.
◆ You have heart problems.
◆ You have high blood pressure.
◆ You suffer from constipation.
◆ You have a bone disease.
◆ You have porphyria.
◆ You are taking other medications.

Pregnancy Safety in pregnancy not estab-lished. Discuss with your doctor.
Breast-feeding No evidence of risk.
Infants and children Not recommended under 6 years except on the advice of a doctor.
Over 60 Increased likelihood of adverse effects. Reduced dose may therefore be necessary.
Driving and hazardous work No known prob-lems.
Alcohol No known problems.

PROLONGED USE
Aluminium hydroxide should not be used for longer than 4 weeks without consulting your doctor. Prolonged high doses may deplete blood phosphate and calcium levels, leading to weakening of the bones and fractures.

Amantadine

Brand name Symmetrel
Used in the following combined preparations
None

QUICK REFERENCE
Drug group Drug for parkinsonism (p.18) and antiviral drug (p.67)
Overdose danger rating Low
Dependence rating Low
Prescription needed Yes
Available as generic No

GENERAL INFORMATION
Amantadine was first used in the 1960s as an antiviral drug, originally for prevention and treatment of influenza A. As a preventative against influenza A, it protects some 70 per cent of those not receiving vaccination. As treatment, it is effective in reducing the severity of symptoms when given within 48 hours of the onset of flu. It can also reduce pain following herpes zoster (shingles).

In 1969 amantadine was found to be help-ful in parkinsonism, except when the condi-tion is caused by drugs. Amantadine usually produces improvement of symptoms during the first few weeks, but its effectiveness usu-ally wears off over six to eight weeks, requir-ing replacement by another drug. It is sometimes given with levodopa (see p.273), another drug for parkinsonism.

INFORMATION FOR USERS
Your drug prescription is tailored for you. Do not alter dosage without checking with your doctor.
How taken Capsules, liquid.
Frequency and timing of doses 1–2 x daily. The second dose should not be taken after 4pm.
Adult dosage range 100–200mg daily.
Onset of effect The full effect may not be felt for up to 2 weeks (parkinsonism). The sever-ity and duration of symptoms is likely to be reduced if the drug is begun within 48 hours of the onset of symptoms (viral infections).
Duration of action Up to 24 hours.
Diet advice None.
Storage Keep in a closed container in a cool, dry place out of reach of children.
Missed dose Take as soon as you remember. If your next dose is due within 2 hours, take a single dose now and skip the next.
Stopping the drug Unless a rash occurs, do not stop taking the drug without consulting your doctor; symptoms may recur.
Exceeding the dose An occasional uninten-tional extra dose is unlikely to be a cause for concern. But if you notice any unusual symptoms, or if a large overdose has been taken, notify your doctor.

POSSIBLE ADVERSE EFFECTS
Adverse effects are uncommon and often wear off with continued treatment. They in-clude agitation, confusion, dizziness, halluci-nations, and blurred vision, which are rarely serious enough to require treatment to be stopped. If you develop a rash, however, stop taking the drug and consult your doctor.

INTERACTIONS

Anticholinergic drugs Amantadine may add to the effects of anticholinergics; your doctor will probably reduce the dosage of these drugs.

SPECIAL PRECAUTIONS

Be sure to tell your doctor if:
◆ You have long-term liver or kidney problems.
◆ You have a peptic ulcer.
◆ You have had epileptic fits.
◆ You have heart disease.
◆ You are taking other medications.

Pregnancy Safety in pregnancy not established. Discuss with your doctor.

Breast-feeding The drug passes into the breast milk and may affect the baby. Discuss with your doctor.

Infants and children Not usually prescribed. Reduced dose necessary.

Over 60 Increased likelihood of adverse effects. Reduced dose necessary.

Driving and hazardous work Avoid such activities until you have learned how amantadine affects you because the drug can cause blurred vision, dizziness, inability to concentrate, hallucinations, agitation, and confusion.

Alcohol No known problems.

PROLONGED USE

The drug's beneficial effects usually diminish during continuous treatment for parkinsonism. When this occurs, another drug may be substituted for, or given together with, amantadine. Sometimes the drug's effectiveness can be restored if it is withdrawn by your doctor and reintroduced a few weeks later.

Amiloride

Brand names Amilospare, Amilamont
Used in the following combined preparations
Burinex A, Co-amilofruse, Co-amilozide, Moduretic, Navispare, and others

QUICK REFERENCE

Drug group Potassium-sparing diuretic (p.30)
Overdose danger rating Low
Dependence rating Low
Prescription needed Yes
Available as generic Yes

GENERAL INFORMATION

Amiloride belongs to a class of drugs known as potassium-sparing diuretics. With thiazide or loop diuretics, it is used in the treatment of hypertension, and of oedema (fluid retention) resulting from heart failure or liver disease.

The effect of amiloride on urine flow may be noticed for several hours. For this reason, the drug should be avoided after about 4 pm; otherwise you may find that you need to pass urine during the night. Amiloride, as with other potassium-sparing diuretics, can be risky for people taking potassium supplements and for those who have unusually high levels of potassium in their blood. Salt substitutes should be avoided, because they contain potassium. Amiloride is prescribed with caution to people with a kidney disorder.

INFORMATION FOR USERS

Your drug prescription is tailored for you. Do not alter dosage without checking with your doctor.

How taken Tablets, liquid.

Frequency and timing of doses Once daily, usually in the morning.

Adult dosage range 5–20mg daily.

Onset of effect Within 2–4 hours.

Duration of action 12–24 hours.

Diet advice Avoid foods that are high in potassium(e.g., dried fruit and salt substitutes).

Storage Keep in a closed container in a cool, dry place out of reach of children.

Missed dose Take as soon as you remember. However, if it is late in the day, do not take the missed dose, or you may need to get up at night to pass urine. Take the next scheduled dose as usual.

Stopping the drug Unless a rash occurs, do not stop taking the drug without consulting your doctor; symptoms may recur.

Exceeding the dose An occasional unintentional extra dose is unlikely to cause problems. If you notice any symptoms, or if a large overdose has been taken, notify your doctor.

POSSIBLE ADVERSE EFFECTS

Amiloride has few adverse effects but may cause digestive disturbance, thirst, confusion, or rash. The main problem is the possibility of potassium being retained by the body, causing muscle weakness and numbness. If you develop a rash, stop taking the drug and consult your doctor.

INTERACTIONS

Lithium Amiloride may increase the blood levels of lithium, leading to an increased risk of lithium poisoning.

ACE inhibitors, ciclosporin, and NSAIDs These drugs may increase the risk of potassium retention if they are taken with amiloride.

SPECIAL PRECAUTIONS

Be sure to tell your doctor if:
◆ You have long-term liver or kidney problems.
◆ You have diabetes.
◆ You are taking other medications.

Pregnancy Not usually prescribed. May cause a reduction in the blood supply to the developing baby. Discuss with your doctor.

Breast-feeding Not usually prescribed during breast-feeding. Discuss with your doctor.

Infants and children Not recommended.

Over 60 Increased likelihood of adverse effects. Reduced dose necessary.

Driving and hazardous work Avoid such activities until you have learned how amiloride affects you because the drug can cause confusion.

Alcohol No special problems.

PROLONGED USE

Monitoring Blood tests may be carried out to monitor levels of body salts.

Amiodarone

Brand name Amidox, Cordarone X
Used in the following combined preparations
None

QUICK REFERENCE

Drug group Anti-arrhythmic drug (p.32)
Overdose danger rating Medium
Dependence rating Low
Prescription needed Yes
Available as generic Yes (tablets)

GENERAL INFORMATION

Introduced in the 1950s, amiodarone is used to treat a variety of abnormal heart rhythms (arrhythmias). It works by slowing nerve impulses in the heart muscle.

Amiodarone is given to prevent recurrent atrial and ventricular fibrillation and to treat ventricular and supraventricular tachycardias and Wolff-Parkinson-White Syndrome. The drug is not usually first choice, especially when used for long-term treatment, because it has potentially serious adverse effects including a light-sensitive rash, liver or lung damage, thyroid problems, and eye damage.

Treatment should be started only under specialist supervision or in hospital, and the dosage is carefully controlled to achieve the desired effect using the lowest possible dose.

INFORMATION FOR USERS

Your drug prescription is tailored for you. Do not alter dosage without checking with your doctor.

How taken Tablets, injection.

Frequency and timing of doses 3 x daily or by injection initially, then reduced to twice daily, then once daily or every other day (maintenance dose).

Adult dosage range 600mg daily, reduced to 400mg, then 100–200mg daily.

Onset of effect Some effects may be noticed within 72 hours, but full benefits may not be felt for some weeks (by mouth); effects may be noticed within 30 minutes (injection)

Duration of action Up to 1 month.

Diet advice None.

Storage Keep in a closed container in a cool, dry place out of reach of children. Protect from light.

Missed dose Take as soon as you remember. If your next dose is due within 12 hours, do not take the missed dose, but take your next scheduled dose as usual.

Stopping the drug Do not stop taking the drug without consulting your doctor; symptoms may recur.

Exceeding the dose An occasional unintentional extra dose is unlikely to cause problems. But if you notice any unusual symptoms or if a large overdose has been taken, notify your doctor at once.

POSSIBLE ADVERSE EFFECTS

Amiodarone has a number of unusual adverse effects, including a metallic taste in the mouth, increased sensitivity of the skin to sunlight (photosensitivity), and a greyish skin colour. The drug can also cause nausea, headache, disturbed vision, and liver, lung, and thyroid problems. If you experience nervousness, tremor, weight loss, or shortness of breath, or if you develop jaundice, consult your doctor.

INTERACTIONS

General note Amiodarone can interact with many drugs. Consult your doctor or pharmacist before taking any other medications.

Diuretics The potassium loss caused by these drugs may increase the toxic effects of amiodarone.

Other anti-arrhythmic drugs Amiodarone may increase the effects of drugs such as beta blockers, digoxin, diltiazem, or verapamil.

Warfarin Amiodarone may increase the anticoagulant effect of warfarin.

SPECIAL PRECAUTIONS

Be sure to tell your doctor if:
◆ You have long-term liver or kidney problems.
◆ You have a lung disorder such as asthma or bronchitis.
◆ You have eye disease.
◆ You have a thyroid disorder.
◆ You are sensitive to iodine.
◆ You are taking other medications.

Pregnancy Not prescribed. Discuss with your doctor.

Breast-feeding The drug passes into the breast milk and may affect the baby. Discuss with your doctor.

Infants and children Not recommended.

Over 60 Increased likelihood of adverse effects. Reduced dose necessary.

Driving and hazardous work Avoid such activities until you have learned how amiodarone affects you because the drug can cause dazzling of the eyes by bright light.

Alcohol No known problems.

PROLONGED USE

Prolonged use of this drug may cause a number of adverse effects on the eyes, lungs, thyroid gland, and liver.

Monitoring A chest X-ray may be taken before treatment starts. Blood tests are carried

out before treatment starts and then every 6 months to check thyroid and liver function. Regular eye examinations are required.

Amisulpride/sulpiride

Brand names Solian [amisulpride] Dolmatil, Sulparex, Sulpitil [sulpiride]
Used in the following combined preparations None

QUICK REFERENCE

Drug group Antipsychotic drug (p.15)
Overdose danger rating Medium
Dependence rating Low
Prescription needed Yes
Available as generic No

GENERAL INFORMATION

Amisulpride and sulpiride are antipsychotic drugs that are used to treat acute and chronic schizophrenia, in which there are "positive" symptoms such as delusions, hallucinations, and thought disorders) and/or "negative" symptoms such as emotional and social withdrawal. Higher doses of amisulpride and sulpiride are needed to control the positive symptoms; lower doses result in increased alertness and elevation of mood. Sulpiride has also been used to treat Tourette's syndrome (an inherited neurological disorder), anxiety disorders, and vertigo.

An advantage of these antipsychotics is that they are less likely than the older drugs to cause parkinsonism or tardive dyskinesia (involuntary movements of the tongue and face).

INFORMATION FOR USERS

Your drug prescription is tailored for you. Do not alter dosage without checking with your doctor.

How taken Tablets.

Frequency and timing of doses 1–2 x daily. (doses of up to 300mg may be once daily).

Dosage range Amisulpride 400–1,200mg daily. Sulpiride 400–1,200mg daily (acute psychosis); 50–300mg daily (predominantly negative symptoms).

Onset of effect 1 hour.

Duration of action 12–24 hours.

Diet advice None.

Storage Keep in a closed container in a cool, dry place out of reach of children.

Missed dose Take as soon as you remember. If your next dose is due within 2 hours, take a single dose now and skip the next dose.

Stopping the drug Unless palpitations or dizziness occur, do not stop taking the drug without consulting your doctor; symptoms may recur.

Exceeding the dose An occasional unintentional extra dose is unlikely to cause problems. Large overdoses may cause drowsiness and low blood pressure. Notify your doctor immediately.

POSSIBLE ADVERSE EFFECTS

Most of the side effects of antipsychotic drugs like amisulpride and sulpiride are mild. Insomnia is the most common problem, but agitation, drowsiness, nausea, breast swelling, weight gain, parkinsonism, palpitations, and dizziness may also occur. If you experience palpitations or dizziness, stop taking the drug and call your doctor immediately.

INTERACTIONS

Antihypertensive drugs Amisulpride and sulpiride may reduce the blood-pressure lowering effect of certain of these drugs.

Central nervous system depressants These drugs may all increase the sedative effects of amisulpride and sulpiride.

SPECIAL PRECAUTIONS

Be sure to tell your doctor if:
◆ You have liver or kidney problems.
◆ You have heart problems or hypertension.
◆ You have epilepsy.
◆ You have Parkinson's disease.
◆ You have phaeochromocytoma.
◆ You have a pituitary tumour or breast cancer.
◆ You have porphyria.
◆ You have had blood problems.
◆ You are taking other medications.

Pregnancy Safety not established. Discuss with your doctor.

Breast-feeding Safety not established. Discuss with your doctor.

Infants and children Not recommended.

Over 60 Reduced dose may be necessary.

Driving and hazardous work Avoid. These drugs can slow reaction times and may occasionally cause drowsiness or loss of concentration.

Alcohol Avoid. Alcohol increases the sedative effects of these drugs.

PROLONGED USE

Tardive dyskinesia may rarely occur during long-term use.

Amitriptyline

Brand names Domical, Elavil, Lentizol, Tryptizol

Used in the following combined preparation
Triptafen

QUICK REFERENCE

Drug group Tricyclic antidepressant drug (p.14)
Overdose danger rating High
Dependence rating Low
Prescription needed Yes
Available as generic Yes

GENERAL INFORMATION

Amitriptyline belongs to a class of antidepressant drugs known as the tricyclics. Used mainly in the long-term treatment of depression, it elevates mood, increases physical activity, improves appetite, and restores interest in everyday activities.

More sedating than similar drugs, amitriptyline is useful when depression is accompanied by anxiety or insomnia. Taken at night, amitriptyline encourages sleep and helps to eliminate the need to take additional sleeping drugs. It is sometimes used to treat nocturnal enuresis (bedwetting) in children.

In overdose, amitriptyline may cause coma, fits, and abnormal heart rhythms.

INFORMATION FOR USERS

Your drug prescription is tailored for you. Do not alter dosage without checking with your doctor.

How taken Tablets, SR-capsules, liquid, injection.
Frequency and timing of doses 1–4 x daily, often as a single dose at night.
Adult dosage range 50–150mg daily.
Onset of effect Sedation can occur within hours, although full antidepressant effect may not be felt for 2–4 weeks.

Duration of action The antidepressant effect may last 6 weeks, but adverse effects may only last a few days.

Diet advice None.

Storage Keep in a closed container in a cool, dry place out of reach of children. Protect from light.

Missed dose Take as soon as you remember. If your next dose is due within 3 hours, take a single dose now and skip the next.

Stopping the drug Unless severe adverse effects occur (see below), do not stop taking the drug without consulting your doctor. He or she may supervise a gradual reduction in dosage; stopping the drug abruptly can cause withdrawal symptoms and a recurrence of the original trouble.

OVERDOSE ACTION
Seek immediate medical advice in all cases. Take emergency action if palpitations are noted or consciousness is lost.

POSSIBLE ADVERSE EFFECTS
The possible adverse effects of this drug are mainly the result of its anticholinergic action and its blocking action on the transmission of signals through the heart. Drowsiness, blurred vision, dry mouth, and sweating may occur. If you have difficulty in passing urine, a sore throat, or palpitations, stop taking the drug and consult your doctor immediately.

INTERACTIONS
MAOIs In the rare cases where these drugs are given with amitriptyline, there is a possibility of serious interactions.

Sedatives All drugs that have sedative effects intensify those of amitriptyline.

Antiarrhythmic drugs There is an increased risk of abnormal heart rhythms when these drugs are taken with amitriptyline.

Antiepileptics The effects of these drugs are reduced by amitriptyline.

SPECIAL PRECAUTIONS
Be sure to tell your doctor if:
◆ You have heart problems.
◆ You have had epileptic fits.
◆ You have long-term liver or kidney problems.
◆ You have glaucoma.

◆ You have prostate trouble.
◆ You have had mania or a psychotic illness.
◆ You have thyroid disease.
◆ You are taking other medications.

Pregnancy Safety in pregnancy not established. Discuss with your doctor.

Breast-feeding The drug passes into the breast milk and may affect the baby. Discuss with your doctor.

Infants and children Not recommended under 16 years for depression, or under 6 years for enuresis.

Over 60 Reduced dose may be necessary.

Driving and hazardous work Avoid such activities until you have learned how amitriptyline affects you because the drug may cause blurred vision and reduced alertness.

Alcohol Avoid excessive amounts. Alcohol may increase the sedative effects of this drug.

Surgery and general anaesthetics Amitriptyline treatment may need to be stopped before you have a general anaesthetic. Discuss with your doctor or dentist before any operation.

PROLONGED USE
No problems expected.

Amlodipine

Brand name Istin
Used in the following combined preparations
None

QUICK REFERENCE
Drug group Anti-angina drug (p.33), antihypertensive drug (p.34)
Overdose danger rating Medium
Dependence rating Low
Prescription needed Yes
Available as generic No

GENERAL INFORMATION
Amlodipine belongs to the group of drugs known as the calcium channel blockers, which interfere with electrical signals in the muscles of the heart and blood vessels.

Amlodipine is used in the treatment of angina to help prevent attacks of chest pain. Unlike some other anti-angina drugs (e.g., beta blockers), it can be used safely by asthmatics and noninsulin-dependent diabetics.

It is often successful when other treatments have failed. Amlodipine is also used to reduce raised blood pressure.

In common with other drugs of its class, amlodipine may cause blood pressure to fall too low at the start of treatment, and, in rare cases, angina may become worse at the start of treatment. The drug may sometimes cause mild to moderate leg and ankle swelling.

INFORMATION FOR USERS
Your drug prescription is tailored for you. Do not alter dosage without checking with your doctor.
How taken Tablets.
Frequency and timing of doses Once daily.
Adult dosage range 5–10mg daily.
Onset of effect 6–12 hours.
Duration of action 24 hours.
Diet advice None.
Storage Keep in a closed container in a cool, dry place out of reach of children.
Missed dose If you miss a dose and you remember it within 12 hours, take it as soon as you remember. However, if you do not remember until later, do not take the missed dose and do not double up the next one. Instead, go back to your regular schedule.
Stopping the drug Unless serious adverse effects occur (see below), do not stop taking the drug without consulting your doctor; stopping the drug may lead to worsening of the underlying condition.
Exceeding the dose An occasional unintentional extra dose is unlikely to cause problems. Large overdoses may markedly lower blood pressure. Notify your doctor immediately.

POSSIBLE ADVERSE EFFECTS
Amlodipine can cause a variety of minor adverse effects, including leg and ankle swelling, headache, flushing, dizziness, fatigue, and nausea. Dizziness, especially on rising, may be due to relaxation of muscles in the walls of blood vessels in the legs, which do not contract sufficiently when you stand up. Palpitations should be discussed with your doctor. If you develop shortness of breath, stop taking the drug and consult your doctor. The most serious effect is the rare possibility of angina worsening after treatment. starts. and should be reported to your doctor imme-

diately. A rash is an unusual adverse effect. Stop taking the drug and seek medical advice.

INTERACTIONS
Beta blockers Amlodipine may increase the effect of these drugs and vice versa.
Antidiabetic drugs These drugs may reduce the effect of amlodipine.

SPECIAL PRECAUTIONS
Be sure to tell your doctor if:
◆ You have long-term liver or kidney problems.
◆ You have heart failure.
◆ You have diabetes.
◆ You are taking other medications.
Pregnancy Safety in pregnancy not established. Discuss with your doctor.
Breast-feeding It is not known if the drug passes into the breast milk. Discuss with your doctor.
Infants and children Not recommended.
Over 60 No special problems.
Driving and hazardous work Avoid such activities until you have learned how amlodipine affects you because the drug can cause dizziness owing to lowered blood pressure.
Alcohol Keep consumption low. Alcohol may further reduce blood pressure, causing dizziness or other symptoms.

PROLONGED USE
No problems expected.

Amoxicillin
Brand names Almodan, Amix, Amoram, Amoxil, Galenamox, Rimoxallin
Used in the following combined preparations Augmentin, Co-amoxiclav

QUICK REFERENCE
Drug group Penicillin antibiotic (p.60)
Overdose danger rating Low
Dependence rating Low
Prescription needed Yes
Available as generic Yes

GENERAL INFORMATION
Amoxicillin is an antibiotic related to penicillin. It is prescribed to treat a variety of

infections but is particularly useful for ear, nose, throat, and respiratory tract infections, cystitis, uncomplicated gonorrhea, and certain skin and soft tissue infections. Taken by mouth, the drug is absorbed well by the body and works quickly and effectively.

The most common side effect of this drug is a rash, which does not necessarily mean that the patient is allergic to penicillin. This drug can also provoke a more severe allergic reaction with fever, swelling of the mouth and tongue, itching, and breathing difficulties. This usually means that the patient is allergic to all penicillin antibiotics.

INFORMATION FOR USERS
Your drug prescription is tailored for you. Do not alter dosage without checking with your doctor.
How taken Tablets, capsules, liquid, powder (dissolved in water), injection
Frequency and timing of doses Normally 3 x daily.
Dosage range *Adults* 750mg–1.5g daily. In some cases a short course of up to 6g daily is given. A single dose of 3g may be given as a preventative. *Children* Reduced dose according to age and weight.
Onset of effect 1–2 hours.
Duration of action Up to 8 hours.
Diet advice None.
Storage Keep in a closed container in a cool, dry place out of reach of children.
Missed dose Take as soon as you remember, then take your next scheduled dose.
Stopping the drug Unless an allergic reaction occurs, take the full course. Even if you feel better, the original infection may still be present and symptoms may recur.
Exceeding the dose An occasional unintentional extra dose is unlikely to be a cause for concern. But if you notice any unusual symptoms, or if a large overdose has been taken, notify your doctor.

POSSIBLE ADVERSE EFFECTS
Nausea and diarrhoea are common. If a rash or joint swelling occur, inform your doctor. Wheezing, shortness of breath, an itching rash, or fever may indicate an allergic reaction; stop taking the drug and call your doctor immediately.

INTERACTIONS
Oral contraceptives Amoxicillin may reduce the effectiveness of the oral contraceptive pill and also increase the risk of breakthrough bleeding. Discuss with your doctor.

SPECIAL PRECAUTIONS
Be sure to tell your doctor if:
◆ You have a long-term kidney problem.
◆ You have an allergy (for example, hay fever, asthma, or eczema).
◆ You have had a previous allergic reaction to a penicillin or cephalosporin antibiotic.
◆ You have ulcerative colitis.
◆ You have glandular fever.
◆ You have chronic leukaemia.
◆ You are taking other medications.
Pregnancy No evidence of risk.
Breast-feeding The drug passes into the breast milk, but at normal doses adverse effects on the baby are unlikely. Discuss with your doctor.
Infants and children Reduced dose necessary.
Over 60 No known problems.
Driving and hazardous work No known problems.
Alcohol No known problems.

PROLONGED USE
Amoxicillin is usually given only for short courses of treatment.

Amphotericin

Brand names Abelcet, AmBisome, Amphocil, Fungilin, Fungizone
Used in the following combined preparations
None

QUICK REFERENCE
Drug group Antifungal drug (p.74)
Overdose danger rating Low (oral)
Dependence rating Low
Prescription needed Yes
Available as generic Yes

GENERAL INFORMATION
Amphotericin is a highly effective and powerful antifungal drug. It is given by injection to treat serious systemic fungal infections and by mouth to treat candida (thrush) infections

of the mouth or intestines, but it is not used in vaginal candidiasis.

Treatment administered by injection is carefully supervised, usually in hospital, because of potentially serious adverse effects. A test dose for allergy may be given before a full injection. The new, recently introduced formulations of this drug appear to be less toxic than the original injection. Adverse reactions to the oral forms are rare.

INFORMATION FOR USERS

Your drug prescription is tailored for you. Do not alter dosage without checking with your doctor.

How taken Tablets, lozenges, liquid, injection.

Frequency and timing of doses Every 6 hours (by mouth); daily, usually over a 6-hour period (injection).

Dosage range 400–800mg daily (tablets and liquid); 40–80mg daily (lozenges); dosage for injection is determined individually.

Onset of effect Improvement may be noticed after 2–4 days.

Duration of action 3–6 hours.

Diet advice When given by injection, this drug may reduce the levels of potassium and magnesium in the blood. To correct this, mineral supplements may be recommended.

Storage Keep in a closed container in a cool, dry place out of reach of children.

Missed dose Take oral dose as soon as you remember, then take your next scheduled dose.

Stopping the drug Take the full course. Even if symptoms improve, the original infection may still be present and symptoms may recur if treatment is stopped too soon.

Exceeding the dose An occasional unintentional extra oral dose is unlikely to be a cause for concern. But if you notice unusual symptoms, notify your doctor.

POSSIBLE ADVERSE EFFECTS

Adverse effects from oral amphotericin are very unusual. Injections are given only under close medical supervision, so adverse effects such as nausea, headache, or muscle pain are carefully monitored and promptly treated.

INTERACTIONS

Digitalis drugs Amphotericin may increase the toxicity of digoxin.

Diuretics Amphotericin increases the risk of low potassium levels with diuretics.

Aminoglycoside antibiotics Taken with amphotericin, these drugs increase the likelihood of kidney damage.

Corticosteroids may increase loss of potassium from the body caused by amphotericin.

Ciclosporin increases the likelihood of kidney damage.

SPECIAL PRECAUTIONS

Be sure to tell your doctor if:
◆ You have a long-term kidney problem.
◆ You have previously had an allergic reaction to amphotericin.
◆ You are taking other medications.

Pregnancy There is no evidence of risk from the oral forms of the drug. Injections are given only when the infection very serious.

Breast-feeding No evidence of risk from oral forms of the drug. It is not known whether the drug passes into the breast milk when given by injection. Discuss with your doctor.

Infants and children Reduced dose may be necessary.

Over 60 No special problems.

Driving and hazardous work No known problems.

Alcohol No known problems.

PROLONGED USE

Given by injection, the drug may cause a reduction in blood levels of potassium and magnesium. It may also damage the kidneys and cause blood disorders.

Monitoring Regular blood tests to monitor liver and kidney function, blood cell counts, and potassium and magnesium levels are advised during treatment by injection.

Aspirin

Brand names Angettes, Aspro, Caprin, Disprin, Nu-Seals Aspirin, and others

Used in the following combined preparations
Anadin, Aspav, Codis, Equagesic, Veganin, and others

QUICK REFERENCE

Drug group Non-opioid analgesic (p.9), antiplatelet drug (p.36), and antipyretic

Overdose danger rating High

Dependence rating Low
Prescription needed No
Available as generic Yes

GENERAL INFORMATION

In use for over 80 years, aspirin relieves pain, reduces fever, and alleviates the symptoms of arthritis. In low doses, it helps to prevent blood clots, particularly in atherosclerosis or angina due to coronary artery disease. It also reduces the risk of heart attacks and strokes in people with known medical problems.

It is present in many medicines for colds, flu, headaches, menstrual period pains, and joint or muscular aches.

Aspirin may irritate the stomach and even cause stomach ulcers or bleeding. It can also cause Reye's syndrome, a rare brain and liver disorder usually occurring in children. For this reason, aspirin should not be given to children under 12 except under close medical supervision. Another drawback of aspirin is that it can provoke asthma attacks.

INFORMATION FOR USERS

Follow instructions on the label. Call your doctor if symptoms worsen.
How taken Tablets, SR-capsules, suppositories.
Frequency and timing of doses Relief of pain or fever Every 4–6 hours, as necessary, with or after food or milk.
Prevention of blood clots Once daily.
Adult dosage range Relief of pain or fever 300–900mg per dose.
Prevention of blood clots 75–300mg daily.
Onset of effect 30–60 minutes (tablets); $1\frac{1}{2}$–8 hours (coated tablets/SR-capsules).
Duration of action Up to 12 hours. Effect persists for several days when used to prevent blood clotting.
Diet advice None.
Storage Keep in a closed container in a cool, dry place out of reach of children.
Missed dose Take as soon as you remember. If your next dose is due within 2 hours, take a single dose now and skip the next.
Stopping the drug Taken in the short term, aspirin can be safely stopped as soon as you no longer need it. Seek medical advice before stopping long-term treatment unless severe adverse effects occur (see below).

OVERDOSE ACTION

Seek immediate medical advice. Take emergency action if there is restlessness, stomach pain, ringing noises in the ears, blurred vision, or vomiting .

POSSIBLE ADVERSE EFFECTS

Adverse effects are more likely to occur with high doses of aspirin, but these may be reduced by taking the drug with food or in buffered or enteric coated forms. If you experience indigestion, rash, or wheezing, stop taking aspirin. If you vomit blood, have black bowel movements, or develop ringing noises in the ears, stop taking the drug and contact your doctor urgently.

INTERACTIONS

Anticoagulants Aspirin may add to the anticoagulant effect of such drugs, leading to an increased risk of abnormal bleeding.
Drugs for gout Aspirin may reduce the effect of these drugs.
Corticosteroids These drugs may increase the risk of stomach bleeding with aspirin.
NSAIDs These drugs may increase the likelihood of stomach irritation with aspirin.
Methotrexate Aspirin may increase the toxicity of this drug.
Oral antidiabetic drugs Aspirin may increase the effect of these drugs.

SPECIAL PRECAUTIONS

Be sure to consult your doctor or pharmacist before taking this drug if:
◆ You have long-term liver or kidney problems.
◆ You have asthma.
◆ You are allergic to aspirin.
◆ You have a blood clotting disorder.
◆ You have had a stomach ulcer.
◆ You are taking other medications.
Pregnancy Not usually recommended. An alternative drug may be safer. Discuss with your doctor.
Breast-feeding The drug passes into breast milk. Discuss with your doctor.
Infants and children Not recommended under 12 years.
Over 60 Adverse effects more likely.
Driving and hazardous work No special problems.

Alcohol Keep consumption low. Alcohol increases the likelihood of stomach irritation with this drug.

Surgery and general anaesthetics Regular treatment with aspirin may need to be stopped about one week before surgery. Discuss with your doctor or dentist before any operation.

PROLONGED USE

Except for low doses to help prevent blood clotting, aspirin should not be taken for longer than 2 days except on your doctor's advice. Prolonged use of aspirin may worsen asthma and lead to bleeding in, and ulcers of, the stomach.

Atenolol

Brand names Antipressan, Atenix, Tenormin, Totamol
Used in the following combined preparations
Beta-Adalat, Co-tenidone, Kalten, Tenchlor, Tenif, Tenoret, Tenoretic, Totaretic

QUICK REFERENCE

Drug group Beta blocker (p.28)
Overdose danger rating Medium
Dependence rating Low
Prescription needed Yes
Available as generic Yes

GENERAL INFORMATION

Atenolol belongs to the group of drugs known as the beta blockers. It prevents the heart from beating too quickly and is used mainly to treat irregular heart rhythms, angina, and high blood pressure. Atenolol may also be given after a heart attack to protect the heart from further damage.

Atenolol is a cardioselective beta blocker (see p.28) and is less likely to provoke breathing difficulties. However, it should still be used with caution by people suffering from asthma, bronchitis, or other forms of respiratory disease. The drug is sometimes prescribed together with a diuretic for high blood pressure.

Atenolol does not cure heart disease; it only controls the symptoms. Therefore, it may have to be taken regularly over a long period of time, even for life.

INFORMATION FOR USERS

Your drug prescription is tailored for you. Do not alter dosage without checking with your doctor.

How taken Tablets, liquid, injection.
Frequency and timing of doses 1–2 x daily.
Adult dosage range 25–100mg daily.
Onset of effect 2–4 hours.
Duration of action 20–30 hours.
Diet advice None.
Storage Keep in a tightly closed container in a cool, dry place out of reach of children. Protect from light.
Missed dose Take as soon as you remember. If your next dose of atenolol is due within 6 hours, do not take the missed dose but take the next scheduled dose as usual.
Stopping the drug Unless you experience wheezing or difficulty in breathing, do not stop taking atenolol without consulting your doctor. Sudden withdrawal of atenolol may lead to dangerous worsening of the underlying condition; the drug should be withdrawn gradually.
Exceeding the dose An occasional unintentional extra dose is unlikely to be a cause for concern. But if you notice any unusual symptoms, or if a large overdose has been taken, notify your doctor.

POSSIBLE ADVERSE EFFECTS

Atenolol has adverse effects that are common to most beta blockers and include aching muscles, dry eyes, and cold hands and feet. Symptoms tend to diminish with long-term use. If wheezing or difficulty in breathing occur, stop taking the drug and consult your doctor immediately.

INTERACTIONS

Anti-arrhythmic drugs Used together with atenolol, these may increase the risk of adverse effects on the heart.
Antidiabetic drugs Used with atenolol, these may increase the risk and/or mask many symptoms of low blood sugar.
Decongestants Used with atenolol, these may increase blood pressure and heart rate.
Calcium channel blockers Taken with atenolol, some of these drugs may further decrease blood pressure and/or heart rate and may reduce the force of the heart's pumping action.

NSAIDs These drugs may reduce the anti-hypertensive effect of atenolol.

SPECIAL PRECAUTIONS
Be sure to tell your doctor if:
◆ You have a long-term kidney problem.
◆ You have diabetes.
◆ You have a lung disorder such as asthma or bronchitis.
◆ You are taking other medications.

Pregnancy Safety in pregnancy not established. Discuss with your doctor.
Breast-feeding The drug passes into the breast milk. Discuss with your doctor.
Infants and children Not recommended.
Over 60 No special problems. Reduced dose may be necessary if there is impaired kidney function.
Driving and hazardous work Avoid such activities until you have learned how atenolol affects you because the drug can cause dizziness.
Alcohol No special problems with small intake.
Surgery and general anaesthetics Atenolol may need to be stopped before you have a general anaesthetic. Discuss this with your doctor or dentist before any surgery.

PROLONGED USE
No special problems expected.

Atorvastatin

Brand name Lipitor
Used in the following combined preparations
None

Drug group Lipid-lowering drug (p.35)
Overdose danger rating Low
Dependence rating Low
Prescription needed Yes
Available as generic No

GENERAL INFORMATION
Atorvastatin is a member of the statin group of lipid-lowering drugs. It is used to treat hypercholesterolaemia (high blood cholesterol levels) in patients who have not responded to other treatments, such as a special diet, and are at risk of developing heart disease.

Atorvastatin blocks the action, in the liver, of an enzyme that is needed for the manufacture of cholesterol. As a result, blood levels of cholesterol are lowered, which can help to prevent coronary heart disease.

Rarely, atorvastatin can cause muscle pain, inflammation, and muscle damage. The risk is increased if the drug is given with a fibrate (another kind of lipid-lowering drug).

INFORMATION FOR USERS
Your drug prescription is tailored for you. Do not alter dosage without checking with your doctor.
How taken Tablets.
Frequency and timing of doses Once daily.
Adult dosage range 10–40mg; up to 80mg (inherited hypercholesterolaemia).
Onset of effect Within 2 weeks. Full beneficial effects may not be felt for 4–6 weeks.
Duration of action 20–30 hours.
Diet advice A low-fat diet is usually recommended.
Storage Keep in a closed container in a cool, dry place out of reach of children.
Missed dose Take as soon as you remember. If your next dose is due within 8 hours, do not take the missed dose, but take the next one on schedule.
Stopping the drug Do not stop taking atorvastatin without consulting your doctor. Stopping the drug may lead to recurrence of the original condition.
Exceeding the dose An occasional unintentional extra dose is unlikely to cause problems. Large overdoses may cause liver problems. Notify your doctor.

POSSIBLE ADVERSE EFFECTS
Adverse effects of atorvastatin, which include nausea, headache, and insomnia, are usually mild and transient. Muscle damage is a rare side effect, and muscle aching or weakness or a rash should be reported to your doctor at once.

INTERACTIONS
Anticoagulant drugs Atorvastatin may increase the effect of anticoagulants.
Antifungal drugs Itraconazole, ketoconazole, and possibly other antifungals, may increase the risk of muscle damage with atorvastatin.

Other lipid-lowering drugs Taken with atorvastatin, these drugs may increase the risk of muscle damage.
Ciclosporin and other immunosuppressant drugs Atorvastatin is not usually prescribed with these drugs because of the increased risk of muscle damage.

SPECIAL PRECAUTIONS
Be sure to tell your doctor if:
◆ You have had liver problems.
◆ You are a heavy drinker.
◆ You are taking other medications.
Pregnancy Not usually prescribed. Safety not established. Discuss with your doctor.
Breast-feeding Safety not established. Discuss with your doctor.
Infants and children Not recommended.
Over 60 No special problems.
Driving and hazardous work No special problems.
Alcohol Avoid excessive amounts. Alcohol may increase the risk of developing liver problems with atorvastatin.

PROLONGED USE
Long-term use of atorvastatin can affect liver function.
Monitoring Regular blood tests to check liver and muscle function are needed.

Atropine

Brand name Minims Atropine
Used in the following combined preparations
Actonorm, Co-phenotrope, Isopto Atropine, Lomotil

QUICK REFERENCE
Drug group Anticholinergic drug for irritable bowel syndrome (p.43) and mydriatic drug (p.112)
Overdose danger rating High
Dependence rating Low
Prescription needed Yes
Available as generic Yes

GENERAL INFORMATION
Atropine is an anticholinergic drug. Because of its antispasmodic action, which relaxes the muscle wall of the intestine, the drug has been used to relieve abdominal cramps in irritable bowel syndrome. Atropine may also

be prescribed in combination with diphenoxylate, an antidiarrhoeal drug. This combination can be dangerous in overdosage, however, particularly in young children.

Atropine eye drops, used to enlarge the pupil during eye examinations, are part of the treatment for uveitis.

Atropine may be used as part of the premedication before a general anaesthetic. It is occasionally injected to restore normal heart beat in heart block (p.32).

Atropine must be used with caution in children and the elderly due to their sensitivity to the drug's effects.

INFORMATION FOR USERS
Your drug prescription is tailored for you. Do not alter dosage without checking with your doctor.
How taken Tablets, injection, eye ointment, eye drops.
Frequency and timing of doses Once only, or up to 4 times daily according to condition (eye drops); as directed (other forms).
Adult dosage range 1–2 drops as directed (eye drops); as directed (other forms).
Onset of effect Varies according to method of administration. 30 minutes (eye drops).
Duration of action 7 days or longer (eye drops); several hours (other forms).
Diet advice None.
Storage Keep in a closed container in a cool, dry place out of reach of children. Protect from light.
Missed dose Take as soon as you remember. If your next dose is due within 2 hours, take a single dose now and skip the next.
Stopping the drug Do not stop taking the drug without consulting your doctor.

OVERDOSE ACTION
Seek immediate medical advice in all cases. Take emergency action if palpitations, tremor, delirium, fits, or loss of consciousness occur.

POSSIBLE ADVERSE EFFECTS
The use of this drug is limited by the frequency of its anticholinergic effects. These include blurred vision, dry mouth, constipation, difficulty in passing urine, palpitations, and confusion, which should be reported to

your doctor at once. In addition to these effects, atropine eye drops may cause stinging.

INTERACTIONS

Anticholinergic drugs Atropine increases the risk of side effects from drugs that also have anticholinergic effects.

Ketoconazole Atropine reduces the absorption of ketoconazole from the digestive tract. Increased dose may be necessary.

SPECIAL PRECAUTIONS

Be sure to tell your doctor if:
◆ You have long-term liver or kidney problems.
◆ You have glaucoma.
◆ You have urinary difficulties.
◆ You have ulcerative colitis.
◆ You wear contact lenses (eye drops).
◆ You have heart problems or high blood pressure.
◆ You are taking other medications.

Pregnancy Safety in pregnancy not established. Discuss with your doctor.

Breast-feeding The drug passes into the breast milk and may affect the baby. Discuss with your doctor.

Infants and children Combination with diphenoxylate not recommended under 4 years; reduced dose necessary in older children.

Over 60 Increased likelihood of adverse effects.

Driving and hazardous work Avoid such activities until you have learned how atropine affects you because the drug can cause blurred vision and may impair concentration.

Alcohol No special problems.

PROLONGED USE

No problems expected.

Azathioprine

Brand names Azamune, Immunoprin, Imuran, Oprisine

Used in the following combined preparations
None

QUICK REFERENCE

Drug group Antirheumatic drug (p.50) and immunosuppressant drug (p.96)

Overdose danger rating Medium

Dependence rating Low

Prescription needed Yes

Available as generic Yes

GENERAL INFORMATION

Azathioprine is an immunosuppressant drug that is used to prevent the rejection of transplanted organs by the immune system. The drug is also given for severe rheumatoid arthritis that has failed to respond to conventional drug therapy.

Autoimmune and collagen diseases (including polymyositis, systemic lupus erythematosus, myasthenia gravis, and dermatomyositis) may be treated with azathioprine, usually when corticosteroids have not been effective.

Azathioprine is administered only under close supervision because of the risk of serious adverse effects. These include suppression of the production of white blood cells, thereby increasing the risk of infection as well as the risk of excessive or prolonged bleeding.

INFORMATION FOR USERS

Your drug prescription is tailored for you. Do not alter dosage without checking with your doctor.

How taken Tablets, injection.

Frequency and timing of doses Usually once daily with or after food.

Dosage range Initially according to body weight and the condition being treated and then adjusted according to response.

Onset of effect 2–4 weeks. Antirheumatic effect may not be felt for 8 weeks or more.

Duration of action The immunosuppressant effects may last for several weeks after the drug is stopped.

Diet advice None.

Storage Keep in a closed container in a cool, dry place out of reach of children. Protect from light.

Missed dose Take as soon as you remember, then return to your normal schedule. If more than 2 doses are missed, consult your doctor.

Stopping the drug Do not stop taking the drug without consulting your doctor. If taken to prevent graft transplant rejection, stopping treatment could provoke the rejection of the transplant.

Exceeding the dose An occasional unintentional extra dose is unlikely to cause problems. Large overdoses may cause nausea, vomiting, abdominal pains, and diarrhoea. Seek urgent medical advice.

POSSIBLE ADVERSE EFFECT

The most common effects of azathioprine are nausea, loss of appetite, thinning hair, weakness, and fatigue. The drug may also cause adverse effects on the blood which could lead to sore throat and fever; unusual bleeding or bruising may be a sign of reduced levels of platelets in the blood. In either case, call your doctor urgently.

INTERACTIONS

Allopurinol Allopurinol increases the effects and toxicity of azathioprine; dosage of one or both drugs will need to be reduced.

Warfarin Azathioprine may reduce the effect of warfarin.

Co-trimoxazole and trimethoprim These drugs may increase the risk of blood problems if taken with azathioprine.

SPECIAL PRECAUTIONS

Be sure to tell your doctor if:
◆ You have long-term liver or kidney problems.
◆ You have had a previous allergic reaction to azathioprine or 6-mercaptopurine.
◆ You have recently had shingles or chickenpox.
◆ You have an infection.
◆ You have a blood disorder.
◆ You are taking other medications.

Pregnancy Azathioprine has been taken in pregnancy without problems. Discuss with your doctor.

Breast-feeding A small amount of the drug passes into the breast milk. Discuss with your doctor.

Infants and children No special problems.

Over 60 Increased likelihood of adverse effects. Reduced dose necessary.

Driving and hazardous work Avoid such activities until you have learned how azathioprine affects you because the drug can cause weakness and fatigue.

Alcohol No special problems.

PROLONGED USE

There may be a slightly increased risk of some cancers with long-term use of azathioprine. Blood changes may also occur. Avoidance of exposure to sunlight may help to prevent adverse skin effects.

Monitoring Regular checks on blood composition are usually carried out.

Baclofen

Brand names Baclospas, Balgifen, Lioresal
Used in the following combined preparations
None.

QUICK REFERENCE
Drug group Muscle-relaxant drug (p.52)
Overdose danger rating Medium
Dependence rating Low
Prescription needed Yes
Available as generic Yes

GENERAL INFORMATION

Baclofen is a muscle-relaxant drug that acts on the central nervous system, including the spinal cord. The drug relieves the spasms, cramping, and rigidity of muscles caused by a variety of disorders, including multiple sclerosis and spinal cord injury. Baclofen is also used to treat the spasticity that results from brain injury, cerebral palsy, or stroke. Although this drug does not cure any of these disorders, it increases mobility, allowing other treatment, such as physiotherapy, to be carried out.

Baclofen is less likely to cause muscle weakness than similar drugs, and its side effects, such as dizziness or drowsiness, are usually temporary. Elderly people are more susceptible to side effects, however, especially during the early stages of treatment.

INFORMATION FOR USERS

Your drug prescription is tailored for you. Do not alter dosage without checking with your doctor.
How taken Tablets, liquid, injection (specialist use).
Frequency and timing of doses 3 x daily with food or milk.
Adult dosage range 15mg daily (starting dose). Daily dose may be increased by 15mg every 3 days as necessary. Maximum daily dose: 100mg.
Onset of effect Some benefits may appear after 1–3 hours, but full beneficial effects may not be felt for several weeks. A dose 1 hour before a specific task will improve mobility.
Duration of action Up to 8 hours.
Diet advice None.

Storage Keep in a closed container in a cool, dry place out of reach of children. Protect liquid from light.
Missed dose Take as soon as you remember. If your next dose is due within 2 hours, take a single dose now and skip the next.
Stopping the drug Do not stop taking the drug without consulting your doctor, who will supervise a gradual reduction in dosage. Abrupt cessation of the drug may cause hallucinations, fits, and worsening spasticity.
Exceeding the dose An occasional unintentional extra dose is unlikely to cause problems. Large overdoses may cause weakness, vomiting, and severe drowsiness. Notify your doctor.

POSSIBLE ADVERSE EFFECTS

Common adverse effects, such as confusion, dizziness, or drowsiness, are related to the drug's sedative effects. Such effects are minimized by starting with a low dose, which is gradually increased. Muscle weakness and difficulty in passing urine may also occur.

INTERACTIONS
Antihypertensive and diuretic drugs Baclofen may increase the blood-pressure lowering effect of such drugs.
Drugs for parkinsonism Some drugs used for parkinsonism may cause confusion and hallucinations if taken with baclofen. Sedatives All drugs with a sedative effect on the central nervous system may increase sedative properties of baclofen.
Tricyclic antidepressants may increase the effects of baclofen, leading to muscle weakness.

SPECIAL PRECAUTIONS
Be sure to tell your doctor if:
◆ You have long-term liver or kidney problems.
◆ You have difficulty in passing urine.
◆ You have had a peptic ulcer.
◆ You have had epileptic fits.
◆ You have diabetes.
◆ You suffer with breathing problems.
◆ You are taking other medications.
Pregnancy Safety in pregnancy not established. Discuss with your doctor.
Breast-feeding The drug passes into the breast milk, but at normal doses adverse effects are unlikely. Discuss with your doctor.

Infants and children Reduced dose necessary.
Over 60 Increased likelihood of adverse effects. Reduced dose may therefore be necessary.
Driving and hazardous work Avoid such activities until you have learned how baclofen affects you because the drug can cause confusion and drowsiness.
Alcohol Avoid excessive amounts. Alcohol may increase the sedative effects of this drug.
Surgery and general anaesthetics Be sure to inform your doctor or dentist that you are taking baclofen before you have a general anaesthetic.

PROLONGED USE
No problems expected.

Beclometasone

Brand names Beclazone, Becloforte, Becodisks, Beconase, Becotide, Filair, Qvar, and others
Used in the following combined preparation Ventide

QUICK REFERENCE
Drug group Corticosteroid (p.78) and Topical corticosteroid (p.116)
Overdose danger rating Low
Dependence rating Low
Prescription needed No (some preparations)
Available as generic Yes

GENERAL INFORMATION
Beclometasone is a corticosteroid drug prescribed to relieve the symptoms of allergic rhinitis (as a nasal spray) and to control asthma (as an inhalant). It controls nasal symptoms by reducing inflammation and mucus production in the nose. It also helps to reduce chest symptoms, such as wheezing and coughing. Asthma sufferers may take beclometasone regularly to reduce the severity and frequency of attacks. Once an attack has started, however, the drug does not relieve symptoms.

Beclometasone is given primarily to people whose asthma has not responded to bronchodilators alone (p.23). Beclometasone is also used as the main ingredient in some skin creams and ointments but is not usually used on the face.

Few serious adverse effects are associated with beclometasone as it is given topically by nasal spray or inhaler. Fungal infections causing mouth and throat irritation are a possible side effect of inhaling it. These can be avoided to some degree by using a spacer device (see p.23) and by rinsing the mouth and gargling with water after each inhalation.

INFORMATION FOR USERS
Your drug prescription is tailored for you. Do not alter dosage without checking with your doctor.
How taken Cream, ointment, inhaler, nasal spray.
Frequency and timing of doses 2–4 x daily.
Dosage range *Adults* 1–2 puffs 3–4 x daily according to preparation used (asthma); 1–2 sprays in each nostril 2–4 x daily (allergic rhinitis); as directed (skin conditions). *Children* Reduced dose according to age and weight.
Onset of effect Within 1 week (asthma); 1–3 days (allergic rhinitis). Full benefit may not be felt for up to 4 weeks.
Duration of action Several days after stopping the drug.
Diet advice None.
Storage Keep in a closed container in a cool, dry place out of reach of children. Protect from light.
Missed dose Take as soon as you remember. If your next dose is due within 2 hours, take a single dose now and skip the next.
Stopping the drug Do not stop taking the drug without consulting your doctor; symptoms may recur. Sometimes a gradual reduction in dosage is recommended.
Exceeding the dose An occasional unintentional extra dose is unlikely to cause problems. But if you notice any unusual symptoms, or if a large overdose has been taken, notify your doctor. Adverse effects may occur if the recommended dose is regularly exceeded over a prolonged period.

POSSIBLE ADVERSE EFFECTS
The main side effects of the nasal spray and inhaler are irritation of the nasal passages and fungal infection of the throat and mouth, which may lead to sore throat or hoarseness. More serious side effects, such as

permanent skin changes, may be seen with the ointment, which should not normally be used on the face.

INTERACTIONS

None.

SPECIAL PRECAUTIONS

Be sure to tell your doctor if:
◆ You have had tuberculosis or another nasal or respiratory infection.
◆ You have a skin infection (cream/ointment).
◆ You have varicose ulcers (cream/ointment).
◆ You are taking other medications.
Pregnancy No evidence of risk.
Breast-feeding No evidence of risk.
Infants and children Reduced dose necessary. Avoid prolonged use of ointment in infants and children.
Over 60 No known problems.
Driving and hazardous work No known problems.
Alcohol No known problems.

PROLONGED USE

No problems expected when used for asthma or rhinitis, but high doses of nasal spray can give systemic effects. Prolonged use of cream or ointment should be avoided where possible because it can cause permanent skin changes, especially on the face, and high doses can suppress the body's own corticosteroid production.
Monitoring Periodic checks to ensure that the adrenal glands are functioning healthily may be required if large doses are being used.

Bendroflumethiazide (Bendrofluazide)

Brand names Aprinox, Berkozide, Neo-Bendromax, Neo-NaClex
Used in the following combined preparations Corgaretic, Inderetic, Inderex, Neo-NaClex-K, Prestim

QUICK REFERENCE

Drug group Thiazide diuretic (p.30)
Overdose danger rating Low
Dependence rating Low
Prescription needed Yes
Available as generic Yes

GENERAL INFORMATION

Bendroflumethiazide belongs to the group of drugs known as the thiazide diuretics, which remove excess water from the body. It is frequently used as a treatment for high blood pressure (see Antihypertensive drugs, p.34). It is also used in higher doses to reduce oedema (water retention) caused by heart conditions, and for treating premenstrual oedema.

As with all thiazides, the drug increases the loss of potassium in the urine, which can cause a variety of symptoms (see p.31), and increases the likelihood of irregular heart rhythms, particularly in people taking drugs such as digoxin for heart failure. Potassium supplements are often given with bendroflumethiazide to counteract this effect.

INFORMATION FOR USERS

Your drug prescription is tailored for you. Do not alter dosage without checking with your doctor.
How taken Tablets.
Frequency and timing of doses Once daily, early in the day. (Sometimes 1–3 x per week.)
Adult dosage range 2.5–10mg daily.
Onset of effect Within 2 hours.
Duration of action 6–12 hours.
Diet advice This drug may reduce potassium in the body, so you should eat plenty of fresh fruit and vegetables. Discuss with your doctor the advisability of reducing salt intake as a further precaution for hypertension.
Storage Keep in a closed container in a cool, dry place out of reach of children.
Missed dose No cause for concern, but take as soon as you remember; but if it is late in the day, do not take the missed dose or you may need to get up during the night to pass urine. Take the next scheduled dose as usual.
Stopping the drug Do not stop taking the drug without consulting your doctor; symptoms may recur.
Exceeding the dose An occasional unintentional extra dose is unlikely to be a cause for concern. But if you notice any unusual symptoms, or if a large overdose has been taken, notify your doctor.

POSSIBLE ADVERSE EFFECTS

Some adverse effects, such as nausea, fatigue, and leg cramps, are the result of excessive loss of potassium but can usually be corrected by taking a potassium supplement. Impotence is a recognized adverse effect. Bendroflumethiazide may precipitate gout in susceptible people, and certain forms of diabetes may become more difficult to control. The blood cholesterol level may rise.

INTERACTIONS

NSAIDs These drugs may reduce the diuretic effect of bendroflumethiazide, which, conversely, may increase kidney toxicity of NSAIDs.

Digoxin The effects of digoxin may be increased if excessive potassium is lost.

Anti-arrhythmic drugs Low potassium levels may increase the toxicity of these drugs.

Lithium Bendroflumethiazide may increase lithium levels in the blood.

Corticosteroids These drugs further increase the loss of potassium from the body when taken with bendroflumethiazide. Potassium supplements may be necessary.

SPECIAL PRECAUTIONS

Be sure to tell your doctor if:
◆ You have long-term liver or kidney problems.
◆ You have had gout.
◆ You have diabetes.
◆ You have Addison's disease.
◆ You have systemic lupus erythematosus (SLE)
◆ You are taking other medications.

Pregnancy Not usually prescribed. Safety in pregnancy not established. May affect the baby adversely. Discuss with your doctor.

Breast-feeding The drug passes into the breast milk and may reduce your milk supply. Discuss with your doctor.

Infants and children Not usually prescribed. Reduced dose necessary.

Over 60 Reduced dose may be necessary.

Driving and hazardous work No special problems.

Alcohol No problems expected if consumption is kept low.

PROLONGED USE

Prolonged use of this drug can lead to excessive loss of potassium and imbalances of other salts.

Monitoring Blood tests may be performed periodically to check kidney function and levels of potassium and other salts.

Benzoyl Peroxide

Brand names Acnecide, Nericur, Panoxyl
Used in the following combined preparations
Acnidazil, Benzamycin, Quinoderm, Quinoped

QUICK REFERENCE

Drug group Drug for acne (p.119) and fungal skin infections (p.74)
Overdose danger rating Low
Dependence rating Low
Prescription needed No
Available as generic No

GENERAL INFORMATION

Benzoyl peroxide is used in a variety of topical preparations for the treatment of acne and some fungal skin infections, particularly of the feet. Available over the counter, it comes in concentrations of varying strengths for moderate acne.

Benzoyl peroxide works by removing the top layer of skin and unblocking the sebaceous glands. The drug reduces inflammation of blocked hair follicles by killing bacteria that infect them.

Benzoyl peroxide may cause irritation due to its drying effect on the skin, but this generally diminishes with time. The drug should be applied to the affected areas as directed on the label. Washing the area prior to application greatly enhances the drug's beneficial effects. Side effects are less likely if treatment is started with a preparation containing a low concentration of benzoyl peroxide, and changed to a stronger preparation only if necessary. Marked dryness and peeling of the skin may occur but can usually be controlled by reducing the frequency of application. Care should be taken to avoid contact of the drug with the eyes, mouth, and mucous membranes. Preparations of benzoyl peroxide may bleach clothing.

INFORMATION FOR USERS

Follow instructions on the label. Call your doctor if symptoms worsen.

How taken Cream, lotion, gel.
Frequency and timing of doses 1–2 x daily.
Dosage range Apply sparingly to affected skin, as instructed on the label.
Onset of effect Reduces oiliness of skin immediately. Acne usually improves within 4–6 weeks.
Duration of action 24–48 hours.
Diet advice None.
Storage Keep in a closed container in a cool, dry place out of reach of children.
Missed dose Apply as soon as you remember.
Stopping the drug Can be safely stopped as soon as you no longer need it.
Exceeding the dose A single extra application is unlikely to cause problems. Regular overuse may result in extensive irritation, peeling, redness, and swelling.

POSSIBLE ADVERSE EFFECTS

Application of benzoyl peroxide may cause temporary burning or stinging of the skin. Redness, peeling, and swelling may result from excessive drying of the skin and usually clears up if the treatment is stopped or used less frequently. If severe burning, blistering, or crusting occur, stop using benzoyl peroxide and consult your doctor.

INTERACTIONS

Skin-drying preparations Medicated cosmetics, soaps, toiletries, and other anti-acne preparations increase the likelihood of dryness and irritation of the skin with benzoyl peroxide.

SPECIAL PRECAUTIONS

Be sure to consult your doctor or pharmacist before using this drug if:
◆ You have eczema.
◆ You have sunburn.
◆ You have had a previous allergic reaction to benzoyl peroxide.
◆ You are taking other medications.
Pregnancy No evidence of risk.
Breast-feeding No evidence of risk.
Infants and children Not recommended under 12 years except under medical supervision.
Over 60 Not usually required.
Driving and hazardous work No known problems.
Alcohol No known problems.

PROLONGED USE

Benzoyl peroxide should not be used for longer than 6 weeks except on the advice of your doctor.

Betahistine

Brand name Serc
Used in the following combined preparations
None

QUICK REFERENCE

Drug group Drug for Ménière's disease (p.21)
Overdose danger rating High
Dependence rating Low
Prescription needed Yes
Available as generic No

GENERAL INFORMATION

Betahistine, a drug that resembles the naturally occurring substance histamine in some of its effects, was introduced in the 1970s as a treatment for Ménière's disease, which is caused by the pressure of excess fluid in the inner ear.

Taken regularly, betahistine reduces the frequency and severity of the nausea and vertigo attacks that characterize this condition. It is also effective in treating tinnitus (ringing in the ears). The drug is thought to work by reducing pressure in the inner ear, possibly by improving blood flow in the small blood vessels. Drug treatment is not successful in all cases, and surgery may be needed.

INFORMATION FOR USERS

Your drug prescription is tailored for you. Do not alter dosage without checking with your doctor.
How taken Tablets.
Frequency and timing of doses 3 x daily after food.
Adult dosage range 24–48mg daily.
Onset of effect Within 1 hour.
Duration of action 6–12 hours.
Diet advice None.
Storage Keep in a closed container in a cool, dry place out of reach of children.
Missed dose Take as soon as you remember. If your next dose is due within 2 hours, take a single dose now and skip the next.

Stopping the drug Do not stop taking the drug without consulting your doctor; symptoms may recur.

OVERDOSE ACTION
Seek immediate medical advice in all cases. Large overdoses may cause collapse requiring emergency action.

POSSIBLE ADVERSE EFFECTS
Adverse effects of betahistine are minor and rarely cause problems. Nausea, indigestion, and headache may occur.

INTERACTIONS
None.

SPECIAL PRECAUTIONS
Be sure to tell your doctor if:
◆ You have asthma.
◆ You have a peptic ulcer.
◆ You have phaeochromocytoma.
◆ You are taking other medications.
Pregnancy Safety in pregnancy not established. Discuss with your doctor.
Breast-feeding The drug passes into the breast milk, but at normal doses adverse effects on the baby are unlikely. Discuss with your doctor.
Infants and children Not recommended.
Over 60 No special problems.
Driving and hazardous work No special problems.
Alcohol No special problems.

PROLONGED USE
No special problems.

Betamethasone

Brand names Betacap, Betnelan, Betnesol, Betnovate, Bettamousse, Diprosone, Vista-Methasone
Used in the following combined preparations
Betnesol-N, Betnovate-C, Betnovate-N, Diprosalic, Fucibet, Lotriderm

QUICK REFERENCE
Drug group Corticosteroid (p.78)
Overdose danger rating Low
Dependence rating Low
Prescription needed Yes
Available as generic Yes

GENERAL INFORMATION
Betamethasone is a corticosteroid drug used to treat a variety of conditions. When injected directly into the joints it relieves joint inflammation and the pain and stiffness of rheumatoid arthritis. It is also given by mouth or injection to treat certain endocrine conditions affecting the pituitary and adrenal glands, and some blood disorders. It is also used topically to treat skin complaints, such as eczema and psoriasis.

When taken for short periods, low or moderate doses rarely cause serious side effects. High dosages or prolonged use can lead to symptoms such as peptic ulcers, weak bones, muscle weakness, and thin skin, and may retard growth in children.

INFORMATION FOR USERS
Your drug prescription is tailored for you. Do not alter dosage without checking with your doctor.
How taken Tablets, injection, cream, ointment, lotion, scalp solution, eye ointment, eye/ear/nose drops.
Frequency and timing of doses Usually once daily in the morning (systemic). Otherwise varies according to disorder being treated.
Dosage range Varies; follow your doctor's instructions.
Onset of effect
Within 30 minutes (injection); within 48 hours (other forms).
Duration of action Up to 24 hours.
Diet advice A low-sodium and high potassium diet may be recommended when the oral form of the drug is prescribed for extended periods. Follow the advice of your doctor.
Storage Keep in a closed container in a cool, dry place out of reach of children. Protect from light.
Missed dose Take as soon as you remember. If your next dose is due within 2 hours, take a single dose now and skip the next.
Stopping the drug Do not stop tablets without consulting your doctor, who may supervise gradual reduction dosage. Stopping abruptly after long-term treatment may cause pituitary and adrenal gland problems.
Exceeding the dose An occasional unintentional extra dose is unlikely to cause problems. However, if you notice any unusual

symptoms, or if a large overdose has been taken, notify your doctor.

POSSIBLE ADVERSE EFFECTS
Topical preparations are unlikely to cause adverse effects unless overused. Serious adverse effects usually occur only with high doses taken by mouth for long periods. They include indigestion, peptic ulcers, acne, mood changes, skin thinning, and muscle weakness.

INTERACTIONS
Insulin, antidiabetic drugs, and oral anticoagulant drugs Betamethasone may alter insulin requirements and the effects of these drugs.
Vaccines Serious reactions can occur when certain vaccinations are given during betamethasone treatment.
Antihypertensive drugs and drugs used in myasthenia gravis Betamethasone may reduce the effects of these drugs.
Anticonvulsants These drugs may reduce the effects of betamethasone.

SPECIAL PRECAUTIONS
Be sure to tell your doctor if:
◆ You suffer from a mental disorder.
◆ You have a heart condition.
◆ You have glaucoma.
◆ You have high blood pressure.
◆ You have a history of epilepsy.
◆ You have had a peptic ulcer.
◆ You have had tuberculosis.
◆ You have any infection.
◆ You have diabetes.
◆ You have liver or kidney problems.
◆ You are taking other medications.
Avoid exposure to chickenpox, measles, or shingles if you are on systemic treatment.
Pregnancy No evidence of risk with topical preparations. Low doses of tablets are unlikely to harm the baby. Discuss with your doctor.
Breast-feeding No evidence of risk with topical preparations. In normal doses taken by mouth, adverse effects on the baby are unlikely. Discuss with your doctor.
Infants and children Reduced dose necessary.
Over 60 Reduced dose may be necessary.
Driving and hazardous work No known problems.
Alcohol Keep consumption low. Betamethasone tablets increase the risk of peptic ulcers.

PROLONGED USE
People taking betamethasone tablets regularly should carry a "steroid treatment card". Prolonged use by mouth can lead to peptic ulcers, thin skin, fragile bones, muscle weakness, and adrenal gland suppression; it can also retard growth in children.

Bezafibrate

Brand names Bezalip, Bezalip-Mono
Used in the following combined preparations
None

QUICK REFERENCE
Drug group Lipid-lowering drug (p.35)
Overdose danger rating Low
Dependence rating Low
Prescription needed Yes
Available as generic No

GENERAL INFORMATION
Bezafibrate belongs to the group of drugs, usually called fibrates, that lower lipid levels in the blood. Fibrates are particularly effective in decreasing levels of triglycerides in the blood. They also reduce blood levels of cholesterol. Raised levels of lipids (fats) in the blood are associated with atherosclerosis (deposition of fat in blood vessel walls). This can lead to coronary heart disease (for example, angina and heart attacks) and cerebrovascular disease (for example, stroke). When bezafibrate is taken with a diet low in saturated fats, there is good evidence that the chances of a heart attack are reduced.

INFORMATION FOR USERS
Your drug prescription is tailored for you. Do not alter dosage without checking with your doctor.
How taken Tablets.
Frequency and timing of doses 1–3 x daily with a little liquid after a meal.
Adult dosage range 400–600mg daily.
Onset of effect A beneficial effect on blood fat levels may not be produced for some weeks, and it takes months or years for fat deposits in the arteries to be reduced. Treatment should be withdrawn if no adequate response is obtained within 3–4 months.

Duration of action About 6–24 hours. This may vary according to the individual.

Diet advice A low-fat diet will have been recommended. Follow your doctor's advice.

Storage Keep in a closed container in a cool, dry place out of reach of children.

Missed dose Take as soon as you remember. If your next dose is due within 4 hours (and you take it once daily), take a single dose now and skip the next. If you take 2–3 times daily, take the next dose as normal.

Stopping the drug Do not stop taking the drug without consulting your doctor.

Exceeding the dose An occasional unintentional extra dose is unlikely to be a cause for concern. But if you notice unusual symptoms, notify your doctor.

POSSIBLE ADVERSE EFFECTS

The most common adverse effects are on the gastrointestinal tract (e.g., loss of appetite and nausea) but normally diminish as treatment continues. If headache, muscle pain, dizziness, or rash occur, consult your doctor.

INTERACTIONS

Anticoagulants Bezafibrate may increase the effect of anticoagulants such as warfarin. Your doctor will reduce the dosage of your anticoagulant when starting bezafibrate.

MAOIs There is a risk of liver damage when bezafibrate is taken with an MAOI.

Antidiabetic drugs Bezafibrate may interact with these drugs to lower blood sugar levels.

Pravastatin, simvastatin, and other lipid lowering drugs whose names end in 'statin' There is an increased risk of muscle damage if bezafibrate is taken with these drugs.

SPECIAL PRECAUTIONS

Be sure to tell your doctor if:
◆ You have long-term liver or kidney problems.
◆ You have a history of gallbladder disease.
◆ You are taking other medications.

Pregnancy Safety in pregnancy not established. Discuss with your doctor.

Breast-feeding The drug may pass into the breast milk and may affect the baby. Discuss with your doctor.

Infants and children Not usually prescribed.

Over 60 No special problems expected.

Driving and hazardous work No special problems.

Alcohol Keep consumption low. Heavy intake of alcohol raises triglyceride levels, counteracting the effect of bezafibrate.

PROLONGED USE

No problems expected.

Monitoring Blood tests will be performed occasionally to monitor the effect of the drug on lipids in the blood.

Bromocriptine

Brand name Parlodel
Used in the following combined preparations
None

QUICK REFERENCE

Drug group Drug for parkinsonism (p.18) and pituitary agent (p.83)
Overdose danger rating Low
Dependence rating Low
Prescription needed Yes
Available as generic Yes

GENERAL INFORMATION

By inhibiting secretion of the hormone prolactin from the pituitary gland, bromocriptine is used in the treatment of conditions associated with excessive prolactin production. These include some types of female infertility and occasionally male infertility and impotence. Bromocriptine is effective in treating some benign breast conditions and other symptoms of menstrual disorders. The drug may also be used to suppress lactation in women who do not wish to breast-feed.

Bromocriptine reduces the release of growth hormone, and therefore is used in the treatment of acromegaly (see p.83).

Bromocriptine is also effective in relieving the symptoms of parkinsonism. The drug is now widely used to treat people who are in the advanced stages of parkinsonism when other drugs have failed or are unsuitable.

Serious adverse effects are uncommon with low doses. The most common problems, nausea and vomiting, can be minimized by taking bromocriptine with meals. In rare cases it may cause ulceration of the stomach.

INFORMATION FOR USERS

Your drug prescription is tailored for you. Do not alter dosage without checking with your doctor.

How taken Tablets, capsules.

Frequency and timing of doses 1–4 x daily with food.

Adult dosage range Dose given depends on the condition being treated and your response. In most cases treatment starts with a daily dose of 1–1.25mg, gradually increased until a satisfactory response is achieved.

Onset of effect Variable depending on the condition.

Duration of action About 8 hours.

Diet advice None.

Storage Keep in a closed container in a cool, dry place out of reach of children. Protect from light.

Missed dose Take as soon as you remember. If your next dose is due within 2 hours, take a single dose now and skip the next.

Stopping the drug Do not stop taking the drug without consulting your doctor; symptoms may recur.

Exceeding the dose An occasional unintentional extra dose is unlikely to be a cause for concern. If you notice any unusual symptoms, or if a large overdose has been taken, notify your doctor.

POSSIBLE ADVERSE EFFECTS

Adverse effects, such as nausea or vomiting and constipation, are usually dose-related. When used for parkinsonism, the drug may cause abnormal movements. If you experience dizziness, drowsiness, or headaches, consult your doctor.

INTERACTIONS

Antipsychotic drugs These drugs oppose the action of bromocriptine and increase the risk of parkinsonism.

Domperidone and metoclopramide These drugs may reduce some of bromocriptine's effects.

Sympathomimetic drugs These drugs increase the risk of toxic effects from bromocriptine.

SPECIAL PRECAUTIONS

Be sure to tell your doctor if:
◆ You have a stomach ulcer.
◆ You have a history of psychiatric disorders.

◆ You have heart problems.
◆ You have porphyria.
◆ You are taking other medications.

Pregnancy Safety in pregnancy not established. Discuss with your doctor.

Breast-feeding The drug suppresses milk production, and prevents it completely if given within 12 hours of delivery. If you wish to breast-feed, consult your doctor.

Infants and children Not usually prescribed under 15 years.

Over 60 Reduced dose may be necessary.

Driving and hazardous work Avoid such activities until you have learned how bromocriptine affects you because the drug may cause dizziness and drowsiness.

Alcohol Avoid. Alcohol increases the likelihood of confusion and reduces tolerance to bromocriptine.

PROLONGED USE

No special problems.

Monitoring Periodic blood tests may be performed to check hormone levels. Gynaecological tests may be carried out annually (or every six months in post-menopausal women). Monitoring for other, rare, adverse effects (e.g., peptic ulcer in acromegaly) may also be carried out.

Budesonide

Brand names Entocort, Pulmicort, Rhinocort Aqua
Used in the following combined preparations None

QUICK REFERENCE

Drug group Corticosteroid (p.78)
Overdose danger rating Low
Dependence rating Low
Prescription needed Yes
Available as generic No

GENERAL INFORMATION

Budesonide is a corticosteroid drug used in the form of slow-release capsules to relieve the symptoms of Crohn's disease and as an enema to treat ulcerative colitis. It is also used as an inhaler to prevent attacks of asthma but will not stop an existing attack. Like other corticosteroids, budesonide is used by people whose asthma is not controlled by bronchodilators (p.23) alone. It is also used as a nasal spray to relieve the symptoms of allergic rhinitis and for nasal polyps.

Budesonide controls symptoms by reducing inflammation, whether it is in the nose, lungs, or intestine.

There are fewer, usually less serious, side effects with the inhaler or nasal spray, since the drug is absorbed in much smaller quantities than when it is taken by mouth. Fungal infections causing irritation of the mouth and throat may occur, however. These can be avoided to some degree by using a spacer device (see p.23) and by rinsing the mouth and gargling with water after each inhalation.

INFORMATION FOR USERS
Your drug prescription is tailored for you. Do not alter dosage without checking with your doctor.
How taken SR-capsules, enema, inhaler, powder for inhalation, nasal spray.
Frequency and timing of doses Once daily before breakfast (capsules); once daily at bedtime (enema); twice daily (inhaler); once or twice daily (nasal spray).
Dosage range 3–9mg (capsules); 2mg (enema); 200–1,600 micrograms (inhaler), 100–200 micrograms (nasal spray).
Onset of effect *Asthma* Within 1 week. *Other conditions* 1–3 days.
Duration of action 12–24 hours.
Diet advice None.
Storage Keep in a closed container in a cool, dry place out of reach of children.
Missed dose Take as soon as you remember. If your next dose is due within 2 hours, take a single dose now and skip the next.
Stopping the drug Do not stop taking the drug without consulting your doctor; symptoms may recur. The SR-capsules used in Crohn's disease should be withdrawn gradually.
Exceeding the dose An occasional extra dose is unlikely to be a cause for concern. If you notice any unusual symptoms, or if a large overdose has been taken, notify your doctor.

POSSIBLE ADVERSE EFFECTS
The main side effects of inhalers and spray are irritation of the nasal passages and fungal infection of the mouth and throat, which may

cause hoarseness. High doses by mouth can cause weight gain, high blood pressure, indigestion, peptic ulcers, acne, mood changes, and muscle weakness.

INTERACTIONS
None.

SPECIAL PRECAUTIONS
Be sure to tell your doctor if:
◆ You have had tuberculosis or another respiratory infection.
◆ You are taking other medications.
Pregnancy No special problems.
Breast-feeding No evidence of risk.
Infants and children Reduced dose necessary.
Over 60 No special problems.
Driving and hazardous work No special problems.
Alcohol No special problems.

PROLONGED USE
Prolonged use may be required for asthma prevention. There may be a small risk of glaucoma, cataracts, and effects on bone with high doses inhaled for a prolonged period.
Monitoring If the drug is being taken in large doses, periodic checks may be needed to ensure that the adrenal glands are working properly. Children using inhalers may have their growth (height) monitored regularly.

Bumetanide

Brand names Burinex, Betinex
Used in the following combined preparations
Burinex A, Burinex K

QUICK REFERENCE
Drug group Loop diuretic (p.30)
Overdose danger rating Low
Dependence rating Low
Prescription needed Yes
Available as generic Yes

GENERAL INFORMATION
Bumetanide is a powerful, short-acting loop diuretic used to treat oedema (fluid retention) resulting from heart failure, nephrotic syndrome, and cirrhosis of the liver. Bumetanide is particularly useful in treating

people with impaired kidney function who do not respond well to thiazide diuretics. Because it is fast-acting, it is often injected in an emergency to relieve pulmonary oedema.

Bumetanide increases potassium loss in the urine, which can result in a wide variety of symptoms (see p.31). For this reason, potassium supplements or a diuretic that conserves potassium within the body are often given with the drug.

INFORMATION FOR USERS

Your drug prescription is tailored for you. Do not alter dosage without checking with your doctor.

How taken Tablets, liquid, injection.

Frequency and timing of doses Usually once daily in the morning; twice daily in some cases.

Dosage range 0.5–5mg daily. Dose may be increased if kidney function is impaired.

Onset of effect Within 30 minutes by mouth; more quickly by injection.

Duration of action 2–4 hours.

Diet advice Use of this drug may reduce potassium in the body. Eat plenty of fresh fruit and vegetables.

Storage Keep in a closed container in a cool, dry place out of reach of children. Protect from light.

Missed dose No cause for concern, but take as soon as you remember. If it is late in the day, however, do not take the missed dose, or you may need to get up during the night to pass urine. Take the next scheduled dose as usual.

Stopping the drug Do not stop taking the drug without consulting your doctor; symptoms may recur.

Exceeding the dose An occasional unintentional extra dose is unlikely to be a cause for concern. But if you notice any unusual symptoms, or if a large overdose has been taken, notify your doctor.

POSSIBLE ADVERSE EFFECTS

Adverse effects are due mainly to the rapid fluid loss produced by bumetanide, which can lead to dizziness and fainting. These diminish as the body adjusts. The drug may precipitate gout in susceptible people and can affect control of diabetes. If you experience lethargy, severe muscle cramps, nausea, vomiting, or a rash, consult your doctor.

INTERACTIONS

Anti-arrhythmic drugs Low potassium levels may increase the toxicity of these drugs with bumetanide.

Antibacterials Bumetanide increases the ear damage caused by some antibiotics.

Digoxin Excessive potassium loss may increase the adverse effects of digoxin.

NSAIDs These drugs may reduce the diuretic effect of bumetanide.

Lithium Bumetanide may increase the blood levels of lithium, leading to an increased risk of lithium toxicity.

Pimozide Low potassium levels increase the risk of abnormal heart rhythms with this antipsychotic drug.

SPECIAL PRECAUTIONS

Be sure to tell your doctor if:
◆ You have long-term liver or kidney problems.
◆ You have diabetes.
◆ You have prostate trouble.
◆ You have gout.
◆ You are taking other medications.

Pregnancy Not usually prescribed. May cause a reduction in blood supply to the developing baby. Discuss with your doctor.

Breast-feeding This drug may reduce your milk supply. Discuss with your doctor.

Infants and children Not usually prescribed. Reduced dose necessary.

Over 60 Dosage is often reduced.

Driving and hazardous work Avoid such activities until you have learned how bumetanide affects you because the drug may cause dizziness and fainting.

Alcohol Keep consumption low. The drug increases the likelihood of dehydration and hangovers after drinking alcohol.

PROLONGED USE

Serious problems are unlikely, but the levels of certain salts in the body may occasionally become abnormal during prolonged use.

Monitoring Regular blood tests may be performed to check kidney function and levels of body salts.

Calcipotriol

Brand name Dovonex
Used in the following combined preparations
None

QUICK REFERENCE
Drug group Drug for psoriasis (p.120)
Overdose danger rating Low
Dependence rating Low
Prescription needed Yes
Available as generic No

GENERAL INFORMATION

Calcipotriol is used for scalp psoriasis and in the treatment of plaque psoriasis affecting up to 40 per cent of the patient's skin area.

Calcipotriol is similar to vitamin D. It is thought to work by reducing production of the skin cells that cause skin thickening and scaling, which are the most common symptoms of psoriasis. Because this drug is related to vitamin D, excessive use (more than 100g per week) can lead to a rise in calcium levels in the body; otherwise calcipotriol is unlikely to cause any serious adverse effects.

The drug is applied to the affected areas in in the form of cream, ointment, or scalp solution. It should not be used on the face, and it is important that the hands are washed after application to avoid accidental transfer to unaffected areas. Local irritation may occur during the early stages of treatment.

INFORMATION FOR USERS

Your drug prescription is tailored for you. Do not alter dosage without checking with your doctor.
How taken Cream, ointment, scalp solution.
Frequency and timing of doses 1–2 x daily.
Adult dosage range Maximum 100g each week. Scalp solution, maximum 60ml each week.
Onset of effect Improvement is seen within 2 weeks.
Duration of action One application lasts up to 12 hours. Beneficial effects are longer lasting.
Diet advice None.
Storage Store at room temperature out of reach of children.
Missed dose Apply the next dose at the scheduled time.

Stopping the drug Do not stop taking the drug without consulting your doctor; symptoms may recur.
Exceeding the dose Excessive prolonged use of calcipotriol may lead to an increase in blood calcium levels, which can cause nausea, constipation, thirst, and frequent urination. Notify your doctor.

POSSIBLE ADVERSE EFFECTS
Temporary local irritation may occur when treatment is started. Other effects, such as thirst, frequent urination, constipation, and nausea, are usually due to heavy or prolonged use, leading to high calcium levels in the blood. If you develop a rash on light-exposed areas, consult your doctor.

INTERACTIONS
None known.

SPECIAL PRECAUTIONS
Be sure to tell your doctor if:
◆ You have a metabolic disorder.
◆ You have previously had a hypersensitivity reaction to the drug.
◆ You are taking other medications.
Pregnancy No evidence of risk, but discuss with your doctor.
Breast-feeding No evidence of risk, but discuss with your doctor.
Infants and children Not recommended.
Over 60 No problems expected.
Driving and hazardous work No problems expected.
Alcohol No problems expected.

PROLONGED USE
No problems expected from low doses.
Monitoring Regular checks on calcium levels in the blood or urine are required during prolonged or heavy use.

Captopril

Brand names Acepril, Capoten, Kaplon
Used in the following combined preparations
Acezide, Capozide

QUICK REFERENCE
Drug group ACE inhibitor (p.30)

Overdose danger rating Medium
Dependence rating Low
Prescription needed Yes
Available as generic Yes

GENERAL INFORMATION

Captopril belongs to the ACE (angiotensin converting enzyme) inhibitor group of drugs and is used to treat high blood pressure (p.34) and heart failure (in which the heart is unable to deal with its workload). It may also be given to patients following a heart attack and is sometimes used to prevent or delay kidney damage in patients with diabetes. It is also often given with a diuretic to increase its effect on high blood pressure and heart failure. Captopril works by relaxing the muscles in blood vessel walls, allowing the vessels to dilate (widen), which enables the blood to circulate more easily and helps to lower blood pressure. The first dose is usually very small and should be taken while lying down because there is a risk of a sudden fall in blood pressure.

A variety of minor side effects may occur with captopril; many people develop a persistent dry cough, while others experience taste disturbance, which a reduction in dose may help to minimize.

INFORMATION FOR USERS

Your drug prescription is tailored for you. Do not alter dosage without checking with your doctor.
How taken Tablets.
Frequency and timing of doses 2–3 x daily.
Adult dosage range 12.5–25mg daily initially, gradually increased to 50–150mg daily.
Onset of effect 30–60 minutes.
Duration of action 6–8 hours.
Diet advice None.
Storage Keep in a closed container in a cool, dry place out of reach of children.
Missed dose Take as soon as you remember. If your next dose is due within 2 hours, take a single dose now and skip the next.
Stopping the drug Unless severe adverse effects occur (see below), do not stop taking the drug without consulting your doctor; stopping the drug may lead to worsening of the underlying condition.

Exceeding the dose An occasional unintentional extra dose is unlikely to cause problems. Large overdoses may cause dizziness or fainting. Notify your doctor.

POSSIBLE ADVERSE EFFECTS

Dizziness on standing is likely to occur after the first dose. Nausea and headache are common but are usually mild and transient. A persistent dry cough is the most common adverse effect, but this can be minimized by taking smaller, more frequent, doses; some people may have to stop taking the drug. Rash or itching may occur. If dizziness or fainting, runny nose or sore throat, confusion or mood changes, or chest pain or palpitations occur, consult your doctor. If you develop jaundice, facial swelling, or breathing difficulties, stop taking the drug and seek urgent medical advice.

INTERACTIONS

NSAIDs Some of these drugs may reduce the effectiveness of captopril. There is also a risk of kidney damage when they are taken with it.
Lithium Blood levels of lithium may be raised by captopril.
Vasodilators (e.g., nitrates) These drugs may reduce blood pressure even further.
Potassium supplements and potassium-sparing diuretics Taken with captopril, these drugs increase the risk of high blood potassium levels.
Ciclosporin This drug increases the risk of high potassium levels in the blood when taken with captopril.
Diuretics Starting captopril while taking these drugs can cause a rapid fall in blood pressure, but the two drugs are often given together.

SPECIAL PRECAUTIONS

Be sure to tell your doctor if:
◆ You have suffered from severe allergies.
◆ You have long-term kidney problems.
◆ You have coronary artery disease.
◆ You peripheral vascular disease.
◆ You are on a low sodium diet
◆ You are allergic to other ACE inhibitors.
◆ You are taking other medications.
Pregnancy Not prescribed. May cause defects in the developing baby.
Breast-feeding The drug passes into the breast milk, but at normal doses adverse

effects on the baby are unlikely. Discuss with your doctor.

Infants and children Not usually prescribed.

Over 60 Reduced dose may be necessary.

Driving and hazardous work Avoid such activities until you have learned how captopril affects you because the drug can cause dizziness and fainting.

Alcohol Avoid excessive amounts. Alcohol may increase the blood-pressure lowering and adverse effects of this drug.

Surgery and general anaesthetics Notify your doctor or dentist that you are taking captopril.

PROLONGED USE

Rarely, prolonged use can lead to changes in the blood count or kidney function.

Monitoring Periodic checks on potassium levels, white blood cell count, kidney function, and urine are usually performed.

Carbamazepine

Brand names Tegretol, Epimaz, Teril CR, Timoril Retard

Used in the following combined preparations
None

QUICK REFERENCE

Drug group Anticonvulsant drug (p.16) and antipsychotic drug (p.15)

Overdose danger rating Medium

Dependence rating Low

Prescription needed Yes

Available as generic Yes

GENERAL INFORMATION

Carbamazepine's main use is as an anticonvulsant because it reduces the likelihood of fits caused by abnormal nerve signals in the brain (epilepsy).

Carbamazepine is also prescribed to relieve the intermittent severe pain caused by damage to the cranial nerves in trigeminal neuralgia. Carbamazepine is also occasionally prescribed to treat manic depression and diabetes insipidus and is used for pain relief in diabetic neuropathy.

To avoid side effects, the drug is usually started at a low dose and gradually increased until the required blood level is achieved.

INFORMATION FOR USERS

Your drug prescription is tailored for you. Do not alter dosage without checking with your doctor.

How taken Tablets, chewable tablets, liquid, suppositories.

Frequency and timing of doses 1–4 x daily.

Adult dosage range *Epilepsy* 100–1,200mg daily (low starting dose slowly increased every 2 weeks). *Pain relief* 100–1,600mg daily. *Psychiatric disorders* 400–1,600mg daily.

Onset of effect Within 4 hours.

Duration of action 12–24 hours.

Diet advice None.

Storage Keep in a closed container in a cool, dry place out of reach of children.

Missed dose Take as soon as you remember. If your next dose is due within 2 hours, take a single dose now and skip the next.

Stopping the drug Unless severe adverse effects occur (see below), do not stop taking the drug without consulting your doctor; symptoms may recur.

Exceeding the dose An occasional unintentional extra dose is unlikely to cause problems. Large overdoses may cause tremor, convulsions, and coma. Notify your doctor.

POSSIBLE ADVERSE EFFECTS

Most people experience very few adverse effects with this drug, but when blood levels get too high adverse effects, including dizziness, drowsiness, poor coordination, clumsiness, nausea, ankle swelling, and blurred vision, are common and the dose may need to be reduced. If you develop a rash, sore throat, or hoarseness, stop taking the drug and consult your doctor promptly.

INTERACTIONS

Anticoagulant drugs, analgesic drugs, and oral contraceptives Carbamazepine may reduce the effects of these drugs.

Analgesic drugs, cimetidine, verapamil, co-proxamol, some antibiotics, and isoniazid These drugs may increase carbamazepine's effects.

Antidepressant and antipsychotic drugs These drugs may antagonize the anticonvulsant effects of carbamazepine.

Other anti-epileptic drugs Complex and variable interactions can occur between these drugs and carbamazepine.

SPECIAL PRECAUTIONS
Be sure to tell your doctor if:
◆ You have long-term liver or kidney problems.
◆ You have heart problems.
◆ You have had blood problems with other drugs.
◆ You are taking other medications.

Pregnancy May be associated with abnormalities in the unborn baby. Folic acid supplements are usually recommended. Discuss with your doctor.

Breast-feeding The drug passes into the breast milk, but at normal doses adverse effects on the baby are unlikely. Discuss with your doctor.

Infants and children Reduced dose necessary.

Over 60 May cause confused or agitated behaviour in the elderly. Reduced dose may be necessary.

Driving and hazardous work Your underlying condition, and the possibility of reduced alertness while taking the drug, may make such activities inadvisable. Discuss with your doctor.

Alcohol Avoid. Alcohol may increase the sedative effects of this drug.

PROLONGED USE
There is a slight risk of changes in liver function or of skin or blood abnormalities occurring during prolonged use.

Monitoring Periodic blood tests may be performed to monitor levels of the drug, blood cell counts, and liver and kidney function.

Carbaryl

Brand names Carylderm
Used in the following combined preparations
None

QUICK REFERENCE
Drug group Drugs to treat skin parasites (p.118)
Overdose danger rating Low
Dependence rating Low
Prescription needed Yes
Available as generic No

GENERAL INFORMATION
Carbaryl is an insecticide used in the treatment of head and crab lice. It kills the lice by interfering with the functioning of their nervous system, causing paralysis and death.

The drug is applied topically either as water-based liquid or alcohol-based lotion. All members of a household should be treated at the same time, at the first sign of infestation. Liquid is more suitable for small children and asthmatics, who may be affected by the alcoholic fumes of lotion. Lotion is unsuitable for treating crab lice because it causes genital irritation.

Because lice develop resistance to insecticides, it is possible that carbaryl (or alternatives such as malathion) may not clear the lice. If the drug does not work for you, consult your pharmacist or doctor. You will need a prescription to obtain carbaryl.

INFORMATION FOR USERS
Your drug prescription is tailored for you. Do not alter dosage without checking with your doctor.

How taken Topical liquid, lotion.

Frequency and timing of doses Once, repeating after a week.

Adult dosage range As directed.

Onset of effect Lotion or liquid should be left on for 12 hours before being washed off.

Duration of action Until washed off.

Diet advice None.

Storage Keep in closed container in a cool, dry place out of reach of children. Protect from light.

Missed dose If you forget the second application, use it as soon as you remember.

Stopping the drug Carbaryl should be applied as a single application or as a short course of treatment.

Exceeding the dose An occasional unintentional extra application is unlikely to be a cause for concern. Take emergency action if accidentally swallowed.

POSSIBLE ADVERSE EFFECTS
Used correctly, carbaryl preparations are unlikely to produce adverse effects, although skin irritation may occur, and the alcoholic fumes given off by some lotions may cause wheezing in asthmatics.

INTERACTIONS
None.

SPECIAL PRECAUTIONS
Be sure to tell your doctor if:
◆ You have asthma.
Pregnancy No evidence of risk. It is unlikely that enough carbaryl would be absorbed after occasional application to affect the developing fetus.
Breast-feeding No evidence of risk. It is unlikely that enough carbaryl would be absorbed after occasional application to affect the baby.
Infants and children No special problems.
Over 60 No special problems.
Driving and hazardous work No special problems.
Alcohol No special problems.

PROLONGED USE
Carbaryl is intended for intermittent use only. It should not be used for prolonged periods.

Carbimazole

Brand name Neo-Mercazole
Used in the following combined preparations
None

QUICK REFERENCE
Drug group Antithyroid drug (p.82)
Overdose danger rating Medium
Dependence rating Low
Prescription needed Yes
Available as generic No

GENERAL INFORMATION
Carbimazole is an antithyroid drug used to suppress the formation of thyroid hormones in people with an overactive thyroid gland (hyperthyroidism). In some people, particularly those with Graves' disease (the most common form of hyperthyroidism), drug treatment alone may relieve the disorder.

Carbimazole is also used in more serious cases, for example, to restore the normal function of the thyroid gland before its partial removal by surgery, or to intensify the absorption of the cell-destroying drug radioactive iodine when that is used. Carbimazole also prevents the harmful release of thyroid hormone that can sometimes follow the use of radioactive iodine. Because the full benefits of this medication are not felt for several weeks, beta blockers may be given during this period to help control symptoms. Maintenance treatment may be continued for as long as 18 months unless surgery or radioactive iodine are used. Occasionally the dose of carbimazole is kept high (often around 30mg per day), and thyroxine is also prescribed as thyroid function diminishes. This approach may be more effective and may prevent a goitre from developing.

INFORMATION FOR USERS
Your drug prescription is tailored for you. Do not alter dosage without checking with your doctor.
How taken Tablets.
Frequency and timing of doses 2–3 x daily.
Adult dosage range 20–60mg daily. Once control is achieved, dosage is reduced gradually to a maintenance dose of 5–15mg for about 18 months.
Onset of effect Some improvement is usually felt within 1–3 weeks. Full beneficial effects usually take 4–8 weeks.
Duration of action 12–24 hours.
Diet advice Your doctor may advise you to avoid foods that are high in iodine.
Storage Keep in a closed container in a cool, dry place out of reach of children.
Missed dose Take as soon as you remember. If your next dose is due, take both doses together.
Stopping the drug Do not stop taking the drug without consulting your doctor; symptoms may recur.
Exceeding the dose An occasional unintentional extra dose is unlikely to cause problems. Large overdoses may cause nausea, vomiting, and headache. Notify your doctor.

POSSIBLE ADVERSE EFFECTS
Serious side effects are rare. Headache, dizziness, nausea, hair loss, and joint pain may occur. A sore throat or mouth ulcers may indicate adverse effects on the blood and require prompt medical attention.

INTERACTIONS
None.

SPECIAL PRECAUTIONS
Be sure to tell your doctor if:
◆ You have long-term liver or kidney problems.
◆ You are taking other medications.
Pregnancy May be associated with defects in the baby. Discuss with your doctor.
Breast-feeding The drug passes into the breast milk, but mothers may breast-feed as long as the lowest effective dose is used and the baby is carefully monitored. Discuss with your doctor.
Infants and children Reduced dose necessary.
Over 60 No special problems.
Driving and hazardous work Usually no problems, but carbimazole may cause dizziness.
Alcohol No known problems.

PROLONGED USE
Carbimazole may stop or reduce the production of blood cells by the bone marrow.
Monitoring Blood cell counts are carried out, and periodic tests of thyroid function are usually required.

Cefalexin

Brand names Ceporex, Keflex, Kiflone, Tenkorex
Used in the following combined preparations
None

QUICK REFERENCE
Drug group Cephalosporin antibiotic (p.60)
Overdose danger rating Low
Dependence rating Low
Prescription needed Yes
Available as generic Yes

GENERAL INFORMATION
Cefalexin is a cephalosporin antibiotic that is prescribed for a variety of mild to moderate infections. Cefalexin does not have such a wide range of uses as some other antibiotics, but it is helpful in treating cystitis, and certain skin and soft tissue infections. In some cases it is prescribed as follow-up treatment for severe infections after a more powerful cephalosporin has been given by injection.

Diarrhoea is the most common side effect of cefalexin, although it tends to be less severe than with other cephalosporin antibiotics. In addition, some people may find that they are allergic to this drug, especially if they are sensitive to penicillin.

INFORMATION FOR USERS
Your drug prescription is tailored for you. Do not alter dosage without checking with your doctor.
How taken Tablets, capsules, liquid.
Frequency and timing of doses 2–4 x daily.
Dosage range *Adults* 1–6g daily.
Children Reduced dose according to age and weight.
Onset of effect Within 1 hour.
Duration of action 6–12 hours.
Diet advice None.
Storage Keep tablets and capsules in a closed container in a cool, dry place out of reach of children. Refrigerate liquid, but do not freeze, and keep for no longer than 10 days. Protect from light.
Missed dose Take as soon as you remember. If your next dose is due at this time, take both doses now.
Stopping the drug Take the full course. Even if you feel better, the original infection may still be present and may recur if treatment is stopped too soon.
Exceeding the dose An occasional unintentional extra dose is unlikely to be a cause for concern. But if you notice any unusual symptoms, or if a large overdose has been taken, notify your doctor.

POSSIBLE ADVERSE EFFECTS
Most people suffer do not suffer any serious adverse effects while taking cefalexin. Diarrhoea is common, but it tends not to be severe. Nausea and abdominal pain may occur. Rare adverse effects, such as rash, itching, and wheezing, are usually the result of an allergic reaction and may necessitate stopping the drug urgently.

INTERACTIONS
Probenecid This drug increases the level of cefalexin in the blood. The dosage of cefalexin may need to be adjusted accordingly.
Oral contraceptives Cefalexin may reduce the contraceptive effect of these drugs. Discuss with your doctor.

SPECIAL PRECAUTIONS
Be sure to tell your doctor if:

◆ You have a long-term kidney problem.
◆ You have had a previous allergic reaction to a penicillin or cephalosporin antibiotic.
◆ You have a history of blood disorders.
◆ You are taking other medications.

Pregnancy No evidence of risk to the developing baby.

Breast-feeding The drug passes into the breast milk but at normal doses adverse effects on the baby are unlikely. Discuss with your doctor.

Infants and children Reduced dose necessary.

Over 60 No special problems.

Driving and hazardous work No known problems.

Alcohol No known problems.

PROLONGED USE
Cefalexin is usually given only for short courses of treatment.

Cetirizine

Brand name Zirtek
Used in the following combined preparations
None

QUICK REFERENCE
Drug group Antihistamine (p.56)
Overdose danger rating Medium
Dependence rating Low
Prescription needed No (tablets); yes (liquid)
Available as generic No

GENERAL INFORMATION
Cetirizine is a long-acting antihistamine. The drug's main use is in the treatment of allergic rhinitis, particularly hay fever.

Cetirizine is also used to treat allergic skin conditions, such as urticaria (hives).

The principal difference between this drug and traditional antihistamines such as chlorphenamine (chlorpheniramine) is that it has less sedative effect on the central nervous system. It may therefore be suitable for people when they need to avoid sleepiness – for example, when driving or at work. However, because cetirizine can cause drowsiness in some people, you should learn how the drug affects you before you undertake any activities that require concentration.

INFORMATION FOR USERS
Follow instructions on the label. Call your doctor if symptoms worsen.

How taken Tablets, liquid.
Frequency and timing of doses 1–2 x daily.
Adult dosage range 10mg daily.
Onset of effect 1–3 hours. Some effect may not be felt for 1–2 days.
Duration of action Up to 24 hours.
Diet advice None.
Storage Keep in a closed container in a cool, dry place out of reach of children.
Missed dose No cause for concern, but take as soon as you remember. If your next dose is due within 8 hours, take a single dose now and skip the next.
Stopping the drug Can be safely stopped as soon as you no longer need it.
Exceeding the dose An occasional unintentional extra dose is unlikely to cause problems. Large overdoses may cause nausea or drowsiness and have adverse effects on the heart. Notify your doctor.

POSSIBLE ADVERSE EFFECTS
The most common adverse effects are dry mouth and fatigue; drowsiness is rare. Side effects may be reduced if the dose is taken as 5mg twice a day.

INTERACTIONS
Anticholinergic drugs The anticholinergic effects of cetirizine may be increased by all drugs that have anticholinergic effects, including antipsychotics and tricyclic antidepressants.

Sedatives Cetirizine may increase the sedative effects of anti-anxiety drugs, sleeping drugs, antidepressants, and antipsychotics.

Allergy tests Antihistamines should be discontinued approximately 48 hours before allergy skin testing.

SPECIAL PRECAUTIONS
Be sure to consult your doctor or pharmacist before taking this drug if:
◆ You have long-term liver or kidney problems.
◆ You have glaucoma.

◆ You are taking other medications.

Pregnancy Safety in pregnancy not established. Discuss with your doctor.

Breast-feeding The drug passes into the breast milk. Discuss with your doctor.

Infants and children Not recommended under 2 years.

Over 60 No problems expected.

Driving and hazardous work Avoid such activities until you have learned how cetirizine affects you because the drug can cause drowsiness in some people.

Alcohol Keep consumption low.

PROLONGED USE
No problems expected.

Chloramphenicol

Brand names Chloromycetin, Kemicetine, Minims Chloramphenicol, Sno-Phenicol
Used in the following combined preparation Actinac

QUICK REFERENCE
Drug group Antibiotic (p.60)
Overdose danger rating Low
Dependence rating Low
Prescription needed Yes
Available as generic Yes

GENERAL INFORMATION
Chloramphenicol is an antibiotic used topically to treat eye and ear infections. Given by mouth or injection, the drug is used in the treatment of meningitis and brain abscesses. Chloramphenicol is also effective in treating acute infections such as typhoid, pneumonia, epiglottitis, or meningitis caused by bacteria that is resistant to other antibiotics.

Most people experience few adverse effects since not enough of the drug is absorbed to cause harm when applied topically. However, it occasionally causes serious or even fatal blood disorders and, for this reason, chloramphenicol by mouth or injection is normally only given to treat life-threatening infections that do not respond to safer drugs.

INFORMATION FOR USERS
Your drug prescription is tailored for you.

Do not alter dosage without checking with your doctor.

How taken Capsules, liquid, injection, cream, eye and ear drops, eye ointment.

Frequency and timing of doses Every 6 hours (by mouth or injection); every 2–6 hours (eye preparations); 3 x daily (ear drops).

Adult dosage range Varies according to preparation and condition. Follow your doctor's instructions.

Onset of effect 1–3 days, depending on the condition and preparation.

Duration of action 6–8 hours.

Diet advice None.

Storage Keep in a closed container in a cool, dry place out of reach of children. Protect from light.

Missed dose Take as soon as you remember (capsules, liquid). If your next dose is due, double the dose to make up the missed dose. For skin, eye, and ear preparations, apply as soon as you remember.

Stopping the drug Unless severe adverse effects occur (see below), take the full course. Even if you feel better the infection may still be present and may recur if treatment is stopped too soon.

Exceeding the dose An occasional unintentional extra dose is unlikely to be a cause for concern. But if you notice any unusual symptoms, or if a large overdose has been taken, notify your doctor.

POSSIBLE ADVERSE EFFECTS
Transient irritation may occur with eye or ear drops. If you are receiving the drug by mouth or injection, and numbness in the hands or feet, blurred vision, or rash occur, stop taking the drug and consult your doctor. Sore throat, fever, and unusual tiredness with any form of the drug may be signs of blood abnormalities and should be reported to your doctor without delay, even if treatment has been stopped.

INTERACTIONS
General note Chloramphenicol by mouth or injection may increase the effect of certain other drugs, including phenytoin, oral anticoagulants, and oral antidiabetics. Phenobarbital or rifampicin may reduce the effect of chloramphenicol.

Antidiabetic drugs Chloramphenicol by mouth or injection may increase the effect of antidiabetic drugs.

SPECIAL PRECAUTIONS
Be sure to tell your doctor if:
◆ You have long-term liver or kidney problems.
◆ You have a blood disorder.
◆ You are taking other medications.
Pregnancy No evidence of risk with eye or ear preparations. Safety in pregnancy, of other methods of administration, not established. Discuss with your doctor.
Breast-feeding No evidence of risk with eye or ear preparations. Taken by mouth, the drug passes into the breast milk and may increase the risk of blood disorders in the baby. Discuss with your doctor.
Infants and children Reduced dose necessary.
Over 60 No problems expected.
Driving and hazardous work No known problems.
Alcohol No known problems.

PROLONGED USE
Prolonged use of this drug may increase the risk of serious blood disorders and eye damage.
Monitoring Periodic blood cell counts and eye tests may be performed. Blood levels of the drug are usually monitored in infants given chloramphenicol by mouth or injection.

Chlordiazepoxide

Brand names Librium, Tropium
Used in the following combined preparations
None

QUICK REFERENCE
Drug group Benzodiazepine anti-anxiety drug (p.13)
Overdose danger rating Medium
Dependence rating Medium
Prescription needed Yes
Available as generic Yes

GENERAL INFORMATION
Chlordiazepoxide was introduced in the mid-1960s and belongs to the group of anti-anxiety drugs known as the benzodiazepines. These drugs are used to help relieve tension

and nervousness, relax muscles, and encourage sleep. The actions and the adverse effects of this drug group are described more fully on page 13.

Prescribed primarily to treat anxiety, chlordiazepoxide is also used to relieve the symptoms of alcohol withdrawal.

Chlordiazepoxide may lead to dependence and withdrawal symptoms if taken regularly over a long period, and it may also lose effectiveness with time. For these reasons, courses of treatment are usually limited to two to four weeks.

INFORMATION FOR USERS
Your drug prescription is tailored for you. Do not alter dosage without checking with your doctor.
How taken Tablets, capsules.
Frequency and timing of doses 1–4 x daily.
Adult dosage range 10–100mg daily. The dosage varies considerably from person to person.
Onset of effect 1–2 hours.
Duration of action 12–24 hours, but some effect may last up to 4 days.
Diet advice None.
Storage Keep in a closed container in a cool, dry place out of reach of children.
Missed dose No cause for concern, but take when you remember. If your next dose is due within 2 hours, take a single dose now and skip the next.
Stopping the drug If you have been taking the drug for less than 2 weeks, it can be safely stopped as soon as you feel you no longer need it. However, if you have been taking the drug for longer, consult your doctor, who may supervise a gradual reduction in dosage. Stopping abruptly may lead to withdrawal symptoms.
Exceeding the dose An occasional unintentional extra dose is unlikely to cause problems. Large overdoses may cause unusual drowsiness or coma. Notify your doctor.

POSSIBLE ADVERSE EFFECTS
The principal adverse effects of this drug are related to its sedative properties and include drowsiness, dizziness, and forgetfulness. These effects normally diminish after the first few days of treatment.

INTERACTIONS

Anticonvulsant drugs These drugs' side effects may be increased with chlordiazepoxide.

Sedatives All drugs that have a sedative effect are likely to increase the sedative properties of chlordiazepoxide.

SPECIAL PRECAUTIONS

Be sure to tell your doctor if:
◆ You have long-term liver or kidney problems.
◆ You have a history of breathing problems.
◆ You have had problems with alcohol or drug abuse.
◆ You are taking other medications.

Pregnancy Safety in pregnancy not established. Discuss with your doctor.

Breast-feeding The drug passes into the breast milk and may affect the baby. Discuss with your doctor.

Infants and children Not recommended.

Over 60 Reduced dose may be necessary.

Driving and hazardous work Avoid such activities until you have learned how chlordiazepoxide affects you because the drug can cause reduced alertness and slowed reactions.

Alcohol Avoid. Alcohol may increase the sedative effects of this drug.

PROLONGED USE

Regular use of chlordiazepoxide over several weeks can lead to a reduction in its effect as the body adapts. The drug may also be habit-forming when taken for extended periods, especially if it is taken in doses that are larger than average.

Chloroquine

Brand names Avloclor, Nivaquine
Used in the following combined preparation
Paludrine/Avloclor

QUICK REFERENCE

Drug group Antimalarial drug (p.73) and antirheumatic drug (p.50)
Overdose danger rating High
Dependence rating Low
Prescription needed No (malaria prevention); Yes (other uses)
Available as generic Yes

GENERAL INFORMATION

Chloroquine was introduced for the prevention and treatment of malaria. It usually clears an attack of the disease within three days. Injections may be given when an attack is severe. As a preventative treatment, a low dose is given once weekly, starting one week before visiting a high-risk area and continuing for four weeks after leaving. Chloroquine is not suitable for use in all parts of the world as resistance to the drug may have developed in some areas. The other main use is in the treatment of autoimmune diseases, such as rheumatoid arthritis and lupus erythematosus.

Common side effects include nausea, headache, diarrhoea, and abdominal cramps. Occasionally a rash develops. More seriously, the drug can damage the retina during prolonged treatment, causing blurred vision that sometimes progresses to blindness. Regular eye checks are needed to detect early changes.

INFORMATION FOR USERS

Follow instructions on the label. Call your doctor if symptoms worsen.

How taken Tablets, liquid, injection.

Frequency and timing of doses *By mouth* 1 x weekly (prevention of malaria); 1–4 x daily (treatment of malaria); 1 x daily (arthritis).

Adult dosage range *Prevention of malaria* 300mg (2 tablets) as a single dose on the same day each week. Start 1 week before entering endemic area, and continue for 4 weeks after leaving. *Treatment of malaria* Initial dose 600mg (4 tablets) and following doses 300mg. *Rheumatoid arthritis* 150mg (1 tablet) per day.

Onset of effect 2–3 days. In rheumatoid arthritis, full effect may not be felt for up to 6 months.

Duration of action Up to 1 week.

Diet advice None.

Storage Keep in a closed container in a cool, dry, place out of reach of children. Protect from light.

Missed dose Take as soon as you remember. If your next dose is due within 24 hours (1 x weekly schedule), or 6 hours (1–2 x daily schedule), take a single dose now and skip the next.

Stopping the drug Unless severe adverse effects occur (see below), do not stop taking the drug without consulting your doctor.

OVERDOSE ACTION

Seek immediate medical advice in all cases. Take emergency action if breathing difficulties, fits, or loss of consciousness occur.

POSSIBLE ADVERSE EFFECTS

Side effects such as nausea, diarrhoea, and abdominal pain might be avoided by taking the drug with food. Headache and dizziness may also occur. If you develop a rash or any change in vision, stop taking the drug and consult your doctor promptly.

INTERACTIONS

Anticonvulsant drugs Chloroquine may reduce the anticonvulsant effect of these drugs.

Digoxin The level of digoxin in the blood may be increased by chloroquine.

Ciclosporin Chloroquine increases the blood level of ciclosporin.

Amiodarone Chloroquine may increase the risk of abnormal heart rhythms if taken with this drug.

SPECIAL PRECAUTIONS

Be sure to consult your doctor or pharmacist before taking this drug if:

◆ You have liver or kidney problems.

◆ You have glucose-6-phosphate dehydrogenase (G6PD) deficiency.

◆ You have eye or vision problems.

◆ You have psoriasis.

◆ You have a history of epilepsy.

◆ You suffer from porphyria.

◆ You are taking other medications.

Pregnancy No evidence of risk with low doses. High doses may affect the baby. Discuss with your doctor.

Breast-feeding The drug may pass into breast milk in small amounts. At normal doses effects on the baby are unlikely. Discuss with your doctor.

Infants and children Reduced dose necessary.

Over 60 No special problems, except that it may be difficult to tell between changes in eyesight due to ageing, and those that are drug induced.

Driving and hazardous work Avoid such activities until you have learned how chloroquine affects you because the drug may cause dizziness.

Alcohol Keep consumption low.

PROLONGED USE

Prolonged use of chloroquine may cause eye damage and blood disorders.

Monitoring Periodic eye tests (which are often self-tests) and blood counts must be carried out.

Chlorphenamine (Chlorpheniramine)

Brand names Calimal, Piriton
Used in the following combined preparations
Contac 400, Dristan, Expulin, Galpseud Plus, Haymine, Tixylix Cough and Cold

QUICK REFERENCE

Drug group Antihistamine (p.56)
Overdose danger rating Medium
Dependence rating Low
Prescription needed No (tablets and liquid); yes (injection)
Available as generic Yes

GENERAL INFORMATION

Chlorphenamine has been used for more than 30 years to treat allergies such as hay fever, allergic conjunctivitis, urticaria (hives), insect bites and stings, and angioedema (allergic swellings). It is included in several over-the-counter cold remedies (see p.25).

Like other antihistamines, chlorphenamine relieves allergic skin symptoms such as itching, swelling, and redness. It also reduces sneezing and the runny nose and itching eyes of hay fever. Chlorphenamine also has a mild anticholinergic action, which suppresses mucus secretion.

Chlorphenamine may also be used to prevent or treat allergic reactions to blood transfusions or X-ray contrast material and can be given with epinephrine (adrenaline) injections for acute allergic shock (anaphylaxis).

INFORMATION FOR USERS

Follow instructions on the label. Call your doctor if symptoms worsen.

How taken Tablets, liquid, injection.
Frequency and timing of doses 4–6 x daily (tablets, liquid); single dose as needed (injection).

Dosage range *Adults* 12–24mg daily (by mouth); up to 40mg daily (injection). *Children* Reduced dose according to age and weight.
Onset of effect Within 60 minutes (by mouth); within 20 minutes (injection).
Duration of action 4–6 hours (tablets, liquid, injection).
Diet advice None.
Storage Keep in a closed container in a cool, dry place out of reach of children.
Missed dose Take as soon as you remember. If your next dose is due within 2 hours, take a single dose now and skip the next.
Stopping the drug Can be safely stopped as soon as you no longer need it.
Exceeding the dose An occasional unintentional extra dose is unlikely to cause problems. Large overdoses may cause drowsiness or agitation. Notify your doctor.

POSSIBLE ADVERSE EFFECTS
Drowsiness is the most common adverse effect; dizziness may also occur, but other adverse effects are rare. Some of these, such as dryness of the mouth, blurred vision, and difficulty passing urine, are due to its anticholinergic effects, and children may become excitable. Gastrointestinal irritation may be reduced by taking the tablets or liquid with food or drink. If you develop a rash, stop taking the drug and consult your doctor.

INTERACTIONS
Sedatives All drugs that have a sedative effect are likely to increase the sedative properties of chlorphenamine.
Phenytoin The effects of phenytoin may be enhanced by chlorphenamine.
Anticholinergic drugs All drugs that have an anticholinergic effect, including certain drugs for treating parkinsonism, are likely to add to the anticholinergic effect of chlorphenamine.

SPECIAL PRECAUTIONS
Be sure to consult your doctor or pharmacist before taking this drug if:
◆ You have a long-term liver problem.
◆ You have had epileptic fits.
◆ You have glaucoma.
◆ You have urinary difficulties.
◆ You are taking other medications.

Pregnancy Safety in pregnancy not established. Discuss with your doctor.
Breast-feeding The drug passes into the breast milk, but at normal doses adverse effects on the baby are unlikely. Discuss with your doctor.
Infants and children Reduced dose necessary.
Over 60 Reduced dose may be necessary. Increased likelihood of adverse effects.
Driving and hazardous work Avoid such activities until you have learned how chlorphenamine affects you because the drug can cause drowsiness, dizziness, and blurred vision.
Alcohol Avoid. Alcohol may increase the sedative effects of this drug.

PROLONGED USE
The effect of chlorphenamine may become weaker with prolonged use over a period of weeks or months as the body adapts to the treatment. Transfer to a different antihistamine may be recommended.

Chlorpromazine

Brand names Chloractil, Largactil
Used in the following combined preparations None

QUICK REFERENCE
Drug group Phenothiazine antipsychotic (p.15) and anti-emetic drug (p.21)
Overdose danger rating Medium
Dependence rating Low
Prescription needed Yes
Available as generic Yes

GENERAL INFORMATION
The first antipsychotic drug to be marketed, chlorpromazine remains one of the most widely used of this drug group. It is effective in reducing aggression, suppressing abnormal behaviour, and producing a generally tranquillizing effect.

Chlorpromazine is prescribed for the treatment of schizophrenia, mania, and other disorders where confused, aggressive, or abnormal behaviour may occur and a degree of sedation is beneficial. Other uses of this drug include the treatment of nausea and vomiting, especially when caused by drug or radiation treatment; and treating severe, prolonged hiccoughs.

The main drawback of chlorpromazine is that it can produce many side effects (see below), some of which may be serious.

INFORMATION FOR USERS

Your drug prescription is tailored for you. Do not alter dosage without checking with your doctor.

How taken Tablets, liquid, injection, suppositories.

Frequency and timing of doses 1–4 x daily.

Adult dosage range *Mental illness* 75–300mg daily; dose is started low and gradually increased. Larger doses may be used in severe illness. *Nausea and vomiting* 40–150mg daily.

Onset of effect 30–60 minutes (by mouth); 15–20 minutes (injection); up to 30 minutes (suppository).

Duration of action 8–12 hours (by mouth or injection); 3–4 hours (suppository). Some effect may persist for up to 3 weeks when stopping the drug after regular use.

Diet advice None.

Storage Keep in a closed container in a cool, dry place out of reach of children. Protect from light.

Missed dose Take as soon as you remember. If your next dose is due within 2 hours, do not take the missed dose. Take your next scheduled dose as usual.

Stopping the drug Unless severe adverse effects occur (see below), do not stop taking the drug without consulting your doctor; symptoms may recur.

Exceeding the dose An occasional unintentional extra dose is unlikely to cause problems. Larger overdoses may cause unusual drowsiness, fainting, abnormal heart rhythms, muscle rigidity, and agitation. Notify your doctor.

POSSIBLE ADVERSE EFFECTS

Chlorpromazine commonly causes mild drowsiness and has an anticholinergic effect, which can cause symptoms such as blurring of vision. It may also cause dizziness or fainting and infrequent periods. The most significant adverse effect is parkinsonism. If you develop jaundice, or a rash on light exposed areas, stop taking the drug and consult your doctor urgently.

INTERACTIONS

Drugs for parkinsonism Chlorpromazine may reduce the effect of these drugs.

Anticholinergic drugs These drugs may add to the anticholinergic properties of chlorpromazine.

Sedatives All drugs that have a sedative effect on the central nervous system are likely to increase the sedative properties of chlorpromazine.

SPECIAL PRECAUTIONS

Be sure to tell your doctor if:
◆ You have long-term liver or kidney problems.
◆ You have had heart problems.
◆ You have had epileptic fits.
◆ You have thyroid disease.
◆ You have Parkinson's disease.
◆ You have glaucoma.
◆ You are taking other medications.

Pregnancy Not usually prescribed. Taken near the time of delivery it can prolong labour and may cause drowsiness in the newborn baby. Discuss with your doctor.

Breast-feeding The drug passes into the breast milk and may affect the baby. Discuss with your doctor.

Infants and children Not recommended for infants under 1 year. Reduced dose necessary for older children.

Over 60 Initial dosage is low; it may be increased if there are no adverse reactions, such as abnormal limb movements or low blood pressure.

Driving and hazardous work Avoid such activities until you have learned how chlorpromazine affects you as the drug can cause drowsiness and slowed reactions.

Alcohol Avoid excessive amounts. Alcohol may increase the sedative effects of this drug.

Surgery and general anaesthetics Chlorpromazine treatment may need to be stopped before you have a general anaesthetic. Discuss this with your doctor or dentist before any operation.

PROLONGED USE

If used for more than a few months, chlorpromazine may cause movement disorders. Occasionally, jaundice may occur due to an allergic effect of the drug.

Chorionic gonadotrophin

Brand names Choragon, Pregnyl, Profasi
Used in the following combined preparations
None

QUICK REFERENCE

Drug group Drug for infertility (p.105)
Overdose danger rating Low
Dependence rating Low
Prescription needed Yes
Available as generic No

GENERAL INFORMATION

Produced by the placenta, human chorionic gonadotrophin (HCG) is a hormone that stimulates the ovaries to produce two other hormones, oestrogen and progesterone, that are essential to the conception and early growth of the fetus. The hormone is extracted from the urine of pregnant women and has several medical purposes.

The principal value is in the treatment of female infertility. Given by injection, usually with another hormone, HCG encourages the ovaries to release an egg (ovulation) so that it can be fertilized. Ovulation usually occurs 18 hours after injection, and intercourse should follow within 48 hours. The likelihood of multiple births increases because several eggs may be released by the ovaries at once.

In rare cases the drug is also given to young boys to treat undescended testes.

The drug is occasionally given to men to improve sperm production; treatment may take as long as six to nine months.

INFORMATION FOR USERS

This drug is given only under medical supervision and is not for self-administration.
How taken Injection.
Frequency and timing of doses 1–3 x per week.
Dosage range Dosage varies from person to person, and may need adjustment during treatment.
Onset of effect 1–8 days (female infertility); 6–9 months (male infertility).
Duration of action 2–3 days.
Diet advice None.
Storage Not applicable. This drug is not kept in the home.
Missed dose Arrange to receive the missed dose as soon as possible. More than 24 hours' delay may reduce the chance of conception.
Stopping the drug Complete the course of treatment as directed. Stopping the drug prematurely reduces the chance of conception.
Exceeding the dose The drug is always injected under close medical supervision. Overdose is unlikely.

POSSIBLE ADVERSE EFFECTS

When HCG is taken for fertility problems, the more common adverse effects, including headache, tiredness, and mood changes, are rarely severe and tend to diminish with time. Women who take large doses may experience abdominal pain or swelling due to overstimulation of the ovaries; men may experience breast enlargement and swollen ankles and should consult their doctor.

INTERACTIONS

None.

SPECIAL PRECAUTIONS

Be sure to tell your doctor if:
◆ You have a long-term kidney problem.
◆ You have asthma.
◆ You have had epileptic fits.
◆ You suffer from migraine.
◆ You have a heart disorder.
◆ You have had a previous allergic reaction to this drug.
◆ You have prostate trouble.
◆ You are taking other medications.
Pregnancy Not prescribed.
Breast feeding Not prescribed.
Infants and children HCG is safely prescribed to treat undescended testes in boys.
Over 60 Not usually required.
Driving and hazardous work Usually no problems, but the drug can cause tiredness.
Alcohol Avoid excessive amounts. Alcohol increases tiredness and, if taken in excess, may reduce fertility.

PROLONGED USE

No special problems.
Monitoring Women taking HCG to improve fertility usually have regular pelvic examinations and checks on cervical mucus to confirm that ovulation is taking place. Men are given regular sperm counts.

Ciclosporin

Brand names Neoral, Sandimmun
Used in the following combined preparations
None

QUICK REFERENCE

Drug group Immunosuppressant drug (p.96)
Overdose danger rating Medium
Dependence rating Low
Prescription needed Yes
Available as generic No

GENERAL INFORMATION

Introduced in 1984, ciclosporin is one of the immunosuppressants, a group of drugs that suppress the body's natural defences against infection and foreign cells. This action is of particular use following organ transplants, when the recipient's immune system may reject the transplanted organ unless the immune system is controlled.

Ciclosporin is widely used after many types of transplant, such as heart, bone marrow, kidney, liver, and pancreas; its use has considerably reduced the risk of rejection. It is sometimes used to treat rheumatoid arthritis, some severe types of dermatitis, and severe psoriasis when other treatments have failed.

Because the drug reduces the immune system's effectiveness, people taking it are more susceptible than usual to infections. It can also cause high blood pressure and kidney damage.

It is important not to make dose changes on your own. Ask your pharmacist for a patient information leaflet printed by the manufacturer. Owing to the differences in blood levels of the drug between the brands, it is important that the brand to be used is specified. If your doctor wants to transfer you from one brand to the other, the change will be made in a controlled way.

INFORMATION FOR USERS

Your drug prescription is tailored for you. Do not alter dosage without checking with your doctor.

How taken Capsules, liquid, injection.
Frequency and timing of doses 1–2 x daily.
Dosage range Dosage is calculated on an individual basis according to age and weight.
Onset of effect Within 12 hours.

Duration of action Up to 3 days.
Diet advice Avoid high-potassium foods and potassium supplements.
Storage Capsules should be left in the blister pack until required. Keep in a closed container in a cool, dry place out of reach of children. Do not refrigerate.
Missed dose Take as soon as you remember. If your dose is more than 36 hours late, consult your doctor.
Stopping the drug Do not stop taking the drug without consulting your doctor; stopping the drug may lead to transplant rejection.
Exceeding the dose An occasional unintentional extra dose is unlikely to cause problems. Large overdoses may cause vomiting and diarrhoea and may affect kidney function. Notify your doctor.

POSSIBLE ADVERSE EFFECTS

The most common adverse effects are gum swelling, excessive growth of body hair, nausea and vomiting, tremor, and high blood pressure. Headache and muscle cramps may also occur. Less common effects are diarrhoea, facial swelling, flushing, "pins and needles" sensation, rash, and itching.

INTERACTIONS

General note Ciclosporin may interact with a large number of drugs. Check with your doctor or pharmacist before taking any new prescription or over-the-counter medications.

SPECIAL PRECAUTIONS

Ciclosporin is prescribed only under close medical supervision, taking account of your present condition and medical history.

Pregnancy Not usually prescribed. Safety in pregnancy not established. Discuss with your doctor.
Breast-feeding Not recommended. The drug passes into the breast milk and safety has not been established. Discuss with your doctor.
Infants and children Safety not established; used only with great caution.
Over 60 Reduced dose may be necessary.
Driving and hazardous work No known problems.
Alcohol No known problems.
Sunlight Avoid prolonged, unprotected exposure.

PROLONGED USE

Long-term use, especially in high doses, can affect kidney and/or liver function. It may reduce numbers of white blood cells, thus increasing susceptibility to infection.

Monitoring Regular blood tests are normally carried out to measure drug levels and to monitor blood pressure and blood composition, as well as liver and kidney function.

Cimetidine

Brand names Acitak, Dyspamet, Galenamet, Peptimax, Phimetin, Tagamet, Ultec, Zita
Used in the following combined preparations Algitec, Tagamet Dual Action

QUICK REFERENCE

Drug group Anti-ulcer drug (p.41)
Overdose danger rating Low
Dependence rating Low
Prescription needed No (some preparations)
Available as generic Yes

GENERAL INFORMATION

Introduced in the 1970s, cimetidine was the first of a new group of anti-ulcer drugs. It reduces secretion of gastric acid and pepsin, an enzyme that helps in the digestion of protein. By reducing levels of acid and pepsin, it promotes ulcer healing in the stomach and duodenum (see p.41). It is also used for reflux oesophagitis, in which acid stomach contents may flow up the oesophagus. Treatment is usually given in four- to eight-week courses, with further short courses if symptoms recur.

Cimetidine also affects the actions of certain enzymes in the liver, where many drugs are broken down. It is therefore prescribed with caution to people who are receiving other drugs, particularly anticoagulants and anticonvulsants, whose levels need to be carefully controlled. Since cimetidine promotes healing of the stomach lining, it may mask the symptoms of stomach cancer and delay diagnosis. It is therefore prescribed with caution if symptoms persist.

INFORMATION FOR USERS

Follow instructions on the label. Call your doctor if symptoms worsen.

How taken Tablets, liquid, injection.
Frequency and timing of doses
1–4 x daily (after meals and at bedtime).
Adult dosage range 800–1,600mg daily (occasionally increased to 2,400mg daily).
Onset of effect Within 90 minutes.
Duration of action 2–6 hours.
Diet advice None.
Storage Keep in a closed container in a cool, dry place out of reach of children. Protect from light.
Missed dose Do not take the missed dose. Take your next dose as usual.
Stopping the drug If cimetidine has been prescribed by your doctor, unless a rash occurs, do not stop taking the drug without consulting him or her because symptoms may recur.
Exceeding the dose An occasional unintentional extra dose is unlikely to be a cause for concern. But if you notice any unusual symptoms, or if a large overdose has been taken, notify your doctor.

POSSIBLE ADVERSE EFFECTS

Adverse effects of cimetidine are uncommon but include dizziness, confusion, tiredness, and muscle pain. They are usually related to dosage level and almost always disappear when the drug is stopped. Impotence and breast enlargement may occur in men. If you develop a rash, stop taking the drug and consult your doctor.

INTERACTIONS

Benzodiazepines Cimetidine may increase the blood levels of some of these drugs, increasing the risk of adverse effects.
Theophylline/aminophylline Cimetidine may increase the blood levels of these drugs and their dose may need to be reduced.
Sildenafil Cimetidine may increase the blood level of this drug.
Beta blockers and antiarrhythmic drugs Cimetidine may increase the blood levels of these drugs.
Anticonvulsant drugs Cimetidine may increase the blood levels of these drugs, and their dose may need to be reduced.
Anticoagulant drugs Cimetidine may increase the effect of anticoagulants and their dose may need to be reduced.

SPECIAL PRECAUTIONS

Be sure to consult your doctor or pharmacist before taking this drug if:

◆ You have long-term liver or kidney problems.

◆ You are taking other medications.

Pregnancy Safety in pregnancy not established. Discuss with your doctor.

Breast-feeding The drug passes into the breast milk, but at normal doses adverse effects on the baby are unlikely. Discuss with your doctor.

Infants and children Reduced dose necessary.

Over 60 No special problems unless kidney function is reduced, in which case dosage is decreased.

Driving and hazardous work No special problems.

Alcohol Avoid. Alcohol may aggravate the underlying condition and counter the beneficial effects of cimetidine.

PROLONGED USE

Courses of longer than 8 weeks are not usually necessary.

Cinnarizine

Brand names Cinaziere, Stugeron, Stugeron Forte
Used in the following combined preparations
None

QUICK REFERENCE

Drug group Antihistamine anti-emetic drug (p.56)
Overdose danger rating Medium
Dependence rating Low
Prescription needed No
Available as generic Yes

GENERAL INFORMATION

Introduced in the 1970s, cinnarizine is an antihistamine drug used mainly to control nausea and vomiting, especially motion (travel) sickness. The drug is also used to control the symptoms (nausea and vertigo) of inner ear disorders such as labyrinthitis and Ménière's disease.

Taken in high doses, cinnarizine has a vasodilator effect and is used to improve circulation in Raynaud's disease and peripheral vascular disease.

Cinnarizine has adverse effects similar to those of most other antihistamines. Drowsiness, the most common problem, is usually less severe than with other antihistamines.

INFORMATION FOR USERS

Follow instructions on the label. Call your doctor if symptoms worsen.

How taken Tablets, capsules.

Frequency and timing of doses 2–3 x daily. For the prevention of motion sickness, the first dose should be taken 2 hours before travel.

Dosage range *Adults* 45–90mg daily (nausea/vomiting); 150–225mg daily (circulatory disorders); 30mg, then 15mg every 8 hours as needed (motion sickness). *Children* aged 5–12, 15mg, then 7.5mg every 8 hours as needed (motion sickness).

Onset of effect Within 30 minutes. Several weeks (circulation diseases).

Duration of action Up to 8 hours.

Diet advice None.

Storage Keep in a closed container in a cool, dry place out of reach of children.

Missed dose Take as soon as you remember. If your next dose is due within 2 hours, take a single dose now and skip the next.

Stopping the drug If you are taking cinnarizine to treat an inner ear disorder or circulatory condition, unless a rash occurs, do not stop taking the drug without consulting your doctor; symptoms may recur. When taken for motion sickness, the drug can be safely stopped as soon as you no longer need it.

Exceeding the dose An occasional unintentional extra dose is unlikely to cause problems. Large overdoses may cause drowsiness or agitation. Notify your doctor.

POSSIBLE ADVERSE EFFECTS

Drowsiness or lethargy are the main adverse effects of this drug. Anticholinergic effects, such as blurred vision and dry mouth, may also occur occasionally. If you develop a rash, stop taking the drug and consult your doctor.

INTERACTIONS

General note All drugs that have a sedative effect on the central nervous system, including sleeping drugs, antidepressants, antianxiety drugs, and opioid analgesics, may increase cinnarizine's sedative properties.

SPECIAL PRECAUTIONS

Be sure to consult your doctor or pharmacist before taking this drug if:

◆ You have low blood pressure.
◆ You have glaucoma.
◆ You have an enlarged prostate.
◆ You are taking other medications.

Pregnancy Safety in pregnancy not established. Discuss with your doctor.

Breast-feeding Safety not established. Discuss with your doctor.

Infants and children Reduced dose necessary.

Over 60 No special problems.

Driving and hazardous work Avoid such activities until you have learned how cinnarizine affects you because the drug can cause drowsiness.

Alcohol Avoid. Alcohol may increase the sedative effects of this drug.

PROLONGED USE

No special problems.

Ciprofloxacin

Brand name Ciproxin
Used in the following combined preparations
None

QUICK REFERENCE

Drug group Antibacterial (p.64)
Overdose danger rating Medium
Dependence rating Low
Prescription needed Yes
Available as generic No

GENERAL INFORMATION

Ciprofloxacin, a quinolone antibacterial, is used to treat several types of bacteria resistant to other commonly used antibiotics. It is especially useful for intestine and urinary tract infections and is also used to treat gonorrhoea.

When taken by mouth, ciprofloxacin is well absorbed by the body and works quickly and effectively. In more severe systemic bacterial infections, however, it may be necessary to administer the drug by injection.

Ciprofloxacin has a long duration of action and needs to be taken only once or twice daily. Its most common side effect is gastrointestinal disturbance.

INFORMATION FOR USERS

Your drug prescription is tailored for you. Do not alter dosage without checking with your doctor.

How taken Tablets, liquid, injection.

Frequency and timing of doses 2 x daily with plenty of fluids.

Adult dosage range 500mg–1.5g daily (tablets); 200–400mg daily (injection).

Onset of effect Within a few hours; full beneficial effect may not be felt for several days.

Duration of action About 12 hours.

Diet advice Do not get dehydrated; ensure that you drink fluids regularly.

Storage Keep in a closed container in a cool, dry place out of reach of children. The injection must be protected from light.

Missed dose Take as soon as you remember, and take your next dose as usual.

Stopping the drug Unless severe adverse effects occur (see below), take the full course. Even if you feel better the original infection may still be present, and symptoms may recur if treatment is stopped too soon.

Exceeding the dose An occasional unintentional extra dose is unlikely to cause problems. Large overdoses may cause mental disturbance and fits. Notify your doctor.

POSSIBLE ADVERSE EFFECTS

Ciprofloxacin commonly causes nausea and vomiting; other side effects are less common, except when very high doses are given. These include dizziness, confusion, sleep disturbance, and a rash on light-exposed areas. Painful or inflamed tendons should be reported to your doctor at once, treatment should be discontinued, and the affected limbs rested.

INTERACTIONS

Oral iron preparations and antacids containing magnesium or aluminium hydroxide interfere with absorption of ciprofloxacin. Do not take antacids within 2 hours of taking ciprofloxacin tablets.

Anticoagulants and oral antidiabetics Blood levels of these drugs may be increased; their dosage may need adjusting.

Theophylline Ciprofloxacin may increase blood levels of this drug; its dose may need adjusting and its blood levels monitored.

Phenytoin Ciprofloxacin may increase the blood levels of this drug.

NSAIDs These drugs increase the risk of epileptic fits.

SPECIAL PRECAUTIONS
Be sure to tell your doctor if:
◆ You have long-term liver or kidney problems.
◆ You have had epileptic fits.
◆ You have glucose-6-phosphate dehydrogenase (G6PD) deficiency.
◆ You are taking other medications.

Pregnancy Safety in pregnancy not established. Discuss with your doctor.

Breast-feeding The drug passes into the breast milk and may affect the baby adversely. Discuss with your doctor.

Infants and children Not usually recommended.

Over 60 No special problems.

Driving and hazardous work Avoid such activities until you have learned how ciprofloxacin affects you because the drug can cause dizziness.

Alcohol Avoid. Alcohol may increase the sedative effects of this drug.

Sunlight Avoid excessive exposure.

PROLONGED USE
No problems expected.

Monitoring Blood tests may be necessary to monitor kidney and liver function.

Cisplatin

Brand names None
Used in the following combined preparations
None

QUICK REFERENCE
Drug group Anticancer drug (p.94)
Overdose danger rating High
Dependence rating Low
Prescription needed Yes
Available as generic Yes

GENERAL INFORMATION
Cisplatin is one of the most effective drugs available to treat cancer of the ovaries or testes. People with cancer of the head, neck, bladder, cervix, and lung have also responded well to the drug. Recent research indicates that cisplatin may be an effective treatment against bone cancer in children. It is often given together with other anti-cancer drugs.

The most common and serious adverse effect of cisplatin is impaired kidney function. To reduce the risk of permanent kidney damage, the drug is usually given only once every four weeks, which allows the kidneys time to recover between courses of treatment. Nausea and vomiting may occur following administration of cisplatin. They usually start within an hour and last for up to 24 hours. In some cases, they can persist for up to a week, and because they may be quite severe, anti-emetic drugs are given to reduce them.

Damage to hearing is common and may be more severe in children. Use of cisplatin may also increase the risk of anaemia, blood clotting disorders, and infection during treatment. Some of the unwanted effects of cisplatin may be avoided by using carboplatin instead.

INFORMATION FOR USERS
This drug is given only under medical supervision and is not for self-administration.

How taken Injection.

Frequency and timing of doses Once daily for 5 days every 3 weeks (on its own or in combination with other anticancer drugs; once every 3–4 weeks (on its own).

Adult dosage range Dosage is determined individually according to body height, weight, and response.

Onset of effect Some adverse effects, such as nausea and vomiting, may appear within 1 hour of starting treatment.

Duration of action Some adverse effects may last for up to 1 week after treatment has stopped.

Diet advice Prior to treatment it is important that the body is well hydrated. Therefore, 1–2 litres of fluid are usually given by infusion over 8–12 hours.

Storage Not applicable. The drug is not normally kept in the home.

Missed dose Not applicable. Cisplatin is given only in hospital under medical supervision.

Stopping the drug Not applicable. The drug will be stopped under medical supervision.

Exceeding the dose Overdosage is unlikely since treatment is carefully monitored, and the drug is given intravenously only under close supervision.

POSSIBLE ADVERSE EFFECTS

Most adverse effects of cisplatin, such as nausea, vomiting, loss of appetite or taste, ringing in the ears, and hearing loss, appear within a few hours of injection and are carefully monitored in hospital after each dose. Some of these effects wear off within 24 hours. Nausea and loss of appetite may last for up to a week. Your doctor will monitor you for effects causing hearing loss, rash, or wheezing.

INTERACTIONS

General note A number of drugs (e.g., antibacterials such as gentamicin) increase the adverse effects of cisplatin. Because cisplatin is given only under close medical supervision, these interactions are carefully monitored and the dosage is adjusted accordingly.

SPECIAL PRECAUTIONS

Cisplatin is prescribed only under close medical supervision, taking account of your present condition and your medical history.

Pregnancy Not usually prescribed. Cisplatin may cause birth defects or premature birth. Discuss with your doctor.

Breast-feeding Not advised. The drug passes into the breast milk and may affect the baby adversely. Discuss with your doctor.

Infants and children The risk of hearing loss is increased. Reduced dose used.

Over 60 Reduced dose may be necessary. Increased likelihood of adverse effects.

Driving and hazardous work No known problems.

Alcohol No known problems.

PROLONGED USE

Prolonged use of this drug increases the risk of damage to the kidneys, nerves, and bone marrow, and to hearing.

Monitoring Hearing tests and blood checks to monitor kidney function and bone marrow activity are carried out regularly.

Citalopram

Brand name Cipramil
Used in the following combined preparations
None

QUICK REFERENCE

Drug group Antidepressant drug (p.14)
Overdose danger rating Medium
Dependence rating Low
Prescription needed Yes
Available as generic No

GENERAL INFORMATION

Citalopram is a member of the selective serotonin re-uptake inhibitor (SSRI) group of antidepressant drugs. It gradually improves the patient's mood, increases physical activity, and restores interest in everyday activities.

Citalopram is generally well tolerated, and any gastrointestinal adverse effects, such as nausea, vomiting, or diarrhoea, are related to the dose and usually diminish with continued use of the drug.

Like other SSRIs, citalopram causes fewer anticholinergic side effects, and it is less sedating than the tricyclic antidepressants. It is also less likely to be harmful if it is taken in overdose. Citalopram can, however, cause drowsiness and can impair the performance of tasks such as driving.

INFORMATION FOR USERS

Your drug prescription is tailored for you. Do not alter dosage without checking with your doctor.

How taken Tablets.

Frequency and timing of doses Once daily in the morning or evening.

Adult dosage range
Depressive illness 20–60mg.
Panic attacks 10mg (starting dose); 20–30mg (usual range).

Onset of effect Some benefit may appear within 7 days, but full benefits may not be felt for 2–4 weeks.

Duration of action Antidepressant effect may persist for some weeks following prolonged treatment.

Diet advice None.

Storage Keep in a closed container in a cool, dry place out of reach of children.

Missed dose Take as soon as you remember. If your next dose is due within 8 hours, take a single dose now and skip the next.

Stopping the drug Unless severe adverse effects occur (see below), do not stop taking the drug without consulting your doctor, who will supervise a gradual reduction in dosage. You may experience withdrawal symptoms such as headaches, nausea, dizziness, a "pins-and-needles" sensation, and anxiety.

Exceeding the dose An occasional unintentional extra dose is unlikely to be a cause for concern. If you notice any unusual symptoms, or if a large overdose has been taken, notify your doctor.

POSSIBLE ADVERSE EFFECTS
Common adverse effects, such as nausea, indigestion, and diarrhoea, usually diminish with a reduction in dosage. Some people may experience a dry mouth, sweating, anxiety, insomnia, headache, tremor, or drowsiness. If palpitations or rapid heart rate, confusion, convulsions, or rash occur, stop taking the drug and consult your doctor urgently.

INTERACTIONS
Sumatriptan and other 5HT$_1$ agonists and lithium There is an increased risk of adverse effects when citalopram is taken with these drugs.

MAOIs These drugs may cause a severe reaction if taken with citalopram; avoid citalopram if MAOIs have been taken in the last 14 days.

Anticoagulants The effect of these drugs may be increased by citalopram.

Drugs for epilepsy Citalopram may oppose the effect of these drugs.

SPECIAL PRECAUTIONS
Be sure to tell your doctor if:
◆ You have epilepsy.
◆ You have liver or kidney problems.
◆ You have had a manic-depressive illness.
◆ You have had heart problems.
◆ You have been taking MAOIs or other antidepressants.
◆ You are taking other medications.

Pregnancy Safety in pregnancy not established. Discuss with your doctor.

Breast-feeding The drug may pass into breast milk and may affect the baby. Discuss with your doctor.

Infants and children Not recommended.

Over 60 Reduced dose necessary.

Driving and hazardous work Avoid such activities until you have learned how citalopram affects you because it can cause drowsiness.

Alcohol Avoid. Alcohol may increase the sedative effects of citalopram.

PROLONGED USE
No problems expected. However, mild withdrawal symptoms may occur if the drug is not stopped gradually.

Clobetasol

Brand name Dermovate
Used in the following combined preparation Dermovate-NN

QUICK REFERENCE
Drug group Topical corticosteroid (p.116)
Overdose danger rating Low
Dependence rating Low
Prescription needed Yes
Available as generic No

GENERAL INFORMATION
Clobetasol is a corticosteroid drug (p.78) used in the short-term treatment of severe skin conditions such as discoid lupus erythematosus, lichen planus and lichen simplex, eczema, and psoriasis. The drug is generally considered the strongest topical corticosteroid and is therefore used only when the disorder has not responded to treatment with another topical corticosteroid.

It is important to apply clobetasol thinly and sparingly to affected areas because it can cause systemic adverse effects such as suppression of the pituitary and adrenal glands and Cushing's syndrome. Other side effects include irreversible changes to the structure of skin in treated areas. Also, clobetasol can exacerbate eczema infected with a virus such as herpes simplex. The drug should not be applied to the face, genital area, or between the toes.

INFORMATION FOR USERS
Your drug prescription is tailored for you. Do not alter dosage without checking with your doctor.

How taken Cream, ointment, scalp application.
Frequency and timing of doses 1 x 2 times daily. If treating the face, use for no more than 5 days.
Dosage range No more than 50g weekly.
Onset of effect
12 hours. Full beneficial effect after 48 hours.
Duration of action Up to 24 hours.
Diet advice None.
Storage Keep in a closed container, in a cool, dry place out of reach of children.
Missed dose Use as soon as you remember. If your next application is due within 8 hours, apply the usual amount now and skip the next application.
Stopping the drug Do not stop using the drug without consulting your doctor; symptoms may recur.
Exceeding the dose An occasional unintentional extra application is unlikely to cause problems. But if you notice any unusual symptoms, notify your doctor.

POSSIBLE ADVERSE EFFECTS

Most people who use clobetasol as directed have no problems. Adverse effects, including thinning of the skin, stretch marks, and loss of pigmentation, mainly affect the skin when high doses are used; some cannot be reversed. Mood changes, high blood pressure, and weight gain may occur if the drug is used in high doses and is absorbed through the skin.

INTERACTIONS

None.

SPECIAL PRECAUTIONS

Be sure to tell your doctor if:
◆ You have a cold sore or chickenpox.
◆ You have any other infection.
◆ You have acne or rosacea.
◆ You are taking other medications.
Pregnancy Safety in pregnancy not established. Discuss with your doctor.
Breast-feeding The drug passes into the breast milk and may affect the baby. Discuss with your doctor.
Infants and children Not recommended for infants under 1 year. Used only with great caution for short periods in older children because overuse can slow growth.
Over 60 No special problems.

Driving and hazardous work No special problems.
Alcohol No special problems.

PROLONGED USE

Clobetasol is not normally used for more than 4 weeks. If the condition has not improved in 2 to 4 weeks, notify your doctor.

Clomifene

Brand names Clomid, Serophene
Used in the following combined preparations
None

QUICK REFERENCE

Drug group Drug for infertility (p.105)
Overdose danger rating Low
Dependence rating Low
Prescription needed Yes
Available as generic No

GENERAL INFORMATION

Clomifene increases the output of hormones by the pituitary gland, thereby stimulating ovulation (egg release) in women. If hormone levels in the blood fail to rise after the drug is taken, the gland is not working as it should.

For female infertility, tablets are taken within about five days of the onset of each menstrual cycle. This stimulates ovulation. If the drug does not stimulate ovulation after several months, other drugs may be prescribed.

Multiple pregnancies (usually twins) occur more commonly in women treated with clomifene than in those who have not been treated. Adverse effects include an increased risk of ovarian cysts and ectopic pregnancy.

INFORMATION FOR USERS

Your drug prescription is tailored for you. Do not alter dosage without checking with your doctor.
How taken Tablets.
Frequency and timing of doses Once daily for 5 days during each menstrual cycle.
Dosage range 50mg daily initially; dose may be increased up to 100mg daily.
Onset of effect Ovulation occurs 4–10 days after the last dose in any cycle. However, ovulation may not occur for several months.

Duration of action 5 days.
Diet advice None.
Storage Keep in a closed container in a cool, dry place out of reach of children. Protect from light.
Missed dose Take as soon as you remember. If your next dose is due, take the missed dose and the next scheduled dose together.
Stopping the drug Unless severe adverse effects occur (see below), take as directed by your doctor. Stopping the drug will reduce the chances of conception.
Exceeding the dose An occasional unintentional extra dose is unlikely to be a cause for concern. But if you notice any unusual symptoms, or if a large overdose has been taken, notify your doctor.

POSSIBLE ADVERSE EFFECTS

Most side effects are dose-related. These include hot flushes, nausea, vomiting, 'breakthrough' bleeding, abdominal discomfort, dizziness, and breast tenderness. Ovarian enlargement and cyst formation can occur. If this happens the problem usually resolves within a few weeks of stopping the drug. If you experience blurred vision, severe pain in the chest or abdomen, convulsions, or you develop a rash, stop taking the drug and consult your doctor.

INTERACTIONS

None.

SPECIAL PRECAUTIONS

Be sure to tell your doctor if:
◆ You have a long-term liver problem.
◆ You are taking other medications.
Pregnancy Not prescribed. The drug is stopped as soon as pregnancy occurs.
Breast-feeding Not prescribed.
Infants and children Not prescribed.
Over 60 Not prescribed.
Driving and hazardous work No special problems.
Alcohol Keep consumption low.

PROLONGED USE

Prolonged use of clomifene may cause visual impairment. Also, no more than 6 courses of treatment are recommended since this may lead to an increased risk of ovarian cancer.

Monitoring Eye tests may be recommended if symptoms of visual impairment are noticed. Monitoring of body temperature and blood or urine hormone levels is performed to detect signs of ovulation and pregnancy.

Clomipramine

Brand names Anafranil, Anafranil SR
Used in the following combined preparations
None

QUICK REFERENCE

Drug group Tricyclic antidepressant (p.14)
Overdose danger rating High
Dependence rating Low
Prescription needed Yes
Available as generic Yes

GENERAL INFORMATION

Clomipramine belongs to the class of antidepressant drugs known as the tricyclics. It is used mainly in the long-term treatment of depression. It elevates the patient's mood, improves appetite, increases physical activity, and restores interest in everyday activities.

Clomipramine is particularly useful in the treatment of irrational fears and obsessive behaviour. Unlike most other tricyclics, it can be given by injection in severe illness.

In overdose, the drug may cause coma and dangerously abnormal heart rhythms.

Tricyclic antidepressant drugs have been linked with an increase in dental caries in long-term use.

INFORMATION FOR USERS

Your drug prescription is tailored for you. Do not alter dosage without checking with your doctor.
How taken SR-tablets, capsules, liquid, injection.
Frequency and timing of doses 1–4 x daily.
Adult dosage range 10–250mg daily.
Onset of effect Some effects may be felt within a few days, but full antidepressant effect may not be felt for up to 4 weeks.
Duration of action During prolonged treatment antidepressant effect may last up to 2 weeks.
Diet advice None.

Storage Keep in a closed container in a cool, dry place out of reach of children.

Missed dose Take as soon as you remember. If your next dose is due within 3 hours, take a single dose now and skip the next.

Stopping the drug Stopping abruptly can cause withdrawal symptoms and recurrence of the original trouble. Consult your doctor, who may supervise gradual dosage reduction.

OVERDOSE ACTION

Seek immediate medical advice in all cases. Take emergency action if palpitations are noted or consciousness is lost.

POSSIBLE ADVERSE EFFECTS

The possible adverse effects of clomipramine are mainly the result of its anticholinergic action, and include drowsiness and dizziness, dry mouth, constipation, blurred vision, and urinary difficulties. If you experience palpitations, consult your doctor urgently.

INTERACTIONS

Sedatives All drugs that have a sedative effect may intensify those of clomipramine.

Antihypertensives Clomipramine may enhance the effect of some of these drugs.

Anticonvulsants Clomipramine may reduce the effects of these drugs and vice versa.

MAOIs A serious reaction may occur if these drugs are given with clomipramine.

Quinidine There is an increased risk of abnormal heart rhythms if this drug is taken with clomipramine.

SPECIAL PRECAUTIONS

Be sure to tell your doctor if:
◆ You have heart problems.
◆ You have had epileptic fits.
◆ You have long-term liver or kidney problems.
◆ You have had glaucoma.
◆ You have thyroid disease.
◆ You have had prostate trouble.
◆ You are taking other medications.

Pregnancy Safety in pregnancy not established. Discuss with your doctor.

Breast-feeding The drug passes into the breast milk and may affect the baby. Discuss with your doctor.

Infants and children Not usually prescribed.

Over 60 Reduced dose may be necessary. Increased likelihood of adverse effects.

Driving and hazardous work Avoid such activities until you have learned how clomipramine affects you because the drug may cause blurred vision, drowsiness, and dizziness.

Alcohol Avoid. Alcohol may increase the sedative effects of this drug.

Surgery and general anaesthetics
Clomipramine treatment may need to be stopped before you have a general anaesthetic. Discuss this with your doctor or dentist before any operation.

PROLONGED USE

No problems expected.

Monitoring Regular checks on liver function are recommended. Regular dental check-ups are also advised because prolonged use of clomipramine can lead to dental caries.

Clonazepam

Brand name Rivotril
Used in the following combined preparations
None

QUICK REFERENCE

Drug group Benzodiazepine anticonvulsant drug (p.16)
Overdose danger rating Medium
Dependence rating Medium
Prescription needed Yes
Available as generic No

GENERAL INFORMATION

Clonazepam belongs to a group of drugs known as the benzodiazepines, which are mainly used in the treatment of anxiety and insomnia (see p.13). However, clonazepam is used almost exclusively as an anticonvulsant to prevent and treat epileptic fits. It is particularly useful for the prevention of brief muscle spasms and absence seizures (petit mal) in children but other forms of epilepsy, such as sudden flaccidity or fits induced by bright lights, also respond to clonazepam treatment. Being a benzodiazepine, the drug also has tranquillizing and sedative effects.

Clonazepam is used either alone or together with other anticonvulsant drugs. Its anticonvulsant effect may begin to wear off after a few months.

INFORMATION FOR USERS

Your drug prescription is tailored for you. Do not alter dosage without checking with your doctor.

How taken Tablets, injection.
Frequency and timing of doses 1–4 x daily.
Dosage range *Adults* 1mg daily (starting dose), increased gradually to 4–8 mg daily (maintenance dose).
Children Reduced dose according to age and weight.
Onset of effect Within 1 hour.
Duration of action Approximately 30 hours.
Diet advice None.
Storage Keep in a closed container in a cool, dry place out of reach of children.
Missed dose No cause for concern, but take as soon as you remember. Take your next dose when it is due.
Stopping the drug Do not stop taking the drug without consulting your doctor because withdrawal symptoms may occur, and your illness may recur.
Exceeding the dose An occasional unintentional extra dose is unlikely to cause problems. Larger overdoses may cause unusual drowsiness and confusion. Notify your doctor.

POSSIBLE ADVERSE EFFECTS

The principal adverse effects of this drug are related to its sedative and tranquillizing properties and include drowsiness, dizziness, forgetfulness, and muscle weakness. Increased salivation may also occur. These effects normally diminish after the first few days of treatment and can often be reduced by medically supervised adjustment of dosage.

INTERACTIONS

Sedatives All drugs that have a sedative effect on the central nervous system are likely to add to the sedative properties of clonazepam. Such drugs include anti-anxiety and sleeping drugs, antihistamines, opioid analgesics, antidepressants, and antipsychotics.
Other anticonvulsants Clonazepam may alter the effects of other anticonvulsants you are taking, and adjustment of dosage or change of drug may be necessary.

SPECIAL PRECAUTIONS

Be sure to tell your doctor if:
◆ You have severe respiratory disease.
◆ You have long-term liver or kidney problems.
◆ You are taking other medications.
Pregnancy Safety in pregnancy not established. Discuss with your doctor.
Breast-feeding The drug passes into the breast milk and may affect the baby adversely. Discuss with your doctor.
Infants and children Reduced dose necessary.
Over 60 Reduced dose may be necessary.
Driving and hazardous work Your underlying condition, as well as the possibility of drowsiness while taking clonazepam, may make such activities inadvisable. Discuss with your doctor.
Alcohol Avoid. Alcohol may increase the sedative effects of this drug.

PROLONGED USE

Both beneficial and adverse effects of clonazepam may become less marked during prolonged treatment as the body adapts to the drug.

Clopidogrel

Brand name Plavix
Used in the following combined preparations
None

QUICK REFERENCE

Drug group Antiplatelet drug (p.36)
Overdose danger rating Medium
Dependence rating Low
Prescription needed Yes
Available as generic No

GENERAL INFORMATION

Clopidogrel is an antiplatelet drug that is used to prevent blood clots from forming. It is prescribed to patients who have a tendency to form clots in the fast-flowing blood of the arteries and heart, or those who have had a stroke or a heart attack.

Clopidogrel may be suitable for people who cannot take aspirin for its antiplatelet effects. It reduces the tendency of platelets to stick together when blood flow is disrupted.

However, this can lead to abnormal bleeding. You should, therefore, report any unusual bleeding to your doctor a once, and, if you require dental treatment, you should tell your dentist that you are taking the drug.

Adverse effects are not common; they are usually associated with bleeding.

INFORMATION FOR USERS
Your drug prescription is tailored for you. Do not alter dosage without checking with your doctor.

How taken Tablets.
Frequency and timing of doses Once daily.
Dosage range 75mg.
Onset of effect 1 hour.
Duration of action 24 hours.
Diet advice None.
Storage Keep in a closed container in a cool, dry place out of reach of children.
Missed dose Take as soon as you remember. If your next dose is due within 4 hours, take a single dose now and skip the next.
Stopping the drug Unless you develop a sore throat or a bleeding problem, do not stop taking the drug without consulting your doctor.
Exceeding the dose An occasional unintentional extra dose is unlikely to be a cause for concern. But if you notice any unusual symptoms, or if a large overdose has been taken, notify your doctor.

POSSIBLE ADVERSE EFFECTS
The principal adverse effects of clopidogrel are bleeding and bruising. These may include nosebleeds, bleeding from a stomach ulcer, or blood in the urine. Any unusual bleeding or bruising should be reported to your doctor without delay. Nausea, vomiting, abdominal pain, and diarrhoea are less common adverse effects of clopidogrel. Headache and dizziness may also occur. If you experience a rash or itching, seek medical advice. If you develop a sore throat, stop taking the drug and consult your doctor urgently.

INTERACTIONS
Aspirin and other NSAID Clopidogrel increases the effect of aspirin on platelets. The risk of gastrointestinal bleeding is increased when clopidogrel is used with these drugs.

Anticoagulant drugs (e.g., warfarin) The anticoagulant effect of these drugs is increased if they are taken with clopidogrel.

SPECIAL PRECAUTIONS
Be sure to tell your doctor if:
◆ You have liver or kidney problems.
◆ You have a condition, such as a peptic ulcer, that makes you more likely to bleed.
◆ You are taking other medications.
Pregnancy Safety in pregnancy not established. Discuss with your doctor.
Breast-feeding The drug passes into the breast milk and may affect the baby. Discuss with your doctor.
Infants and children Not recommended.
Over 60 No special problems.
Driving and hazardous work No special problems.
Alcohol Excessive intake of alcohol may irritate the stomach and increase the risk of bleeding.
Surgery and general anaesthetics Clopidogrel may need to be stopped a week before surgery. Discuss this with your doctor or dentist.

PROLONGED USE
No special problems.

Clotrimazole

Brand names Canesten, Masnoderm, Mycil Gold
Used in the following combined preparations Canesten HC, Lotriderm

QUICK REFERENCE
Drug group Antifungal drug (p.74)
Overdose danger rating Low
Dependence rating Low
Prescription needed No
Available as generic Yes

GENERAL INFORMATION
Clotrimazole is an antifungal drug that is commonly used to treat fungal and yeast infections. It is used for treating tinea (ringworm) infections of the skin, and candida (thrush) infections of the mouth, vagina, or penis. The drug is applied in the form of a cream, spray, topical solution, or dusting

powder to the affected area and inserted as pessaries or cream for vaginal conditions such as candida.

Adverse effects from clotrimazole are very rare, although some people may experience burning and irritation on the skin surface in the area where the drug has been applied.

INFORMATION FOR USERS

Follow instructions on the label. Call your doctor if symptoms worsen.

How taken Pessaries, cream, spray, dusting powder, topical solution.

Frequency and timing of doses 2–3 x daily (skin cream, spray, solution); once daily at bedtime (pessaries); 1–2 x daily (vaginal cream).

Dosage range *Vaginal infections* One applicatorful (5g) per dose (vaginal cream); 100–500mg per dose (pessaries). *Skin infections* (skin cream, spray, solution) as directed.

Onset of effect Within 2–3 days.

Duration of action Up to 12 hours.

Diet advice None.

Storage Keep in a closed container in a cool, dry place out of reach of children.

Missed dose No cause for concern, but make up the missed dose or application as soon as you remember.

Stopping the drug Unless a rash occurs, apply the full course. Even if symptoms disappear, the original infection may still be present and may recur if treatment is stopped too soon.

Exceeding the dose An occasional unintentional extra dose is unlikely to cause problems. But if you notice unusual symptoms or if a large amount has been swallowed, notify your doctor.

POSSIBLE ADVERSE EFFECTS

Clotrimazole rarely causes adverse effects. Skin preparations and vaginal applications may occasionally cause localized stinging or irritation. If you develop a rash, stop using the drug.

INTERACTIONS

None known.

SPECIAL PRECAUTIONS

Be sure to tell your doctor or pharmacist if:
◆ You are taking other medications.

Pregnancy No evidence of risk to developing baby.

Breast-feeding No evidence of risk.

Infants and children No special problems.

Over 60 No special problems.

Driving and hazardous work No known problems.

Alcohol No known problems.

PROLONGED USE

No problems expected.

Clozapine

Brand name Clozaril
Used in the following combined preparations None

QUICK REFERENCE

Drug group Antipsychotic (p.15)
Overdose danger rating Medium
Dependence rating Low
Prescription needed Yes
Available as generic No

GENERAL INFORMATION

Clozapine is a new type of antipsychotic drug used to treat schizophrenia. It is prescribed only for patients who have not responded to other treatments or those who have experienced intolerable side effects with other drugs. Clozapine helps control severe resistant schizophrenia, helping the patient to re-establish a more normal lifestyle. The improvement is gradual, and relief of severe symptoms can take more than three weeks.

All treatment is started and supervised by a hospital, because all patients must be registered with the Clozaril Patient Monitoring Service (CPMS). The drug can cause a very serious side effect, agranulocytosis (a large decrease in the number of white blood cells). Blood tests are done before treatment and regularly thereafter; the drug is supplied only if results are normal.

Clozapine is less likely than other antipsychotics to cause parkinsonism.

INFORMATION FOR USERS

This drug is given only under strict medical supervision and continual monitoring.

How taken Tablets.
Frequency and timing of doses 1–3 x daily; a larger dose may be given at night.
Adult dosage range 25–900mg daily.
Onset of effect Gradual. Some effect may appear within 3–5 days, but the full beneficial effect may not be felt for over 3 weeks.
Duration of action Up to 16 hours.
Diet advice None.
Storage Keep in a closed container in a cool, dry place out of reach of children.
Missed dose Take as soon as you remember. If your next dose is due within 2 hours, take a single dose now and skip the next.
Stopping the drug Do not stop taking the drug without consulting your doctor because symptoms may recur.
Exceeding the dose An occasional unintentional extra dose is unlikely to cause problems. Large overdoses may cause unusual drowsiness, fits, and agitation. Notify your doctor.

POSSIBLE ADVERSE EFFECTS
Clozapine is less likely to cause parkinsonian side effects (tremor and stiffness), which occur with other antipsychotic drugs, but may cause drowsiness, tiredness, dry mouth, fast heartbeat, or blurred vision, and it occasionally causes dizziness or fainting. Clozapine may, rarely, cause epileptic fits requiring urgent medical attention. The most serious side effect is agranulocytosis, and strict monitoring of the white blood cell count is necessary. Drowsiness or tiredness may be signs of this; if they occur, seek urgent medical advice.

INTERACTIONS
General note A number of drugs increase the risk of adverse effects on the blood. Do not take other medication without checking with your doctor or pharmacist.
Sedatives All drugs that have a sedative effect on the central nervous system are likely to increase the sedative properties of clozapine.

SPECIAL PRECAUTIONS
Be sure to tell your doctor if:
◆ You have long-term liver or kidney problems.
◆ You have a history of blood disorders.
◆ You have had epileptic fits.
◆ You are taking other medications.

Pregnancy Not usually prescribed. Safety not established. Discuss with your doctor.
Breast-feeding The drug passes into the breast milk and may affect the baby adversely. Discuss with your doctor.
Infants and children Not prescribed.
Over 60 Adverse effects are more likely. Initial dose is low and is slowly increased.
Driving and hazardous work Avoid such activities until you have learned how clozapine affects you because the drug can cause drowsiness, dizziness, and blurred vision.
Alcohol Avoid. Alcohol may increase the sedative effects of this drug.

PROLONGED USE
There is a risk of agranulocytosis (see Introduction, above) and occasionally liver function may be upset.
Monitoring Test to measure the white blood cell count are carried out weekly for the first 18 weeks, fortnightly until the end of the first year, and, if blood counts are stable, at four-weekly intervals thereafter. Liver function tests may also be performed.

Codeine
Used in the following combined preparations
Benylin with Codeine, Co-codamol, Codafen Continus, Codis, Diarrest, Migraleve, Panadol Ultra, Solpadeine, Solpadol, Syndol, Terpoin, Tylex, Veganin, and others

QUICK REFERENCE
Drug group Opioid analgesic (p.9), antidiarrhoeal drug (p.42), and cough suppressant (p.25)
Overdose danger rating High
Dependence rating Medium
Prescription needed Yes (some preparations)
Available as generic Yes

GENERAL INFORMATION
Codeine is a mild opioid analgesic that is similar to, but weaker than, morphine. It has been in common medical use since the beginning of this century.

Codeine is prescribed primarily to relieve mild to moderate pain and is often combined with a non-opioid analgesic such as paracetamol. It is also an effective cough suppressant and, for this reason, is included as an ingredient in many non-prescription cough syrups and cold relief preparations.

Like the other opioid, codeine is constipating, which sometimes makes it useful in the short-term control of diarrhoea.

Although codeine is habit-forming, addiction seldom occurs if the drug is used for a limited period of time and at the recommended dosage.

Constipation is common with codeine. Other, rare, adverse effects include breathing difficulties, which should be reported to your doctor without delay.

INFORMATION FOR USERS
Your drug prescription is tailored for you. Do not alter dosage without checking with your doctor.

How taken Tablets, liquid, injection.
Frequency and timing of doses 4–6 x daily (pain); 3–4 x daily when necessary (cough); every 4–6 hours when necessary (diarrhoea).
Adult dosage range 120–240mg daily (pain); 45–120mg daily (cough); 30–180mg daily (diarrhoea).
Onset of effect 30–60 minutes.
Duration of action 4–6 hours.
Diet advice None.
Storage Keep in a closed container in a cool, dry place out of reach of children. Protect from light.
Missed dose Take as soon as you remember if needed for relief of symptoms. If not needed, do not take the missed dose, and return to your normal dose schedule when necessary.
Stopping the drug Can be safely stopped as soon as you no longer need it.

OVERDOSE ACTION
Seek immediate medical advice in all cases. Take emergency action if there are symptoms such as slow or irregular breathing, severe drowsiness, or loss of consciousness.

POSSIBLE ADVERSE EFFECTS
Serious adverse effects are rare with codeine. Constipation occurs, especially with prolonged use, but other side effects such as nausea, vomiting, dizziness, and drowsiness are not usually troublesome at recommended doses, and usually disappear if the dose is reduced. If you experience agitation or restlessness,

stop taking the drug. If you develop a rash, hives, wheezing, or breathlessness, stop taking it and seek urgent medical attention.

INTERACTIONS
Sedatives All drugs, including alcohol, that have a sedative effect on the central nervous system are likely to increase sedation with codeine. Such drugs include sleeping drugs, antidepressants, and antihistamines.

SPECIAL PRECAUTIONS
Be sure tell your doctor if:
◆ You have long-term liver or kidney problems.
◆ You have a lung disorder such as asthma or bronchitis.
◆ You are taking other medications.
Pregnancy No evidence of risk, but may adversely affect the baby's breathing if taken during labour.
Breast-feeding The drug passes into the breast milk, but at normal doses adverse effects on the baby are unlikely. Discuss with your doctor.
Infants and children Reduced dose necessary.
Over 60 Reduced dose may be necessary.
Driving and hazardous work Avoid such activities until you have learned how codeine affects you because the drug may cause dizziness and drowsiness.
Alcohol Avoid. Alcohol may increase the sedative effects of this drug.

PROLONGED USE
Codeine is normally used only for short-term relief of symptoms. It can be habit-forming if taken for extended periods, especially if higher-than-average doses are taken.

Colchicine

Brand names None
Used in the following combined preparations
None

QUICK REFERENCE
Drug group Drug for gout (p.51)
Overdose danger rating High
Dependence rating Low
Prescription needed Yes
Available as generic Yes

GENERAL INFORMATION

Colchicine, a drug originally extracted from the autumn crocus flower and later synthesized, has been used since the 18th century for gout. Although it has now, to some extent, been superseded by newer drugs, it is still often used to relieve joint pain and inflammation in flare-ups of gout. Colchicine is most effective when taken at the first sign of symptoms, and almost always produces an improvement. The drug is also often given during the first few months of treatment with allopurinol (another drugs used for treating gout), because it may at first increase the frequency of gout attacks.

Colchicine is also prescribed for the relief of the symptoms of familial Mediterranean fever (a rare congenital condition).

INFORMATION FOR USERS

Your drug prescription is tailored for you. Do not alter dosage without checking with your doctor.

How taken Tablets.

Frequency and timing of doses *Prevention of gout attacks* 2–3 x daily.
Relief of gout attacks Every 2–3 hours.

Adult dosage range *Prevention of gout attacks* 1–1.5mg daily.
Relief of gout attacks 1mg initially, followed by 0.5mg every 2–3 hours, until relief of pain, vomiting, or diarrhoea occurs, or until a total dose of 6mg is reached. This course must not be repeated within 3 days.

Onset of effect Relief of symptoms in an attack of gout may be felt in 6–24 hours. Full effect in gout prevention may not be felt for several days.

Duration of action Up to 2 hours. Some effect may last longer.

Diet advice Certain foods are known to make gout worse. Discuss with your doctor.

Storage Keep in a closed container in a cool, dry place out of reach of children. Protect from light.

Missed dose Take as soon as you remember. If your next dose is due within 30 minutes, take a single dose now and skip the next.

Stopping the drug When taking colchicine frequently during an acute attack of gout, stop taking it if diarrhoea or abdominal pain develop.

OVERDOSE ACTION

Seek immediate medical advice in all cases. Some reactions can be fatal. Take emergency action if severe nausea, vomiting, bloody diarrhoea, severe abdominal pain, or loss of consciousness occur.

POSSIBLE ADVERSE EFFECTS

The appearance of any symptom that may be an adverse effect of colchicine is a sign that you should stop taking the drug until you have received further medical advice. These symptoms include nausea, vomiting, diarrhoea, abdominal pain, numbness and tingling, unusual bleeding or bruising, and a rash.

INTERACTIONS

Ciclosporin Taking ciclosporin with colchicine may lead to adverse effects on the kidneys.

SPECIAL PRECAUTIONS

Be sure to tell your doctor if:
◆ You have long-term liver or kidney problems.
◆ You have heart problems.
◆ You have a blood disorder.
◆ You have stomach ulcers.
◆ You have chronic inflammation of the bowel.
◆ You are taking other medications.

Pregnancy Not usually prescribed. May cause defects in the unborn baby. Discuss with your doctor.

Breast-feeding The drug passes into the breast milk and may affect the baby. Discuss with your doctor.

Infants and children Not recommended.

Over 60 Increased likelihood of adverse effects.

Driving and hazardous work No special problems.

Alcohol Avoid. Alcohol may increase stomach irritation caused by colchicine.

PROLONGED USE

Prolonged use of this drug may lead to hair loss, rash, tingling in the hands and feet, muscle pain and weakness, and blood disorders.

Monitoring Periodic blood checks are usually required.

Colestyramine

Brand names Questran, Questran Light
Used in the following combined preparations
None

QUICK REFERENCE

Drug group Lipid-lowering drug (p.35)
Overdose danger rating Low
Dependence rating Low
Prescription needed Yes
Available as generic No

GENERAL INFORMATION

Colestyramine is a resin that binds bile acids in the intestine, preventing their reabsorption. Cholesterol in the body is normally converted to bile acids. Therefore, the use of colestyramine results in a reduction of cholesterol levels in the blood. This action on the bile acids makes bowel movements bulkier, creating an antidiarrhoeal effect. The action on cholesterol helps people with hyperlipidaemia (high levels of fat in the blood) who have not responded to dietary measures, and who are at particular risk from heart disease as a result of diabetes or a family history of death from heart attacks.

In liver disorders such as primary biliary cirrhosis, bile salts sometimes accumulate in the bloodstream, and colestyramine may be prescribed to alleviate any itching that occurs.

Taken in large doses, the drug often causes bloating, mild nausea, and constipation. It may also interfere with the body's ability to absorb fat and certain fat-soluble vitamins, causing pale, bulky, foul-smelling faeces.

INFORMATION FOR USERS

Your drug prescription is tailored for you. Do not alter dosage without checking with your doctor.
How taken Powder mixed with water, juice, or soft food.
Frequency and timing of doses 1–4 x daily before meals and at bedtime.
Adult dosage range 4–36g daily.
Onset of effect Full beneficial effects may not be felt for several weeks.
Duration of action 12–24 hours.
Diet advice A low-fat, low-calorie diet may be advised for patients who are overweight. Use of this drug may deplete levels of certain vitamins. Supplements may be advised.
Storage Keep in a closed container in a cool, dry place out of reach of children.
Missed dose Take as soon as you remember.
Stopping the drug Do not stop taking the drug without consulting your doctor.
Exceeding the dose An occasional unintentional extra dose is unlikely to cause problems. But if you notice any unusual symptoms, or if a large overdose has been taken, notify your doctor.

POSSIBLE ADVERSE EFFECTS

Adverse effects are more likely if large doses are taken by people over 60. Minor side effects such as indigestion and abdominal discomfort are rarely a cause for concern. Nausea, vomiting, and constipation may also occur. High doses may cause diarrhoea. More serious adverse effects, such as bruising or increased bleeding, are usually the result of vitamin deficiency.

INTERACTIONS

General note Colestyramine reduces the body's ability to absorb other drugs. It may be necessary to organize a schedule in consultation with your doctor whereby you take other medications at a fixed time before you take colestyramine. Usually, taking other medications 30 to 60 minutes prior to colestyramine, or 4 to 6 hours after, solves the problem. The dosage of other drugs may need to be adjusted.

SPECIAL PRECAUTIONS

Be sure to tell your doctor if:
◆ You have jaundice.
◆ You have a peptic ulcer.
◆ You suffer from haemorrhoids.
◆ You are taking other medications.
Pregnancy Safety in pregnancy not established. Discuss with your doctor.
Breast-feeding Safety not established. The drug binds fat-soluble vitamins long term and may cause vitamin deficiency in the baby. Discuss with your doctor.
Infants and children Not recommended under 6 years. Reduced dose necessary in older children.
Over 60 Increased likelihood of adverse effects.

Driving and hazardous work No special problems.

Alcohol Although this drug does not interact with alcohol, your underlying condition may make it inadvisable to take alcohol.

PROLONGED USE

As this drug reduces vitamin absorption, supplements of vitamins A, D, and K may be advised.

Monitoring Periodic blood checks are usually required to monitor the level of cholesterol in the blood.

Conjugated estrogens

Brand name Premarin
Used in the following combined preparation
Prempak-C

QUICK REFERENCE

Drug group Female sex hormone (p.86) and drug for bone disorders (p.54)
Overdose danger rating Low
Dependence rating Low
Prescription needed Yes
Available as generic Yes

GENERAL INFORMATION

Preparations of conjugated estrogens consist of naturally occurring estrogens similar to those found in the urine of pregnant mares.

Given by mouth, they are used to relieve menopausal symptoms such as hot flushes and sweating. They are also used to prevent osteoporosis (brittle bones), which may occur after the menopause.

As replacement therapy, conjugated estrogens are usually taken on a cyclic dosing schedule, usually in conjunction with a progestogen, to simulate the hormonal changes that occur in a normal menstrual cycle. They may also be prescribed in the form of vaginal cream to relieve pain and dryness of the vagina or vulva after the menopause.

INFORMATION FOR USERS

Your drug prescription is tailored for you. Do not alter dosage without checking with your doctor.
How taken Tablets, cream.

Frequency and timing of doses 1–3 x daily (tablets). Once daily (cream).
Adult dosage range *Replacement therapy* 0.625–1.25mg daily (tablets); 1–2g daily (cream).
Onset of effect 5–20 days.
Duration of action 1–2 days.
Diet advice None.
Storage Keep in a closed container in a cool, dry place out of reach of children.
Missed dose Take as soon as you remember.
Stopping the drug Do not stop taking the drug without consulting your doctor because symptoms may recur.
Exceeding the dose An occasional unintentional extra dose is unlikely to be a cause for concern. But if you notice any unusual symptoms, or if a large overdose has been taken, notify your doctor.

POSSIBLE ADVERSE EFFECTS

The most common adverse effects of conjugated estrogens, such as nausea, vomiting, weight increase or decrease, and breast swelling or tenderness, are similar to symptoms that occur in the early stages of pregnancy. These generally diminish or disappear after 2–3 months of treatment. If you have vaginal bleeding, consult your doctor; and seek urgent medical advice if reduced sex drive or depression occur. Swelling or pain in the legs, sudden shortness of breath, or pain in the chest may indicate an abnormal blood clot requiring urgent medical attention.

INTERACTIONS

Tobacco smoking Smoking increases the risk of serious adverse effects on the heart and circulation with conjugated estrogens.
Oral anticoagulant drugs Conjugated estrogens reduce the anticoagulant effect of these drugs.

SPECIAL PRECAUTIONS

Be sure to tell your doctor if:
◆ You have heart failure or high blood pressure.
◆ You have had blood clots or a stroke.
◆ You have a history of breast disease.
◆ You have had fibroids in the uterus.
◆ You suffer from migraine or epilepsy.
◆ You are taking other medications.

◆ You have long-term liver or kidney problems.

Pregnancy Not prescribed. May affect the baby adversely. Discuss with your doctor.

Breast-feeding Not prescribed. The drug passes into the breast milk and may inhibit the flow of milk. Discuss with your doctor.

Infants and children Not prescribed.

Over 60 No special problems.

Driving and hazardous work No known problems.

Alcohol No known problems.

Surgery and general anaesthetics Conjugated estrogens may need to be stopped several weeks before you have surgery. Discuss with your doctor.

PROLONGED USE
There is a slightly higher risk of cancer of the uterus when estrogens are used long term. The risk of gallbladder disease is also increased, and the risk of blood clots is also increased in susceptible people.

Monitoring Physical examinations and blood pressure checks may be needed.

Co-Proxamol

Brand names Cosalgesic, Distalgesic
Used in the following combined preparations
(Co-proxamol is a combination of two drugs)

QUICK REFERENCE
Drug group Opioid analgesic (p.9)
Overdose danger rating High
Dependence rating Medium
Prescription needed Yes
Available as generic Yes

GENERAL INFORMATION
Co-proxamol is the generic name for a combination of the non-opioid analgesic drug paracetamol and a mild opioid analgesic, dextropropoxyphene. Co-proxamol is widely used for the relief of mild to moderate pain, but research does not show it to be more effective than paracetamol alone.

Because the drug contains an opioid, it can cause a variety of side effects that are common to drugs of that group: dizziness, mild euphoria, nausea, and constipation.

Co-proxamol may also be habit-forming if taken regularly for an extended period. Overdose with co-proxamol is dangerous because dextropropoxyphene may interfere with breathing if it is taken in excess, and overdose of paracetamol may cause irreversible damage to the liver and kidneys.

INFORMATION FOR USERS
Your drug prescription is tailored for you. Do not alter dosage without checking with your doctor.

How taken Tablets.

Frequency and timing of doses 3–4 x daily as necessary.

Adult dosage range 2 tablets per dose, up to a maximum of 8 tablets daily.

Onset of effect 30–60 minutes.

Duration of action 6 hours.

Diet advice None.

Storage Keep in a closed container in a cool, dry place out of reach of children.

Missed dose Take as soon as you remember if needed for the relief of pain. Do not take doses less than 4 hours apart.

Stopping the drug If you have been taking the drug regularly for less than 4 weeks, it can be safely stopped as soon as you no longer need it. If you have been regularly taking the drug longer than this, your doctor may recommend a gradual reduction in dosage.

OVERDOSE ACTION
Seek immediate medical advice in all cases. Take emergency action if irregular breathing, drowsiness or loss of consciousness occur.

POSSIBLE ADVERSE EFFECTS
Serious adverse effects are rare with this drug. However, dizziness, drowsiness, nausea, vomiting, and constipation occur in some people. If you become euphoric or you develop hallucinations, stop taking the drug. If you develop a rash, stop taking the drug and consult your doctor.

INTERACTIONS
General note All drugs, including alcohol, that have a sedative effect are likely to increase the sedative properties of co-proxamol. These include sleeping drugs, anti-anxiety drugs, and antidepressants.

Carbamazepine Co-proxamol can enhance the effects of carbamazepine.
Oral anticoagulant drugs Co-proxamol may increase the anticoagulant effect of these drugs.

SPECIAL PRECAUTIONS

Be sure to tell your doctor if:
◆ You have long-term liver or kidney problems.
◆ You have had problems with drug or alcohol abuse.
◆ You have a lung disorder such as asthma or bronchitis.
◆ You suffer from depression.
◆ You are taking other medications.
Pregnancy Safety in pregnancy not established. Discuss with your doctor.
Breast-feeding The drug passes into the breast milk and may affect the baby. Discuss with your doctor.
Infants and children Not recommended.
Over 60 Reduced dose necessary.
Driving and hazardous work Avoid such activities until you have learned how co-proxamol affects you because the drug can cause drowsiness and dizziness.
Alcohol Avoid. Alcohol will dangerously increase the toxicity of this drug.

PROLONGED USE

Co-proxamol is not usually prescribed for long-term use. It can be habit forming if taken for extended periods and a higher dose may be needed to produce the same effect as your body adapts to the drug.

Co-trimoxazole

Brand names Bactrim, Chemotrim, Comixco, Fectrim, Laratrim, Septrin
Used in the following combined preparations
(Co-trimoxazole is a combination of trimethoprim and sulfamethoxazole)

QUICK REFERENCE

Drug group Antibacterial drug (p.64)
Overdose danger rating Medium
Dependence rating Low
Prescription needed Yes
Available as generic Yes

GENERAL INFORMATION

Co-trimoxazole is a mixture of two antibacterial drugs in the ratio of one part trimethoprim and five parts sulfamethoxazole. It is prescribed for serious respiratory and urinary tract infections only when they cannot be treated with other drugs. Co-trimoxazole is also used to prevent and treat pneumocystis pneumonia, and to treat toxoplasmosis and the fungal infection nocardiasis. The drug may also be used for otitis media in children if no safer drug is suitable. Although co-trimoxazole was widely prescribed in the past, its use has now greatly declined with the introduction of new, more effective, and safer drugs.

The drug's side effects are a combination of those caused by the antibacterial drugs it contains; they include nausea, vomiting, rash, sore tongue, and rarely jaundice, rash, blood disorders, and serious liver or kidney damage.

INFORMATION FOR USERS

Your drug prescription is tailored for you. Do not alter dosage without checking with your doctor.
How taken Tablets, liquid, injection.
Frequency and timing of doses Normally 2 x daily, preferably with food.
Adult dosage range Usually 4–6 tablets daily (each standard tablet is 480mg). Higher doses are required for the treatment of pneumocystis pneumonia.
Onset of effect 1–4 hours.
Duration of action 12 hours.
Diet advice Drink plenty of fluids, particularly in warm weather.
Storage Keep in a closed container in a cool, dry place out of reach of children. Protect from light.
Missed dose Take as soon as you remember. If your next dose is due at this time, double the usual dose to make up the missed dose.
Stopping the drug Unless severe adverse effects occur occur (see below), take the full course. Even if you feel better, the original infection may still be present and symptoms may recur if treatment is stopped too soon.
Exceeding the dose An occasional unintentional extra dose is unlikely to be a cause for concern. Large overdoses may cause nausea, vomiting, dizziness, and confusion. Notify your doctor.

POSSIBLE ADVERSE EFFECTS

Side effects can be caused by either the trimethoprim or the sulfamethoxazole ingredient of this preparation. The most common problems are nausea or vomiting and diarrhoea. A sore tongue and a headache are less common and should be discussed with your doctor. If you develop itching or a rash or you become jaundiced, stop taking the drug and seek urgent medical attention as some types of adverse effect are potentially serious.

INTERACTIONS

Warfarin Co-trimoxazole may increase its anticoagulant effect; the dose of warfarin may have to be reduced.

Phenytoin Co-trimoxazole may cause a build-up of phenytoin in the body; the dose of phenytoin may have to be reduced.

Oral antidiabetic drugs Co-trimoxazole may increase the blood sugar lowering effect of these drugs.

Ciclosporin Taking ciclosporin with co-trimoxazole can impair kidney function.

SPECIAL PRECAUTIONS

Be sure to tell your doctor if:
◆ You have long-term liver or kidney problems.
◆ You have a blood disorder.
◆ You have glucose-6-phosphate dehydrogenase (G6PD) deficiency.
◆ You are allergic to sulphonamide drugs.
◆ You suffer from porphyria.
◆ You are taking other medications.

Pregnancy Not usually prescribed. May cause defects in the baby. Discuss with your doctor.

Breast-feeding The drug passes into the breast milk, but at normal levels adverse effects on the baby are unlikely. Discuss with your doctor.

Infants and children Not recommended in infants under 6 weeks old. Reduced dose necessary in older children.

Over 60 Side effects are more likely. Used only when necessary, often in reduced dosage.

Driving and hazardous work No known problems.

Alcohol No known problems.

PROLONGED USE

Long-term use of this drug may lead to folic acid deficiency which, in turn, can cause a

blood abnormality. Folic acid supplements may be prescribed.

Monitoring Periodic blood tests to monitor blood composition are usually carried out.

Cyclopenthiazide

Brand name Navidrex
Used in the following combined preparations
Navispare, Trasidrex

QUICK REFERENCE

Drug group Thiazide diuretic (p.30)
Overdose danger rating Low
Dependence rating Low
Prescription needed Yes
Available as generic No

GENERAL INFORMATION

Cyclopenthiazide belongs to the thiazide diuretic group of drugs, which remove excess water from the body and reduce oedema (fluid retention) in people with congestive heart failure and liver and kidney disorders. The drug may occasionally be used on a short-term basis to treat fluid retention in premenstrual syndrome.

Cyclopenthiazide is most commonly used to treat high blood pressure (see Antihypertensive drugs, p.34). The drug increases loss of potassium in the urine, which can cause a variety of symptoms (see p.31) and increases the likelihood of irregular heart rhythms, particularly if you are taking drugs such as digoxin. Therefore, a potassium supplement or a diet rich in potassium is often recommended for patients taking cyclopenthiazide.

INFORMATION FOR USERS

Your drug prescription is tailored for you. Do not alter dosage without checking with your doctor

How taken Tablets.
Frequency and timing of doses Once daily (preferably in the morning).
Adult dosage range 0.25–1mg daily.
Onset of effect Within 2 hours.
Duration of action 6–12 hours.
Diet advice Use of this drug may reduce potassium in the body. Eat plenty of fresh fruit and vegetables.

Storage Keep in a closed container in a cool, dry place out of reach of children.

Missed dose No cause for concern, but take as soon as you remember. However, if it is late in the day do not take the missed dose, or you may need to get up during the night to pass urine. Take the next scheduled dose as usual.

Stopping the drug Unless a rash occurs, do not stop taking the drug without consulting your doctor; symptoms may recur.

Exceeding the dose An occasional unintentional extra dose is unlikely to be a cause for concern. But if you notice any unusual symptoms, or if a large overdose has been taken, notify your doctor.

POSSIBLE ADVERSE EFFECTS

Some adverse effects are caused by excessive loss of potassium and can usually be put right by taking a potassium supplement. Nausea and loss of appetite are common, and diarrhoea or constipation may also occur. If you experience headache, dizziness, muscle weakness, or leg cramps, consult your doctor. In rare cases gout may occur in susceptible people, and certain forms of diabetes may become more difficult to control. If you develop a rash, stop taking the drug and consult your doctor.

INTERACTIONS

NSAIDs Some of these drugs may reduce the diuretic effect of cyclopenthiazide, the dosage of which may need to be adjusted.

ACE inhibitors and other antihypertensive drugs Cyclopenthiazide may cause a further decrease in blood pressure when taken in combination with these drugs.

Corticosteroids These drugs further increase the loss of potassium from the body when taken with cyclopenthiazide.

Lithium Cyclopenthiazide may increase lithium levels in the blood, leading to a risk of serious adverse effects.

Digoxin The effects of digoxin may be increased if excessive potassium is lost.

SPECIAL PRECAUTIONS

Be sure to tell your doctor if:
◆ You have long-term liver or kidney problems.

◆ You have had gout.
◆ You have diabetes.
◆ You are taking other medications.

Pregnancy Safety in pregnancy not established. Discuss with your doctor.

Breast-feeding The drug passes into the breast milk, but at normal doses adverse effects on the baby are unlikely. Discuss with your doctor.

Infants and children Not usually prescribed. Reduced dose necessary.

Over 60 Increased likelihood of adverse effects.

Driving and hazardous work No special problems.

Alcohol Keep consumption low. Cyclopenthiazide increases the likelihood of dehydration and hangovers after consumption of alcohol.

PROLONGED USE

Excessive loss of potassium may result in irregular heart rhythms. Cyclopenthiazide occasionally causes reduced levels of red blood cells and platelets.

Monitoring Blood tests may be performed periodically to check kidney function and levels of potassium.

Cyclophosphamide

Brand name Endoxana
Used in the following combined preparations
None

QUICK REFERENCE

Drug group Anticancer drug (p.94)
Overdose danger rating Medium
Dependence rating Low
Prescription needed Yes
Available as generic Yes

GENERAL INFORMATION

Cyclophosphamide belongs to a group of anticancer drugs known as alkylating agents. It is used for a wide range of cancers, including lymphomas (lymph gland cancers), leukaemias, and solid tumours, particularly of the breast and lung. It is commonly given together with radio therapy or other drugs. Cyclophosphamide has also been used for autoimmune diseases.

Cyclophosphamide causes nausea, vomiting, and hair loss, and can affect the heart, lungs, and liver. It can also cause bladder damage in susceptible people because it produces a toxic substance called acrolein. To reduce toxicity, people considered to be at risk may be given a drug called mesna before and after each dose of cyclophosphamide. Also, because the drug often reduces production of blood cells, it may lead to abnormal bleeding, increased risk of infection, and reduced fertility in men.

INFORMATION FOR USERS

Your drug prescription is tailored for you. Do not alter dosage without checking with your doctor.

How taken Tablets, injection.

Frequency and timing of doses Varies from once daily to every 20 days, depending on the condition being treated.

Dosage range Dosage is determined individually according to the nature of the condition, body weight, and response.

Onset of effect Some effects may appear within hours of starting treatment. Full beneficial effects may not be felt for up to 6 weeks.

Duration of action Several weeks.

Diet advice High fluid intake with frequent bladder emptying is recommended. This will usually prevent the drug causing bladder irritation.

Storage Keep in a closed container in a cool, dry place out of reach of children. Protect from light.

Missed dose Injections are given only in hospital. If you are taking tablets, take the missed dose as soon as you remember. If your next dose is due within 6 hours, take a single dose now and skip the next. Tell your doctor that you missed a dose.

Stopping the drug The drug will be stopped under medical supervision (injection). Do not stop taking the drug without consulting your doctor (tablets); stopping the drug may lead to worsening of the underlying condition.

Exceeding the dose An occasional unintentional extra dose is unlikely to cause problems. Large overdoses may cause nausea, vomiting, and bladder damage. Notify your doctor.

POSSIBLE ADVERSE EFFECTS

Cyclophosphamide often causes nausea and vomiting, which usually diminish as your body adjusts. Hair loss is a common sign that the drug is having an effect on growing cells. Mouth ulcers may also occur, and women often experience irregular periods. Cloudy or bloodstained urine may be a sign of bladder damage and requires prompt medical attention. Those people thought to be at risk of bladder damage may be given mesna before and after doses of cyclophosphamide.

INTERACTIONS

Allopurinol may increase the risk of toxic effects caused by cyclophosphamide.

SPECIAL PRECAUTIONS

Cyclophosphamide is prescribed only under close medical supervision, taking account of your present condition and medical history.

Pregnancy Not usually prescribed. May cause birth defects. Discuss with your doctor.

Breast-feeding Not advised. The drug passes into the breast milk and may affect the baby adversely. Discuss with your doctor.

Infants and children Reduced dose necessary.

Over 60 No special problems.

Driving and hazardous work No known problems.

Alcohol No problems expected, but avoid excessive amounts.

PROLONGED USE

Prolonged use of this drug may reduce the production of blood cells.

Monitoring Periodic checks on blood composition and on all effects of the drug are usually required.

Danazol

Brand name Danol
Used in the following combined preparations
None

QUICK REFERENCE

Drug group Drug for menstrual disorders (p.100)
Overdose danger rating Low
Dependence rating Low
Prescription needed Yes
Available as generic Yes

GENERAL INFORMATION

Danazol is a synthetic steroid hormone that inhibits hormones called pituitary gonado-trophins. It is used in a range of conditions, including endometriosis (fragments of endometrial tissue growing outside the uterus), menorrhagia, and, in men, to reduce gynaecomastia (breast swelling). It has also been used long term to treat hereditary angioedema (a rare allergic disorder that causes facial swelling).

Danazol is also used to relieve pain, tenderness, and lumpiness in the breasts caused by fibrocystic disease. Treatment commonly disrupts normal menstrual periods and in some cases periods may cease altogether. Women taking high doses of the drug may notice unusual hair growth and deepening of the voice.

INFORMATION FOR USERS

Your drug prescription is tailored for you. Do not alter dosage without checking with your doctor.
How taken Capsules.
Frequency and timing of doses 2–4 x daily.
Dosage range 200–800mg daily, depending on the condition being treated, its severity, and the response to the drug.
Onset of effect Some effects occur after a few days. Full beneficial effects may take some months.
Duration of action 1–2 days.
Diet advice None.
Storage Keep in a closed container in a cool, dry place out of reach of children.
Missed dose Take as soon as you remember. If your next dose is due within 2 hours, take a single dose now and skip the next.

Stopping the drug Do not stop taking the drug without consulting your doctor; symptoms may recur.
Exceeding the dose An occasional unintentional extra dose is unlikely to cause problems. But if you notice any unusual symptoms, or if a large overdose has been taken, notify your doctor.

POSSIBLE ADVERSE EFFECTS

Danazol rarely causes adverse effects in low doses. Adverse effects from higher doses, including acne, weight gain, ankle swelling, muscle cramps, and nausea, are the result of hormonal changes. Reduced breast size, voice changes, and unusual hair growth in women are largely reversed after treatment. If you develop blurred vision or headaches, consult your doctor.

INTERACTIONS

Oral anticoagulant drugs Danazol may increase the effects of these drugs.
Immunosuppressants Danazol may increase the effects of ciclosporin and tacrolimus.
Oral antidiabetic drugs Danazol may reduce the effects of these drugs.
Anticonvulsant drugs The effects of these drugs may be altered by danazol.

SPECIAL PRECAUTIONS

Be sure to tell your doctor if:
◆ You have long-term liver or kidney problems.
◆ You have heart disease.
◆ You have had epileptic fits.
◆ You suffer from migraine.
◆ You suffer from unexplained vaginal bleeding.
◆ You have diabetes mellitus.
◆ You are taking other medications.
Pregnancy Not prescribed. May cause masculine characteristics in a female baby. Non-hormonal methods of contraception should be used for women of childbearing age; and pregnancy should be avoided for 3 months after cessation of treatment.
Breast-feeding The drug passes into the breast milk and may affect the baby. Discuss with your doctor.
Infants and children Not recommended.
Over 60 Unlikely to be required.

Driving and hazardous work No known problems.

Alcohol No known problems.

PROLONGED USE

The drug is normally taken for 3–9 months depending on the condition being treated. There is a slight risk of liver damage. See also Possible adverse effects, p.193.

Monitoring Periodic liver function tests may be carried out.

Desmopressin

Brand names DDAVP, Desmospray, Desmotabs
Used in the following combined preparations
None

QUICK REFERENCE

Drug group Drug for diabetes insipidus (p.83)
Overdose danger rating Medium
Dependence rating Low
Prescription needed Yes
Available as generic No

GENERAL INFORMATION

Desmopressin is a synthetic form of vasopressin, a hormone adjusted in response to the concentration of salts in the blood. Deficiency causes diabetes insipidus, in which frequent urination and continual thirst occur because the kidneys cannot concentrate the urine.

Desmopressin controls urine production by correcting the deficiency of vasopressin. It is also used to test for diabetes insipidus, to check kidney function, and to treat nocturnal enuresis (bedwetting) in both children and adults. When given by injection, it helps to boost clotting factors in haemophilia.

Important side effects include low blood sodium and fluid retention (which may require control of the amount of fluid consumed and, sometimes, monitoring of body weight and blood pressure to check the body's water balance).

INFORMATION FOR USERS

Your drug prescription is tailored for you. Do not alter dosage without checking with your doctor.

How taken Tablets, injection, nasal solution, nasal spray.

Frequency and timing of doses *Diabetes insipidus* 3 x daily (tablets); 1–2 x daily (nasal spray/solution).
Nocturnal enuresis At bedtime (tablets, nasal spray/solution).

Dosage range Diabetes insipidus: *Adults* 300–600 micrograms daily (tablets); 1–4 puffs (nasal spray); 10–40 micrograms daily (nasal solution). *Children* 300–600 micrograms daily (tablets); up to 2 puffs (nasal spray); 20 micrograms (nasal solution).
Nocturnal enuresis: 200–400 micrograms for children over 5 years only (tablets); 20–40 micrograms (nasal solution); 2–4 puffs (nasal spray).

Onset of effect Begins within a few minutes with full effects in a few hours (injection, nasal solution, and nasal spray); 30–90 minutes (tablets).

Duration of action Tablets 8 hours; injection and nasal solutions 8–12 hours; nasal spray 10–12 hours.

Diet advice Your doctor may advise you to monitor your fluid intake.

Storage Keep in a cool, dry place (tablets) or in a refrigerator, without freezing (nasal solution and nasal spray), out of reach of children. Protect from light.

Missed dose Take as soon as you remember. If your next dose is due within 2 hours, take a single dose now and skip the next.

Stopping the drug Unless vomiting or diarrhoea occur, do not stop taking the drug without consulting your doctor; symptoms of diabetes insipidus may recur.

Exceeding the dose An occasional unintentional extra dose is unlikely to cause problems. Large overdoses may prevent the kidneys from eliminating fluid, with ensuing problems including convulsions. Notify your doctor immediately.

POSSIBLE ADVERSE EFFECTS

Desmopressin can cause fluid retention and low blood sodium, especially if fluid intake is too high (in serious cases this can lead to convulsions). Headache, nausea, vomiting, and epistaxis (nosebleeds) also occur. If vomiting or diarrhoea occur, stop taking the drug and consult your doctor.

INTERACTIONS

Antidepressants, chlorpropamide, and carbamazepine These drugs may increase the effects of desmopressin.

Indomethacin This anti-inflammatory drug may increase the body's response to desmopressin.

SPECIAL PRECAUTIONS

Be sure to tell your doctor if:
◆ You have heart problems.
◆ You have high blood pressure.
◆ You have kidney problems.
◆ You have cystic fibrosis.
◆ You have asthma or allergic rhinitis.
◆ You have epilepsy.
◆ You are taking other medications.

Pregnancy Used with caution in pregnancy.

Breast-feeding The drug passes into breast milk, in small amounts, but at normal doses adverse effects on the baby are unlikely.

Infants and children No special problems in children; infants may need monitoring to ensure that fluid balance is correct.

Over 60 May need monitoring to ensure that fluid balance is correct.

Driving and hazardous work No known problems.

Alcohol Your doctor may advise on your fluid intake.

PROLONGED USE

Diabetes insipidus: No problems expected. Nocturnal enuresis: The drug will be withdrawn for at least a week after 3 months for assessment of the need to continue treatment.

Dexamethasone

Brand name Decadron
Used in the following combined preparations
Dexa-Rhinaspray, Maxidex, Maxitrol, Otomize, Sofradex

QUICK REFERENCE

Drug group Corticosteroid (p.79)
Overdose danger rating Low
Dependence rating Low
Prescription needed Yes
Available as generic Yes

GENERAL INFORMATION

Dexamethasone is a long-acting corticosteroid prescribed for a variety of skin and soft tissue conditions caused by allergy or inflammation. It can also be injected into joints to relieve joint pain and stiffness due to rheumatoid arthritis (see p.51). It is injected into a vein for the emergency treatment of shock and brain swelling (due to head injury, stroke, or a tumour), asthma, and emphysema. Eye drops are used for eye inflammation.

Low doses of the drug taken for short periods rarely cause serious side effects. But, as with other corticosteroids, long-term treatment with high doses can cause unpleasant or dangerous side effects, and some infections such as chickenpox may be more severe.

INFORMATION FOR USERS

Your drug prescription is tailored for you. Do not alter dosage without checking with your doctor.

How taken Tablets, injection, eye drops, ear drops/spray.

Frequency and timing of doses 2–4 x daily (with food when taking by mouth); 1–6 hourly (eye drops).

Dosage range Usually 0.5–10mg daily.

Onset of effect 1–4 days.

Duration of action Some effects may last several days.

Diet advice None.

Storage Keep in a closed container in a cool, dry place out of reach of children. Protect from light.

Missed dose Take as soon as you remember. If your next dose is due within 2 hours, take a single dose now and skip the next.

Stopping the drug Do not stop taking the drug without consulting your doctor, who will supervise a gradual reduction in dosage. Stopping abruptly can cause adrenal failure, with possible weakness and collapse.

Exceeding the dose An occasional unintentional extra dose is unlikely to be a cause for concern. But if you notice any unusual symptoms, or if a large overdose has been taken, notify your doctor.

POSSIBLE ADVERSE EFFECTS

Indigestion and weight gain occur commonly. The more serious adverse effects of dexamethasone only occur with high doses of the drug taken for long periods. These effects, including acne and skin thinning, raised blood pressure, muscle weakness, and mood changes, are carefully monitored during prolonged treatment.

INTERACTIONS

Antidiabetic drugs Dexamethasone reduces the action of these drugs. Dosage may need to be adjusted accordingly to prevent abnormally high blood sugar.

Barbiturates, phenytoin, rifampicin, and carbamazepine These drugs may reduce the effectiveness of dexamethasone. The dosage may need to be adjusted accordingly.

Oral anticoagulant drugs Dexamethasone may increase the effects of these drugs.

NSAIDs These drugs may increase the likelihood of indigestion from dexamethasone.

Antacids These drugs may reduce the effectiveness of, and should be taken at least 2 hours apart from, dexamethasone.

Vaccines Dexamethasone can interact with some vaccines. Discuss with your doctor before having any vaccinations.

SPECIAL PRECAUTIONS

Be sure to tell your doctor if:
◆ You have had a peptic ulcer.
◆ You have glaucoma.
◆ You have had tuberculosis.
◆ You have suffered from depression or mental illness.
◆ You have a herpes infection.
◆ You are taking other medications.
Avoid exposure to chickenpox or shingles if you are on systemic treatment.

Pregnancy Safety in pregnancy not established. Discuss with your doctor.

Breast-feeding The drug passes into the breast milk, but at normal doses adverse effects on the baby are unlikely. Discuss with your doctor.

Infants and children Reduced dose necessary.

Over 60 No known problems.

Driving and hazardous work No known problems.

Alcohol Avoid. Alcohol may increase the risk of peptic ulcer with this drug.

Surgery and general anaesthetics The dose of dexamethasone needs to be increased during operations. Discuss with your doctor or dentist before any surgery.

PROLONGED USE

Prolonged use of this drug can lead to glaucoma, cataracts, diabetes, mental disturbances, muscle wasting, fragile bones, and thin skin, and can retard growth in children. If you are receiving long-term treatment, you are advised to carry a 'steroid treatment' card, which can be obtained from your doctor or pharmacist.

Diazepam

Brand names Atensine, Dialar, Diazemuls, Rimapam, Stesolid, Tensium, Valclair, Valium
Used in the following combined preparations None

QUICK REFERENCE

Drug group Benzodiazepine anti-anxiety drug (p.13), muscle relaxant (p.52), and anticonvulsant (p.16)
Overdose danger rating Medium
Dependence rating High
Prescription needed Yes
Available as generic Yes

GENERAL INFORMATION

Introduced in the early 1960s, diazepam is the best known and most widely used of the benzodiazepine group of drugs. The benzodiazepines help relieve tension and nervousness, relax muscles, and encourage sleep. Their actions and adverse effects are described more fully on page 13.

Diazepam has a wide range of uses. Besides being commonly used in the treatment of anxiety and anxiety-related insomnia, it is prescribed as a muscle relaxant, in the treatment of alcohol withdrawal, and for the relief of epileptic fits. Given intravenously, diazepam is used to sedate people who are undergoing certain uncomfortable medical procedures.

Diazepam can be habit-forming if it is taken regularly over a long period of time. The effects of the drug may also diminish with time. For these reasons, courses of treatment with diazepam are limited to two weeks whenever possible.

INFORMATION FOR USERS

Your drug prescription is tailored for you. Do not alter dosage without checking with your doctor.

How taken Tablets, liquid, injection, suppositories, rectal solution.

Frequency and timing of doses 1–4 x daily.

Adult dosage range *Anxiety* 6–30mg daily. *Muscle spasm* 2–60mg daily.

Onset of effect Immediate effect (injection, rectal solution); 30 minutes–2 hours (other methods of administration).

Duration of action Up to 24 hours. Some effect may last up to 4 days.

Diet advice None.

Storage Keep in a closed container in a cool, dry place out of reach of children.

Missed dose Take as soon as you remember. If your next dose is due within 2 hours, take a single dose now and skip the next.

Stopping the drug If you have been taking the drug continuously for less than 2 weeks, it can be safely stopped as soon as you no longer need it. However, if you have been taking it for longer, consult your doctor, who will supervise a gradual reduction in dosage. Stopping abruptly may lead to withdrawal symptoms.

Exceeding the dose An occasional unintentional extra dose is unlikely to cause problems. Larger overdoses may cause unusual drowsiness. Notify your doctor.

POSSIBLE ADVERSE EFFECTS

The principal adverse effects of this drug are related to its sedative properties. They include daytime drowsiness, dizziness or unsteadiness, headache, blurred vision, and forgetfulness or confusion. These effects normally diminish after a few days and can often be reduced by adjustment of dosage. However, if you develop a rash, consult your doctor.

INTERACTIONS

Sedatives All drugs that have a sedative effect on the central nervous system can increase the sedative properties of diazepam.

Cimetidine Breakdown of diazepam in the liver may be inhibited by cimetidine. This can cause a build-up of diazepam in the blood, which increases the likelihood of adverse effects.

SPECIAL PRECAUTIONS

Be sure to tell your doctor if:
◆ You have severe respiratory disease.
◆ You have long-term liver or kidney problems.
◆ You have had problems with alcohol or drug abuse.
◆ You are taking other medications.

Pregnancy Safety in pregnancy not established. Discuss with your doctor.

Breast-feeding The drug passes into the breast milk and may affect the baby. Discuss with your doctor.

Infants and children Reduced dose necessary.

Over 60 Reduced dose may be necessary. Increased likelihood of adverse effects.

Driving and hazardous work Avoid such activities until you have learned how diazepam affects you because the drug can cause reduced alertness, slowed reactions, and increased aggression.

Alcohol Avoid. Alcohol may increase the sedative effects of this drug.

PROLONGED USE

Regular use of this drug over several weeks can lead to a reduction in its effect as the body adapts. It may also be habit-forming when taken for extended periods, and severe withdrawal reactions can occur.

Diclofenac

Brand names Diclomax SR, Motifene, Rhumalgan, Volraman, Voltarol, and others
Used in the following combined preparation Arthrotec

QUICK REFERENCE

Drug group Non-steroidal anti-inflammatory drug (p.48), analgesic (p.9), and drug for gout (p.51)
Overdose danger rating Low
Dependence rating Low
Prescription needed Yes
Available as generic Yes

GENERAL INFORMATION

Taken as a single dose, diclofenac has analgesic properties similar to those of paracetamol. It is taken to relieve mild to moderate headache, menstrual pain, and pain following minor surgery. When diclofenac is given regularly over a long period, it exerts an anti-inflammatory effect and is used to relieve the pain and stiffness associated with rheumatoid arthritis and advanced osteoarthritis. Some formulations are slow release (SR) and can be taken less frequently, while still relieving pain effectively. Diclofenac may also be prescribed to treat acute attacks of gout.

The combined preparation, Arthrotec, contains diclofenac and misoprostol (see p.306). Misoprostol helps to prevent gastroduodenal ulceration and may be particularly useful in patients at risk of developing this problem.

INFORMATION FOR USERS
Your drug prescription is tailored for you. Do not alter dosage without checking with your doctor.

How taken Tablets, dispersible tablets, SR-tablets, capsules, SR-capsules, injection, suppositories, gel.

Frequency and timing of doses 1–3 x daily with food.

Adult dosage range 75–150mg daily.

Onset of effect Approximately 1 hour (pain relief); full anti-inflammatory effect may take 2 weeks.

Duration of action Up to 12 hours; up to 24 hours (SR-preparations).

Diet advice None.

Storage Keep in a closed container in a cool, dry place out of reach of children.

Missed dose Take as soon as you remember. If your next dose is due within 2 hours, take a single dose now and skip the next.

Stopping the drug When taken for short-term pain relief, diclofenac can be safely stopped as soon as you no longer need it. Seek medical advice before stopping long-term treatment of arthritis unless serious adverse effects occur (see below).

Exceeding the dose An occasional unintentional extra dose is unlikely to be a cause for concern. But if you notice any unusual symptoms or if a large overdose has been taken, notify your doctor.

POSSIBLE ADVERSE EFFECTS
Dizziness and headache and gastrointestinal side effects, such as nausea and indigestion, are not generally serious. Discuss symptoms such as abdominal pain and swollen feet or ankles with your doctor. If rash, wheezing or breathlessness, bruising, or bleeding or black bowel movements occur, stop taking the drug and call your doctor immediately.

INTERACTIONS
General note Diclofenac interacts with many drugs including other NSAIDs, oral anticoagulants, and corticosteroids.

Antihypertensive drugs and diuretics The beneficial effects of these drugs may be reduced with diclofenac.

Ciclosporin Diclofenac may increase the risk of kidney problems.

Lithium, digoxin, and methotrexate Diclofenac may increase the blood levels of these drugs.

Indigestion remedies These should not be taken at the same time of the day as enteric coated diclofenac preparations because they disrupt this coating.

SPECIAL PRECAUTIONS
Be sure to tell your doctor if:
◆ You have long-term liver or kidney problems.
◆ You have a bleeding disorder.
◆ You have had a peptic ulcer or oesophagitis.
◆ You have porphyria.
◆ You suffer from indigestion.
◆ You are allergic to aspirin.
◆ You suffer from asthma.
◆ You have heart problems or high blood pressure.
◆ You are taking other medications.

Pregnancy Not usually prescribed in the last 3 months of pregnancy as it may increase the risk of adverse effects on the baby's heart and may prolong labour. Discuss with your doctor.

Breast-feeding Small amounts of the drug pass into the breast milk, but adverse effects on the baby are unlikely. Discuss with your doctor.

Infants and children Reduced dose necessary.

Over 60 Increased risk of adverse effects. Reduced dose may therefore be necessary.

Driving and hazardous work No problems expected.

Alcohol Keep consumption low. Alcohol may increase the risk of stomach irritation.

Surgery and general anaesthetics Discuss with your doctor or dentist before any surgery.

PROLONGED USE
There is an increased risk of bleeding from peptic ulcers and in the bowel with prolonged use of diclofenac.

Dicycloverine (Dicyclomine)

Brand name Merbentyl
Used in the following combined preparations
Diarrest, Kolanticon

QUICK REFERENCE
Drug group Drug for irritable bowel syndrome (p.43)
Overdose danger rating Medium
Dependence rating Low
Prescription needed No (doses of 10mg or less) Yes (doses of more than 10mg)
Available as generic No

GENERAL INFORMATION
Dicycloverine is a mild anticholinergic antispasmodic drug that relieves painful abdominal cramps caused by spasm in the gastrointestinal tract. It is used to treat irritable bowel syndrome, indigestion not associated with ulcers, and colicky conditions in babies. Because the drug has anticholinergic properties, it is also included in some combined preparations used to treat flatulence, indigestion, and diarrhoea. It relieves symptoms but does not cure the underlying condition. Additional treatment with other drugs and self-help measures, such as dietary changes, may be recommended by your doctor.

Side effects with dicycloverine are rare, but they include headaches, constipation, urinary difficulties, and palpitations.

INFORMATION FOR USERS
Follow instructions on the label. Call your doctor if symptoms worsen.
How taken Tablets, liquid.
Frequency and timing of doses
3 x daily before or after meals.
Dosage range Adults 30–60mg daily. Children Reduced dose according to age and weight.
Onset of effect Within 1–2 hours.

Duration of action 4–6 hours.
Diet advice None.
Storage Keep in a closed container in a cool, dry place out of reach of children. Protect from light.
Missed dose Take as soon as you remember. If your next dose is due within 2 hours, take a single dose now and skip the next.
Stopping the drug Do not stop taking the drug without consulting your doctor; symptoms may recur.
Exceeding the dose An occasional unintentional extra dose is unlikely to cause problems. Large overdoses may cause drowsiness, dizziness, and difficulty in swallowing. Notify your doctor.

POSSIBLE ADVERSE EFFECTS
Most people notice no adverse effects. Those effects that do occur are related to the drug's anticholinergic properties and include drowsiness, dry mouth, and constipation. These may be overcome by adjusting the dosage or may disappear after a few days as your body adjusts. If you experience severe headache or blurred vision, or have palpitations or difficulty in passing urine, consult your doctor.

INTERACTIONS
Sedatives All drugs that have a sedative effect on the central nervous system may increase the sedative properties of dicycloverine.
Anticholinergic drugs These drug may increase the adverse effects of dicycloverine.

SPECIAL PRECAUTIONS
Be sure to consult your doctor or pharmacist before taking this drug if:
◆ You have glaucoma.
◆ You have urinary problems.
◆ You have hiatus hernia.
◆ You are taking other medications.
Pregnancy No evidence of risk.
Breast-feeding The drug passes into the breast milk, but at normal doses adverse effects on the baby are unlikely. Discuss with your doctor.
Infants and children Reduced dose necessary.
Over 60 Reduced dose necessary. The elderly are more susceptible to the drug's anticholinergic side effects.
Driving and hazardous work Avoid such activities until you have learned how dicycloverine

affects you because the drug can cause drowsiness and blurred vision.

Alcohol Avoid. Alcohol may increase the sedative effects of this drug.

PROLONGED USE
No problems expected.

Didanosine (DdI)

Brand name Videx
Used in the following combined preparations
None

QUICK REFERENCE
Drug group Antiviral drug for AIDS (p.97)
Overdose danger rating Medium
Dependence rating Low
Prescription needed Yes
Available as generic No

GENERAL INFORMATION
Didanosine is an antiviral agent used in the treatment of HIV infection, usually in combination with two other drugs. Like zidovudine (AZT), didanosine works by blocking the action of the reverse transcriptase enzyme, which is central to the action of the virus which causes AIDS.

Didanosine delays the progression of AIDS by temporarily boosting immunity, thereby reducing the frequency and severity of infections, which helps AIDS patients to gain weight. However, didanosine is not a cure for HIV infection, and patients may continue to be afflicted by the illnesses associated with AIDS.

The major adverse effects of this drug are pancreatitis (inflammation of the pancreas) and peripheral neuropathy (impaired function of the nerves in the hands and feet).

INFORMATION FOR USERS
Your drug prescription is tailored for you. Do not alter dosage without checking with your doctor.

How taken Chewable/dispersible tablets. The tablets should not be swallowed whole: they should be thoroughly chewed, crushed, or dispersed in water or clear apple juice before swallowing.

Frequency and timing of doses *Adults* Every 12 hours on an empty stomach.

Adult dosage range 250–400mg daily.
Onset of effect Usually within 48 hours.
Duration of action 8–12 hours.
Diet advice None.
Storage Keep in a closed container in a cool, dry place out of reach of children. Protect from light.
Missed dose Take as soon as you remember. If your next dose is due within 4 hours, take a single dose now and skip the next.
Stopping the drug Unless severe adverse effects occur (see below), do not stop taking the drug without consulting your doctor; symptoms may recur.
Exceeding the dose An occasional unintentional extra dose is unlikely to cause problems. Large overdoses may cause diarrhoea and abdominal pain. Notify your doctor immediately.

POSSIBLE ADVERSE EFFECTS
Many patients experience headache, insomnia, vomiting, diarrhoea, fatigue, and weakness. Some have joint or muscle pain. The major adverse effects are pancreatitis and peripheral neuropathy. Symptoms of pancreatitis include abdominal pain, nausea, and vomiting (but nausea, vomiting, and diarrhoea are also common side effects of the drug). Symptoms of peripheral neuropathy include tingling, burning, pain, or numbness in hands or feet. If you think you have any of the major adverse effects, or if you develop a cough, breathlessness, chills, fever, or a rash, stop taking the drug and consult your doctor urgently.

INTERACTIONS
General note A wide range of drugs may increase the harmful effects or decrease the absorption of didanosine; and didanosine tablets contain antacids which may interfere with the absorption of other drugs. Obtain full information from a doctor or pharmacist.

SPECIAL PRECAUTIONS
Be sure to tell your doctor if:
◆ You are taking any other drugs to treat HIV infection or AIDS complications.
◆ You have long-term liver, kidney, or respiratory problems.

DIETHYLSTILBESTROL

◆ You have raised uric acid levels.
◆ You have had pancreatitis.
◆ You are taking other medications.

Pregnancy Safety in pregnancy not established. Discuss with your doctor.

Breast-feeding Not recommended. Discuss with your doctor.

Infants and children Not recommended under 3 months of age. Safety in children not established. Discuss with your doctor.

Over 60 Reduced dose may be necessary. Increased likelihood of adverse effects.

Driving and hazardous work No special problems.

Alcohol Avoid. May increase the possibility of adverse effects.

PROLONGED USE
The long-term effects of didanosine are unknown at this time.

Monitoring Regular blood checks and liver function tests are required during treatment. Eye examinations may be recommended.

Diethylstilbestrol

Brand name Apstil
Used in the following combined preparation
Tampovagan

QUICK REFERENCE
Drug group Female sex hormone (p.86) and anticancer drug (p.94)
Overdose danger rating Low
Dependence rating Low
Prescription needed Yes
Available as generic Yes

GENERAL INFORMATION
Diethylstilbestrol is a powerful synthetic oestrogen. Although the drug has been used for many years for a wide range of conditions, including hormone deficiency and menopausal symptoms, its main use these days is in the treatment of prostate cancer and post-menopausal breast cancer. In these conditions diethylstilbestrol works by suppressing the effects of male sex hormones. Newer drugs are used nowadays for treating the other conditions that were previously treated with diethylstilbestrol.

Because side effects are common, the drug is now less widely used. In men, impotence is often a problem and gynaecomastia (abnormal breast development) can occur. In women, withdrawal bleeding often occurs.

INFORMATION FOR USERS
Your drug prescription is tailored for you. Do not alter dosage without checking with your doctor.

How taken Tablets, pessaries.
Frequency and timing of doses *Tablets* Once daily. *Pessaries* Once daily.
Adult dosage range *Prostate cancer* 1–3mg daily. *Breast cancer* 10–20mg daily.
Onset of effect 10–20 days.
Duration of action Up to 24 hours. Some effects may last a few weeks.
Diet advice A low sodium diet is advised.
Storage Keep in a closed container in a cool, dry place out of reach of children.
Missed dose Take as soon as you remember. If your next dose is due within 6 hours, take a single dose now and skip the next.
Stopping the drug Unless severe adverse effects occur (see below), do not stop taking the drug without consulting your doctor.
Exceeding the dose An occasional unintentional extra dose is unlikely to cause problems. If you notice unusual symptoms, or if a large overdose has been taken, notify your doctor.

POSSIBLE ADVERSE EFFECTS
The most common adverse effects are similar to the symptoms of early pregnancy but improve after 2–3 months of treatment. Sudden breathlessness, a cough, sharp pain in the chest, or a swollen or painful leg may indicate an abnormal blood clot. Stop taking the drug and seek urgent medical attention. Diethystilbestrol may also affect the cornea in patients who wear contact lenses.

INTERACTIONS
Tobacco smoking Smoking increases the risk of serious adverse effects on the heart and circulation with diethylstilbestrol.
Anticonvulsants, rifampicin, and certain antibiotics These drugs may reduce the effectiveness of diethylstilbestrol.
Antihypertensives and diuretics Diethylstilbestrol may reduce the blood pressure

lowering effect of these drugs by causing fluid retention.

SPECIAL PRECAUTIONS

Be sure to tell your doctor if:
◆ You have a long-term liver problem.
◆ You have porphyria.
◆ You have heart failure or high blood pressure.
◆ You have had blood clots or a stroke.
◆ You have diabetes.
◆ You have thyroid disease.
◆ You suffer from migraine or epilepsy.
◆ You are taking other medications.

Pregnancy Not prescribed.

Breast-feeding The drug passes into the breast milk and may affect the baby. The drug may also have adverse effects on lactation. Discuss with your doctor.

Infants and children Not recommended.

Over 60 No special problems.

Driving and hazardous work No known problems.

Alcohol No known problems.

PROLONGED USE

The risk of gallstones is increased with long-term use of this drug.

Monitoring Periodic general physical examinations and checks on blood pressure are usually required.

Digoxin

Brand name Lanoxin
Used in the following combined preparations
None

QUICK REFERENCE

Drug group Digitalis drug (p.27)
Overdose danger rating High
Dependence rating Low
Prescription needed Yes
Available as generic Yes

GENERAL INFORMATION

Digoxin is the most widely used form of digitalis, a drug extracted from the leaves of the foxglove plant. It is sometimes given in the treatment of congestive heart failure and certain alterations of heart rhythm.

Digoxin slows down the heart rate, making each beat pump blood more effectively. In congestive heart failure it also helps to control tiredness, breathlessness, and fluid retention.

For digoxin to be effective, the dose must be close to the toxic dose, and the treatment must be monitored carefully. Adverse effects are not infrequent and may suggest that the dose should be reduced. Consult your doctor, who can check the level of digoxin in your blood and find the correct dose for you.

INFORMATION FOR USERS

Your drug prescription is tailored for you. Do not alter dosage without checking with your doctor.

How taken Tablets, liquid, injection.

Frequency and timing of doses Up to 3 x daily (starting dose); once daily, or divided to reduce nausea, (maintenance dose).

Adult dosage range 62.5–250 micrograms daily (by mouth).

Onset of effect Within a few minutes (injection); within 1–2 hours (by mouth).

Duration of action Up to 4 days.

Diet advice This drug may be more toxic if potassium levels are depleted, so your diet should include fresh fruit and vegetables.

Storage Keep in a closed container in a cool, dry place out of reach of children. Protect from light.

Missed dose Take as soon as you remember. If your next dose is due within 8 hours, take a dose now and skip the next.

Stopping the drug Unless palpitations occur, do not stop taking the drug without consulting your doctor; stopping the drug may lead to worsening of the underlying condition.

OVERDOSE ACTION

Seek immediate medical advice in all cases. Take emergency action if palpitations, severe weakness, chest pain, or loss of consciousness occur.

POSSIBLE ADVERSE EFFECTS

The possible adverse effects are usually due to increased blood levels of the drug. Common adverse effects include tiredness, confusion, loss of appetite, nausea or vomiting, and visual disturbances. Report any symptoms to your doctor without delay. The drug is often given for disorders in which palpitations are experienced. If you experience palpitations accompanied by breathlessness, chest pain, lightheadedness, or collapse, stop taking the drug and seek immediate medical attention.

INTERACTIONS

General note Many drugs interact with digoxin. Do not take any medication without your doctor's or pharmacist's advice.

Diuretics may increase the risk of adverse effects from digoxin.

Antacids may reduce the effects of digoxin. The effect of digoxin may increase when such drugs are stopped.

Anti-arrhythmic drugs may increase blood levels of digoxin.

SPECIAL PRECAUTIONS

Be sure to tell your doctor if:
◆ You have a long-term liver problem.
◆ You have thyroid trouble.
◆ You are taking other medications.

Pregnancy No evidence of risk, but adjustment in dose may be necessary.

Breast-feeding The drug passes into the breast milk, but at normal doses adverse effects on the baby are unlikely. Discuss with your doctor.

Infants and children Reduced dose necessary.

Over 60 Reduced dose may be necessary. Increased likelihood of adverse effects.

Driving and hazardous work Special problems are unlikely, but do not undertake these activities until you know how digoxin affects you.

Alcohol No special problems.

PROLONGED USE

No problems expected.

Monitoring Periodic checks on blood levels of digoxin and body salts may be advised.

Diltiazem

Brand names Adizem, Calcicard, Dilzem, Slozem, Tildiem, and others
Used in the following combined preparations None

QUICK REFERENCE

Drug group Calcium channel blocker (p.33) and antihypertensive drug (p.34)

Overdose danger rating Medium
Dependence rating Low
Prescription needed Yes
Available as generic Yes

GENERAL INFORMATION

Diltiazem belongs to the group of drugs known as calcium channel blockers (p.33). These drugs interfere with the conduction of electrical signals in the muscles of the heart and blood vessels. Diltiazem is used in the treatment of angina and high blood pressure.

When taken regularly, diltiazem reduces the frequency of angina attacks but does not work quickly enough to reduce the pain of an angina attack already in progress.

Diltiazem does not adversely affect breathing and is of particular value for people with asthma, for whom other anti-angina drugs may not be suitable. Adverse effects include headache, ankle swelling, and tiredness.

INFORMATION FOR USERS

Your drug prescription is tailored for you. Do not alter dosage without checking with your doctor.

How taken Tablets, SR-tablets, capsules, SR-capsules.

Frequency and timing of doses 3 x daily (tablets/capsules); 1–2 x daily (SR-tablets/SR-capsules).

Adult dosage range 180–480mg daily.

Onset of effect 2–3 hours.

Duration of action 6–8 hours.

Diet advice None.

Storage Keep in a closed container in a cool, dry place out of reach of children.

Missed dose Take as soon as you remember. If your next dose is due within 2 hours, take a single dose now and skip the next.

Stopping the drug Unless a rash occurs, do not stop taking the drug without consulting your doctor; symptoms may recur. Stopping suddenly may worsen angina.

Exceeding the dose An occasional unintentional extra dose is unlikely to cause problems. Large overdoses may cause dizziness. Notify your doctor.

POSSIBLE ADVERSE EFFECTS

Diltiazem can cause various minor symptoms that are common to other calcium channel blockers. These include headache, nausea, dry mouth, and swelling of the leg or ankle. The most serious effect is the possibility of a slowed heart beat, which may cause tiredness or dizziness. These effects can sometimes be controlled by an adjustment in dosage. If you develop a rash, stop taking the drug and seek medical attention.

INTERACTIONS

Antihypertensive drugs Diltiazem increases the effects of these drugs, leading to a further reduction in blood pressure. However, this interaction is often desired for better control of blood pressure.

Anticonvulsant drugs Levels of these drugs may be altered by diltiazem.

Anti-arrhythmic drugs There is a risk of side effects on the heart if these drugs are taken with digoxin.

Digoxin Blood levels and adverse effects of this drug may be increased if it is taken with diltiazem. The dosage of digoxin may need to be reduced.

Theophylline/aminophylline Diltiazem may increase the levels of this drug.

Beta blockers These drugs increase the risk of the heart slowing.

SPECIAL PRECAUTIONS

Be sure to tell your doctor if:
◆ You have long-term liver or kidney problems.
◆ You have heart failure.
◆ You are taking other medications.
Pregnancy Not usually prescribed. Discuss with your doctor.
Breast-feeding The drug passes into the breast milk and may affect the baby. Discuss with your doctor.
Infants and children Not recommended.
Over 60 Reduced dose may be necessary. Increased likelihood of adverse effects.
Driving and hazardous work Avoid such activities until you have learned how diltiazem affects you because the drug can cause dizziness due to lowered blood pressure.
Alcohol Avoid excessive amounts. Alcohol may lower blood pressure, causing dizziness.

PROLONGED USE

No problems expected.

Diphenoxylate

Brand names None
Used in the following combined preparations
Co-phenotrope, Diarphen, Lomotil, Tropergen

QUICK REFERENCE

Drug group Opioid antidiarrhoeal drug (p.42)
Overdose danger rating Medium
Dependence rating Medium
Prescription needed Yes
Available as generic No

GENERAL INFORMATION

Diphenoxylate is an antidiarrhoeal drug chemically related to the opiate analgesics. It reduces bowel contractions and, therefore, the fluidity and frequency of bowel movements. Available in the form of tablets, diphenoxylate is prescribed for the relief of sudden or recurrent bouts of diarrhoea.

The drug is not suitable for diarrhoea that is caused by infection, poisons, or antibiotics as it may delay recovery by slowing expulsion of harmful substances from the bowel. Diphenoxylate can cause toxic megacolon, a dangerous dilation of the bowel that shuts off the blood supply to the wall of the bowel and increases the risk of perforation.

At recommended doses, serious adverse effects are rare. To guard against addiction, atropine is added to diphenoxylate tablets. If these are taken in excessive amounts, the atropine will cause highly unpleasant anticholinergic effects. Diphenoxylate is especially dangerous for young children; be sure to store the drug out of their reach.

INFORMATION FOR USERS

Your drug prescription is tailored for you. Do not alter dosage without checking with your doctor.
How taken Tablets.
Frequency and timing of doses 3–4 x daily.
Dosage range *Adults* 10mg initially, followed by doses of 5mg. *Children* Reduced dose necessary according to age and weight.
Onset of effect Within 1 hour. Control of diarrhoea may take some hours.
Duration of action Up to 24 hours.
Diet advice Ensure adequate fluid intake during an attack of diarrhoea.

Storage Keep in a closed container in a cool, dry place out of reach of children. Protect from light.

Missed dose Take as soon as you remember. If your next dose is due within 3 hours, take a single dose now and skip the next.

Stopping the drug Can be safely stopped as soon as you no longer need it.

Exceeding the dose An occasional unintentional extra dose is unlikely to cause problems. Large overdoses may cause unusual drowsiness, dryness of the mouth and skin, restlessness, and in extreme cases, loss of consciousness. Symptoms of overdose may be delayed. Notify your doctor.

POSSIBLE ADVERSE EFFECTS

Side effects, including drowsiness, restlessness, headache, and dizziness, occur infrequently with diphenoxylate. Abdominal pain or distension, nausea, or vomiting may be part of your illness, but, if they worsen or begin after treatment has started, notify your doctor. If you develop a rash, stop taking the drug and seek medical attention.

INTERACTIONS

Sedatives All drugs that have a sedative effect on the central nervous system may increase the sedative effect of diphenoxylate.

MAOIs There is a risk of a dangerous rise in blood pressure if MAOIs are taken together with diphenoxylate.

SPECIAL PRECAUTIONS

Be sure to tell your doctor if:
◆ You have a long-term liver problem.
◆ You have severe abdominal pain.
◆ You have bloodstained diarrhoea.
◆ You have recently taken antibiotics.
◆ You have ulcerative colitis.
◆ You have recently travelled abroad.
◆ You are taking other medications.

Pregnancy Safety in pregnancy not established. Discuss with your doctor.

Breast-feeding The drug passes into the breast milk and may cause drowsiness in the baby. Discuss with your doctor.

Infants and children Not recommended under 4 years. Reduced dose necessary for older children.

Over 60 Reduced dose may be necessary.

Driving and hazardous work Avoid such activities until you have learned how diphenoxylate affects you because the drug may cause drowsiness and dizziness.

Alcohol Avoid. Alcohol may increase the sedative effects of this drug.

PROLONGED USE

Not usually recommended.

Dipyridamole

Brand names Cerebrovase, Modaplate, Persantin
Used in the following combined preparation
Asasantin Retard

QUICK REFERENCE

Drug group Antiplatelet drug (p.36)
Overdose danger rating Medium
Dependence rating Low
Prescription needed Yes
Available as generic Yes

GENERAL INFORMATION

Dipyridamole was introduced in the late 1970s as an anti-angina drug, to improve the capability of people with angina to exercise. Although more effective drugs are now available, dipyridamole is still prescribed as an antiplatelet drug. It "thins" the blood in patients who have had heart valve replacement surgery, a heart attack, or a stroke, reducing the possibility of blood clots in the circulation.

Dipyridamole is usually given together with other drugs such as warfarin or aspirin. It can also be given by injection during certain types of diagnostic test on the heart.

Side effects may occur, especially in the early days of treatment. If they persist, your doctor may advise a reduction in dosage.

INFORMATION FOR USERS

Your drug prescription is tailored for you. Do not alter dosage without checking with your doctor.

How taken Tablets, capsules, SR-capsules, liquid, injection (for diagnostic tests only).

Frequency and timing of doses 3–4 x daily, 1 hour before meals (tablets, capsules, liquid). 2 x daily with food (SR-capsules).

Adult dosage range 300–600mg daily.

Onset of effect Within 1 hour. Full therapeutic effect may not be felt for 2–3 weeks.
Duration of action Up to 8 hours. Up to 12 hours (SR-capsules)
Diet advice None.
Storage Keep in a closed container in a cool, dry place out of reach of children. Protect from light.
Missed dose Take as soon as you remember. If your next dose is due within 2 hours, take a single dose now and skip the next.
Stopping the drug Unless severe adverse effects occur (see below), do not stop taking the drug without consulting your doctor; withdrawal could lead to abnormal blood clotting.
Exceeding the dose An occasional unintentional extra dose is unlikely to be a cause for concern. Large overdoses may cause dizziness or vomiting. Notify your doctor.

POSSIBLE ADVERSE EFFECTS
Adverse effects are rare. Possible symptoms include dizziness, headache, fainting, nausea, diarrhoea, and rash. If you experience dizziness or fainting, or you develop a rash, stop taking the drug and consult your doctor urgently. Rarely, the drug may aggravate angina.

INTERACTIONS
Anticoagulants The effect of these drugs may be increased by dipyridamole, increasing the risk of uncontrolled bleeding. The dosage of the anticoagulant should be reduced.
Antacids These may reduce the effectiveness of dipyridamole.

SPECIAL PRECAUTIONS
Be sure to tell your doctor if:
◆ You have low blood pressure.
◆ You suffer from migraine.
◆ You have angina.
◆ You have had a recent heart attack.
◆ You are taking other medications.
Pregnancy Safety in pregnancy not established. Discuss with your doctor.
Breast-feeding The drug passes into the breast milk but at normal doses adverse effects on the baby are unlikely. Discuss with your doctor.
Infants and children Reduced dose necessary.
Over 60 No special problems.
Driving and hazardous work No problems expected.

Alcohol No known problems.

PROLONGED USE
No known problems.

Disulfiram
Brand name Antabuse
Used in the following combined preparations
None

QUICK REFERENCE
Drug group Alcohol abuse deterrent
Overdose danger rating Medium
Dependence rating Low
Prescription needed Yes
Available as generic No

GENERAL INFORMATION
Disulfiram is used to help alcoholics abstain from alcohol. It does not cure alcoholism but provides a powerful deterrent to drinking.

If you are taking disulfiram and drink even a small amount of alcohol, highly unpleasant reactions follow, such as flushing, throbbing headache, nausea, thirst, breathlessness, palpitations, dizziness, and fainting. Such reactions may last from 30 minutes to several hours, leaving you feeling drowsy and sleepy. Because the reactions can also include unconsciousness, it is wise to carry a card stating the person to be notified in an emergency.

When disulfiram and alcohol are taken together, acetaldehyde (a toxic breakdown product of alcohol) builds up in the blood, triggering the unwanted symptoms. It is important not to drink any alcohol for at least 24 hours before beginning disulfiram treatment, and for at least a week after stopping. Foods, medicines, and even toiletries that contain alcohol should also be avoided.

INFORMATION FOR USERS
Your drug prescription is tailored for you. Do not alter dosage without checking with your doctor.
How taken Tablets.
Frequency and timing of doses Once daily.
Adult dosage range 800mg initially, gradually reduced over 5 days to 100–200mg (maintenance dose).

Onset of effect Interaction with alcohol occurs within a few minutes of taking alcohol.

Duration of action Interaction with alcohol can occur for up to 6 days after the last dose of disulfiram.

Diet advice Avoid all alcoholic drinks, even in very small amounts. Food, fermented vinegar, medicines, mouthwashes, and lotions containing alcohol should also be avoided.

Storage Keep in a closed container in a cool, dry place out of reach of children. Protect from light.

Missed dose Take as soon as you remember. If your next dose is due within 2 hours, take a single dose now and skip the next.

Stopping the drug Do not stop taking the drug without consulting your doctor.

Exceeding the dose An occasional unintentional extra dose is unlikely to cause problems. Large overdoses may cause a temporary increase in adverse effects. Notify your doctor.

POSSIBLE ADVERSE EFFECTS
Adverse effects, such as drowsiness, nausea, and reduced libido, usually disappear with continued treatment. If they persist or become severe, the dosage may need to be adjusted. The most important and potentially severe effects are due to the interaction of the drug with alcohol (see General information, above).

INTERACTIONS
General note A number of drugs can produce an adverse reaction when taken with disulfiram. Check with your doctor or pharmacist before taking any other medication.

Phenytoin Disulfiram increases the blood levels of this drug.

Anticoagulant drugs Disulfiram increases the effect of these drugs.

Metronidazole A severe reaction can occur if this drug is taken with disulfiram.

Theophylline Disulfiram may increase the toxic effects of this drug.

SPECIAL PRECAUTIONS
Be sure to tell your doctor if:
◆ You have long-term liver or kidney problems.
◆ You have heart problems, coronary artery disease, or high blood pressure.
◆ You have had epileptic fits.

◆ You have diabetes.
◆ You have breathing problems. You are taking other medications.

Pregnancy Safety in pregnancy not established. Discuss with your doctor.

Breast-feeding The drug passes into the breast milk and may affect the baby adversely. Discuss with your doctor.

Over 60 Reduced dose may be necessary.

Driving and hazardous work Avoid such activities until you have learned how disulfiram affects you because the drug can cause drowsiness and dizziness.

Alcohol Never drink alcohol while under treatment with disulfiram, and avoid all foods, medicines, and toiletries containing alcohol. Alcohol may interact dangerously with disulfiram.

PROLONGED USE
Not usually prescribed for longer than 6 months without review. It is wise to carry a card indicating you are taking disulfiram with instructions as to who should be notified in an emergency.

Domperidone

Brand name Motilium
Used in the following combined preparations
Domperamol

QUICK REFERENCE
Drug group Anti-emetic drug (p.21)
Overdose danger rating Medium
Dependence rating Low
Prescription needed No
Available as generic No

GENERAL INFORMATION
Domperidone is an anti-emetic drug that was first introduced in the early 1980s. It is particularly effective for treating the nausea and vomiting that are caused by gastrointestinal disorders, such as gastroenteritis, or that occur as a side effect of other drug treatment (especially anticancer drugs) or radiation therapy. Domperidone is not effective for motion sickness or nausea that is caused by inner ear disorders such as Ménière's disease.

The main advantage of domperidone over other anti-emetics is that it does not usually cause sedation or other adverse effects such as abnormal movement. The drug is not suitable for long-term treatment of gastrointestinal disorders, however, for which alternative drug treatment, is often prescribed.

Domperidone may also be used to relieve dyspepsia (indigestion and heartburn); and, in combination with paracetamol, it is sometimes used to treat acute attacks of migraine.

INFORMATION FOR USERS

Follow instructions on the label. Call your doctor if symptoms worsen.

How taken Tablets, liquid, suppositories.
Frequency and timing of doses *Nausea/vomiting* Every 4–8 hours as required. *Dyspepsia* 3 x daily with water before meals and at night (tablets only).
Adult dosage range 10–20mg (by mouth); 30–60mg (rectally).
Onset of effect Within 1 hour. The effects of the drug may be delayed if taken after the onset of nausea.
Duration of action Approximately 6 hours.
Diet advice None.
Storage Keep in a closed container in a cool, dry place out of reach of children. Protect from light.
Missed dose Take as soon as you remember for dyspepsia. If your next dose is due within 4 hours, take a single dose now and skip the next. Then return to your normal dosing schedule.
Stopping the drug Can be safely stopped as soon as you no longer need it.
Exceeding the dose An occasional unintentional extra dose is unlikely to cause problems. Large overdoses may cause dizziness. Notify your doctor.

POSSIBLE ADVERSE EFFECTS

Adverse effects from this drug are rare. However, if you begin to experience muscle spasms or tremors, breast enlargement or milk secretion, reduced libido, or if you develop a rash, consult your doctor.

INTERACTIONS

Anticholinergic drugs These may reduce the beneficial effects of domperidone.

Opioid analgesics These may reduce the beneficial effects of domperidone.
Bromocriptine and cabergoline Domperidone may reduce the effects of these drugs in some people.

SPECIAL PRECAUTIONS

Be sure to tell your doctor if:
◆ You have a long-term kidney problem.
◆ You have thyroid disease.
◆ You are taking other medications.
Pregnancy Safety in pregnancy not established. Discuss with your doctor.
Breast-feeding The drug may pass into the breast milk, but at normal doses adverse effects on the baby are unlikely. Discuss with your doctor.
Infants and children Prescribed only to treat nausea and vomiting caused by anticancer drugs or radiation therapy. Reduced dose necessary.
Over 60 No special problems.
Driving and hazardous work No special problems.
Alcohol No special problems, but alcohol is best avoided in cases of nausea and vomiting.

PROLONGED USE

Not prescribed for long-term treatment.

Donepezil

Brand name Aricept
Used in the following combined preparations None

QUICK REFERENCE

Drug group Drug for dementia (p.19)
Overdose danger rating Medium
Dependence rating Low
Prescription needed Yes
Available as generic No

GENERAL INFORMATION

Donepezil is an inhibitor of the enzyme acetylcholinesterase. This enzyme breaks down the natural neurotransmitter acetylcholine to limit its effects. Blocking the enzyme raises the levels of acetylcholine which, in the brain, increases alertness.

Donepezil has been found to reduce the progression of dementia due to Alzheimer's disease in up to half of the patients given the drug, and it is used to diminish deterioration in that disease. It is therefore ineffective in many patients with Alzheimer's disease, and it has no effect on dementia due to other causes. It is usual for an expert to start you on the treatment and assess you after about three months to decide whether the drug is helping and whether it is worth continuing treatment. Side effects may include bladder outflow obstruction and psychiatric problems, such as agitation and aggression, which might be thought due to the disease.

INFORMATION FOR USERS
Your drug prescription is tailored for you. Do not alter dosage without checking with your doctor.
How taken Tablets.
Frequency and timing of doses Once daily at bedtime.
Adult dosage range 5–10mg.
Onset of effect 1 hour. Full effects might take up to 3 months.
Duration of action 1–2 days.
Diet advice None.
Storage Keep in a closed container in a cool, dry place out of reach of children.
Missed dose Take as soon as you remember. A carer should be overseeing the taking of the tablets.
Stopping the drug Do not stop taking the drug without consulting your doctor; symptoms may recur.
Exceeding the dose An occasional unintentional extra dose is unlikely to be a cause for concern. But if you notice any unusual symptoms, or if a large overdose has been taken, notify your doctor.

POSSIBLE ADVERSE EFFECTS
Adverse effects include agitation, fatigue insomnia, and problems such as accidents, which are common in this group of people, even those not treated. Other adverse effects include nausea, vomiting, diarrhoea, muscle cramps, and headache. If you experience dizziness or fainting or have palpitations or difficulty in passing urine, consult your doctor urgently.

INTERACTIONS
Aminoglycoside antibiotics, clindamycin, and colistin These drugs block the effect of donepezil.
Antimalarials and anti-arrhythmics Certain of these drugs may block donepezil's effects.
Muscle relaxants used in surgery Donepezil may increase the effect of some muscle relaxants, but it may also block some others.

SPECIAL PRECAUTIONS
Be sure to tell your doctor if:
◆ You have a heart problem.
◆ You have asthma or respiratory problems.
◆ You have had a peptic ulcer.
◆ You are taking an NSAID regularly.
◆ You are taking other medications.
Pregnancy Not prescribed.
Breast-feeding Not prescribed.
Infants and children Not prescribed.
Over 60 No special problems.
Driving and hazardous work Your underlying condition may make such activities inadvisable. Discuss with your doctor.
Alcohol Avoid. Alcohol may reduce the effect of donepezil.
Surgery and general anaesthetics Treatment with donepezil may need to be stopped before you have a general anaesthetic. Discuss this with your doctor or dentist before any operation.

PROLONGED USE
May be continued for as long as there is benefit. Stopping the drug leads to a gradual loss of the improvements.
Monitoring Periodic checks may be performed to test whether the drug is still providing some benefit.

Dorzolamide

Brand name Trusopt
Used in the following combined preparation Cosopt

QUICK REFERENCE
Drug group Drug for Glaucoma (p.110)
Overdose danger rating Low
Dependence rating Low
Prescription needed Yes
Available as generic No

GENERAL INFORMATION

Dorzolamide is a carbonic anhydrase inhibitor (a kind of diuretic) used, in the form of eye drops only, to treat glaucoma and for ocular hypertension (high blood pressure inside the eye). The drug relieves the pressure by reducing production of aqueous humour, the fluid in the front chamber of the eye.

Dorzolamide may be used with a beta blocker in a combined preparation but is also used on its own by people resistant to the effects of beta blockers or for whom beta blockers are unsuitable.

Most side effects of dorzolamide are local to the eye, but systemic effects may occur if enough of the drug is absorbed by the body.

INFORMATION FOR USERS

Your drug prescription is tailored for you. Do not alter dosage without checking with your doctor.

How taken Eye drops.
Frequency and timing of doses 3 x daily (on its own); 2 x daily (combined).
Adult dosage range 1 drop in the affected eye(s) or as directed.
Onset of effect 15–30 minutes.
Duration of action 4–8 hours.
Diet advice None.
Storage Keep in a closed container in a cool, dry place out of reach of children. Protect from light. Discard eye drops 4 weeks after opening.
Missed dose Take as soon as you remember. If your next dose is due, skip the missed dose then go back to your normal dosing schedule.
Stopping the drug Unless severe adverse effects occur (see below), do not stop taking the drug without consulting your doctor; symptoms may recur.
Exceeding the dose An occasional unintentional extra application is unlikely to cause problems. Excessive use may provoke side effects as described below.

POSSIBLE ADVERSE EFFECTS

Local side effects include conjunctivitis and keratitis (inflammation of the cornea, the transparent part of the eye). This may lead to burning, stinging, or runny eyes; inflammation or soreness of the eyes or blurred vision; or a bitter taste in the mouth. Systemic side effects, such as nausea, dizziness, tiredness, and headache may also occur. If you develop a rash or breathing difficulties, stop taking the drug and consult your doctor urgently.

INTERACTIONS

General note Dorzolamide may interact with the following drugs, but there appear to be no published reports of problems. Consult your doctor.
Thiazide diuretics Excessive loss of potassium may occur when these drugs are taken with dorzolamide.
Aspirin This drug may increase dorzolamide levels and also the risk of adverse effects.
Lithium Dorzolamide may reduce blood levels of lithium.

SPECIAL PRECAUTIONS

Be sure to tell your doctor if:
◆ You have liver or kidney problems.
◆ You are allergic to sulphonamide drugs.
◆ You are allergic to benzalkonium chloride.
You are taking other medications.
Pregnancy Not prescribed. Discuss with your doctor.
Breast-feeding Not recommended. Discuss with your doctor.
Infants and children Not recommended.
Over 60 No special problems.
Driving and hazardous work Avoid such activities until you have learned how dorzolamide affects you because the drug can cause dizziness and blurred vision.
Alcohol No special problems.

PROLONGED USE

No special problems.

Dosulepin (Dothiepin)

Brand names Dothapax, Prepadine, Prothiaden
Used in the following combined preparations
None

QUICK REFERENCE

Drug group Tricyclic antidepressant drug (p.14)
Overdose danger rating High
Dependence rating Low
Prescription needed Yes
Available as generic Yes

GENERAL INFORMATION

Dosulepin belongs to the tricyclic class of antidepressants and is used in the long-term treatment of depression. It is particularly useful when the depression is accompanied by anxiety and insomnia. Dosulepin has a number of effects; it elevates mood, increases physical activity, improves appetite, and restores interest in everyday activities. Taken at night, it encourages sleep and helps to eliminate the need for additional sleeping drugs.

Dosulepin takes several weeks to achieve its full antidepressant effect. It has adverse effects that are common to all tricyclics. These include a risk of causing dangerous heart rhythms, fits, and coma if it builds up in the body or is taken in overdose.

INFORMATION FOR USERS

Your drug prescription is tailored for you. Do not alter dosage without checking with your doctor.

How taken Tablets, capsules.
Frequency and timing of doses 2–3 x daily or once at night.
Adult dosage range 75–150mg daily.
Onset of effect Full antidepressant effect may not be felt for 2–4 weeks, but adverse effects may be noticed within a day or two.
Duration of action Several days.
Diet advice None.
Storage Keep in a closed container in a cool, dry place out of reach of children.
Missed dose Take as soon as you remember. If your next dose is due within 2 hours, take a single dose now and skip the next.
Stopping the drug Unless severe adverse effects occur (see below), do not stop taking the drug without consulting your doctor, who may supervise gradual dosage reduction. Abrupt cessation may cause withdrawal symptoms and recurrence of the original problem.

OVERDOSE ACTION

Seek immediate medical advice in all cases. Take emergency action if palpitations or loss of consciousness occur.

POSSIBLE ADVERSE EFFECTS

The drug's adverse effects are mainly the result of its anticholinergic action. They include drowsiness, dry mouth, sweating, and blurred vision and are more common in the early days of treatment. If you experience dizziness, fainting, rash, difficulty in passing urine, palpitations, or loss of consciousness, stop taking the drug and consult your doctor urgently.

INTERACTIONS

Sedatives All drugs that have a sedative effect on the central nervous system increase the sedative properties of dosulepin.
Heavy smoking This may reduce the antidepressant effect of dosulepin.
Antiepileptic drugs dosulepin may reduce the effectiveness of these drugs.
MAOIs In the rare cases where these drugs are given with dosulepin, serious interactions may occur.

SPECIAL PRECAUTIONS

Be sure to tell your doctor if:
◆ You have heart problems.
◆ You have had epileptic fits.
◆ You have long-term liver or kidney problems.
◆ You have glaucoma.
◆ You have prostate trouble.
◆ You are taking other medications.
Pregnancy Safety in pregnancy not established. Discuss with your doctor.
Breast-feeding The drug passes into the breast milk, but effects on the baby are unlikely. Discuss with your doctor.
Infants and children Not recommended.
Over 60 Reduced dose may be necessary.
Driving and hazardous work Avoid such activities until you have learned how dosulepin affects you because the drug can reduce alertness and may cause blurred vision, dizziness, and drowsiness.
Alcohol Avoid. Alcohol may increase the sedative effects of this drug.
Surgery and general anaesthetics Treatment with dosulepin may need to be stopped before you have a general anaesthetic. Discuss this with your doctor or dentist before any operation.

PROLONGED USE

No problems expected.
Monitoring Elderly people who experience drowsiness, confusion, or convulsions should be monitored for low blood sodium levels.

Doxazosin

Brand name Cardura
Used in the following combined preparations
None

QUICK REFERENCE
Drug group Vasodilator (p.30) and antihypertensive drug (p.34)
Overdose danger rating Medium
Dependence rating Low
Prescription needed Yes
Available as generic No

GENERAL INFORMATION

Doxazosin is an antihypertensive vasodilator drug that relieves hypertension (high blood pressure) by relaxing muscles in the blood vessel walls, allowing them to dilate. Because doxazosin is eliminated slowly from the body, it is usually given only once daily. Doxazosin may be administered together with other antihypertensive drugs, including beta blockers, because its effects on blood pressure are increased when it is combined with most other antihypertensives.

Given in low doses, doxazosin is also used to relieve symptoms caused by an enlarged prostate gland.

Dizziness and fainting may occur at the onset of treatment with doxazosin, because the first dose may cause a marked fall in blood pressure. For this reason, the initial dose is usually low.

INFORMATION FOR USERS

Your drug prescription is tailored for you. Do not alter dosage without checking with your doctor.
How taken Tablets.
Frequency and timing of doses Once daily.
Adult dosage range *Hypertension* 1mg (starting dose), increased gradually as necessary up to 16mg. *Enlarged prostate* 1mg (starting dose), increased gradually at 1–2-week intervals up to 8mg.
Onset of effect Within 2 hours.
Duration of action 24 hours.
Diet advice None.
Storage Keep in a closed container in a cool, dry place out of reach of children.
Missed dose Take as soon as you remember. If your next dose is due within 6 hours, take a single dose now and skip the next.
Stopping the drug Do not stop taking the drug without consulting your doctor; stopping the drug may lead to a rise in blood pressure.
Exceeding the dose An occasional unintentional extra dose is unlikely to be a cause for concern. Larger overdoses may cause dizziness or fainting. Notify your doctor.

POSSIBLE ADVERSE EFFECTS

Nausea, stuffy nose, headache, drowsiness, and weakness are common adverse effects with doxazosin. The main problem, however, is that it may cause dizziness or fainting when you stand up. Urinary incontinence may occur in women. Consult your doctor if you develop a rash.

INTERACTIONS
Antihypertensive drugs Any drugs that can reduce the blood pressure are likely to have an increased effect when taken with doxazosin; this interaction is often desired for better control of blood pressure.

SPECIAL PRECAUTIONS
Be sure to tell your doctor if:
◆ You have long-term liver or kidney problems.
◆ You are taking other medications.
Pregnancy Safety in pregnancy not established. Discuss with your doctor.
Breast-feeding The drug passes into the breast milk. Discuss with your doctor.
Infants and children Not recommended.
Over 60 Reduced dose may be necessary. You should take extra care when standing up until you have learned how doxazosin affects you.
Driving and hazardous work Avoid such activities until you have learned how doxazosin affects you because the drug can cause drowsiness, dizziness, and fainting.
Alcohol Avoid excessive amounts. Alcohol may increase some of the adverse effects of doxazosin, such as dizziness, drowsiness, and fainting.

PROLONGED USE
No known problems.

Doxorubicin

Brand name Caelyx
Used in the following combined preparations
None

QUICK REFERENCE

Drug group Cytotoxic anticancer drug (p.94)
Overdose danger rating Medium
Dependence rating Low
Prescription needed Yes
Available as generic Yes

GENERAL INFORMATION

Doxorubicin is one of the most effective anticancer drugs. It is prescribed to treat a wide variety of cancers, usually in conjunction with other anticancer drugs. It is used in acute leukaemia and cancer of the lymph nodes (Hodgkin's disease), lung, breast, bladder, stomach, thyroid, and reproductive organs. It is also used to treat Kaposi's sarcoma in AIDS patients.

Nausea and vomiting after injection are the most common side effects of doxorubicin. Although these symptoms are unpleasant, they tend to be less severe as the body adjusts to the treatment. Doxorubicin may stain the urine bright red, but this is not harmful. More seriously, because the drug interferes with the production of blood cells, blood clotting disorders, anaemia, and infections may occur. Therefore, effects on the blood are carefully monitored. Hair loss is also a common side effect of the drug. Rarely, heart rhythm disturbance and heart failure are dose-dependent side effects that may also occur.

INFORMATION FOR USERS

This drug is given only under medical supervision and is not for self-administration.
How taken Injection, bladder instillation.
Frequency and timing of doses Every 1–3 weeks.
Adult dosage range Dosage is determined individually according to body height, weight, and response.
Onset of effect Some adverse effects may appear within one hour, but full beneficial effects may not be felt for up to 4 weeks.
Duration of action Adverse effects can persist for up to 2 weeks after stopping treatment.

Diet advice None.
Storage Not applicable. The drug is not normally kept in the home.
Missed dose The drug is administered in hospital under close medical supervision. If for some reason you skip your dose, contact your doctor as soon as you can.
Stopping the drug Do not stop taking the drug without consulting your doctor. Stopping abruptly may lead to a worsening of the underlying condition.
Exceeding the dose Overdosage is unlikely since treatment is carefully monitored and supervised.

POSSIBLE ADVERSE EFFECTS

Nausea and vomiting generally occur within an hour of injection. Hair loss, loss of appetite, and diarrhoea are common. Mouth ulcers and skin irritation or ulcers may also occur. Palpitations may indicate an adverse effect of the drug on the heart. Since treatment is closely supervised in hospital, all adverse effects are monitored.

INTERACTIONS

Ciclosporin Administration of ciclosporin while receiving doxorubicin can lead to adverse effects on the nervous system.

SPECIAL PRECAUTIONS

Doxorubicin is prescribed only under close medical supervision, taking account of your present condition and medical history.
Pregnancy Not usually prescribed. The drug may cause birth defects or premature birth. Discuss with your doctor.
Breast-feeding Not advised. The drug passes into the breast milk and may affect the baby adversely. Discuss with your doctor.
Infants and children Reduced dose necessary.
Over 60 Increased risk of adverse effects. Reduced dose may be necessary.
Driving and hazardous work No known problems.
Alcohol No known problems.

PROLONGED USE

Prolonged use of doxorubicin may reduce the activity of the bone marrow, leading to reduced production of all types of blood cell. It may also affect the heart adversely.

Monitoring Periodic checks on blood composition are usually required. Regular heart examinations are also carried out.

Doxycycline

Brand names Cyclodox, Demix, Doxylar, Ramysis, Vibramycin
Used in the following combined preparations None

QUICK REFERENCE
Drug group Tetracycline antibiotic (p.60)
Overdose danger rating Low
Dependence rating Low
Prescription needed Yes
Available as generic Yes

GENERAL INFORMATION
Doxycycline is a tetracycline antibiotic drug that is longer acting than some other drugs in this group. It is used mainly in the treatment of infections of the urinary, respiratory, and gastrointestinal tracts and of the skin, eye, and prostate. Doxycycline is often used in the treatment of acne and may be recommended for malaria prevention in some parts of the world (see p.73).

Doxycycline is less likely to cause diarrhoea as a side effect than other tetracyclines, and its absorption is not significantly impaired by milk and food. The drug can therefore be taken with meals to reduce side effects such as nausea or indigestion. Unlike most other tetracyclines, however, doxycycline is also safe for people whose kidney function is impaired. Like other tetracyclines, it can stain developing teeth and may affect bone development. Doxycycline is therefore usually avoided in young children or pregnant women.

INFORMATION FOR USERS
Your drug prescription is tailored for you. Do not alter dosage without checking with your doctor.
How taken Tablets, capsules.
Frequency and timing of doses 1–2 x daily with water, or with or after food, in a sitting or standing position.
Dosage range 100–200mg daily.

Onset of effect 4–12 hours; several weeks (acne).
Duration of action Up to 24 hours; several weeks (acne).
Diet advice None.
Storage Keep in closed container in a cool, dry place out of reach of children.
Missed dose Take as soon as you remember. If your next dose is due within 6 hours, take a single dose now and skip the next.
Stopping the drug Take the full course. Even if you feel better, the original infection may still be present and symptoms may recur if treatment is stopped too soon.
Exceeding the dose An occasional unintentional extra dose is unlikely to be a cause for concern. But if you notice any unusual symptoms, or if a large overdose has been taken, notify your doctor.

POSSIBLE ADVERSE EFFECTS
Adverse effects are rare, but some people may experience nausea, vomiting, or diarrhoea. Other rare adverse effects include rash, itching, and increased sensitivity of the skin to sunlight, which may cause a rash to develop. If you experience headaches or visual disturbances, consult your doctor.

INTERACTIONS
Oral anticoagulant drugs Doxycycline may increase the anticoagulant action of these drugs.
Barbiturates, carbamazepine, and phenytoin All of these drugs reduce the effectiveness of doxycycline. Doxycycline dosage may need to be increased.
Oral contraceptives A slight risk exists of doxycycline reducing the effectiveness of oral contraceptives. Discuss with your doctor.
Antacids and preparations containing iron, calcium, or magnesium These may impair absorption of this drug. Do not take within 2–3 hours of doxycycline.
Ciclosporin Doxycycline may increase the blood levels of this drug.

SPECIAL PRECAUTIONS
Be sure to tell your doctor if:
◆ You have a long-term liver problem.
◆ You have previously suffered an allergic reaction to a tetracycline antibiotic.

◆ You have porphyria.
◆ You are taking other medications.

Pregnancy Not usually prescribed. Is laid down in bones, but this is not harmful; it may discolour the teeth of the developing baby. Discuss with your doctor.

Breast-feeding The drug passes into the breast milk and may lead to discoloration of the baby's teeth and may also have other adverse effects. Discuss with your doctor.

Infants and children Not recommended under 12 years. Reduced dose necessary for older children.

Over 60 No special problems. Dispersible tablets should be used as they are less likely to cause oesophageal irritation or ulceration.

Driving and hazardous work No known problems.

Alcohol No known problems, but avoid excessive amounts.

PROLONGED USE
Not usually prescribed long term, except for acne.

Dydrogesterone

Brand names Duphaston, Duphaston HRT
Used in the following combined preparations
Femoston, Femapak

QUICK REFERENCE
Drug group Female sex hormone (p.86)
Overdose danger rating Low
Dependence rating Low
Prescription needed Yes
Available as generic No

GENERAL INFORMATION
Dydrogesterone is a progestogen, a synthetic hormone similar to the natural female sex hormone progesterone. The drug is widely used to treat a variety of menstrual disorders that are thought to result from a deficiency of progesterone. These include premenstrual syndrome and absent, irregular, or painful periods (see also p.100).

Dydrogesterone is also prescribed together with an oestrogen as part of hormone replacement therapy following the menopause. It may be prescribed for endometriosis (p.100),

and is also given to prevent miscarriage in women who have had repeated miscarriages.

Dydrogesterone is usually taken on selected days during the menstrual cycle, depending on the disorder that is being treated.

INFORMATION FOR USERS
Your drug prescription is tailored for you. Do not alter dosage without checking with your doctor.

How taken Tablets.
Frequency and timing of doses 1–3 x daily. In many conditions, this drug is taken at certain times in the menstrual cycle.
Adult dosage range 10–30mg daily.
Onset of effect Beneficial effects of this drug may not be felt for several months.
Duration of action 12 hours.
Diet advice None.
Storage Keep in a closed container in a cool, dry place out of reach of children. Protect from light.
Missed dose Take as soon as you remember. If your next dose is due within 2 hours, take a single dose now and skip the next.
Stopping the drug Do not stop taking the drug without consulting your doctor; symptoms may recur.
Exceeding the dose An occasional unintentional extra dose is unlikely to be a cause for concern. But if you notice any unusual symptoms, or if a large overdose has been taken, notify your doctor.

POSSIBLE ADVERSE EFFECTS
Irregular periods and "breakthrough" bleeding are the most common adverse effects but may be helped by dosage adjustment. Fluid retention, leading to swollen feet or ankles, weight gain, nausea or vomiting, breast tenderness, headache or dizziness may also occur. Consult your doctor if any of these become severe or if you develop a rash.

INTERACTIONS
Ciclosporin Dydrogesterone increases the effects of this drug.

SPECIAL PRECAUTIONS
Be sure to tell your doctor if:
◆ You have a long-term liver or kidney problem.

- You have heart or circulatory problems.
- You have diabetes.
- You have high blood pressure.
- You have porphyria.
- You are taking other medications.

Pregnancy No evidence of risk at normal dosage. The drug is used to prevent miscarriage.

Breast-feeding The drug passes into the breast milk, but at normal doses adverse effects on the baby are unlikely. High doses may suppress milk production.

Infants and children Not prescribed.

Over 60 No special problems.

Driving and hazardous work Avoid such activities until you have learned how dydrogesterone affects you because the drug may rarely cause dizziness.

Alcohol No special problems.

PROLONGED USE

No special problems.

Enalapril

Brand names Innovace, Innovace Melt
Used in the following combined preparation
Innozide

QUICK REFERENCE

Drug group Ace inhibitor vasodilator (p.30)
Overdose danger rating Medium
Dependence rating Low
Prescription needed Yes
Available as generic No

GENERAL INFORMATION

Enalapril belongs to the ACE (angiotensin converting enzyme) inhibitor group of drugs and is used to treat high blood pressure (p.34) and heart failure (in which the heart is unable to deal with its workload). It may also be given to patients following a heart attack and is sometimes used to prevent or delay kidney damage in patients with diabetes. It is also often given with a diuretic to increase its effect on high blood pressure and heart failure. Enalapril works by relaxing the muscles in blood vessel walls, allowing the vessels to dilate (widen), which enables the blood to circulate more easily and helps to lower blood pressure. The drug is long acting and is taken once or twice daily. The first dose may cause a sudden drop in blood pressure, especially in patients taking a diuretic. For this reason, you should lie down for 2–3 hours afterwards.

A variety of minor side effects may occur with enalapril; many people develop a persistent dry cough, while others experience taste disturbance, which a reduction in dose may help to minimize.

INFORMATION FOR USERS

Your drug prescription is tailored for you. Do not alter dosage without checking with your doctor.
How taken Tablets, wafers.
Frequency and timing of doses 1–2 x daily.
Adult dosage range 2.5–5mg daily (starting dose), increased to 10–40mg daily (maintenance dose).
Onset of effect Within 1 hour.
Duration of action 24 hours.
Diet advice None.

Storage Keep in a closed container in a cool, dry place out of reach of children. Protect from light.
Missed dose Take as soon as you remember. If your next dose is due within 8 hours, take a single dose now and skip the next.
Stopping the drug Unless severe adverse effects occur (see below), do not stop taking the drug without consulting your doctor; stopping the drug may lead to worsening of the underlying condition.
Exceeding the dose An occasional unintentional extra dose is unlikely to be a cause for concern. Large overdoses may cause dizziness or fainting. Notify your doctor.

POSSIBLE ADVERSE EFFECTS

Dizziness on standing is likely to occur after the first dose. Nausea and headache are common but are usually mild and transient. A persistent dry cough is the most common adverse effect, but this can be minimized by taking smaller, more frequent, doses; some people may have to stop taking the drug. Rash or itching may occur. If dizziness or fainting, runny nose or sore throat, confusion or mood changes, or chest pain or palpitations occur, consult your doctor. If you develop jaundice, swelling of the face, or breathing difficulties, stop taking the drug and seek urgent medical advice.

INTERACTIONS

Antihypertensive drugs and NSAIDs These drugs are likely to enhance the blood pressure-lowering effect of enalapril.
Lithium Enalapril increases the levels of lithium in the blood, and serious adverse effects from lithium excess may occur.
Ciclosporin Taken with enalapril, this drug may increase blood levels of potassium.
Potassium supplements and potassium-sparing diuretics Enalapril may add to the effect of these drugs, leading to raised levels of potassium in the blood.
NSAIDs Some of these drugs may reduce the effectiveness of enalapril. There is also risk of kidney damage when they are taken with it.

SPECIAL PRECAUTIONS

Be sure to tell your doctor if:
◆ You have suffered from severe allergies.

◆ You have long-term kidney problems.
◆ You have coronary artery disease.
◆ You peripheral vascular disease.
◆ You are on a low sodium diet
◆ You are allergic to other ACE inhibitors.
◆ You are taking other medications.

Pregnancy Not prescribed. May cause defects in the developing baby.

Breast-feeding The drug passes into the breast milk, but at normal doses adverse effects on the baby are unlikely. Discuss with your doctor.

Infants and children Not usually prescribed.

Over 60 Reduced dose may be necessary.

Driving and hazardous work Avoid such activities until you have learned how enalapril affects you because the drug can cause dizziness and fainting.

Alcohol Avoid excessive amounts. Alcohol may increase the blood-pressure lowering and adverse effects of this drug.

Surgery and general anaesthetics Notify your doctor or dentist that you are taking enalapril.

PROLONGED USE
No problems expected.

Ephedrine

Brand name CAM
Used in the following combined preparations
Do-Do, Do-Do Chesteze, Expulin, Franol, Haymine, and others

QUICK REFERENCE
Drug group Bronchodilator (p.23) and decongestant (p.24)
Overdose danger rating Medium
Dependence rating Low
Prescription needed No
Available as generic Yes

GENERAL INFORMATION
In use for more than 50 years, ephedrine promotes the release of norephedrine, a neurotransmitter. It was once widely prescribed as a bronchodilator to relax the muscles surrounding the airways, easing the breathing difficulty caused by asthma, and to help some patients suffering from chronic bronchitis or emphysema. Newer, more effective drugs have largely replaced ephedrine for these purposes. Its main use now is as a decongestant in nasal drops and cough preparations.

Adverse effects are unusual from nasal drops used in moderation, but taken by mouth the drug may stimulate the heart and central nervous system, causing palpitations and anxiety. It is not recommended for the elderly, who are more sensitive to ephedrine's effects on the heart, and the drug may also cause urinary retention in elderly men.

INFORMATION FOR USERS
Follow instructions on the label. Call your doctor if symptoms worsen.
How taken Tablets, syrup, injection, nasal drops.
Frequency and timing of doses By mouth 3 x daily. Nasal drops 3–4 x daily.
Dosage range *Adults* 45–180mg daily (by mouth); 1–2 drops into each nostril per dose (drops). Children Reduced dose according to age and weight.
Onset of effect Within 15–60 minutes.
Duration of action 3–6 hours.
Diet advice None.
Storage Keep in a closed container in a cool, dry place out of reach of children. Protect from light.
Missed dose Do not take the missed dose. Take your next dose as usual.
Stopping the drug Can be safely stopped as soon as you no longer need it.
Exceeding the dose An occasional unintentional extra dose is unlikely to cause problems. Large overdoses may cause shortness of breath, high fever, fits, or loss of consciousness. Notify your doctor immediately.

POSSIBLE ADVERSE EFFECTS
Adverse effects from ephedrine nasal drops are uncommon, although local irritation can occur. When taken by mouth, the drug may have adverse effects on the central nervous system (for example, insomnia and anxiety) and the cardiovascular system (palpitations or chest pain), requiring urgent medical attention. However, taking the last dose before 4 pm may prevent insomnia. Other adverse effects include confusion, tremor, dry mouth, and urinary difficulties.

INTERACTIONS

MAOIs Ephedrine may interact with these drugs to cause a dangerous rise in blood pressure.

Beta blockers Ephedrine may interact with these drugs to cause a dangerous rise in blood pressure.

Antihypertensive drugs Ephedrine may counteract the effects of some of these drugs.

SPECIAL PRECAUTIONS

Be sure to consult your doctor or pharmacist before taking this drug if:
◆ You have a long-term kidney problem.
◆ You have heart disease.
◆ You have high blood pressure.
◆ You have diabetes.
◆ You have an overactive thyroid gland.
◆ You have had glaucoma.
◆ You have urinary difficulties.
◆ You are taking other medications.

Pregnancy Safety in pregnancy not established. Discuss with your doctor.

Breast-feeding The drug passes into the breast milk and may affect the baby. Discuss with your doctor.

Infants and children Reduced dose necessary.

Over 60 Not usually prescribed.

Driving and hazardous work Avoid such activities until you have learned how ephedrine affects you. No special problems with nasal drops.

Alcohol No special problems.

Surgery and general anaesthetics Ephedrine may need to be stopped before you have a general anaesthetic. Discuss this with your doctor or dentist before surgery.

PROLONGED USE

Not recommended except on medical advice. Decongestant effects may lessen with nasal drops, and rebound congestion may occur.

Epinephrine (Adrenaline)

Brand names Ana-Guard, EpiPen, Eppy, Mini-I-Jet Epinephrine, Simplene
Used in the following combined preparations
Brovon, Ganda, several local anaesthetics (e.g., Xylocaine with epinephrine)

QUICK REFERENCE

Drug group Drug for glaucoma (p.110), cardiac resuscitation, and anaphylaxis
Overdose danger rating High
Dependence rating Low
Prescription needed Yes
Available as generic Yes

GENERAL INFORMATION

Epinephrine is a neurotransmitter that is produced in the centre (medulla) of the adrenal glands. Synthetic epinephrine has been made since 1900. The drug is given in an emergency to stimulate heart activity and raise low blood pressure. It also narrows blood vessels in the skin and intestine.

Epinephrine is injected to counteract cardiac arrest, or to relieve severe allergic reactions (anaphylaxis) to drugs, food, or insect stings. For patients at risk of anaphylaxis, it is provided as a pre-filled syringe for immediate self-injection at the start of an attack.

Given as eye drops, the drug lowers the pressure within the eye, making it useful in glaucoma and eye surgery.

Because it constricts blood vessels, epinephrine is used to control bleeding and to slow the dispersal, and thereby prolong the effect, of local anaesthetics.

INFORMATION FOR USERS

Your drug prescription is tailored for you. Do not alter dosage without checking with your doctor.

How taken Injection, eye drops.

Frequency and timing of doses As directed according to method of administration and underlying disorder.

Dosage range As directed according to method of administration and underlying disorder.

Onset of effect Within 5 minutes (injection); within 1 hour (eye drops).

Duration of action Up to 4 hours (injection); up to 24 hours (eye drops).

Diet advice None.

Storage Keep in a closed container in a cool, dry place out of reach of children. Protect from light.

Missed dose Do not take the missed dose. Take the next dose as usual.

Stopping the drug Do not stop using the eye drops without consulting your doctor;

stopping the drug may lead to worsening of the underlying condition.

OVERDOSE ACTION

Seek immediate medical advice in all cases. Take emergency action if palpitations, breathing difficulties, or loss of consciousness occur.

POSSIBLE ADVERSE EFFECTS

The drug's main adverse effects are related to its stimulant action on the heart and central nervous system. These effects include palpitations, nervousness or restlessness, dry mouth, and headache or blurred vision. Eye drops may cause local burning or inflammation.

INTERACTIONS

General note A variety of drugs interact with epinephrine to increase the risk of palpitations and/or high blood pressure. Such drugs include monoamine oxidase inhibitors (MAOIs) and tricyclic antidepressants.

Beta blockers Epinephrine can produce a dangerous rise in blood pressure with certain beta blockers, such as propranolol.

Antidiabetic drugs Epinephrine may reduce the effectiveness of these drugs.

SPECIAL PRECAUTIONS

Be sure to tell your doctor if:
◆ You have a heart problem.
◆ You have diabetes.
◆ You have an overactive thyroid gland.
◆ You have a nervous system problem.
◆ You have high blood pressure.
◆ You are taking other medications.

Pregnancy Not usually prescribed. May cause defects in the fetus and prolong labour. Discuss with your doctor.

Breast-feeding Adverse effects on the baby are unlikely. Discuss with your doctor.

Infants and children Reduced dose necessary.

Over 60 Reduced dose may be necessary. Increased likelihood of adverse effects.

Driving and hazardous work No known problems.

Alcohol No known problems.

Surgery and general anaesthetics
Epinephrine may need to be stopped before you have a general anaesthetic. Discuss this with your doctor or dentist before surgery.

PROLONGED USE

Long-term use of epinephrine eye drops with soft contact lenses is not recommended.

Epoetin (Erythropoietin)

Brand names Eprex, NeoRecormon
Used in the following combined preparations None

QUICK REFERENCE

Drug group Kidney hormone (p.78)
Overdose danger rating Low
Dependence rating Low
Prescription needed Yes
Available as generic No

GENERAL INFORMATION

Epoetin is a form of erythropoietin, a naturally occurring hormone produced by the kidneys. Available in two forms (alpha and beta), epoetin stimulates the body to produce red blood cells. The drug is manufactured by a special technique that uses bacteria to make human erythropoietin.

Epoetin is used to treat anaemia in people suffering from chronic kidney failure, including patients on dialysis. People with kidney failure produce very little erythropoietin themselves, so the number of red blood cells is very low. This was previously only treatable by giving the patients regular blood transfusions. When epoetin is injected regularly, more red blood cells are made by the bone marrow, and this relieves the anaemia, making blood transfusions unnecessary. Since it is a natural hormone, epoetin has few side effects, but treatment must be carefully monitored, otherwise patients may produce too many red blood cells, causing high blood pressure, or the blood may start clotting too easily.

The drug has also been given to patients with cancer and AIDS who have anaemia due to these diseases or their treatment; however, this is a trial use and is not yet widely available. Epoetin has also been tried by athletes who wish to improve their performance; but this is not a recognized use and is regarded as an illegal use of drugs by the sports authorities.

INFORMATION FOR USERS

Your drug prescription is tailored for you. Do not alter dosage without checking with your doctor.

How taken Injection.

Frequency and timing of doses 2–3 x weekly.

Dosage range Calculated on individual basis according to body weight. Dosage also varies depending on the form of epoetin used.

Onset of effect The drug is active inside the body within 4 hours, but effects may not be noted for 2–3 months.

Duration of action Some effects may persist for several days.

Diet advice None, but if you have kidney failure, you may have to follow a special diet.

Storage Store at 2–8°C, out of reach of children. Do not freeze or shake. Protect from light.

Missed dose Do not make up any missed doses.

Stopping the drug Discuss with your doctor.

Exceeding the dose A single excessive dose is unlikely to be a cause for concern. Too high a dose over a long period can increase the likelihood of adverse effects.

POSSIBLE ADVERSE EFFECTS

The most common effects are raised blood pressure and problems at the injection site. Other adverse effects include flu-like symptoms, skin reactions, bone pain, a stabbing headache, and epileptic fits. Any unusual symptoms should be discussed with your doctor immediately.

INTERACTIONS

ACE inhibitors These drugs may increase potassium levels in the blood and epoetin may reduce their blood pressure-lowering effect.

Iron This may increase the effect of epoetin if you have a low level of iron in your blood.

SPECIAL PRECAUTIONS

Be sure to tell your doctor if:
◆ You have high blood pressure.
◆ You have a long-term liver problem.
◆ You have previously suffered allergic reactions to any drugs.
◆ You have peripheral vascular disease.
◆ You have had epileptic fits.
◆ You are taking other medications.

Pregnancy Not usually prescribed. Safety in pregnancy not established. Discuss with your doctor.

Breast-feeding Safety not established. Discuss with your doctor.

Infants and children Reduced dose necessary.

Over 60 No known problems.

Driving and hazardous work Not applicable.

Alcohol Follow your doctor's advice.

PROLONGED USE

Long-term effects are still under investigation; problems are unlikely with careful monitoring.

Monitoring Regular blood tests to monitor blood composition and blood pressure monitoring are required.

Ergotamine

Brand names Lingraine, Medihaler-Ergotamine
Used in the following combined preparations Cafergot, Migril

QUICK REFERENCE

Drug group Drug for migraine (p.20)
Overdose danger rating Medium
Dependence rating Medium
Prescription needed Yes
Available as generic Yes

GENERAL INFORMATION

Ergotamine is used in the treatment of migraine. It constricts blood vessels around the skull and is used only when analgesics such as paracetamol or aspirin do not provide enough relief. It is most effective if taken at the first sign of a migraine (the "aura"); once nausea and headache are established, it is less likely to be effective and may cause stomach upset and increase nausea. Ergotamine is also combined with caffeine as tablets and suppositories. These may be more effective for some patients.

Ergotamine causes temporary narrowing of blood vessels throughout the body and is therefore not prescribed to people with poor circulation. If taken too frequently, the drug can dangerously reduce circulation to the hands and feet; it should never be taken regularly. Frequent migraine attacks may indicate the need for a drug to prevent migraine.

INFORMATION FOR USERS

Your drug prescription is tailored for you. Do not alter dosage without checking with your doctor.

How taken Tablets (held under the tongue or swallowed), suppositories, inhaler.

Frequency and timing of doses Once at the onset (all forms), repeated if needed after 30 minutes (tablets) or 5 minutes (inhaler), up to the maximum dose (see below).

Adult dosage range Varies according to product. Generally 1–2mg per dose. Take no more than 6mg in 24 hours or 10mg in 1 week (by mouth); 6 inhalations in 24 hours or 15 inhalations in 1 week (inhaler); 4mg in 24 hours or 8mg in 1 week (rectally). Treatment should not be repeated within 4 days or more than twice a month.

Onset of effect 15–30 minutes.

Duration of action Up to 24 hours.

Diet advice Changes in diet are unlikely to affect this drug's action, but certain foods may provoke migraine attacks in some people.

Storage Keep in a closed container in a cool, dry place out of reach of children. Protect from light.

Missed dose Regular doses of this drug are not necessary and may be dangerous. Take only when you have symptoms of migraine.

Stopping the drug Can be safely stopped as soon as you no longer need it.

Exceeding the dose An occasional unintentional extra dose is unlikely to cause problems. Large overdoses may cause vomiting, dizziness, fits, or coma. Notify your doctor immediately.

POSSIBLE ADVERSE EFFECTS

Digestive disturbances and nausea (for which an anti-emetic may be given) are common. Diarrhoea, vertigo, and muscle pain and stiffness are also recognized adverse effects. Cold or numb fingers and toes are rare but serious effects that may result from arterial spasm. Seek immediate medical advice if this occurs.

INTERACTIONS

Beta blockers These drugs may increase circulatory problems with ergotamine.

Sumatriptan and related drugs The risk of adverse effects on blood circulation is increased if ergotamine is used with these drugs.

Erythromycin Increased likelihood of adverse effects if this drug is taken with ergotamine.

Oral contraceptives There is an increased risk of blood clotting in women taking these with ergotamine.

SPECIAL PRECAUTIONS

Be sure to tell your doctor if:
◆ You have long-term liver or kidney problems.
◆ You have heart problems.
◆ You have poor circulation.
◆ You have high blood pressure.
◆ You have had a recent stroke.
◆ You have an overactive thyroid gland.
◆ You are taking other medications.

Pregnancy Not usually prescribed. Ergotamine can cause contractions of the uterus.

Breast-feeding Not recommended. The drug passes into breast milk and may have adverse effects on the baby. It may also reduce your milk supply.

Infants and children Not usually prescribed.

Over 60 Use with caution. Hidden heart or circulatory problems may be aggravated.

Driving and hazardous work Avoid such activities until you have learned how ergotamine affects you because the drug can cause vertigo.

Alcohol No special problems, but some spirits may provoke migraine in some people.

Surgery and general anaesthetics Notify your doctor if you have used ergotamine within 48 hours prior to surgery.

PROLONGED USE

Reduced circulation to the hands and feet may result if doses near to the maximum are taken for too long. Do not exceed the recommended dosage and length of treatment; rebound headache may occur.

Erythromycin

Brand names Arpimycin, Erycen, Erymax, Erythrocin, Erythromid, Erythroped, Ilosone, Rommix, Stiemycin
Used in the following combined preparation
Zineryt

QUICK REFERENCE

Drug group Antibiotic (p.60)
Overdose danger rating Low

Dependence rating Low
Prescription needed Yes
Available as generic Yes

GENERAL INFORMATION

One of the safest and most widely used antibiotics, erythromycin is effective against many bacteria. It is used instead of penicillins and tetracyclines for people allergic to these drugs.

Erythromycin is used to treat throat, middle ear, and chest (including some rare types of pneumonia such as Legionnaires' disease). The drug is also used to treat sexually transmitted diseases such as chlamydial infections, and some forms of gastroenteritis.

Erythromycin may also be included as part of the treatment for diphtheria and is sometimes given to treat, and reduce the likelihood of infecting others with, pertussis (whooping cough).

When taken by mouth, erythromycin may sometimes cause nausea and vomiting. Other possible adverse effects include rash as well as a rare risk of liver disorders. Oral administration or local application of the drug is sometimes helpful in treating acne.

INFORMATION FOR USERS

Your drug prescription is tailored for you. Do not alter dosage without consulting your doctor.
How taken Tablets, capsules, liquid, injection, topical solution.
Frequency and timing of doses Every 6–12 hours before or with meals.
Dosage range 1–4g daily.
Onset of effect 1–4 hours.
Duration of action 6–12 hours.
Diet advice None.
Storage Keep in a closed container in a cool, dry place out of reach of children.
Missed dose Take as soon as you remember. If your next dose is due within 2 hours, take a single dose now and skip the next.
Stopping the drug Take the full course. Even if you feel better, the original infection may still be present and symptoms may recur if treatment is stopped too soon.
Exceeding the dose An occasional unintentional extra dose is unlikely to be a cause for concern. But if you notice any unusual symptoms, or if a large overdose has been taken, notify your doctor.

POSSIBLE ADVERSE EFFECTS

Nausea and vomiting are the most common adverse effects and are most likely to occur with large doses taken by mouth. Deafness may occur at high doses in people with poor kidney function. Symptoms such as fever, rash, and jaundice may be a sign of a liver disorder and should always be reported to your doctor.

INTERACTIONS

General note Erythromycin interacts with a number of other drugs, particularly:
Carbamazepine Erythromycin may increase blood levels of this drug.
Digoxin Erythromycin may increase blood levels of this drug.
Warfarin Erythromycin increases the risk of bleeding with warfarin.
Mizolastine Erythromycin increases the risk of adverse effects on the heart with this drug.
Ergotamine Erythromycin increases the risk of side effects with this drug.
Theophylline/aminophylline Erythromycin increases the risk of adverse effects with these drugs.

SPECIAL PRECAUTIONS

Be sure to tell your doctor if:
◆ You have a long-term liver or kidney problem.
◆ You have had a previous allergic reaction to erythromycin.
◆ You have porphyria.
◆ You are taking other medications.
Pregnancy No evidence of risk to the developing fetus.
Breast-feeding The drug passes into the breast milk, but at normal doses adverse effects on the baby are unlikely. Discuss with your doctor.
Infants and children Reduced dose necessary.
Over 60 No special problems.
Driving and hazardous work No known problems.
Alcohol No known problems.

PROLONGED USE

Courses of longer than 14 days may increase the risk of liver damage.

Estradiol

Brand names Climaval, Estraderm, FemSeven, Menorest, Oestrogel, Progynova, Zumenon, and others
Used in the following combined preparations
Climagest, Climesse, Estracombi, Femapak, Trisequens, and others

QUICK REFERENCE

Drug group Female sex hormone (p.86)
Overdose danger rating Low
Dependence rating Low
Prescription needed Yes
Available as generic No

GENERAL INFORMATION

Estradiol is a naturally occurring oestrogen (female sex hormone). It is mainly used as hormone replacement therapy (HRT) for menopausal and post-menopausal symptoms such as hot flushes, night sweats, and vaginal atrophy. Other beneficial effects include prevention of the loss of bone tissue that occurs in osteoporosis and possible reduction of the risk of heart attacks. Estradiol is often given with a progestogen, either as separate drugs or a combined product. In certain cases, treatment is for a specific number of days each month; follow your doctor's instructions carefully.

Estradiol is available in a variety of forms, including implants and skin patches. Implants need to be replaced only after four to eight months. Skin patches may cause a local rash and itching at the site of application.

INFORMATION FOR USERS

Your drug prescription is tailored for you. Do not alter dosage without checking with your doctor.
How taken Tablets, pessaries, vaginal rings, skin gel, patches, implants.
Frequency and timing of doses Once daily (tablets, gel); every 1–7 days (skin patches); every 4–8 months (implants); every 1–7 days (pessaries); every 3 months (vaginal ring).
Adult dosage range 1–4mg daily (tablets); 2–4 measures daily (skin gel); 25–100 micrograms daily (skin patches); 25–100mg per dose (implants); 25 micrograms per dose (pessaries); 7.5 micrograms daily (vaginal ring).
Onset of effect 10–20 days.

Duration of action Up to 24 hours; some effects may be longer lasting.
Diet advice None.
Storage Keep in a closed container in a cool, dry place out of reach of children.
Missed dose Take as soon as you remember. If your next daily treatment is due within 4 hours, take a single dose now and skip the next.
Stopping the drug Do not stop taking the drug without consulting your doctor; symptoms may recur.
Exceeding the dose An occasional unintentional extra dose is unlikely to be a cause for concern. But if you notice any unusual symptoms, or if a large overdose has been taken, notify your doctor.

POSSIBLE ADVERSE EFFECTS

The most common adverse effects with estradiol are similar to symptoms in the early stages of pregnancy and generally diminish with time. These include nausea or vomiting, breast swelling or tenderness, and weight gain. Headache and symptoms of depression may also occur. Swelling or pain in the leg, or a sudden sharp pain in the chest, may indicate an abnormal blood clot that needs attention.

INTERACTIONS

Tobacco smoking This increases the risk of serious adverse effects on the heart and circulation with estradiol.
Rifampicin This drug may reduce the effects of estradiol.
Anticonvulsants The effects of estradiol are reduced by carbamazepine, phenytoin, and phenobarbital.
Anticoagulant drugs The effects of these drugs are reduced by estradiol.

SPECIAL PRECAUTIONS

Be sure to tell your doctor if:
◆ You have a long-term liver problem.
◆ You have heart or circulation problems.
◆ You have porphyria.
◆ You have had blood clots or a stroke.
◆ You have diabetes.
◆ You are a smoker.
◆ You suffer from migraine or epilepsy.
◆ You are taking other medications.
Pregnancy Not prescribed.

Breast-feeding Not prescribed. The drug passes into breast milk and may inhibit its flow. Discuss with your doctor.
Infants and children Not usually prescribed.
Over 60 No special problems.
Driving and hazardous work No problems expected.
Alcohol No known problems.
Surgery and general anaesthetics You may need to stop taking estradiol several weeks before major surgery. Discuss with your doctor.

PROLONGED USE
Use of estradiol for longer than 5 years may slightly increase the risk of cancer of the uterus and breast. The risk of gallstones may also be higher.
Monitoring Blood pressure checks and physical examinations, including regular mammograms, may be performed.

Ethambutol

Brand name Myambutol
Used in the following combined preparations
None

QUICK REFERENCE
Drug group Antituberculous drug (p.65)
Overdose danger rating Medium
Dependence rating Low
Prescription needed Yes
Available as generic Yes

GENERAL INFORMATION
Ethambutol is used in the treatment of tuberculosis. Given in conjunction with other antituberculous drugs, it helps to boost their effects.

If resistance to more commonly used drugs is suspected, ethambutol may be used early in treatment. This may apply if the disease might have been caught by contact with a recent immigrant from Africa or Asia, where resistance to other drugs has been increasing. Resistant organisms are likely to emerge if the full course of treatment is not adhered to. Therefore, it is important to take the full course of treatment.

Although the drug has few common adverse effects, it may occasionally cause optic neuritis, a type of eye damage that leads to blurring and fading of vision. As a result, ethambutol is not usually prescribed for children under six years of age or for other patients who are unable to communicate their symptoms adequately. Patients taking this drug are normally advised to have periodic eye checks.

INFORMATION FOR USERS
Your drug prescription is tailored for you. Do not alter dosage without checking with your doctor.
How taken Tablets.
Frequency and timing of doses Once daily.
Adult dosage range According to body weight.
Onset of effect It may take several days for symptoms to improve.
Duration of action Up to 24 hours.
Diet advice None.
Storage Keep in a closed container in a cool, dry, place out of reach of children.
Missed dose Take as soon as you remember. If your next dose is due within 6 hours, take a single dose now and skip the next.
Stopping the drug Take the full course. Even if you feel better the original infection may still be present and may recur (and be more difficult to treat) if treatment is stopped too soon.
Exceeding the dose An occasional unintentional extra dose is unlikely to cause problems. Large overdoses may cause headache and abdominal pain. Notify your doctor.

POSSIBLE ADVERSE EFFECTS
Side effects are uncommon with this drug but are more likely after prolonged treatment at high doses. These include nausea or vomiting, dizziness, and numbness and tingling of the hands or feet. If you develop a rash or itching, consult your doctor. Blurred vision, loss of colour vision, or eye pain require prompt medical attention.

INTERACTIONS
None.

SPECIAL PRECAUTIONS
Be sure to tell your doctor if:
◆ You have a long-term kidney problem.
◆ You have cataracts or other eye problems.

◆ You have gout.
◆ You have had a previous allergic reaction to this drug.
◆ You are taking other medications.

Pregnancy Safety in pregnancy not established. Discuss with your doctor.

Breast-feeding The drug passes into the breast milk, but at normal doses adverse effects on the baby are unlikely. Discuss with your doctor.

Infants and children Not prescribed under 6 years.

Over 60 Increased likelihood of adverse effects. Reduced dose may therefore be necessary.

Driving and hazardous work Avoid such activities until you have learned how ethambutol affects you because the drug may cause dizziness.

Alcohol No known problems.

PROLONGED USE

Prolonged use of ethambutol may increase the risk of eye damage.

Monitoring Periodic eye tests are usually necessary.

Ethinylestradiol

Used in the following combined preparations
Combined oral contraceptives (e.g., Brevinor, Eugynon 30, Femodene, Loestrin, Microgynon 30, Norimin, Ovran 30, Ovranette, Ovysmen), Dianette, Schering PC4

QUICK REFERENCE

Drug group Female sex hormone (p.86) and oral contraceptive (p.101)
Overdose danger rating Low
Dependence rating Low
Prescription needed Yes
Available as generic Yes

GENERAL INFORMATION

Ethinylestradiol is a synthetic oestrogen similar to estradiol, a natural female sex hormone. It is widely used in oral contraceptives, in combination with a synthetic progestogen. The drug is also very occasionally used (often with a progestogen) to supplement oestrogen during the menopause.

Ethinylestradiol is occasionally given to control abnormally heavy bleeding from the uterus and to treat delayed sexual development (hypogonadism) in females. Certain breast and prostate cancers respond to the drug. High doses are sometimes given for postcoital contraception. It is used in conjunction with cyproterone to treat severe acne in women.

INFORMATION FOR USERS

Your drug prescription is tailored for you. Do not alter dosage without checking with your doctor.

How taken Tablets.

Frequency and timing of doses Once daily. Often at certain times of the menstrual cycle.

Adult dosage range *Menopausal symptoms* 10–20 micrograms daily. *Hormone deficiency* 10–50 micrograms daily. *Combined contraceptive pills* 20–50 micrograms daily, depending on preparation. *Acne* 35 micrograms daily. *Breast and prostate cancer* up to 3mg daily.

Onset of effect 10–20 days. Contraceptive protection is effective after 7 days in most cases.

Duration of action 1–2 days.

Diet advice None.

Storage Keep in a closed container in a cool, dry place out of reach of children.

Missed dose Take as soon as you remember. If your next dose is due within 4 hours, take a single dose now and skip the next. If you are taking the drug for contraceptive purposes, see What to do if you miss a pill (p.104).

Stopping the drug Do not stop taking the drug without consulting your doctor. Contraceptive protection is lost unless an alternative is used.

Exceeding the dose An occasional unintentional extra dose is unlikely to be a cause for concern. But if you notice any unusual symptoms, or if a large overdose has been taken, notify your doctor.

POSSIBLE ADVERSE EFFECTS

The most common adverse effects with ethinylestradiol are similar to symptoms in the early stages of pregnancy and generally diminish with time. These include nausea or vomiting, breast swelling or tenderness, and weight gain. Headache and symptoms of depression may also occur. Swelling or pain in the leg or a sudden sharp pain in the chest may indicate an abnormal blood clot that needs attention.

INTERACTIONS

Tobacco smoking This increases the risk of serious adverse effects on the heart and circulation with ethinylestradiol.

Rifampicin and anticonvulsant drugs These drugs significantly reduce the effectiveness of oral contraceptives containing ethinylestradiol, for which a higher dose will be needed.

Antihypertensive drugs and diuretics Ethinylestradiol may reduce the effectiveness of these drugs.

Other antibiotics These drugs may reduce the effectiveness of oral contraceptives containing ethinylestradiol.

SPECIAL PRECAUTIONS

Be sure to tell your doctor if:
◆ You have heart failure or high blood pressure.
◆ You or a close relative have had blood clots or a stroke.
◆ You have a long-term liver problem.
◆ You are a smoker.
◆ You have diabetes.
◆ You suffer from migraine or epilepsy. You are taking other medications.

Pregnancy Not prescribed. May affect the baby adversely. Discuss with your doctor.

Breast-feeding The drug passes into the breast milk; it may also inhibit milk flow. Discuss with your doctor.

Infants and children Not usually prescribed.

Over 60 No special problems.

Driving and hazardous work No known problems.

Alcohol No known problems.

Surgery and general anaesthetics Ethinylestradiol may need to be stopped several weeks before you have major surgery. Discuss this with your doctor.

PROLONGED USE

Use of ethinylestradiol for longer than 5 years may slightly increase the risk of cancer of the uterus after the menopause when used without a progestogen. There may also be an increased risk of gallstones.

Monitoring Physical examinations and periodic blood pressure checks may be performed.

Ethosuximide

Brand names Emeside, Zarontin
Used in the following combined preparations None

QUICK REFERENCE

Drug group Anticonvulsant (p.16)
Overdose danger rating Medium
Dependence rating Low
Prescription needed Yes
Available as generic No

GENERAL INFORMATION

Ethosuximide, introduced in 1960,belongs to the anticonvulsant group of drugs, which are used in the treatment of epilepsy. It is most commonly prescribed for long-term prevention of absence seizures (daydream-like episodes also known as petit mal). The drug is also used to treat myoclonic seizures. Other types of epilepsy do not respond well to the drug. The major drawback to its use is that it can reduce production of blood cells. Minor adverse effects often occur in the early days of treatment, but these diminish with time.

INFORMATION FOR USERS

Your drug prescription is tailored for you. Do not alter dosage without checking with your doctor.

How taken Capsules, liquid.

Frequency and timing of doses 1–2 x daily.

Dosage range *Adults and children over 6 years* 500mg daily (starting dose), gradually increased up to a maximum of 1.5g daily. *Children up to 6 years* 250mg daily (starting dose) gradually increased up to a maximum of 20mg/kg of body weight daily.

Onset of effect Within 1 hour.

Duration of action Approximately 2 days.

Diet advice None.

Storage Keep in a closed container in a cool, dry place out of reach of children.

Missed dose Take as soon as you remember. If your next dose is due within 6 hours, take a single dose now and skip the next.

Stopping the drug Do not stop taking the drug without consulting your doctor; symptoms may recur.

Exceeding the dose An occasional unintentional extra dose is unlikely to be a cause for concern. Larger overdoses may cause unusual drowsiness. Notify your doctor.

POSSIBLE ADVERSE EFFECTS

Most people experience few adverse effects with this drug, but, when blood levels get too high, effects such as loss of appetite, nausea or vomiting, dizziness, drowsiness, and headache are common and the dosage may need to be reduced. Depression and paranoia may also occur. If you develop a sore throat or mouth ulcers, easy bruising or bleeding, or a rash, consult your doctor urgently.

INTERACTIONS

Sedatives All drugs that have a sedative effect on the central nervous system are likely to increase the sedative properties of ethosuximide. Such drugs include sleeping drugs, antihistamines, opioid analgesics, antipsychotics, and antidepressants.

Carbamazepine This drug may reduce levels of ethosuximide in the blood.

Phenytoin and sodium valproate These drugs may alter blood levels of ethosuximide.

SPECIAL PRECAUTIONS

Be sure to tell your doctor if:
◆ You have long-term liver or kidney problems.
◆ You have porphyria.
◆ You are taking other medications.

Pregnancy Safety in pregnancy not established. Discuss with your doctor.

Breast-feeding The drug passes into breast milk and may have effects on the baby. Poor suckling may occur. Discuss with your doctor.

Infants and children Reduced dose necessary.

Over 60 Not usually prescribed.

Driving and hazardous work Your underlying condition, as well as the sedative effects of ethosuximide, may make such activities inadvisable. Discuss with your doctor.

Alcohol Avoid. Alcohol may increase the sedative effect of this drug.

PROLONGED USE

A slight risk of blood abnormalities exists with prolonged use of ethosuximide.

Monitoring Periodic blood counts, liver function tests, and urine examinations may be carried out.

Etidronate

Brand names Didronel, Didronel PMO
Used in the following combined preparations
None

QUICK REFERENCE

Drug group Drug for bone disorders (p.54)
Overdose danger rating Medium
Dependence rating Low
Prescription needed Yes
Available as generic No

GENERAL INFORMATION

Etidronate is given for the treatment of bone disorders such as Paget's disease. It acts only on bones, reducing the activity of bone cells, which stops the progress of the disease. This action also stops calcium being released from the bones into the bloodstream, reducing the amount of calcium in the blood. The drug is also used with calcium tablets to treat osteoporosis in postmenopausal women and prevent and treat steroid-induced osteoporosis.

Generally, the drug's side effects are mild. The most common, diarrhoea, is more likely to occur with higher doses. If taken at high doses (20mg/kg body weight daily), the drug stops new bone being formed properly, which can lead to bone thinning and fractures. High doses must therefore be carefully monitored and used for as short a time as possible. The effect is reversed on stopping the drug.

INFORMATION FOR USERS

Your drug prescription is tailored for you. Do not alter dosage without checking with your doctor.

How taken Tablets.

Frequency and timing of doses Once daily on an empty stomach, 2 hours before or after food.

Dosage range *Paget's disease* 5–20mg/kg body weight daily for a maximum of 3–6 months. There may be repeated cycles.
Osteoporosis 400mg daily for 2 weeks, repeated every 3 months.

Onset of effect Paget's disease/osteoporosis Beneficial effects may not be felt for several months.

Duration of action Some effects may persist for several weeks or months.

Diet advice Absorption of etidronate is reduced by foods, especially those containing calcium (e.g., dairy products), so the drug should be taken on an empty stomach. The diet must contain adequate calcium and vitamin D; supplements may be given.

Storage Keep in a closed container in a cool, dry place out of reach of children. Protect from light.

Missed dose Take as soon as you remember. If your next dose is due within 6 hours, take a single dose now and skip the next.

Stopping the drug Do not stop taking the drug without consulting your doctor. Stopping the drug may lead to worsening of the underlying condition.

Exceeding the dose An occasional unintentional extra dose is unlikely to cause problems. Large overdoses may cause numbness and muscle spasm. Notify your doctor.

POSSIBLE ADVERSE EFFECTS

The most common side effect is diarrhoea, which is more likely to occur if the dosage is increased above 5mg/kg daily. Other effects include nausea, constipation, abdominal pain, and rash or itching. In some patients with Paget's disease, bone pain may be increased initially but usually disappears with further treatment.

INTERACTIONS

Antacids and iron Antacids or iron should be given at least 2 hours before or after etidronate to minimize effects on absorption.

SPECIAL PRECAUTIONS

Be sure to tell your doctor if:
◆ You have a long-term kidney problem.
◆ You have had a previous allergic reaction to etidronate or other bisphosphonates.
◆ You have colitis.
◆ You are taking other medications.

Pregnancy Safety in pregnancy not established. Discuss with your doctor.

Breast-feeding Safety in breast-feeding not established. Discuss with your doctor.

Infants and children Not recommended.

Over 60 No special problems.

Driving and hazardous work No special problems.

Alcohol No special problems.

PROLONGED USE

Courses of treatment longer than 3 to 6 months are not usually prescribed, but repeat courses are commonly given. Continuous use of etidronate is not recommended because it may lead to an increased risk of bone fractures.

Monitoring Blood and urine tests may be carried out.

Felbinac

Brand name Traxam
Used in the following combined preparations
None

QUICK REFERENCE

Drug group Nonsteroidal anti-inflammatory drug, (p.48)
Overdose danger rating Low
Dependence rating Low
Prescription needed Yes
Available as generic No

GENERAL INFORMATION

Felbinac is a member of the non-steroidal anti-inflammatory (NSAID) group of drugs and works in a similar way to aspirin (as an analgesic as well as reducing inflammation).

Felbinac is prescribed for the relief of pain and inflammation in soft-tissue injuries, such as sprains, strains, and bruising. It is applied topically as gel or aerosol foam and is gently massaged into the affected areas of skin.

It is usually only prescribed in the short-term because the risk of adverse effects is increased with prolonged use. Your doctor will usually review the treatment after two weeks.

Rarely, felbinac may cause indigestion, rash, or breathing difficulties.

INFORMATION FOR USERS

Your drug prescription is tailored for you. Do not alter dosage without checking with your doctor.
How taken Gel, aerosol foam.
Frequency and timing of doses 2–4 times daily.
Adult dosage range 1g per application massaged in. This is 2.5cm (1in) of gel or a 4-cm (1.5-in) ball of foam. Maximum 25 grams daily for all areas being treated.
Onset of effect Pain relief; 30 minutes. Full anti-inflammatory effect; 1–2 days.
Duration of action 4–6 hours.
Diet advice None.
Storage Keep in a cool dry place, out of reach of children. Protect the aerosol canister from sunlight. Do not spray foam near naked flame or while smoking.
Missed dose Use as soon as you remember. If it is almost time for the next application, skip the missed one then resume normal schedule.

Stopping the drug The drug can be safely stopped as soon as it is no longer needed.
Exceeding the dose An occasional unintentional extra application is unlikely to cause problems. But if you notice any unusual symptoms, notify your doctor.

POSSIBLE ADVERSE EFFECTS

Side effects, such as skin irritation or redness and itching or dermatitis, are usually localized to the skin. Systemic effects such as heartburn or indigestion, blotchy skin, swelling of the face, and shortness of breath or wheezing, may sometimes occur, however, because small amounts of the drug are absorbed through the skin. If you experience any systemic effects, seek urgent medical advice.

INTERACTIONS

Interactions with other drugs are unlikely because amounts of felbinac in the blood are usually very low.

SPECIAL PRECAUTIONS

Be sure to tell your doctor if:
◆ You have asthma.
◆ You are allergic to aspirin or NSAIDs.
◆ You are taking other medications.
Pregnancy Not recommended. Discuss with your doctor.
Breast-feeding Safety in breast feeding not established. Discuss with your doctor.
Infants and children Safety not established. Discuss with your doctor.
Over 60 No special problems.
Driving and hazardous work No special problems.
Alcohol No special problems.

PROLONGED USE

There is an increased risk of stomach ulcers or intestinal bleeding with prolonged use.

Filgrastim

Brand name Neupogen
Used in the following combined preparations
None

QUICK REFERENCE

Drug group Blood stimulant

Overdose danger rating Medium
Dependence rating High
Prescription needed Yes
Available as generic No

GENERAL INFORMATION

Filgrastim is a synthetic form of G-CSF (granulocyte-colony stimulating factor), a naturally occurring protein responsible for the manufacture of white blood cells. Deficiency of G-CSF increases the risk of bacterial infection. The drug works by stimulating bone marrow to produce white blood cells, thus reducing the risk of infection. It also causes bone marrow cells to move into the bloodstream, where they can be collected to use in the treatment of bone marrow disease, or to replace bone marrow lost during intensive cancer treatment.

Filgrastim is used to treat patients with congenital neutropenia (deficiency of G-CSF from birth), some AIDS patients, and those people who have recently received high doses of chemo- or radiotherapy during bone-marrow transplantation or cancer treatment. Such patients are prone to frequent and severe infections.

Bone pain is a common adverse effect of filgrastim treatment, but can be controlled using painkillers. There is an increased risk of leukaemia if filgrastim is given to patients with certain rare blood disorders.

INFORMATION FOR USERS

The drug is given only under medical supervision and is not for self-administration.
How taken Injection.
Frequency and timing of doses Once daily.
Adult dosage range 5–12 micrograms/kg body weight, depending upon condition being treated and response.
Onset of effect 24 hours (increase); several weeks (recovery of normal numbers).
Duration of action Approximately 2 days.
Diet advice None.
Storage Not applicable. The drug is not normally kept in the home.
Missed dose Not applicable. The drug is given only in hospital under medical supervision.
Stopping the drug Do not stop the drug without consulting your doctor; stopping may lead to worsening of the underlying condition.

Exceeding the dose Overdose is unlikely since the drug is given only under close supervision and treatment is carefully monitored.

POSSIBLE ADVERSE EFFECTS

Adverse effects are unusual with short courses. Most common is bone pain probably linked to the drug's stimulant effect on bone marrow. Urinary difficulty and rash may also occur.

INTERACTIONS

Cytotoxic chemotherapy or radiotherapy should not be administered within 24 hours of taking filgrastim because of the risk of increasing damage on bone marrow.

SPECIAL PRECAUTIONS

Be sure to tell your doctor if:
◆ You suffer from any blood disorders.
◆ You are taking other medications.
Pregnancy Safety in pregnancy not established. Discuss with your doctor.
Breast-feeding Safety in breast-feeding not established. Discuss with your doctor.
Infants and children No special problems.
Over 60 No special problems.
Driving and hazardous work No known problems.
Alcohol No known problems.

PROLONGED USE

Prolonged use may lead to a slightly increased risk of certain leukaemias. Cutaneous vaculitis (inflammation of blood vessels of the skin), osteoporosis (bone weakening), hair thinning, enlargement of the spleen and liver, and bleeding due to a reduction in platelet numbers may also occur.
Monitoring Blood checks and regular physical examinations are performed. X-rays or bone scans may also be carried out to check for bone thinning.

Finasteride

Brand name Proscar
Used in the following combined preparations
None

QUICK REFERENCE
Drug group Drug used for urinary disorders, p.108

Overdose danger rating Low
Dependence rating Low
Prescription needed Yes
Available as generic No

GENERAL INFORMATION

Finasteride is an an anti-androgen drug (see Male sex hormones, p.85) used to treat benign prostatic hyperplasia (BPH), in which the prostate gland increases in size, making urination difficult. The drug works by gradually shrinking the prostate gland, which improves urine flow and other symptoms such as difficulty in starting urination.

Because the drug is excreted in semen and can feminize a male foetus, you should use a condom if your sexual partner may be, or is likely to become, pregnant. Also, women of childbearing age should not handle broken or crushed tablets because small quantities of the drug are absorbed through the skin.

Low doses are used to reverse male-pattern baldness by preventing the hair follicles from becoming inactive. Noticeable improvements may take about three months but disappear within a year of treatment being stopped.

INFORMATION FOR USERS

Your drug prescription is tailored for you. Do not alter dosage without checking with your doctor.
How taken Tablets.
Frequency and timing of doses Once daily.
Adult dosage range 5mg.
Onset of effect Within 1 hour, but full beneficial effects may take several months.
Duration of action 24 hours.
Diet advice None.
Storage Keep in a closed container, in a cool, dry place out of reach of children. Protect from light.
Missed dose Do not take the missed dose, but take your next scheduled dose as usual.
Stopping the drug Do not stop taking the drug without consulting your doctor; stopping the drug may lead to worsening of the underlying condition.
Exceeding the dose An occasional unintentional extra dose is unlikely to cause problems. But if you notice any unusual symptoms, or if a large overdose has been taken, notify your doctor.

POSSIBLE ADVERSE EFFECTS

Most people experience very few adverse effects with finasteride; decreased libido, impotence, and reduced ejaculate volume are the most common. Breast swelling or tenderness occur more rarely. If you develop a blotchy rash, swelling of the lips, or wheezing, seek urgent medical attention.

INTERACTIONS

None.

SPECIAL PRECAUTIONS

Be sure to tell your doctor if:
◆ You are taking other medications.
Pregnancy Not prescribed.
Breast-feeding Not applicable.
Infants and children Not prescribed.
Over 60 No special problems.
Driving and hazardous work No special problems.
Alcohol No special problems.

PROLONGED USE

Treatment is reviewed after about six months to see if it has been effective.

Fluconazole

Brand name Diflucan
Used in the following combined preparations
None

QUICK REFERENCE

Drug group Antifungal drug (p.74)
Overdose danger rating Medium
Dependence rating Low
Prescription needed Yes (except for vaginal infection preparations)
Available as generic No

GENERAL INFORMATION

Fluconazole is an antifungal drug used to treat systemic candida infections and local candida infections ("thrush") of the vagina, mouth, and skin. It is also used to treat more unusual fungal infections, including cryptococcal meningitis. It may also be used to prevent fungal infections in people with defective immunity. Dosage and length of course will depend on the condition being treated.

The drug is generally well tolerated, but side effects such as nausea and vomiting, diarrhoea, and abdominal discomfort are common.

INFORMATION FOR USERS

Your drug prescription is tailored for you. Do not alter dosage without checking with your doctor.

How taken Capsules, liquid, injection.
Frequency and timing of doses Once daily.
Adult dosage range 50–400mg daily.
Onset of effect Within a few hours, but full beneficial effects may take several days.
Duration of action Up to 24 hours.
Diet advice None.
Storage Keep in a closed container in a cool, dry place out of reach of children. Store liquid in a refrigerator (do not freeze) for no longer than 14 days.
Missed dose Take as soon as you remember. If your next dose is due within 6 hours, take a single dose now and skip the next.
Stopping the drug Take the full course. Even if you feel better, the original infection may still be present and may recur if treatment is stopped too soon.
Exceeding the dose An occasional unintentional extra dose is unlikely to be a cause for concern. But if you notice any unusual symptoms, or if a large overdose has been taken, notify your doctor.

POSSIBLE ADVERSE EFFECTS

Fluconazole is generally well tolerated. Most problems affect the gastrointestinal tract and include flatulence, abdominal discomfort, nausea or vomiting, and diarrhoea. If, rarely, a rash occurs, it should be reported to your doctor without delay.

INTERACTIONS

Anticoagulants Fluconazole may increase the effect of oral anticoagulants such as warfarin.
Oral antidiabetic drugs Fluconazole may increase the risk of hypoglycaemia with oral sulphonylureas such as gliclazide, glibenclamide, chlorpropamide, and tolbutamide.
Phenytoin Fluconazole may increase the blood level of phenytoin.
Theophylline/aminophylline Fluconazole may increase the blood level of this drug.
Ciclosporin Fluconazole may increase the

blood level of ciclosporin.
Rifampicin The effect of fluconazole may be reduced by rifampicin.

SPECIAL PRECAUTIONS

Be sure to tell your doctor if:
◆ You have long-term liver or kidney problems.
◆ You have previously had an allergic reaction to antifungal drugs.
◆ You are taking other medications.
Pregnancy Safety in pregnancy not established. Discuss with your doctor.
Breast-feeding Not recommended. The drug passes into the breast milk. Discuss with your doctor.
Infants and children Reduced dose necessary.
Over 60 Normal dose used as long as kidney function is not impaired.
Driving and hazardous work No known problems.
Alcohol No known problems.

PROLONGED USE

Fluconazole is usually given for short courses of treatment. However, to prevent relapse of cryptococcal meningitis in patients with defective immunity, the drug may be administered indefinitely.

Fluoxetine

Brand name Prozac
Used in the following combined preparations
None

QUICK REFERENCE

Drug group Antidepressant (p.14)
Overdose danger rating Medium
Dependence rating Low
Prescription needed Yes
Available as generic No

GENERAL INFORMATION

Fluoxetine belongs a relatively new group of antidepressants called selective serotonin reuptake inhibitors (SSRIs). These drugs tend to cause less sedation and have different side effects to older antidepressants. Fluoxetine elevates mood, increases physical activity, and restores interest in everyday activities.

Fluoxetine is broken down slowly and remains in the body for several weeks after treatment is stopped. Headache, nausea, restlessness, and insomnia are common side effects. The drug is used to treat depression, to reduce binge eating and purging activity (bulimia nervosa), and to treat obsessive-compulsive disorder.

INFORMATION FOR USERS

Your drug prescription is tailored for you. Do not alter dosage without checking with your doctor.

How taken Capsules, liquid.

Frequency and timing of doses Once daily in the morning.

Adult dosage range 20–60mg daily.

Onset of effect Some benefits may appear within 14 days, but full benefits may not be felt for 4 weeks or more.

Duration of action Beneficial effects may last up to 6 weeks following prolonged treatment. Adverse effects may wear off within a few days.

Diet advice None.

Storage Keep in a closed container in a cool, dry place out of reach of children.

Missed dose Take as soon as you remember. If your next dose is due within 8 hours, take a single dose now and skip the next.

Stopping the drug Unless a rash occurs, do not stop taking the drug without consulting your doctor, who may supervise a gradual reduction in dosage.

Exceeding the dose An occasional unintentional extra dose is unlikely to cause problems. Large overdoses may cause adverse effects. Notify your doctor.

POSSIBLE ADVERSE EFFECTS

The most common adverse effects are restlessness, insomnia, headache, and intestinal irregularities such as nausea and diarrhoea. There are fewer anticholinergic side effects than with tricyclics. Although weight loss is a symptom of depression, fluoxetine can also cause weight loss. Drowsiness and sexual dysfunction may also occur. If you develop a rash, stop taking the drug and seek medical advice.

INTERACTIONS

Sedatives All drugs having a sedative effect may increase the sedative effects of fluoxetine.

MAOIs Fluoxetine treatment should not be started less than 14 days after stopping an MAOI (except moclobemide) because serious adverse effects can occur. An MAOI should not be started less than 5 weeks after stopping fluoxetine.

Lithium Fluoxetine increases blood levels and toxicity of lithium.

Other antidepressants Fluoxetine reduces the breakdown of tricyclics and may result in sedation, dry mouth, and constipation.

Tryptophan Taken together, tryptophan and fluoxetine may produce agitation, restlessness, and gastric distress.

SPECIAL PRECAUTIONS

Be sure to tell your doctor if:
◆ You have long-term liver or kidney problems.
◆ You have heart problems.
◆ You have diabetes.
◆ You have had epileptic fits.
◆ You have previously had an allergic reaction to fluoxetine or other SSRIs.
◆ You are taking other medications.

Pregnancy Safety in pregnancy not established. Discuss with your doctor.

Breast-feeding The drug passes into the breast milk. Discuss with your doctor.

Infants and children Safety and effectiveness not established.

Over 60 No special problems.

Driving and hazardous work Avoid such activities until you have learned how fluoxetine affects you because the drug can cause drowsiness and can affect your judgment and coordination.

Alcohol No special problems.

PROLONGED USE

No problems expected. Side effects tend to decrease with time.

Flupentixol

Brand names Depixol, Fluanxol
Used in the following combined preparations
None

QUICK REFERENCE

Drug group Antipsychotic drug (p.15)

Overdose danger rating Medium
Dependence rating Low
Prescription needed Yes
Available as generic No

GENERAL INFORMATION

Flupentixol is an antipsychotic drug used to treat schizophrenia and similar illnesses. It is also used as an antidepressant for mild to moderate depression. Flupentixol's side effects are similar to those of phenothiazines, but it is less sedating. It is not suitable for patients with mania as it may worsen symptoms.

The drug has fewer anticholinergic effects than the phenothiazines but is more likely to cause side effects such as parkinsonism. Control of severe symptoms may take up to six months, after which a lower maintenance dose is prescribed.

INFORMATION FOR USERS

Your drug prescription is tailored for you. Do not alter dosage without checking with your doctor.
How taken Tablets, injection.
Frequency and timing of doses 1–2 x daily no later than 4 pm (tablets); every 2–4 weeks (injection).
Adult dosage range Psychosis 6–18mg daily (tablets); 50mg every 4 weeks 300–400mg every 2 weeks (injection). Depression 1–3mg daily.
Onset of effect 10 days (side effects may appear much sooner).
Duration of action Up to 12 hours (by mouth); 2–4 weeks (by injection).
Diet advice None.
Storage Store at room temperature out of reach of children. Protect injections from light.
Missed dose Take as soon as you remember. If your next dose is due within 2 hours, do not take the missed dose, but take your next scheduled dose as usual.
Stopping the drug Unless severe adverse effects occur (see below), do not stop taking the drug without consulting your doctor, who will supervise a gradual reduction in dosage. Abrupt cessation of the drug may cause withdrawal symptoms and a recurrence of the original problem.
Exceeding the dose An occasional unintentional extra dose is unlikely to cause problems.

Larger overdoses may cause severe drowsiness, fits, low blood pressure, high or low body temperature, or shock. Notify your doctor.

POSSIBLE ADVERSE EFFECTS

The possible adverse effects of this drug are mainly the result of its anticholinergic action. These include blurred vision, rapid heartbeat, dry mouth, and difficulty in passing urine. Drowsiness, nausea, weight gain, and parkinsonism or tremor may also occur. If dizziness, fainting, confusion, epileptic fits, persistent infection or sore throat, jaundice, or rash occur, stop taking the drug and seek urgent medical attention.

INTERACTIONS

Antiarrhythmics Taken with these drugs, flupentixol may increase the risk of arrhythmias.
Anticholinergic drugs Flupentixol may increase the effects of these drugs.
Anticonvulsant drugs Flupentixol may reduce the effects of these drugs.
Sedatives Flupentixol enhances the effect of all sedative drugs.

SPECIAL PRECAUTIONS

Be sure to tell your doctor if:
◆ You have long-term liver or kidney problems.
◆ You have heart problems.
◆ You have porphyria.
◆ You have had epileptic fits.
◆ You have thyroid disease.
◆ You have Parkinson's disease.
◆ You have glaucoma.
◆ You are taking other medications.
Pregnancy Not usually prescribed. May cause lethargy in the baby during labour. Discuss with your doctor.
Breast-feeding The drug passes into the breast milk and may affect the baby. Discuss with your doctor.
Infants and children Not recommended.
Over 60 Reduced dose necessary. Increased risk of late-appearing movement disorders or confusion.
Driving and hazardous work Avoid such activities until you have learned how flupentixol affects you because the drug can cause drowsiness and slowed reactions.

Alcohol Avoid excessive amounts. Flupentixol enhances the sedative effect of alcohol.
Surgery and general anaesthetics Flupentixol may need to be stopped before any surgery. Discuss this with your doctor or dentist.

PROLONGED USE
The risk of late-appearing movement disorders increases as treatment continues. Blood disorders, as well as jaundice and other liver disorders, are seen occasionally.
Monitoring Blood tests may be performed, particularly if there is persistent infection.

Flutamide

Brand names Chimax, Drogenil
Used in the following combined preparations
None

QUICK REFERENCE
Drug group Anticancer drug (p.94)
Overdose danger rating Medium
Dependence rating Low
Prescription needed Yes
Available as generic Yes

GENERAL INFORMATION
Flutamide is an anti-androgen drug used in the treatment of advanced prostate cancer, often in combination with gonadorelin analogues, such as goserelin, that control production of the male sex hormones (androgens). Both drugs are effective because the cancer is dependent on androgens for its continued development. Flutamide is effective on its own but is also given with gonadorelin analogues to block the release of testosterone that occurs at the start of treatment with these drugs. In the UK, flutamide treatment is begun three days before the gonadorelin analogue.

Flutamide may discolour the urine amber or yellow-green. This is harmless and is not an adverse effect. Notify your doctor immediately, however, if your urine becomes dark coloured since this may indicate liver damage.

INFORMATION FOR USERS
Your drug prescription is tailored for you. Do not alter dosage without checking with your doctor.

How taken Tablets.
Frequency and timing of doses 3 x daily, starting 3 days before the gonadorelin analogue and continuing for 3 weeks.
Adult dosage range 250mg.
Onset of effect 1 hour.
Duration of action 8 hours.
Diet advice None.
Storage Keep in a closed container in a cool, dry place out of reach of children.
Missed dose Take as soon as you remember. If your next dose is due within 2 hours, take a single dose now and skip the next.
Stopping the drug Unless you develop jaundice or pass dark urine, do not stop taking the drug without consulting your doctor because the condition may worsen rapidly.
Exceeding the dose An occasional unintentional extra dose is unlikely to be a cause for concern. But if you notice any unusual symptoms, or if a large overdose has been taken, notify your doctor.

POSSIBLE ADVERSE EFFECTS
Nausea and tiredness are common. Breast swelling also occurs when the drug is given in an effective dose; this is usually reversible when treatment stops or dosage is reduced. Other adverse effects include insomnia, tiredness, headache, dizziness, blurred vision, and skin reactions. If you develop jaundice or start to pass dark urine, stop taking the drug and consult your doctor urgently.

INTERACTIONS
Warfarin Flutamide increases the effect of this drug.

SPECIAL PRECAUTIONS
Be sure to tell your doctor if:
◆ You have heart problems.
◆ You have liver problems.
◆ You are taking other medications.
Pregnancy Not prescribed.
Breast-feeding Not prescribed.
Infants and children Not prescribed.
Over 60 No special problems.
Driving and hazardous work Do not undertake such activities until you have learned how flutamide affects you because the drug can cause blurred vision and dizziness.
Alcohol No special problems.

PROLONGED USE
Prolonged use of flutamide may cause liver damage. Because it is an anti-androgen, the drug also reduces sperm count.
Monitoring Periodic liver-function tests are usually performed.

Fluticasone

Brand names Cutivate, Flixonase, Flixotide
Used in the following combined preparation
Seretide

QUICK REFERENCE
Drug group Corticosteroid (p.78)
Overdose danger rating Low
Dependence rating Low
Prescription needed Yes
Available as generic No

GENERAL INFORMATION
Fluticasone is a corticosteroid drug used to control asthma and relieve the symptoms of allergic rhinitis. The drug acts mainly by reducing inflammation. Fluticasone does not produce relief immediately, so it is important to take the drug regularly. For allergic rhinitis, treatment with the nasal spray needs to begin two to three weeks before the hay fever season commences. People who suffer from asthma should take fluticasone regularly by inhaler in order to prevent attacks. Proper instruction is essential to ensure that the inhaler is used correctly. Fluticasone is also prescribed in the form of an ointment or cream to treat dermatitis and eczema (see Topical corticosteroids, p.116).

There are few serious adverse effects associated with fluticasone because it is administered directly into the lungs (by the inhaler) or nasal mucosa (by the nasal spray). Candida infection ("thrush"), causing irritation of the mouth and throat is a possible side effect of the inhaled form but can be minimized by thoroughly rinsing the mouth and gargling with water after each inhalation.

INFORMATION FOR USERS
Your drug prescription is tailored for you. Do not alter dosage without checking with your doctor.

How taken Ointment, cream, inhaler, nasal spray.
Frequency and timing of doses *Allergic rhinitis* 1–2 x daily; asthma 2 x daily.
Adult dosage range *Allergic rhinitis* 2 sprays into each nostril per dose; asthma 100–1,000 micrograms per dose.
Onset of effect 4–7 days (asthma); 3–4 days (allergic rhinitis).
Duration of action The effects can last for several days after stopping the drug.
Diet advice None.
Storage Keep in a cool, dry place out of reach of children.
Missed dose Take as soon as you remember.
Stopping the drug Do not stop taking the drug without consulting your doctor; symptoms may recur.
Exceeding the dose An occasional unintentional extra dose is unlikely to be a cause for concern. Adverse effects may occur if the recommended dose is regularly exceeded over a prolonged period.

POSSIBLE ADVERSE EFFECTS
Adverse effects are unlikely. The main side effects are irritation of the nasal passages or, rarely, nosebleeds (nasal spray), and sore throat or mouth or hoarseness, which are usually due to candida infection of the throat and mouth (inhaler); this can be minimized by thoroughly rinsing the mouth, brushing the teeth, or gargling with water. Skin changes (ointment/cream) and disturbances in taste or smell may also occur. If you develop a rash or facial swelling, breathing difficulties, or wheezing, consult your doctor urgently.

INTERACTIONS
None.

SPECIAL PRECAUTIONS
Be sure to tell your doctor if:
◆ You have chronic sinusitis.
◆ You have had nasal ulcers or surgery.
◆ You have had tuberculosis or another respiratory infection.
◆ You are taking other medications.
Pregnancy Safety in pregnancy not established. Discuss with your doctor.
Breast-feeding Safety in breast-feeding not established. However, fluticasone is unlikely

to pass into breast milk. Discuss with your doctor.

Infants and children Not recommended under 4 years. Reduced dose necessary in older children. Avoid prolonged use of ointment in children.

Over 60 No known problems.

Driving and hazardous work No known problems.

Alcohol No known problems.

PROLONGED USE

No problems expected when used for asthma or rhinitis. Prolonged use of ointment and cream can lead to adrenal suppression and can cause permanent skin changes, particularly in facial skin, and should be avoided whenever possible.

Monitoring Checks to confirm that the adrenal glands are functioning properly may be required if large doses are being taken.

Fosinopril

Brand name Staril
Used in the following combined preparations
None

QUICK REFERENCE

Drug group Ace inhibitor vasodilator (p.30)
Overdose danger rating Medium
Dependence rating Low
Prescription needed Yes
Available as generic No

GENERAL INFORMATION

Fosinopril belongs to the ACE (angiotensin converting enzyme) inhibitor group of drugs and is used to treat high blood pressure (see Antihypertensive drugs, p.34) and heart failure, in which the heart is unable to deal with its workload. The drug may also be given to patients following a heart attack and is sometimes used to prevent or delay kidney damage in patients with diabetes. It is also often given with a diuretic to increase its effect on high blood pressure and heart failure. Fosinopril works by relaxing the muscles in blood vessel walls, allowing the vessels to dilate (widen), which, in turn, enables the blood to circulate more easily and helps to lower blood pressure. The drug is long acting and may be taken once daily. The first dose may cause a sudden drop in blood pressure, especially in patients taking a diuretic. For this reason, you should lie down for 2–3 hours afterwards.

A variety of minor side effects may occur with fosinopril; many people develop a persistent dry cough, while others experience taste disturbance, which a reduction in dose may help to minimize.

INFORMATION FOR USERS

Your drug prescription is tailored for you. Do not alter dosage without checking with your doctor.

How taken Tablets.
Frequency and timing of doses Once daily.
Adult dosage range 10–40mg.
Onset of effect 1 hour.
Duration of action Up to 24 hours.
Diet advice None.
Storage Keep in a closed container in a cool, dry place out of reach of children.
Missed dose Take as soon as you remember. If your next dose is due within 4 hours, take a single dose now and skip the next.
Stopping the drug Unless severe adverse effects occur (see below), do not stop taking the drug without consulting your doctor; symptoms may recur.
Exceeding the dose An occasional unintentional extra dose is unlikely to cause problems. Large overdoses may cause dizziness, fainting, and a fall in blood pressure. Notify your doctor immediately.

POSSIBLE ADVERSE EFFECTS

Dizziness on standing is likely to occur after the first dose of fosinopril. Nausea and headache are common but are usually mild and transient. A persistent dry cough is the most common adverse effect, but this can be minimized by taking smaller, more frequent, doses; some people may have to stop taking the drug. Rash or itching may occur. If dizziness or fainting, runny nose or sore throat, confusion or mood changes, or chest pain or palpitations occur, consult your doctor. If you develop jaundice, facial swelling, or breathing difficulties, stop taking the drug and seek urgent medical advice.

INTERACTIONS

Antacids These drugs may impair absorption of fosinopril and should be taken at least 2 hours before or after.

NSAIDs Some of these drugs may reduce the effect of fosinopril. Used together, there may be a greater risk of kidney damage.

Lithium Blood levels of lithium may be increased by fosinopril.

Vasodilators, diuretics, and other drugs to lower blood pressure These drugs increase the effect of fosinopril.

Potassium supplements, potassium-sparing diuretics, and ciclosporin When taken with fosinopril, these drugs increase the risk of high blood levels of potassium.

SPECIAL PRECAUTIONS

Be sure to tell your doctor if:
◆ You have suffered from severe allergies.
◆ You have long-term kidney problems.
◆ You have coronary artery disease.
◆ You peripheral vascular disease.
◆ You are on a low sodium diet.
◆ You are allergic to other ACE inhibitors.
◆ You are taking other medications.

Pregnancy Not prescribed. May cause defects in the developing baby.

Breast-feeding The drug passes into the breast milk, but at normal doses adverse effects on the baby are unlikely. Discuss with your doctor.

Infants and children Not usually prescribed.

Over 60 Reduced dose may be necessary.

Driving and hazardous work Avoid such activities until you have learned how fosinopril affects you because the drug can cause dizziness and fainting.

Alcohol Avoid excessive amounts. Alcohol may increase the blood-pressure lowering and adverse effects of this drug.

Surgery and general anaesthetics Notify your doctor or dentist that you are taking fosinopril.

PROLONGED USE

Prolonged use of fosinopril can, in rare cases, lead to changes in blood count or kidney function.

Monitoring Periodic checks on potassium levels, white blood cell counts, and urine are usually performed.

Furosemide (Frusemide)

Brand names Dryptal, Froop, Lasix, Rusyde, Frusol
Used in the following combined preparations Co-Amilofruse, Diumide-K Continus, Fru-Co, Frumil, Lasikal, and others

QUICK REFERENCE

Drug group Loop diuretic (p.30) and antihypertensive drug (p.34)
Overdose danger rating Low
Dependence rating Low
Prescription needed Yes
Available as generic Yes

GENERAL INFORMATION

Furosemide, in use for over 20 years, is a powerful, short-acting loop diuretic. Like other diuretics, it is used to treat oedema (fluid retention) caused by heart failure, and certain lung, liver, and kidney disorders.

Because it is fast acting, furosemide is often used in emergencies to relieve pulmonary oedema (shortness of breath due to fluid accumulation in the lungs). Furosemide is particularly useful for people who have impaired kidney function because they do not respond well to thiazide diuretics (see p.31).

Because furosemide increases potassium loss, potassium supplements or a potassium-sparing diuretic are often given with it.

INFORMATION FOR USERS

Your drug prescription is tailored for you. Do not alter dosage without checking with your doctor.

How taken Tablets, liquid, injection.
Frequency and timing of doses Once daily, usually in the morning; 4–6 x hourly (high dose therapy).
Adult dosage range 20–80mg daily. Dose may be increased to a maximum of 2g daily if kidney function is impaired.
Onset of effect Within 1 hour (by mouth); within 5 minutes (by injection).
Duration of action Up to 6 hours.
Diet advice Use of this drug may reduce potassium in the body. Eat plenty of potassium-rich fresh fruits and vegetables.
Storage Keep in a closed container in a cool, dry place out of reach of children. Protect from light.

Missed dose No cause for concern, but take as soon as you remember. However, if it is late in the day do not take the missed dose, or you may need to get up during the night to pass urine. Take the next scheduled dose as usual.

Stopping the drug Do not stop taking the drug without consulting your doctor; symptoms may recur.

Exceeding the dose An occasional unintentional extra dose is unlikely to be a cause for concern. But if you notice any unusual symptoms, or if a large overdose has been taken, notify your doctor.

POSSIBLE ADVERSE EFFECTS

Adverse effects, which include dizziness, nausea, and lethargy, are caused mainly by the rapid fluid loss produced by furosemide. These tend to diminish as the body adjusts to the drug. The disturbance in body salts and water balance can also result in muscle cramps, headaches, and dizziness. If you develop a rash, which may be more marked in light-exposed areas of skin, consult your doctor urgently. Ringing in the ears may occur with high doses given by injection.

INTERACTIONS

NSAIDs Some of these drugs may reduce the diuretic effect of furosemide.

Lithium Furosemide may increase blood levels of lithium, leading to an increased risk of lithium poisoning.

Digoxin Although this drug is often prescribed with furosemide, loss of potassium may lead to digoxin toxicity when they are taken together.

Aminoglycoside antibiotics The risk of hearing and kidney problems may be increased when these drugs are taken with furosemide.

Angiotensin-converting enzyme inhibitors Low blood pressure may occur when these drugs are taken with furosemide. This interaction is often desired for better control of blood pressure.

SPECIAL PRECAUTIONS

Be sure to tell your doctor if:
◆ You have long-term liver problems.
◆ You have gout.
◆ You have diabetes.

◆ You have previously had an allergic reaction to furosemide or sulphonamides.
◆ You have prostate trouble. If you are taking laxatives.
◆ You are taking other medications.

Pregnancy Safety in pregnancy not established. Discuss with your doctor.

Breast-feeding The drug may reduce milk supply, but the amount of it in the milk is unlikely to affect the baby. Discuss with your doctor.

Infants and children Reduced dose necessary.

Over 60 Reduced dose may be necessary.

Driving and hazardous work No problems expected.

Alcohol Keep consumption low. Furosemide increases the likelihood of dehydration and hangovers after alcohol consumption.

PROLONGED USE

Serious problems are unlikely, but levels of salts such as potassium, sodium, and calcium, may become depleted. Low blood pressure, headaches, difficulty in passing urine, or muscle cramps may develop, particularly in the elderly.

Monitoring Periodic tests may be performed to check on kidney function and levels of body salts.

Gamolenic Acid

Brand names Efamast, Epogam
Used in the following combined preparations
Many preparations containing evening primrose oil, including Efamol and EPOC

QUICK REFERENCE
Overdose danger rating Low
Dependence rating Low
Prescription needed No
Available as generic No

GENERAL INFORMATION

Gamolenic acid is an essential fatty acid found in evening primrose oil and starflower oil (borage oil). Essential fatty acids are found in some foods and are necessary for full health. The beneficial effects of evening primrose oil include improving the hair and skin condition and strengthening the nails. Essential fatty acids have numerous functions and contribute to the manufacture of cells and certain important chemicals such as prostaglandins. Administration of gamolenic acid enhances production of these chemicals in the body.

Gamolenic acid has been investigated for use in a variety of conditions, including premenstrual syndrome. The drug is prescribed for eczema and mastitis (breast pain).

INFORMATION FOR USERS

Follow instructions on the label. Call your doctor if symptoms worsen.
How taken Capsules, liquid.
Frequency and timing of doses 2 x daily, if desired. The capsules may be cut open and the contents swallowed.
Adult dosage range Epogam 8–12 capsules daily (eczema); Efamast 6–8 capsules daily (breast pain). For other brands, follow the instructions on the packet.
Onset of effect Normally 8–12 weeks, but some effects may take longer.
Duration of action 12–24 hours, although the beneficial effects will last longer.
Diet advice None.
Storage Keep in a closed container in a cool, dry, place out of reach of children.
Missed dose Take as soon as you remember.
Stopping the drug Symptoms may eventually recur if the drug is stopped.

Exceeding the dose An occasional unintentional extra dose is unlikely to be a cause for concern. Large overdoses may cause loose faeces and abdominal pain. If you notice any unusual symptoms, or if a large overdose has been taken, notify your doctor.

POSSIBLE ADVERSE EFFECTS

Gamolenic acid does not usually cause adverse effects, but nausea and headache may occur.

INTERACTIONS

Phenothiazine antipsychotic drugs (chlorpromazine and prochlorperazine, for example) There is an increased risk of convulsions in people taking phenothiazines with gamolenic acid.

SPECIAL PRECAUTIONS

Be sure to tell your doctor if:
◆ You have a history of epilepsy.
◆ You have ever had a psychiatric illness.
◆ You are taking other medications.
Pregnancy Safety in pregnancy not established. Discuss with your doctor.
Breast-feeding No known problems.
Infants and children Not recommended under 1 year. Reduced dose necessary in older children.
Over 60 No special problems.
Driving and hazardous work No known problems.
Alcohol No known problems.

PROLONGED USE

No problems expected.

Gentamicin

Brand names Cidomycin, Garamycin, Genticin, Minims gentamicin
Used in the following combined preparations
Gentisone HC

QUICK REFERENCE
Drug group Aminoglycoside antibiotic (p.60)
Overdose danger rating Low
Dependence rating Low
Prescription needed Yes
Available as generic Yes

GENERAL INFORMATION

Gentamicin is one of the aminoglycoside antibiotics. The injectable form is usually reserved for treatment, in hospital, of serious or complicated infections. These include infections of the lungs, urinary tract, bones, and joints, and wound infections, as well as peritonitis, septicaemia, and meningitis. This form is also used together with a penicillin for prevention and treatment of heart valve infections (endocarditis).

Gentamicin is also available as drops and ointment and is commonly used to treat infections of the eye and ear. The ointment may in some cases be prescribed for infected burns or ulcers. Resistance is a common problem following treatment with skin preparations of the drug.

Gentamicin given by injection can have serious adverse effects on the ears, which may lead to damage to the balance mechanism and deafness, and on the kidneys. Courses of treatment are therefore limited to the shortest duration necessary and monitoring of blood levels is usually required. Treatment is monitored with particular care when high doses are needed or when kidney function is poor.

INFORMATION FOR USERS

Your drug prescription is tailored for you. Do not alter dosage without checking with your doctor.

How taken Injection, cream, ointment, eye ointment, eye and ear drops.

Frequency and timing of doses 1–3 x daily (injection); 3–4 x daily or as directed (skin preparations, eye and ear drops, eye ointments).

Adult dosage range According to condition and response (injection); according to your doctor's instructions (eye, ear, and skin preparations).

Onset of effect Within 1–2 hours.

Duration of action 8–12 hours.

Diet advice None.

Storage Keep in closed container in a cool, dry place out of reach of children.

Missed dose Apply skin, eye, and ear preparations as soon as you remember.

Stopping the drug Complete the course. Even if you feel better, the original infection may still be present and may recur if treatment is stopped too soon.

Exceeding the dose Overdose by injection is dangerous but unlikely because treatment is carefully monitored. For other preparations, an occasional unintentional extra dose is unlikely cause concern. But if you notice any unusual symptoms, notify your doctor.

POSSIBLE ADVERSE EFFECTS

Adverse effects are rare but those that occur with the injectable form of gentamicin can be serious. Dizziness, loss of balance (vertigo), ringing in the ears, impaired hearing, and changes in the urine should be reported promptly. Nausea or vomiting may also occur. The drug may be absorbed if the ointment or cream is applied to large areas, and could cause hearing loss. Allergic reactions, including rash and itching, may occur with all preparations that contain gentamicin. Blurred vision or eye irritation may occur with the eye preparations and should be reported to your doctor.

INTERACTIONS

General note A wide range of drugs, including furosemide, vancomycin, and cephalosporins, increase the risk of hearing loss and/or kidney failure with gentamicin.

SPECIAL PRECAUTIONS

Be sure to tell your doctor if:
◆ You have a long-term kidney problem.
◆ You have a hearing disorder.
◆ You have myasthenia gravis.
◆ You have Parkinson's disease.
◆ You have previously had an allergic reaction to aminoglycosides.
◆ You are taking other medications.

Pregnancy No evidence of risk with topical preparations. Injections are not prescribed, because they may cause hearing defects in the baby. Discuss with your doctor.

Breast-feeding No evidence of risk with topical preparations. Given by injection, the drug may pass into the breast milk. Discuss with your doctor.

Infants and children Reduced dose necessary for injections.

Over 60 Reduced dose may be necessary. Increased likelihood of adverse effects.

Driving and hazardous work No known problems from skin, eye, or ear preparations.
Alcohol No known problems.

PROLONGED USE
[We need to say something]
Monitoring Blood levels of the drug are usually checked if it is given by injection. Tests on kidney function are also usually carried out.

Glibenclamide

Brand names Daonil, Euglucon, Semi-Daonil
Used in the following combined preparations
None

QUICK REFERENCE
Drug group Oral antidiabetic drug (p.80)
Overdose danger rating High
Dependence rating Low
Prescription needed Yes
Available as generic Yes

GENERAL INFORMATION
Glibenclamide is an oral antidiabetic drug belonging to the sulphonylurea class. Like other drugs of this type, it stimulates the production and secretion of insulin from the islet cells in the pancreas and promotes the uptake of sugar into body cells, thereby lowering the level of sugar in the blood.

This drug is used in the treatment of adult (maturity-onset) diabetes mellitus, in conjunction with a diabetic diet that is low in fat and refined carbohydrate.

In conditions of severe illness, injury, or stress, glibenclamide may lose its effectiveness, which makes insulin injections necessary. Adverse effects are generally mild. However, symptoms of poor diabetic control will occur if the dosage of glibenclamide is not appropriate.

INFORMATION FOR USERS
Your drug prescription is tailored for you. Do not alter dosage without checking with your doctor.
How taken Tablets.
Frequency and timing of doses Once daily in the morning with breakfast.
Adult dosage range 5–15mg daily.

Onset of effect Within 3 hours.
Duration of action 10–15 hours.
Diet advice A low-carbohydrate, low-fat diet must be maintained in order for the drug to be fully effective. Follow the advice of your doctor.
Storage Keep in a closed container in a cool, dry place out of reach of children. Protect from light.
Missed dose Take before your next meal.
Stopping the drug Do not stop taking the drug without consulting your doctor; stopping the drug may lead to worsening of your diabetes.

OVERDOSE ACTION
Seek immediate medical advice in all cases. If any early warning symptoms of excessively low blood sugar (such as fainting, sweating, trembling, confusion, or headache) occur, eat or drink something sugary. Take emergency action if fits or loss of consciousness occur.

POSSIBLE ADVERSE EFFECTS
Serious adverse effects with glibenclamide are rare. Symptoms such as fainting or confusion, weakness or tremor, and sweating may be signs of low blood sugar due to lack of food or too high a dose of the drug; eat or drink something sugary immediately and seek urgent medical assistance. Other adverse effects include nausea or vomiting and weight changes. If you develop a rash or itching or jaundice, consult your doctor.

INTERACTIONS
General note A variety of drugs may reduce the effect of glibenclamide and so may raise blood sugar levels. These include corticosteroids, oestrogens, diuretics, and rifampicin. Other drugs increase the risk of low blood sugar. These include warfarin, sulphonamides and other antibacterials, aspirin, beta blockers, and ACE inhibitors.

SPECIAL PRECAUTIONS
Be sure to tell your doctor if:
◆ You have long-term liver or kidney problems.
◆ You are allergic to sulphonamide drugs. You have thyroid problems.

◆ You have ever had problems with your adrenal glands.
◆ You are taking other medications.
Pregnancy Not usually prescribed. Insulin is generally substituted in pregnancy because it gives better diabetic control.
Breast-feeding The drug passes into the breast milk, but at normal doses adverse effects on the baby are unlikely. Discuss with your doctor.
Infants and children Not prescribed.
Over 60 Reduced dose may be necessary. Greater likelihood of low blood sugar exists when glibenclamide is used.
Driving and hazardous work Usually no problems. Avoid these activities if you have warning signs of low blood sugar.
Alcohol Avoid. Alcoholic drinks may upset diabetic control.
Surgery and general anaesthetics Surgery may alter the effect of this drug on diabetes; insulin treatment may need to be substituted.

PROLONGED USE
No problems expected.
Monitoring Regular monitoring of levels of sugar in the urine or blood is required. Periodic assessment of the eyes, heart, and kidneys may also be advised.

Gliclazide

Brand name Diamicron
Used in the following combined preparations
None

QUICK REFERENCE
Drug group Oral antidiabetic drug (p.80)
Overdose danger rating High
Dependence rating Low
Prescription needed Yes
Available as generic No

GENERAL INFORMATION
Gliclazide is an antidiabetic drug that lowers blood sugar by stimulating insulin secretion from the pancreas. It is used to treat adult (maturity-onset) diabetes mellitus in conjunction with a diabetic diet low in fat and refined carbohydrate. Regular exercise is an important part of the treatment of diabetes.

In conditions of severe illness, injury, stress, or surgery, gliclazide may lose its effectiveness, causing loss of diabetic control and necessitating the use of insulin injections. Adverse effects of gliclazide are generally mild. However, symptoms of poor diabetic control will occur if the dosage is not appropriate.

INFORMATION FOR USERS
Your drug prescription is tailored for you. Do not alter dosage without checking with your doctor.
How taken Tablets.
Frequency and timing of doses 1–2 x daily (in the morning and evening with a meal).
Dosage range 80–320mg daily.
Onset of effect Within 1 hour.
Duration of action 12–24 hours.
Diet advice An individualized, low-fat, low-carbohydrate diet must be maintained for the drug to be fully effective. Follow the advice of your doctor.
Storage Keep in a closed container in a cool, dry place out of reach of children.
Missed dose Take as soon as you remember with the next meal.
Stopping the drug Do not stop taking the drug without consulting your doctor; stopping the drug may lead to worsening of the underlying condition.

OVERDOSE ACTION
Seek immediate medical advice in all cases. If early warning symptoms of excessively low blood sugar such as fainting, sweating, trembling, confusion, or headache occur, eat or drink something sugary at once. Take emergency action if fits or loss of consciousness occur.

POSSIBLE ADVERSE EFFECTS
Serious adverse effects with gliclazide are rare. Symptoms such as fainting or confusion, weakness or tremor, and sweating may be signs of low blood sugar due to lack of food or too high a dose of the drug. You should eat or drink something sugary immediately and seek urgent medical assistance. Other adverse effects include nausea or vomiting and weight changes. If you experience prolonged bleeding or bruising, or if you

develop a rash or itching, jaundice, or a sore throat or fever, consult your doctor urgently.

INTERACTIONS

General note Many drugs (such as cortico-steroids and barbiturates) may oppose the effects of gliclazide, thereby raising blood sugar levels. Other drugs (such as warfarin and aspirin) increase the risk of low blood sugar.

SPECIAL PRECAUTIONS

Be sure to tell your doctor if:
◆ You have or have recently had a serious trauma or infection.
◆ You have long-term liver or kidney problems.
◆ You have thyroid problems.
◆ You do not eat properly.
◆ You are planning a pregnancy.
◆ You have Addison's disease.
◆ You have an allergy to sulphonylureas.
◆ You are taking other medications.

Pregnancy Not recommended. May cause abnormally low blood sugar in the newborn baby. Insulin is generally substituted in pregnancy because it gives better diabetic control.

Breast-feeding The drug passes into the breast milk and may cause low blood sugar in the baby. Discuss with your doctor.

Infants and children Not prescribed.

Over 60 Signs of low blood sugar may be more difficult to recognize. Reduced dose may be necessary.

Driving and hazardous work Avoid such activities until you have learned how gliclazide affects you because it can cause dizziness, drowsiness, and confusion.

Alcohol Avoid. Alcoholic drinks upset diabetic control, and gliclazide may cause intolerance to alcohol.

Surgery and general anaesthetics Notify your doctor or dentist that you are diabetic before undergoing any type of surgery.

PROLONGED USE

No problems expected.

Monitoring Regular testing of sugar levels in the blood and/or urine is required. Periodic assessment of the eyes, heart, and kidneys may also be advised.

Glyceryl Trinitrate

Brand names Coro-Nitro, Deponit, Minitran, Nitro-Dur, Nitrolingual, Suscard, Sustac, Transiderm-Nitro, and others
Used in the following combined preparations
None

QUICK REFERENCE

Drug group Anti-angina drug (p.33)
Overdose danger rating Medium
Dependence rating Low
Prescription needed Yes
Available as generic Yes

GENERAL INFORMATION

Introduced in the late 1800s, glyceryl tri-nitrate is one of the oldest drugs in continual use. It belongs to the group of vasodilator drugs called nitrates that are used to relieve the pain of angina attacks. It is available in short-acting forms (sublingual or buccal tablets and spray), which act very quickly to relieve angina, and in long-acting forms (slow-release tablets and skin patches). It is also given by injection in hospital for severe angina and for controlling blood pressure.

The drug may cause a variety of minor symptoms, such as flushing and headache, most of which can be controlled by adjusting the dosage. It is best taken for the first time while you are sitting, as fainting may follow the drop in blood pressure caused by this medication. If the drug fails to relieve angina, and the attack lasts for more than 20 minutes, this may be a sign of a heart attack and requires urgent medical assistance.

INFORMATION FOR USERS

Your drug prescription is tailored for you. Do not alter dosage without checking with your doctor.

How taken SR-tablets, buccal tablets, sublingual tablets, injection, ointment, skin patches, spray.

Frequency and timing of doses *Prevention* 3 x daily (buccal and SR-tablets); once daily (patches); every 3–4 hours (ointment). *Relief* Use buccal or sublingual tablets or spray at the onset of an attack or immediately prior to exercise. Dose may be repeated within 5 minutes if further relief is required.

Adult dosage range *Prevention* 5.2–30mg daily (SR-tablets); 3–15mg daily (buccal tablets); 2.5–15mg daily (patches); as directed (ointment). *Relief* 0.3–1mg per dose (sublingual tablets); 1–3mg per dose (buccal tablets); 1–2 sprays per dose (spray).

Onset of effect Within minutes (buccal and sublingual tablets and spray); 1–3 hours (SR-tablets, patches, and ointment).

Duration of action 20–30 minutes (sublingual tablets and spray); 3–5 hours (buccal tablets and ointment); 8–12 hours (SR-tablets); up to 24 hours (patches).

Diet advice None.

Storage Keep buccal and sublingual tablets in a tightly closed glass container fitted with a foil-lined, screw-on cap in a cool, dry place out of reach of children. Protect from light. Do not expose to heat. Discard tablets within 8 weeks of opening. Check label of other preparations for storage conditions.

Missed dose Take as soon as you remember, or when needed. If your next dose is due within 2 hours, take a single dose now and skip the next.

Stopping the drug Do not stop taking the drug without consulting your doctor.

Exceeding the dose An occasional unintentional extra dose is unlikely to cause problems. Large overdoses may cause dizziness, vomiting, severe headache, fits, or loss of consciousness. Notify your doctor.

POSSIBLE ADVERSE EFFECTS
The most serious adverse effect is lowered blood pressure, which may cause dizziness. Other adverse effects, such as headache and flushing, usually decrease in severity after regular use but can also be controlled by adjustment in dosage.

INTERACTIONS
Antihypertensive drugs These drugs, which are often used by patients who also need to take glyceryl trintrate, increase the possibility of lowered blood pressure or fainting when the two drugs are taken together.

SPECIAL PRECAUTIONS
Be sure to tell your doctor if:
◆ You have any other heart condition.
◆ You have a lung condition.
◆ You have long-term liver or kidney problems.
◆ You have any blood disorders.
◆ You have glaucoma.
◆ You have thyroid disease.
◆ You are taking other medications.

Pregnancy Safety in pregnancy not established. Discuss with your doctor.

Breast-feeding It is not known whether the drug passes into the breast milk. Discuss with your doctor.

Infants and children Not usually prescribed.

Over 60 No special problems.

Driving and hazardous work Avoid such activities until you have learned how glyceryl trinitrate affects you because the drug can cause dizziness.

Alcohol Avoid excessive intake. Alcohol may increase dizziness due to lowered blood pressure.

PROLONGED USE
The effects of the drug usually become slightly weaker during prolonged use as the body adapts.

Monitoring Periodic checks on blood pressure are usually required.

Goserelin

Brand name Zoladex
Used in the following combined preparations
None

QUICK REFERENCE
Drug group Anticancer drug (p.94)
Overdose danger rating Low
Dependence rating Low
Prescription needed Yes
Available as generic No

GENERAL INFORMATION
Goserelin is a synthetic drug chemically related to the hormone gonadorelin. Like gonadorelin, it stimulates the release of hormones from the pituitary gland, which in turn control production of the sex hormones.

Goserelin is used to suppress the production of sex hormones in cancers of the breast and prostate. It is usually given with an anti-androgen drug such as flutamide (see p.236) at the start of treatment for cancer of the prostate to prevent testosterone release from causing an initial growth spurt of the tumour.

The drug is also used in the management of fibroids, infertility, and endometriosis. The first dose is normally given during menstruation to avoid the possibility that the patient may be pregnant. It is advisable for women of childbearing age to use barrier methods of contraception during treatment.

The injections are usually given by a general practitioner or district nurse.

Loss of bone density is an important side effect in women, so repeat courses of the drug are given only for cancerous conditions.

INFORMATION FOR USERS

Your drug prescription is tailored for you. Do not alter dosage without checking with your doctor

How taken Implant injection, long-acting (LA) implant injection.

Frequency and timing of doses *Endometriosis* Every 28 days, maximum of a single 6-month treatment only (implant). *Fibroids* Implant every 28 days, maximum 3 months' treatment. *Prostate cancer* Every 12 weeks (LA implant).

Adult dosage range 3.6mg every 28 days (endometriosis/fibroids); 10.8mg every 3 months (prostate).

Onset of effect Within 24 hours (endometriosis/fibroids); 1–2 weeks after tumour flare (prostate).

Duration of action 28 days (implant); 12 weeks (long-acting implant).

Diet advice None.

Storage Not applicable. The drug is not kept in the home.

Missed dose No cause for concern. Treatment can be resumed when possible.

Stopping the drug Do not stop treatment without consulting your doctor.

Exceeding the dose Overdosage is unlikely since treatment is not self-administered.

POSSIBLE ADVERSE EFFECTS

Symptoms similar to those of the menopause, such as hot flushes, headache, changes in breast size, and bleeding on stopping goserelin, are common. Rare adverse effects, such as dizziness or fainting, ovarian cysts, rash or wheezing, and reaction at the injection site, should be reported to your doctor straight away.

INTERACTIONS

None.

SPECIAL PRECAUTIONS

Be sure to tell your doctor if:

◆ You have osteoporosis.

◆ You have previously been treated with goserelin (or another gonadorelin analogue) for endometriosis or fibroids.

◆ You have polycystic ovarian disease.

◆ You are allergic to gonadorelin analogues.

◆ You are taking other medications.

Pregnancy Not prescribed.

Breast-feeding Not recommended. Discuss with your doctor.

Infants and children Not recommended.

Over 60 No special problems.

Driving and hazardous work No special problems.

Alcohol No special problems.

PROLONGED USE

Goserelin is only used in the long term for treatment of prostate or breast cancer. Bone density is lost over time in women taking the drug, but this may be partly recoverable once treatment stops.

Monitoring Women may be monitored for changes in bone density.

Haloperidol

Brand names Dozic, Haldol, Serenace
Used in the following combined preparations
None

QUICK REFERENCE

Drug group Butyrophenone antipsychotic drug (p.15)
Overdose danger rating Medium
Dependence rating Low
Prescription needed Yes
Available as generic Yes

GENERAL INFORMATION

Introduced in the 1960s, haloperidol is used to reduce the violent, aggressive manifestations of mental illnesses such as schizophrenia, mania, dementia, and other disorders in which hallucinations are experienced. The drug is also used in the short term for severe anxiety. It does not cure the underlying disorder but relieves the distressing symptoms.

Haloperidol is also used in the control of Tourette's syndrome and may be of benefit in children who have severe behavioural problems for which other drugs are ineffective.

The main drawback of the drug is that it may produce abnormal, involuntary movements and stiffness of the face and limbs.

INFORMATION FOR USERS

Your drug prescription is tailored for you. Do not alter dosage without checking with your doctor.

How taken Tablets, capsules, liquid, injection, depot injection.
Frequency and timing of doses 2–4 x daily.
Adult dosage range *Mental illness* 1.5–20mg daily initially, increased gradually, if necessary, up to a maximum of 100mg daily (or rarely up to 120mg daily). *Severe anxiety* 1mg daily.
Onset of effect 2–3 hours (by mouth); 20–30 minutes (by injection).
Duration of action 6–24 hours (by mouth); 2–4 hours (injection); up to 4 weeks (depot injection).
Diet advice None.
Storage Keep in a closed container in a cool, dry place out of reach of children.
Missed dose Take as soon as you remember. If your next dose is due within 3 hours, take a single dose now and skip the next.

Stopping the drug Unless severe adverse effects occur (see below), do not stop taking the drug without consulting your doctor; symptoms may recur.
Exceeding the dose An occasional unintentional extra dose is unlikely to cause problems. Larger overdoses may cause unusual drowsiness, muscle weakness or rigidity, and/or faintness. Notify your doctor.

POSSIBLE ADVERSE EFFECTS

Haloperidol can cause a variety of minor anticholinergic symptoms, such as dry mouth, blurred vision, and difficulty in passing urine, which often become less marked with time. Loss of appetite, drowsiness or lethargy, and dizziness or fainting may also occur. If you experience stiffness of the tongue, neck, or limbs after the first dose or develop a rash, seek medical advice. If you develop a high fever or confusion, or muscle stiffness, stop taking the drug and consult your doctor urgently. The most significant adverse effect, parkinsonism (abnormal face and limb movements), can be controlled by dosage adjustment .

INTERACTIONS

Sedatives Sedatives are likely to increase the sedative properties of haloperidol.
Rifampicin and anticonvulsants These drugs may reduce the effects of haloperidol, the dosage of which may need to be increased.
Lithium This drug may increase the risk of parkinsonism and effects on the nerves.
Methyldopa This drug may increase the risk of parkinsonism and low blood pressure.
Anticholinergic drugs Haloperidol may increase the side effects of these drugs.

SPECIAL PRECAUTIONS

Be sure to tell your doctor if:
◆ You have long-term liver or kidney problems.
◆ You have heart or circulation problems.
◆ You have had epileptic fits.
◆ You have an overactive thyroid gland.
◆ You have Parkinson's disease.
◆ You have had glaucoma.
◆ You have asthma, bronchitis, or another lung disorder.
◆ You have ever had phaeochromocytoma.
◆ You are taking other medications.

Pregnancy Safety in pregnancy not established. Discuss with your doctor.

Breast-feeding The drug passes into the breast milk and may affect the baby. Discuss with your doctor.

Infants and children Rarely required. Reduced dose necessary.

Over 60 Reduced dose may be necessary.

Driving and hazardous work Avoid such activities until you have learned how haloperidol affects you because the drug may cause drowsiness and slowed reactions.

Alcohol Avoid. Alcohol may increase the sedative effect of this drug.

PROLONGED USE

Use of this drug for more than a few months may lead to tardive dyskinesia (abnormal, involuntary movements of the eyes, face, and tongue). Occasionally, jaundice may occur.

Heparin/Low molecular weight heparins

Brand names Calciparine, Minihep, Monoparin, Multiparin, Uniparin; [LMWH] Alphaparin, Clexane, Fragmin, Innohep

Used in the following combined preparations
None

QUICK REFERENCE

Drug group Anticoagulant (p.36)
Overdose danger rating High
Dependence rating Low
Prescription needed Yes
Available as generic Yes (heparin); no (LMWH)

GENERAL INFORMATION

Heparin is an anticoagulant drug used to prevent formation of, and aid in dispersion of, blood clots. Because it acts quickly, it is particularly useful in emergencies (e.g., to prevent further clotting when a clot has already reached the lungs or brain. People undergoing open heart surgery or kidney dialysis are also given heparin to prevent clotting. Certoparin, dalteparin, enoxaparin, and tinzaparin are new forms of heparin called "low molecular weight heparins" (LMWH). They are now widely used and do not have to be given in hospital. A low dose of a heparin is sometimes given following surgery to prevent deep vein thrombosis (clots forming in the leg veins). Heparins are often given in conjunction with other slower-acting anticoagulants such as warfarin. It is also used to treat unstable angina.

The most serious adverse effect of heparin as with all anticoagulants, is the risk of excessive bleeding, so the ability of the blood to clot is watched very carefully. Bruising may occur around the site of the injection.

INFORMATION FOR USERS

This drug is given only under medical supervision and is not for self-administration.

How taken Injection.

Frequency and timing of doses Every 8–12 hours (continuous intravenous infusion); once daily (LMWH).

Dosage range *Treatment* 5,000 units initially, followed by 40,000 units over 24 hours (heparin); treatment depends on bodyweight (LMWH). *Prevention* 5,000 units.

Onset of effect Within 15 minutes.

Duration of action 4–12 hours after treatment is stopped.

Diet advice None.

Storage Keep in a cool, dry place out of reach of children.

Missed dose Notify your doctor.

Stopping the drug Do not stop taking the drug without consulting your doctor; Stopping may lead to clotting of the blood.

OVERDOSE ACTION

Seek immediate medical advice in all cases. Take emergency action if bleeding, severe headache, or loss of consciousness occur. Overdose can be reversed under medical supervision by a drug called protamine.

POSSIBLE ADVERSE EFFECTS

As with all anticoagulants, bleeding is the most common adverse effect. The less common effects may occur with long-**term** treatment.

INTERACTIONS

Aspirin The anticoagulant effect of heparin may be increased by aspirin, and the drugs may be given together for this reason.

Dipyridamole Heparin's anticoagulant effect may be increased with this drug. The heparin dosage may need to be adjusted accordingly.

SPECIAL PRECAUTIONS

Be sure to tell your doctor if:

◆ You have long-term liver or kidney problems.

◆ You have high blood pressure.

◆ You bleed easily.

◆ You have any allergies.

◆ You have stomach ulcers.

◆ You are taking other medications.

Pregnancy The drug needs careful monitoring; taken near delivery, it may cause the mother to bleed excessively. Discuss with your doctor.

Breast-feeding No evidence of risk.

Infants and children Reduced dose necessary according to age and weight.

Over 60 No special problems.

Driving and hazardous work Avoid risk of injury; excessive bruising and bleeding may occur.

Alcohol No special problems.

Surgery and general anaesthetics Heparin treatment may need to be stopped. Discuss this with your doctor or dentist before having any surgery.

PROLONGED USE

Osteoporosis and hair loss may occur; tolerance to heparin may develop.

Monitoring Periodic blood and liver function tests will be required.

Hydrochlorothiazide

Brand name HydroSaluric
Used in the following combined preparations
Acezide, Capozide, Co-Betaloc, Dyazide, Moducren, Moduretic, and others

QUICK REFERENCE

Drug group Thiazide diuretic (p.30)
Overdose danger rating Low
Dependence rating Low
Prescription needed Yes
Available as generic No

GENERAL INFORMATION

Hydrochlorothiazide belongs to the thiazide group of diuretic drugs, which remove excess water from the body and reduce oedema (fluid retention) in people with congestive heart failure, kidney disorders, cirrhosis of the liver, and premenstrual syndrome. This drug is used to treat high blood pressure (see Antihypertensive drugs, p.34).

Hydrochlorothiazide increases potassium loss in the urine, which can cause a variety of symptoms (see p.30), and increases the likelihood of irregular heart rhythms, particularly in patients taking drugs such as digoxin. For this reason, potassium supplements are often given with hydrochlorothiazide.

INFORMATION FOR USERS

Your drug prescription is tailored for you. Do not alter dosage without checking with your doctor.

How taken Tablets.

Frequency and timing of doses
Once daily, or every 2 days, early in the day.

Adult dosage range 25–50mg daily.

Onset of effect Within 2 hours.

Duration of action 6–12 hours.

Diet advice Use of hydrochlorothiazide may reduce potassium in the body. Eat plenty of fresh fruit and vegetables, and discuss with your doctor the advisability of reducing your salt intake.

Storage Keep in a closed container in a cool, dry place out of reach of children. Protect from light.

Missed dose No cause for concern, but take as soon as you remember. If it is late in the day, however, do not take the missed dose, or you may have to get up during the night to pass urine. Take the next scheduled dose as usual.

Stopping the drug Unless a rash occurs, do not stop taking the drug without consulting your doctor; symptoms may recur.

Exceeding the dose An occasional unintentional extra dose is unlikely to be a cause for concern. But if you notice any unusual symptoms, or if a large overdose has been taken, notify your doctor.

POSSIBLE ADVERSE EFFECTS

The most common problem with hydrochlorothiazide is muscle cramps, which often occur at night. Lethargy, dizziness, digestive disturbances, and impotence may also occur. Some effects are due to excessive loss of potassium. This can sometimes be put right by taking a potassium supplement. Rarely, gout may occur in susceptible people, and certain forms of diabetes may become more difficult to control. If you develop a rash, stop taking the drug and consult your doctor.

INTERACTIONS

NSAIDs Some NSAIDs may reduce the diuretic effect of hydrochlorothiazide, the dosage of which may need to be adjusted.

Digoxin Adverse effects may be increased if excessive potassium is lost.

Corticosteroids These drugs further increase loss of potassium from the body when taken with hydrochlorothiazide.

Lithium Hydrochlorothiazide may increase lithium levels in the blood, leading to a risk of serious adverse effects.

SPECIAL PRECAUTIONS

Be sure to tell your doctor if:
◆ You have long-term liver or kidney problems.
◆ You have had gout.
◆ You have diabetes.
◆ You have Addison's disease or systemic lupus erythematosus.
◆ You are taking other medications.

Pregnancy Not usually prescribed. May cause jaundice in the newborn baby. Discuss with your doctor.

Breast-feeding The drug passes into the breast milk, but at normal doses adverse effects on the baby are unlikely. Discuss with your doctor.

Infants and children Not usually prescribed. Reduced dose necessary.

Over 60 Increased likelihood of adverse effects.

Driving and hazardous work Avoid such activities until you have learned how hydrochlorothiazide affects you because the drug may reduce mental alertness and cause dizziness.

Alcohol Keep consumption low. Hydrochlorothiazide increases the likelihood of dehydration and hangovers after consumption of alcohol.

PROLONGED USE

Excessive loss of potassium and imbalances of other salts may result.

Monitoring Blood tests may be performed periodically to check kidney function and levels of potassium and other salts.

Hydrocortisone

Brand names Colifoam, Corlan, Dioderm, Efcortelan, Efcortesol, Hydrocortistab, Hydrocortisyl, Hydrocortone, Solu-Cortef

Used in the following combined preparations
Alphaderm, Tarcortin, Xyloproct, and many others

QUICK REFERENCE

Drug group Corticosteroid (p.78)
Overdose danger rating Low
Dependence rating Low
Prescription needed Yes (except for some topical preparations)
Available as generic Yes

GENERAL INFORMATION

Hydrocortisone is chemically identical to the hormone cortisol, produced by the adrenal glands. For this reason, the drug is prescribed to replace natural hormones in adrenal insufficiency (Addison's disease). The dose given replaces the body's production of hormone, and side effects should be minimal.

Hydrocortisone's main use is in the treatment of a variety of allergic and inflammatory conditions. Used topically, it provides prompt relief from inflammation of the skin, eye, and outer ear. In oral form it relieves asthma, inflammatory bowel disease, and many rheumatic and allergic disorders. Injected directly into the joints, the drug relieves pain and stiffness (see p.51). Injections may also be given to relieve severe attacks of asthma.

Overuse of skin preparations can lead to permanent thinning of the skin. Taken by mouth, long-term treatment with high doses may cause serious side effects.

INFORMATION FOR USERS

Your drug prescription is tailored for you. Do not alter dosage without checking with your doctor.

How taken Tablets, lozenges, injection, rectal foam, cream, ointment, eye ointment/drops.

Frequency and timing of doses Varies according to condition.

Dosage range Varies according to condition, but should be increased to cover serious injury or surgery.

Onset of effect 4 hours to several days, depending on condition.

Duration of action Up to 12 hours.
Diet advice Salt intake may need to be restricted when the drug is taken by mouth. Potassium supplements may also be necessary.
Storage Keep in a closed container in a cool, dry place out of reach of children.
Missed dose Take as soon as you remember. If your next dose is due within 2 hours, take a single dose now and skip the next.
Stopping the drug Do not stop taking the drug without consulting your doctor. A gradual reduction in dosage is required following prolonged treatment with oral hydrocortisone.
Exceeding the dose An occasional unintentional extra dose is unlikely to be a cause for concern. But if you notice any unusual symptoms, or if a large overdose has been taken, notify your doctor.

POSSIBLE ADVERSE EFFECTS

Taken by mouth, hydrocortisone may cause indigestion, weight gain, acne, fluid retention, and high blood pressure. High doses may lead to muscle weakness and mood changes; consult your doctor. The most serious adverse effects only occur when hydrocortisone is taken by mouth in high doses for long periods of time (see Prolonged use, below). These are carefully monitored during treatment.

INTERACTIONS

Barbiturates, anticonvulsants, and rifampicin These drugs reduce the effectiveness of hydrocortisone.
Antidiabetic drugs Hydrocortisone reduces the action of these drugs.
Antihypertensive drugs Hydrocortisone reduces the effects of these drugs.
Vaccines Severe reactions can occur if this drug is taken with certain vaccines.

SPECIAL PRECAUTIONS

Be sure to tell your doctor if:
◆ You have liver or kidney problems.
◆ You have had a peptic ulcer.
◆ You have had a mental illness or epilepsy.
◆ You have glaucoma.
◆ You have had tuberculosis.
◆ You have diabetes or heart problems.
◆ You are taking other medications.

Avoid exposure to chickenpox, shingles, or measles if you are on systemic treatment.
Pregnancy No evidence of risk with topical preparations. Oral doses may adversely affect the developing baby. Discuss with your doctor.
Breast-feeding The drug passes into the breast milk and may affect the baby. Discuss with your doctor.
Infants and children Reduced dose necessary.
Over 60 Reduced dose may be necessary.
Driving and hazardous work No special problems.
Alcohol Avoid. Alcohol may increase the risk of peptic ulcer when this drug is taken by mouth.

PROLONGED USE

Depending on method of administration, prolonged high dosage may cause diabetes, glaucoma, fragile bones, and thin skin, and may retard growth in children. People having long-term treatment are advised to carry a treatment card.
Monitoring Periodic checks on blood pressure are usually required when the drug is taken by mouth.

Hyoscine

Brand names Buscopan, Joy-Rides, Kwells, Scopoderm TTS, Travel Calm
Used in the following combined preparation Papaveretum and hyoscine

QUICK REFERENCE

Drug group Drug for irritable bowel syndrome (p.43), drug affecting the pupil (p.112), and drug for nausea/vomiting (p.21)
Overdose danger rating Medium
Dependence rating Low
Prescription needed No
Available as generic Yes

GENERAL INFORMATION

Originally derived from the henbane plant, hyoscine is an anticholinergic drug that has both an antispasmodic effect on the intestine and a calming action on the nerve pathways that control nausea and vomiting. By its anticholinergic action, hyoscine also dilates the pupil.

The drug is produced in two forms. Hyoscine butylbromide is prescribed to reduce spasm of the gastrointestinal tract in irritable bowel syndrome. The other form, hyoscine hydrobromide, is used to control motion sickness and the giddiness and nausea caused by disturbances of the inner ear (see Vertigo and Ménière's disease, p.21) and can be administered as skin patches as well as in tablets. This form is also used as a premedication to dry secretions before operations. Eye drops containing the hydrobromide form are used to dilate the pupil during eye examinations and eye surgery.

INFORMATION FOR USERS

Follow instructions on the label. Call your doctor if symptoms worsen.

How taken Tablets, injection, eye drops, skin patches.

Frequency and timing of doses As required up to 4 x daily by mouth (irritable bowel syndrome) or up to 3 x daily (nausea and vomiting); every 3 days (patches).

Adult dosage range *Irritable bowel syndrome* 80mg (hyoscine butylbromide) daily. *Nausea and vomiting* 0.3mg (hyoscine hydrobromide) per dose.

Onset of effect Within 1 hour.

Duration of action Up to 6 hours (by mouth); up to 72 hours (patches).

Diet advice None.

Storage Keep in a closed container in a cool, dry place out of reach of children. Protect from light.

Missed dose Take when you remember. Adjust the timing of your next dose accordingly.

Stopping the drug Can be safely stopped as soon as you no longer need it.

Exceeding the dose An occasional unintentional extra dose is unlikely to cause problems. Large overdoses may cause drowsiness or agitation. Notify your doctor.

POSSIBLE ADVERSE EFFECTS

Taken by mouth or by injection, hyoscine has a strong anticholinergic effect on the body, causing a variety of minor symptoms. These include drowsiness, dry mouth, blurred vision, and constipation and can sometimes be minimized by a reduction in dosage. If you experience difficulty in passing urine, increased heart rate, or palpitations, consult your doctor.

INTERACTIONS

Sedatives All drugs that have a sedative effect on the central nervous system are likely to increase the sedative properties of hyoscine. Such drugs include anti-anxiety and sleeping drugs, antidepressants, opioid analgesics, and antipsychotics.

Anticholinergic drugs Many drugs have either anticholinergic or antimuscarinic effects. Using one of these drugs with hyoscine will increase side effects such as dry mouth, difficulty in passing urine, and constipation.

SPECIAL PRECAUTIONS

Be sure to consult your doctor or pharmacist before taking this drug if:

◆ You have long-term liver or kidney problems.

◆ You have heart problems.

◆ You have myasthenia gravis.

◆ You have megacolon or intestinal obstruction problems.

◆ You have had glaucoma.

◆ You have prostate trouble or urinary retention.

◆ You are taking other medications.

Pregnancy Safety in pregnancy not established. Discuss with your doctor.

Breast-feeding No evidence of risk. Discuss with your doctor.

Infants and children Not recommended under 6 years. Reduced dose necessary in older children.

Over 60 Reduced dose may be necessary.

Driving and hazardous work Avoid such activities until you have learned how hyoscine affects you because the drug can cause drowsiness and blurred vision.

Alcohol Avoid. Alcohol may increase the sedative effect of this drug.

PROLONGED USE

Use of this drug for longer than a few days is unlikely to be necessary.

Ibuprofen

Brand names Arthrofen, Brufen, Ebufac, Fenbid, Ibufac, Ibugel, Ibuleve, Inoven, Motrin, Nurofen, and many others
Used in the following combined preparation Codafen

QUICK REFERENCE

Drug group Analgesic (p.9) and non-steroidal anti-inflammatory drug (p.48)
Overdose danger rating Low
Dependence rating Low
Prescription needed No
Available as generic Yes

GENERAL INFORMATION

Ibuprofen is a non-steroidal anti-inflammatory drug (NSAID) which, like other NSAIDs, reduces pain, stiffness, and inflammation. It is an effective treatment for the symptoms of osteoarthritis, rheumatoid arthritis, and gout. In the treatment of rheumatoid arthritis, ibuprofen may be prescribed with slower-acting drugs. It is also used to relieve mild to moderate headache, menstrual and dental pain, pain resulting from soft tissue injuries, or the pain that may follow an operation.

Ibuprofen has fewer side effects than many of the other NSAIDs. It rarely causes bleeding in the stomach and seems to be safer than aspirin in this respect. Ibuprofen is also available as a cream or gel that can be applied to the skin for muscular aches and sprains.

INFORMATION FOR USERS

Follow instructions on the label. Call your doctor if symptoms worsen.
How taken Tablets, SR-tablets, capsules, liquid, granules, cream, gel.
Frequency and timing of doses 1–2 x daily for SR-tablets or 4–6 x daily (general pain relief); 3–4 x daily with food (arthritis).
Adult dosage range *General pain relief* 600mg–1.8g daily. *Arthritis* 1.2–2.4g daily.
Onset of effect Pain relief begins in 1–2 hours. The full anti-inflammatory effect in arthritic conditions may not be felt for up to 2 weeks.
Duration of action 5–10 hours.
Diet advice None.

Storage Keep in a closed container in a cool, dry place out of reach of children.
Missed dose Take as soon as you remember. If your next dose is due within 2 hours, take a single dose now and skip the next.
Stopping the drug When taken for short-term pain relief, the drug can be safely stopped as soon as you no longer need it. If prescribed for the long-term treatment of arthritis, you should seek medical advice before stopping the drug unless rash, wheezing, or breathlessness occur.
Exceeding the dose An occasional unintentional extra dose is unlikely to be a cause for concern. But if you notice any unusual symptoms, or if a large overdose has been taken, notify your doctor.

POSSIBLE ADVERSE EFFECTS

The most common adverse effects are the result of gastrointestinal disturbances. Heartburn, indigestion, nausea, and vomiting may occur. Black or bloodstained faeces should be reported to your doctor without delay. If you develop a rash, wheezing, or breathlessness, stop taking the drug and consult your doctor immediately. Swollen feet or ankles and ringing in the ears are uncommon adverse effects normally associated with too high a dose.

INTERACTIONS

General note Ibuprofen interacts with a wide range of drugs to increase the risk of bleeding and/or peptic ulcers. Such drugs include other NSAIDs, aspirin, oral anticoagulants, and corticosteroids.
Ciprofloxacin This drug and related antibiotics may increase the risk of seizures.
Antihypertensive drugs and diuretics The beneficial effects of these drugs may be reduced by ibuprofen.
Lithium Ibuprofen may raise blood levels of lithium.
Methotrexate Ibuprofen may raise blood levels of methotrexate.

SPECIAL PRECAUTIONS

Be sure to consult your doctor or pharmacist before taking this drug if:
◆ You have a long-term kidney problem.
◆ You have a long-term liver problem.

◆ You have high blood pressure.
◆ You have had a peptic ulcer, oesophagitis, or acid indigestion.
◆ You are allergic to aspirin.
◆ You have asthma.
◆ You are taking other medications.

Pregnancy Not usually prescribed. May affect the unborn baby and may prolong labour. Discuss with your doctor.

Breast-feeding The drug passes into the breast milk, but at normal doses adverse effects on the baby are unlikely. Discuss with your doctor.

Infants and children Reduced dose necessary.

Over 60 Reduced dose may be necessary.

Driving and hazardous work No problems expected.

Alcohol Avoid. Alcohol may increase the risk of stomach disorders with ibuprofen.

Surgery and general anaesthetics Ibuprofen may prolong bleeding. Discuss the possibility of stopping treatment temporarily with your doctor or dentist.

PROLONGED USE

There is a small, but definite, increase in risk of bleeding from peptic ulcers and in the bowel with prolonged use of ibuprofen.

Imipramine

Brand name Tofranil
Used in the following combined preparations
None

QUICK REFERENCE

Drug group Tricyclic antidepressant (p.14) and drug for urinary disorders (p.108)
Overdose danger rating High
Dependence rating Low
Prescription needed Yes
Available as generic Yes

GENERAL INFORMATION

Imipramine belongs to the tricyclic class of antidepressant drugs. It is used mainly in the long-term treatment of depression to elevate mood, improve appetite, increase physical activity, and restore interest in everyday life. Because imipramine is less sedating than some other antidepressants, it is particularly useful when a depressed person is withdrawn or apathetic, although it can aggravate insomnia if it is taken in the evening.

Imipramine is also prescribed to treat night-time enuresis (bedwetting) in children, although proof of its benefit is not conclusive. Imipramine can cause a variety of side effects. In overdose the drug may cause coma and dangerous heart rhythms.

INFORMATION FOR USERS

Your drug prescription is tailored for you. Do not alter dosage without checking with your doctor.

How taken Tablets, liquid.

Frequency and timing of doses 1–4 x daily.

Dosage range *Adults* Usually 75–200mg daily. *Children* Reduced dose according to age and weight.

Onset of effect Some benefits and effects may appear within hours, but full antidepressant effect may not be felt for 2–6 weeks.

Duration of action Following prolonged treatment, antidepressant effect may persist for up to 6 weeks. Any adverse effects may wear off within days.

Diet advice None.

Storage Keep in a closed container in a cool, dry place out of reach of children.

Missed dose Take as soon as you remember. If your next dose is due within 3 hours, take a single dose now and skip the next.

Stopping the drug Unless giddy spells or palpitations occur, do not stop taking the drug without consulting your doctor, who will supervise gradual reduction dosage. Stopping abruptly may cause withdrawal symptoms.

OVERDOSE ACTION

Seek immediate medical advice in all cases. Take emergency action if consciousness is lost.

POSSIBLE ADVERSE EFFECTS

The drug's possible adverse effects are mainly the result of its anticholinergic action and its effect on the heart's normal rhythm. Sweating, flushing, dry mouth, constipation, difficulty in passing urine, and blurred vision are common, especially at the start of treatment. Dizziness and drowsiness may also occur. If you develop a rash, consult your doctor. If you have giddy spells or palpitations, stop taking the drug and seek urgent medical advice.

INTERACTIONS

Sedatives Imipramine may increase the effects of sedative drugs.

MAOIs There is a possibility of a serious interaction. Such drugs are prescribed with imipramine only under strict supervision.

Antihypertensive drugs Imipramine may reduce the effectiveness of these drugs.

Phenytoin Imipramine may increase levels of phenytoin.

Amiodarone and sotalol These drugs may increase the risk of abnormal heart rhythms.

SPECIAL PRECAUTIONS

Be sure to tell your doctor if:
◆ You have had heart problems.
◆ You have long-term liver or kidney problems.
◆ You have had epileptic fits.
◆ You have had glaucoma.
◆ You have prostate trouble.
◆ You have had mania or a psychotic illness.
◆ You are taking other medications.

Pregnancy Safety in pregnancy not established. Discuss with your doctor.

Breast-feeding The drug passes into the breast milk, but at normal doses adverse effects on the baby are unlikely. Discuss with your doctor.

Infants and children Not recommended under 7 years. Reduced dose necessary in older children.

Over 60 Increased likelihood of adverse effects. Reduced dose may therefore be necessary.

Driving and hazardous work Avoid such activities until you have learned how imipramine affects you because the drug can cause reduced alertness and blurred vision.

Alcohol Avoid. Alcohol may increase the sedative effect of imipramine.

Surgery and general anaesthetics Imipramine treatment may need to be stopped before you have a general anaesthetic. Discuss this with your doctor or dentist before any operation.

PROLONGED USE

No problems expected with prolonged use of imipramine. The drug is not usually prescribed for children as a treatment for bedwetting for longer than three months.

Indapamide

Brand names Natramid, Natrilix, Nindaxa, Opumide,
Used in the following combined preparations
None

QUICK REFERENCE

Drug group Diuretic (p.30)
Overdose danger rating Low
Dependence rating Low
Prescription needed Yes
Available as generic Yes

GENERAL INFORMATION

Indapamide is related in its effects and uses to the thiazide diuretic group of drugs but is used to treat hypertension (high blood pressure).

The drug prevents the hormone norepinephrine (noradrenaline) from constricting blood vessels, thereby allowing them to dilate.

Indapamide is sometimes combined with other antihypertensive drugs but not with other diuretics.

The diuretic effects of indapamide are slight at low doses, but susceptible people need to have blood levels of potassium and uric acid monitored. These include the elderly, those taking digitalis drugs, or those with gout or hyperaldosteronism (overproduction of the hormone aldosterone). Unlike the thiazides, indapamide does not affect diabetic control.

INFORMATION FOR USERS

Your drug prescription is tailored for you. Do not alter dosage without checking with your doctor.

How taken Tablets, SR-tablets.
Frequency and timing of doses Once daily in the morning.
Adult dosage range 1.5–2.5mg.
Onset of effect 1–2 hours, but the full effect may not be felt for several months.
Duration of action 12–24 hours.
Diet advice None.
Storage Keep in a closed container in a cool, dry place out of reach of children.
Missed dose Take as soon as you remember. If your next dose is due within 4 hours, take a single dose now and skip the next.
Stopping the drug Do not stop taking the drug without consulting your doctor; high blood pressure may return.

Exceeding the dose An occasional unintentional extra dose is unlikely to cause problems. But if you notice any unusual symptoms, or if a large overdose has been taken, notify your doctor.

POSSIBLE ADVERSE EFFECTS
Headaches, fatigue, and muscle cramps are common adverse effects. Diarrhoea, constipation, and impotence are less common. If you experience dizziness, fainting, palpitations, tingling, or "pins and needles", consult your doctor. If you develop a sore throat, a rash, or jaundice, seek medical advice.

INTERACTIONS
Diuretics There is a risk of imbalance of salts in the blood if these drugs are taken with indapamide.

Digitalis drugs Loss of potassium may lead to toxicity of these drugs with indapamide.

Lithium Blood levels of lithium are increased when it is taken with indapamide.

Antiarrhythmics Potassium loss may make these drugs less effective if taken with indapamide.

SPECIAL PRECAUTIONS
Be sure to tell your doctor if:
◆ You have had a stroke.
◆ You have liver or kidney problems.
◆ You have gout.
◆ You have hyperaldosteronism or hyperparathyroidism
◆ You are allergic to sulphonamide drugs.
◆ You are taking digitalis drugs.
◆ You are taking other medications.
Pregnancy Safety not established. Discuss with your doctor.
Breast-feeding Safety not established. Discuss with your doctor.
Infants and children Not prescribed.
Over 60 No special problems.
Driving and hazardous work No special problems.
Alcohol No special problems.

PROLONGED USE
Long-term use may lead to potassium loss in the elderly and certain other groups.
Monitoring Blood tests may be performed periodically to check kidney function and levels of potassium and other salts.

Indoramin
Brand names Baratol, Doralese
Used in the following combined preparations
None

QUICK REFERENCE
Drug group Antihypertensive drug (p.34) and drug for urinary retention (p.109)
Overdose danger rating Medium
Dependence rating Low
Prescription needed Yes
Available as generic No

GENERAL INFORMATION
Indoramin is a selective alpha blocker drug that is used to treat hypertension (high blood pressure). It works by relaxing the muscles in the blood vessel walls, dilating (widening) them, thereby easing the flow of blood. Indoramin may be combined with other antihypertensive drugs in order to achieve better control.

Indoramin is also used, in lower doses, to relieve urinary retention caused by an enlarged prostate gland.

The drug works by relaxing the muscle of the prostate, enabling urine to be passed more easily. Because indoramin can initially cause a rapid fall in blood pressure, the first dose is usually low, and should be taken lying down. The drug can also cause drowsiness at the start of treatment and whenever dosage is increased. If unequal sized daily doses are taken, the largest dose is usually prescribed for bedtime.

INFORMATION FOR USERS
Your drug prescription is tailored for you. Do not alter dosage without checking with your doctor.
How taken Tablets.
Frequency and timing of doses *Hypertension* 2–3 x daily. *Urinary retention*: 1–2 x daily.
Adult dosage range *Hypertension* 25mg (starting dose), increased if necessary at 2-week intervals. Maximum daily dose 200mg. *Urinary retention* 20mg (starting dose), increased if necessary at 2-week intervals. Maximum daily dose 100mg.
Onset of effect 1 hour.
Duration of action 6–12 hours.

Diet advice None.

Storage Keep in a closed container in a cool, dry place out of reach of children.

Missed dose Take as soon as you remember. If your next dose is due within 2 hours, take a single dose now and skip the next.

Stopping the drug Do not stop taking the drug without consulting your doctor. Stopping the drug may lead to worsening of the underlying condition.

Exceeding the dose An occasional unintentional extra dose is unlikely to be a cause for concern. Large overdoses may produce deep sedation and fits. Notify your doctor immediately.

POSSIBLE ADVERSE EFFECTS

Drowsiness and dizziness are the most common adverse effects of treatment with indoramin. A dry mouth, nasal congestion, fatigue, and headache may also occur. These effects are often worse at the start of treatment or following an increase in dosage. If you experience depression or develop tremor or abnormal movements, consult your doctor.

INTERACTIONS

Antidepressants, beta-blockers, calcium channel blockers, diuretics, thymoxamine These drugs increase the blood-pressure lowering effect of indoramin.

SPECIAL PRECAUTIONS

Be sure to tell your doctor if:
◆ You have liver or kidney problems.
◆ You have Parkinson's disease.
◆ You have epilepsy.
◆ You have heart failure.
◆ You have a history of depression.
◆ You are taking an MAOI drug.
◆ You are taking other medications.

Pregnancy Safety not established. Discuss with your doctor.

Breast-feeding Safety not established. Discuss with your doctor.

Infants and children Not recommended.

Over 60 Reduced dose may be necessary.

Driving and hazardous work Avoid such activities until you have learned how indoramin affects you because the drug can cause drowsiness and dizziness.

Alcohol Avoid. Alcohol increases the amount of indoramin absorbed, which increases its sedative effects.

Surgery and general anaesthetics Anaesthesia may increase the blood-pressure lowering effect of indoramin. Discuss this with your doctor or dentist before surgery.

PROLONGED USE
No special problems.

Insulin

Brand names Humalog, Human Actrapid, Human Insulatard, Human Mixtard, Human Monotard, Human Ultratard, Human Velosulin, Humulin, Hypurin, Lentard MC, Pork Insulatard, Pork Mixtard, Pork Velosulin, and others

QUICK REFERENCE
Drug group Drug for diabetes (p.80)
Overdose danger rating High
Dependence rating Low
Prescription needed Yes
Available as generic No

GENERAL INFORMATION

Insulin is a hormone manufactured by the pancreas and vital to the body's ability to use sugar. It is given by injection to supplement or replace natural insulin in the treatment of diabetes mellitus. It is the only effective treatment in juvenile (insulin-dependent or Type 1) diabetes and may also be prescribed in adult (maturity-onset or Type 2) diabetes. Insulin should be used with a carefully controlled diet supervised by your practice nurse or a dietitian. Illness, vomiting, or alterations in diet or in exercise levels may require dosage adjustment.

Insulin is available in a wide variety of preparations, which can be short-, medium-, or long-acting. Combinations of these types are often given. People receiving insulin should carry a warning card or tag.

INFORMATION FOR USERS

Your drug prescription is tailored for you. Do not alter dosage without checking with your doctor.

How taken Injection, infusion pump.

Frequency and timing of doses 1–4 x daily. Short-acting insulin usually 15–30 minutes before meals. The exact time of the injections and administration for longer-acting preparations will be tailored to your individual needs; follow the instructions you are given, and be sure to rotate the injection sites.

Dosage range Dose (and type) is determined according to the needs of the individual.

Onset of effect 30–60 minutes (short-acting); 1–2 hours (medium- and long-acting).

Duration of action 6–8 hours (short-acting); 18–26 hours (medium-acting); 28–36 hours (long-acting).

Diet advice A low-carbohydrate diet is necessary. Follow your doctor's advice.

Storage Refrigerate, but do not freeze. Follow the instructions on the container.

Missed dose Discuss with your doctor. Appropriate action depends on dose and type .

Stopping the drug Do not stop taking the drug without consulting your doctor; confusion and coma may occur.

OVERDOSE ACTION

Seek immediate medical advice. You may notice symptoms of low blood glucose, such as faintness, hunger, sweating, trembling. You should at or drink something sugary. Take emergency action if fits or loss of consciousness occur.

POSSIBLE ADVERSE EFFECTS

Symptoms such as dizziness, sweating, weakness, and confusion indicate low blood glucose. Serious allergic reactions such as rash, swelling, and shortness of breath are very rare and require urgent medical attention. If you develop eyesight problems or experience irritation or dimpling at the injection site, consult your doctor.

INTERACTIONS

General note 1 Many drugs, including some antibiotics, MAOIs, and oral antidiabetics, increase the risk of low blood glucose.

Corticosteroids and diuretics may oppose the effect of insulin.

General note 2 Check with your doctor or pharmacist before taking any medicines; some contain sugar and may upset diabetic control.

Beta blockers may affect insulin needs and could mask some signs of low blood glucose.

SPECIAL PRECAUTIONS

Be sure to tell your doctor if:
◆ You have had a previous allergic reaction to insulin.
◆ You are taking other medications, or your other drug treatment is changed.

Pregnancy No evidence of risk to the developing baby from insulin, but poor control of diabetes increases the risk of birth defects. Careful monitoring is required.

Breast-feeding No evidence of risk. Adjustment in dose may be necessary while breast-feeding.

Infants and children Reduced dose necessary.

Over 60 No special problems.

Driving and hazardous work Usually no problem, but strenuous exercise alters requirements of insulin and sugar. Avoid these activities if you have warning signs of low blood glucose.

Alcohol Avoid. Alcohol upsets diabetic control.

Surgery and general anaesthetics Insulin requirements may increase during surgery, and blood glucose levels will need to be monitored during and after an operation. Notify your doctor or dentist that you are diabetic before any surgery.

PROLONGED USE

No problems expected.

Monitoring Regular review by your doctor or diabetic clinic is essential to reduce the risk of your developing long-term complications of diabetes.

Interferon

Brand names Betaferon, Immukin, Intron-A, Roferon-A, Viraferon, Wellferon, Avonex, Rebif

Used in the following combined preparations
None

QUICK REFERENCE

Drug group Antiviral drug (p.67) and anticancer drug (p.94).

Overdose danger rating Medium

Dependence rating Low

Prescription needed Yes

Available as generic No

GENERAL INFORMATION

Interferons are a group of substances produced in human and animal cells that have
been infected with viruses or stimulated by
other substances. They are thought to
promote resistance to several types of viral
infection. Three main types of interferon
(alpha, beta, and gamma) are used to treat a
range of diseases. Interferon alpha is used for
leukaemias, other cancers, and chronic active
hepatitis B. Interferon beta may reduce the
frequency and severity of relapses in some
forms of multiple sclerosis. Interferon
gamma is prescribed in conjunction with antibiotics for patients suffering from chronic
granulomatous disease.

Interferons can cause severe adverse
effects (see below).

INFORMATION FOR USERS

This drug is given only under medical supervision and is not for self-administration.

How taken Injection.

Frequency and timing of doses Once daily or
on alternate days.

Adult dosage range The dosage is calculated
taking account of the body surface area of
the patient and the condition that is being
treated.

Onset of effect The drug is active inside the
body within 1 hour, but its effects may not be
noted for 1–2 months.

Duration of action Effects last for about
12 hours.

Diet advice None.

Storage Store in a refrigerator at 2–8°C
(36–46°F). Do not let it freeze, and protect
from light. Keep out of reach of children.

Missed dose Not applicable. This drug is usually given only in hospital under close medical supervision.

Stopping the drug Discuss with your doctor.

Exceeding the dose Overdosage is unlikely
since treatment is carefully monitored.

POSSIBLE ADVERSE EFFECTS

Headache, lethargy, depression, dizziness,
drowsiness, digestive disturbance, poor
appetite, and weight loss are the most
common problems. All unusual symptoms
should be brought to your doctor's attention
without delay. Some of these are dose-
related, and a reduction in dosage may be
necessary to eliminate them. If you experience fever, muscle-ache, or hair loss, consult
your doctor.

INTERACTIONS

General note A number of drugs increase the
risk of adverse effects on the blood, heart, or
nervous system. This is taken into account
when an interferon is prescribed with other
drugs.

Vaccines Interferon may reduce the effectiveness of vaccines.

Theophylline/aminophylline The effects of this
drug may be enhanced by interferon.

Sedatives All drugs that have a sedative effect
on the central nervous system are likely to
increase the sedative properties of interferons. Such drugs include opioid analgesics,
anti-anxiety drugs, sleeping drugs, antihistamines, antidepressants, and antipsychotics.

SPECIAL PRECAUTIONS

Be sure to tell your doctor if:
◆ You have long-term liver or kidney prob-
lems.
◆ You have heart disease.
◆ You have had epileptic fits.
◆ You have previously suffered allergic reac-
tions to any drugs.
◆ You have had asthma or eczema.
◆ You suffer from depression.
◆ You are taking other medications.

Pregnancy Not usually prescribed. Safety in
pregnancy not established. Discuss with your
doctor.

Breast-feeding It is not known whether the
drug passes into the breast milk. Discuss
with your doctor.

Infants and children Not usually used.

Over 60 Reduced dose may be necessary.
Increased likelihood of adverse effects.

Driving and hazardous work Not applicable.

Alcohol Avoid. Alcohol may increase the
sedative effects of this drug.

PROLONGED USE

There may be an increased risk of liver
damage with prolonged use of this drug.
Blood cell production in the bone marrow
may be reduced. Repeated large doses are

associated with lethargy, fatigue, collapse, and coma.

Monitoring Frequent blood tests are required to monitor blood composition and liver function.

Ipratropium Bromide

Brand names Atrovent, Rinatec, Respontin
Used in the following combined preparations
Combivent, Duovent

QUICK REFERENCE

Drug group Bronchodilator (p.23)
Overdose danger rating Low
Dependence rating Low
Prescription needed Yes
Available as generic Yes

GENERAL INFORMATION

Ipratropium bromide is an anticholinergic bronchodilator that relaxes the muscles surrounding the bronchioles (airways in the lung). It is used primarily in the maintenance treatment of reversible airway disorders, particularly chronic bronchitis. It is given only by inhaler or via a nebulizer for these conditions. Although its effect lasts longer, ipratropium bromide has a slower onset of action than the sympathomimetic bronchodilators. For this reason, it is not as effective in treating acute attacks of wheezing, or in the emergency treatment of asthma, and it is usually used together with the faster-acting drugs. Ipratropium bromide is also prescribed as a nasal spray for the treatment of a continually runny nose as a result of allergy.

Unlike with other anticholinergic drugs, side effects are rare with ipratropium bromide. It is not likely to affect the heart, eyes, bowel, or bladder. The drug must be used with caution by people with glaucoma, but problems are unlikely at normal doses.

INFORMATION FOR USERS

Your drug prescription is tailored for you. Do not alter dosage without checking with your doctor.

How taken Inhaler, nasal spray, liquid for nebulizer.

Frequency and timing of doses 3–4 x daily.

Adult dosage range 80–320 micrograms daily (inhaler); 400–2,000 micrograms daily (nebulizer); 1–2 puffs to the affected nostril 2–3 x daily (nasal spray).

Onset of effect 5–15 minutes.

Duration of action Up to 8 hours.

Diet advice None.

Storage Keep in a cool, dry place out of reach of children. Do not puncture or burn containers.

Missed dose Take as soon as you remember. If your next dose is due within 2 hours, take a single dose now and skip the next.

Stopping the drug Do not stop taking the drug without consulting your doctor; symptoms may recur.

Exceeding the dose An occasional unintentional extra dose is unlikely to be a cause for concern. But if you notice any unusual symptoms, or if a large overdose has been taken, notify your doctor.

POSSIBLE ADVERSE EFFECTS

Side effects are rare with ipratropium bromide. The most common is dry mouth or throat. Constipation and difficulty in passing urine may occur with high doses.

INTERACTIONS

None.

SPECIAL PRECAUTIONS

Be sure to tell your doctor if:
◆ You have glaucoma.
◆ You have prostate problems.
◆ You have difficulty in passing urine.
◆ You are taking other medications.

Pregnancy No evidence of risk, but discuss with your doctor before using ipratropium bromide during the first 3 months of pregnancy.

Breast-feeding No evidence of risk, but discuss with your doctor.

Infants and children Reduced dose necessary.

Over 60 No special problems.

Driving and hazardous work No special problems.

Alcohol No known problems.

PROLONGED USE

No special problems.

Irbesartan

Brand name Aprovel
Used in the following combined preparations
None

QUICK REFERENCE

Drug group Vasodilator (p.30) and antihypertensive drug (p.34)
Overdose danger rating Medium
Dependence rating Low
Prescription needed Yes
Available as generic No

GENERAL INFORMATION

Irbesartan is a member of the group of vasodilator drugs called angiotensin-II blockers. Used to treat hypertension, the drug works by blocking the action of angiotensin-II (a naturally occurring substance that constricts blood vessels). This action causes the blood vessel walls to relax, thereby lowering blood pressure.

Unlike ACE inhibitors, irbesartan does not cause a persistent dry cough.

Along with other angiotensin-II blockers, it is being evaluated for the treatment of other conditions, such as heart failure, for which ACE inhibitors are used.

Irbesartan is prescribed with caution to people with stenosis (narrowing) of the arteries to the kidneys because the drug may make kidney function worse in people with this problem. It is important to notify your doctor if you know that you have this condition.

INFORMATION FOR USERS

Your drug prescription is tailored for you. Do not alter dosage without checking with your doctor.
How taken Tablets.
Frequency and timing of doses Once daily.
Adult dosage range 150–300mg, but 75mg may be used in people over 75 years.
Onset of effect Within 1 hour. Blood pressure is lowered within 1–2 weeks, and maximum beneficial effect is felt 4–6 weeks from start of treatment.
Duration of action 24 hours.
Diet advice None.
Storage Keep in a closed container in a cool, dry place out of reach of children.

Missed dose Take as soon as you remember. If your next dose is due within 8 hours, take a single dose now and skip the next.
Stopping the drug Unless wheezing, itching, or rash occur, do not stop taking the drug without consulting your doctor. Stopping the drug may lead to worsening control of high blood pressure.
Exceeding the dose An occasional unintentional extra dose is unlikely to be a cause for concern. Large overdoses may cause dizziness and fainting. Notify your doctor.

POSSIBLE ADVERSE EFFECTS

Adverse effects are usually mild. Dizziness, fatigue, and flushing are common; headaches are less so. If you develop wheezing, a blotchy rash, or itching, stop taking the drug immediately and consult your doctor urgently.

INTERACTIONS

Diuretics There is a risk of a sudden fall in blood pressure if these drugs are being taken when irbesartan treatment is started.
Potassium supplements, potassium-sparing diuretics, and ciclosporin Irbesartan enhances the effect of these drugs, leading to raised levels of potassium in the blood.
Lithium Irbesartan increases the blood levels and toxicity of lithium.
NSAIDs Certain of these drugs may reduce the blood-pressure lowering effects of irbesartan.

SPECIAL PRECAUTIONS

Be sure to tell your doctor if:
◆ You have kidney problems or renal artery stenosis.
◆ You have heart problems.
◆ You have congestive heart failure.
◆ You have primary aldosteronism.
◆ You are taking other medications.
Pregnancy Not prescribed.
Breast-feeding Safety not established. Discuss with your doctor.
Infants and children Not prescribed.
Over 60 Reduced dose may be necessary in people over 75 years.
Driving and hazardous work Avoid such activities until you have learned how irbesartan affects you because the drug can cause dizziness and fatigue.

Alcohol Avoid. Regular alcohol intake may raise blood pressure and reduce the effectiveness of irbesartan. It may also increase the likelihood of an excessive fall in blood pressure.

PROLONGED USE

No special problems.

Monitoring Blood pressure will be monitored during treatment with irbesartan, as with all antihypertensive drugs. Periodic kidney function tests and checks on blood potassium levels may be performed.

Isoniazid

Brand names None
Used in the following combined preparations
Rifater, Rifinah, Rimactazid

QUICK REFERENCE

Drug group Antituberculous drug (p.65)
Overdose danger rating High
Dependence rating Low
Prescription needed Yes
Available as generic Yes

GENERAL INFORMATION

Isoniazid (also known as INAH and INH) has been in use for over 30 years and remains an effective drug for tuberculosis. It is given alone to prevent tuberculosis and in combination with other drugs for the treatment of the disease. Treatment usually lasts for six months. However, courses lasting nine months or a year may sometimes be prescribed.

One of the side effects of isoniazid is the increased loss of pyridoxine (vitamin B_6) from the body. This effect, which is more likely with high doses, is rare in children but common among people with poor nutrition. Because pyridoxine deficiency can lead to irreversible nerve damage, supplements are usually given.

INFORMATION FOR USERS

Your drug prescription is tailored for you. Do not alter dosage without checking with your doctor.

How taken Tablets, liquid, injection.
Frequency and timing of doses Normally once daily.

Dosage range *Adults* 300mg daily.
Children According to age and weight.
Onset of effect Over 2–3 days.
Duration of action Up to 24 hours.
Diet advice Isoniazid may deplete pyridoxine (vitamin B_6) levels in the body. Supplements may therefore be prescribed.
Storage Keep in a closed container in a cool, dry place out of reach of children. Protect from light.
Missed dose Take as soon as you remember. If your next dose is scheduled within 8 hours, take a single dose now and skip the next.
Stopping the drug Unless serious adverse effects occur (see below), take the full course. Even if you feel better the infection may still be present and may recur if treatment is stopped too soon.

OVERDOSE ACTION

Seek immediate medical advice in all cases. Take emergency action if breathing difficulties, fits, or loss of consciousness occur.

POSSIBLE ADVERSE EFFECTS

Although serious problems are uncommon with this drug, all adverse effects should receive prompt medical attention because of the possibility of nerve or liver damage. Adverse effects that may be experienced include nausea, vomiting, fatigue, weakness, numbness, tingling, and a rash. If you develop blurred vision, jaundice, twitching, or muscle weakness, stop taking the drug and consult your doctor urgently.

INTERACTIONS

Alcohol and rifampicin Large quantities of alcohol may reduce the effectiveness of isoniazid. If the two are taken together, the likelihood of liver damage is increased; if rifampicin is also being taken, the likelihood is increased even further.

Anticonvulsants The effects of these drugs may be increased with isoniazid.

Antacids These drugs may reduce the absorption of isoniazid.

SPECIAL PRECAUTIONS

Be sure to tell your doctor if:
◆ You have long-term liver or kidney problems.

◆ You have had liver damage following isoniazid treatment in the past.

◆ If you have problems with drugs or alcohol abuse.

◆ You have diabetes.

◆ You have had epileptic fits. You are taking other medications.

Pregnancy Safety in pregnancy not established. Discuss with your doctor.

Breast-feeding The drug passes into the breast milk and may affect the baby. The infant should be monitored for signs of toxic effects. Discuss with your doctor.

Infants and children Reduced dose necessary.

Over 60 Increased likelihood of adverse effects.

Driving and hazardous work No special problems.

Alcohol Avoid excessive amounts.

PROLONGED USE

Pyridoxine (vitamin B_6) deficiency may occur with prolonged use and lead to nerve damage. Supplements are usually prescribed. There is also a risk of serious liver damage.

Monitoring Periodic blood tests are sometimes performed to monitor liver function.

Isosorbide dinitrate/ mononitrate

Brand names [Dinitrate] Cedocard, Isocard, Isoket, Isordil, Sorbichew, Sorbid SA, Sorbitrate; [Mononitrate] Elantan, Imdur, Isib 60XL, Ismo, Isotard, Isotrate, MCR-50, Modisal, Monit, Mono-Cedocard, Monomax, Monosorb

Used in the following combined preparation
Imazin XL

QUICK REFERENCE

Drug group Nitrate vasodilator (p.30) and anti-angina drug (p.33)

Overdose danger rating Medium

Dependence rating Low

Prescription needed Yes

Available as generic Yes

GENERAL INFORMATION

Isosorbide dinitrate and mononitrate are vasodilator drugs similar to glyceryl trinitrate. They are usually used to treat patients with angina as well as some cases of heart failure.

Unlike glyceryl trinitrate, however, both forms of isosorbide are stable and can be stored for long periods without losing their effectiveness. They are often sold as slow-release (SR) preparations, which have a longer action.

Headache, flushing, and dizziness are common side effects during the early stages of treatment; small initial doses of the drug minimize these symptoms. The effectiveness of isosorbide dinitrate and mononitrate may be reduced after a few months; if this occurs, an alternative treatment may need to be considered. They are not taken round the clock; it is usual to leave a drug-free interval overnight so that the drugs regain their effectiveness.

INFORMATION FOR USERS

Your drug prescription is tailored for you. Do not alter dosage without checking with your doctor.

How taken *Dinitrate* Tablets (held under the tongue, chewed, or swallowed), SR-tablets, SR-capsules, injection, spray. *Mononitrate* Tablets, SR-tablets, SR-capsules.

Frequency and timing of doses *Relief of angina attacks* Tablets chewed or held under the tongue, or spray, as needed (certain preparations only). *Prevention of angina* 2–4 x daily, not to be taken after 6pm; 1–2 x daily, maximum, to avoid loss of effectiveness (SR-tablets, capsules).

Adult dosage range *Relief of angina attacks* 5–10mg per dose. *Prevention of angina* 30–120mg daily.

Onset of effect 2–3 minutes when chewed or held under the tongue or used as spray (certain preparations only); 30 minutes when swallowed.

Duration of action Up to 2 hours (chewed); up to 5 hours (swallowed); up to 10 hours (SR-capsules).

Diet advice None.

Storage Keep in a closed container in a cool, dry place out of reach of children. Protect from light.

Missed dose Take as soon as you remember. If your next dose is due within 2 hours, take a single dose now and skip the next.

Stopping the drug Do not stop taking the drug without consulting your doctor;

stopping the drug may lead to worsening of the underlying condition.

Exceeding the dose An occasional unintentional extra dose is unlikely to cause problems. Large overdoses may cause dizziness and headache. Notify your doctor.

POSSIBLE ADVERSE EFFECTS

Flushing and headache are common. The most serious adverse effect is excessively lowered blood pressure, which may show itself as dizziness, fainting, or weakness, and should be discussed with your doctor. Other adverse effects of both forms of the drug usually improve after regular use; and an adjustment of dose may help.

INTERACTIONS

Antihypertensives A further lowering of blood pressure occurs when such drugs are taken with isosorbide dinitrate.

SPECIAL PRECAUTIONS

Be sure to tell your doctor if:
◆ You have long-term liver or kidney problems.
◆ You have any blood disorders or anaemia.
◆ You have had glaucoma.
◆ You have low blood pressure.
◆ You have ever had a heart attack.
◆ You have an underactive thyroid.
◆ You are taking other medications.

Pregnancy Safety in pregnancy not established. Discuss with your doctor.

Breast-feeding Safety not established. Discuss with your doctor.

Infants and children Not usually prescribed.

Over 60 No special problems.

Driving and hazardous work Avoid such activities until you have learned how isosorbide dinitrate or mononitrate affect you because these drugs can cause dizziness.

Alcohol Avoid excessive intake. Alcohol may further lower blood pressure, depressing the heart and causing dizziness and fainting.

PROLONGED USE

The initial adverse effects may disappear with prolonged use. The effects of the drug may also become weaker as the body adapts to the treatment, requiring increased dosage or other drugs.

Isotretinoin

Brand names Isotrex, Roaccutane
Used in the following combined preparation
Isotrexin

QUICK REFERENCE

Drug group Drug for acne (p.119)
Overdose danger rating Medium
Dependence rating Low
Prescription needed Yes
Available as generic No

GENERAL INFORMATION

Isotretinoin, a drug that is chemically related to vitamin A, is prescribed for the treatment of severe acne that has failed to respond to other treatments.

The drug reduces production of the skin's natural oils (sebum) and of the horny protein (keratin) in the outer layers of the skin, making it useful in conditions such as ichthyosis, in which the skin thickens abnormally, causing scaling.

A single 16-week course of treatment often clears the acne. The skin may be very dry, flaky, and itchy at first but usually improves as treatment continues. Serious adverse effects include liver damage and bowel inflammation. The drug may harm a developing fetus, and it should never be taken during pregnancy or by women planning pregnancy.

INFORMATION FOR USERS

Your drug prescription is tailored for you. Do not alter dosage without checking with your doctor.

How taken Capsules, gel.

Frequency and timing of doses 1–2 x daily (take capsules with food or milk).

Adult dosage range Dosage is determined individually.

Onset of effect 2–4 weeks. Acne may worsen during the first few weeks of treatment in some people.

Duration of action Effects persist for several weeks after the drug has been stopped. Acne is usually completely cleared.

Diet advice None.

Storage Keep in a closed container in a cool, dry place out of reach of children. Protect from light.

Missed dose Take as soon as you remember. If your next dose is due within 4 hours, take a single dose now and skip the next.

Stopping the drug Can be safely stopped as soon as you no longer need it, but best results are achieved when the course of treatment is completed as prescribed.

Exceeding the dose An occasional unintentional extra dose is unlikely to cause problems. Large overdoses may cause headaches, vomiting, abdominal pain, facial flushing, incoordination, and dizziness. Notify your doctor.

POSSIBLE ADVERSE EFFECTS

Dryness of the nose, mouth, and eyes, inflammation of the lips, and flaking of the skin occur in most cases. Mood changes, muscle or joint pains, and temporary loss or increased growth of hair may also occur. If you experience headache, accompanied by symptoms such as nausea and vomiting, abdominal pain with diarrhoea and/or blood in the faeces, or visual impairment, consult your doctor promptly.

INTERACTIONS

Tetracycline antibiotics These may increase the risk of pressure changes in the fluid around the brain, leading to headaches, nausea, and vomiting.

Skin-drying preparations Medicated cosmetics, soaps, toiletries, and anti- acne preparations increase the likelihood of dryness and irritation of the skin with isotretinoin.

Vitamin A Supplements of this vitamin increase the risk of adverse effects from isotretinoin.

SPECIAL PRECAUTIONS

Do not donate blood during, or for at least a month after, taking oral isotretinoin. Be sure to tell your doctor if:
◆ You have long-term liver or kidney problems.
◆ You suffer from arthritis.
◆ You have diabetes.
◆ You wear contact lenses.
◆ You suffer from gout.
◆ You are taking other medications.

Pregnancy Not prescribed. May cause abnormalities in the developing baby. Effective contraception must be used during treatment and for at least a month before and after.

Breast-feeding The drug passes into the breast milk and may affect the baby. Discuss with your doctor.

Infants and children Not prescribed.

Over 60 Not usually prescribed.

Driving and hazardous work Avoid such activities until you have learned how the drug affects you because it can cause vision problems in dim light or darkness.

Alcohol Regular heavy drinking may raise blood fat levels with isotretinoin.

Sunlight Avoid exposure to the sun and do not use a sunlamp or sunbed.

PROLONGED USE

A course of treatment rarely exceeds 16 weeks. Prolonged use may raise fat levels in the blood, thereby increasing the risk of heart and blood vessel disease. Bone changes may also occur.

Monitoring Liver function tests and periodic checks on fat levels in the blood are usually performed.

Ketoconazole

Brand name Nizoral
Used in the following combined preparations
None

QUICK REFERENCE

Drug group Antifungal drug (p.74)
Overdose danger rating Medium
Dependence rating Low
Prescription needed Yes
Available as generic No

GENERAL INFORMATION

Ketoconazole is prescribed for severe, internal systemic fungal infections. It is also given to treat serious infections of the skin and mucous membranes caused by the Candida yeast. People with rare fungal diseases (for example, paracoccidioidomycosis, histoplasmosis, and coccidioidomycosis) may also be given this antifungal drug.

Ketoconazole is applied as a cream to treat fungal skin infections, and as a shampoo for the treatment of scalp infections and seborrhoeic dermatitis.

The most common side effect with ketoconazole is nausea, which can be reduced by taking the drug at bedtime or with meals. Ketoconazole may also cause liver damage.

INFORMATION FOR USERS

Your drug prescription is tailored for you. Do not alter dosage without checking with your doctor.
How taken Tablets, liquid, cream, shampoo.
Frequency and timing of doses Once daily with food (by mouth); 1–2 x daily (cream); 1–2 times weekly (shampoo used for seborrhoeic dermatitis).
Dosage range *Adults* 200–400mg daily (by mouth). *Children* Reduced dose according to age and weight.
Onset of effect The drug begins to work within a few hours; full beneficial effect may take several days.
Duration of action Up to 24 hours.
Diet advice None.
Storage Keep in a closed container in a cool, dry place out of reach of children.
Missed dose (oral) Take as soon as you remember. If your next dose is due within

6 hours, take a single dose now and skip the next.
Stopping the drug Unless severe adverse effects occur (see below), take the full course. Even if you feel better, the infection may still be present; symptoms may recur if treatment is stopped too soon.
Exceeding the dose An occasional unintentional extra dose is unlikely to be a cause for concern. Large overdoses may cause gastric problems. Notify your doctor.

POSSIBLE ADVERSE EFFECTS

Nausea is the most common side effect of ketoconazole; vomiting, abdominal pain, and headache may also occur. Liver damage is a rare but serious adverse effect, causing jaundice that may necessitate stopping the drug. If you develop itching, a rash, or painful breasts (men), stop taking the drug and consult your doctor.

INTERACTIONS (ADMINISTRATION BY MOUTH ONLY)

Antacids, cimetidine, and ranitidine These drugs may reduce the effectiveness of ketoconazole if they are taken within 2 hours before or after ketoconazole.
Rifampicin This drug reduces the effect of ketoconazole.
Sedatives and warfarin Ketoconazole increases the effects of these drugs.
Ciclosporin, tacrolimus, and theophylline Ketoconazole increases the level of these drugs in the blood.
Phenytoin Levels of ketoconazole may be reduced by phenytoin.
Simvastatin Ketoconazole may increase the risk of muscle damage if it is taken with this drug.

SPECIAL PRECAUTIONS

Be sure to tell your doctor if:
◆ You have long-term liver or kidney problems.
◆ You have porphyria.
◆ You have previously had an allergic reaction to antifungal drugs.
◆ You are taking other medications.
Pregnancy Not usually prescribed. May cause defects in the developing baby. Discuss with your doctor.

Breast-feeding The drug passes into the breast milk and may affect the baby. Discuss with your doctor.
Infants and children Reduced dose necessary.
Over 60 No special problems.
Driving and hazardous work No special problems.
Alcohol Avoid. Alcohol may interact with this drug to cause flushing and nausea.

PROLONGED USE
The risk of liver damage increases with use for more than 14 days.
Monitoring Periodic blood tests are usually performed to check the effect of the drug on the liver.

Ketoprofen

Brand names Fenoket, Ketocid, Ketovail, Ketozip, Larafen, Orudis, Oruvail, Powergel
Used in the following combined preparations
None

QUICK REFERENCE
Drug group Non-steroidal anti-inflammatory drug (p.49)
Overdose danger rating Medium
Dependence rating Low
Prescription needed No
Available as generic No

GENERAL INFORMATION
Ketoprofen is a member of the non-steroidal anti-inflammatory (NSAID) group of drugs. Like other NSAIDs, it relieves pain and reduces inflammation and stiffness in rheumatoid arthritis, osteoarthritis, and ankylosing spondylitis. Ketoprofen does not cure the underlying disease, however.

Ketoprofen is also given to relieve the mild to moderate pain of menstruation and soft tissue injuries, and the pain that occurs following operations.

The most common adverse reactions to ketoprofen, as with all NSAIDs, are gastrointestinal disturbances such as nausea and indigestion. Switching to another NSAID may be recommended by your doctor if unwanted effects are persistent or troublesome.

INFORMATION FOR USERS
Follow instructions on the label. Call your doctor if symptoms worsen.
How taken Tablets, capsules, injection, suppositories, gel.
Frequency and timing of doses 2–4 x daily with food (by mouth). 6 x daily for up to 3 days (injection). 2 x daily (suppositories).
Adult dosage range 100–200mg daily.
Onset of effect Pain relief may be felt in 30 minutes to 2 hours. Full anti-inflammatory effect may not be felt for up to 2 weeks.
Duration of action Up to 8–12 hours.
Diet advice None.
Storage Keep in a closed container in a cool, dry place out of reach of children.
Missed dose Take as soon as you remember. If your next dose is due within 4 hours, take a single dose now and skip the next.
Stopping the drug Unless severe adverse effects occur (see below), seek medical advice before stopping the drug.
Exceeding the dose An occasional unintentional extra dose is unlikely to be a cause for concern. Large overdoses may cause vomiting, confusion, or irritability. Notify your doctor.

POSSIBLE ADVERSE EFFECTS
Gastrointestinal disturbances, such as nausea, abdominal pain, and indigestion, commonly occur with ketoprofen when taken by mouth. Dizziness, drowsiness, and headache or fluid retention (leading to swollen feet or legs and weight gain) may also occur. Suppositories may cause rectal irritation. Black or bloodstained faeces should be reported promptly. If you develop a rash, itching, wheezing, or breathlessness, stop taking the drug and consult your doctor urgently.

INTERACTIONS
General note Ketoprofen interacts with a wide range of drugs, such as other NSAIDs including aspirin, oral anticoagulants, and corticosteroids, to increase the risk of bleeding and/or stomach ulcers.
Methotrexate Ketoprofen may raise blood levels of methotrexate, leading to an increased risk of adverse effects.
Phenytoin Ketoprofen may enhance the effects of phenytoin.

Quinolone antibiotics Ketoprofen may increase the risk of seizures if taken with these drugs.

Antihypertensive drugs Ketoprofen may reduce the beneficial effects of these drugs.

SPECIAL PRECAUTIONS

Be sure to consult your doctor or pharmacist before taking this drug if:

◆ You have long-term liver or kidney problems.

◆ You have heart problems.

◆ You have high blood pressure.

◆ You have asthma.

◆ You have had a peptic ulcer, oesophagitis, or acid indigestion.

◆ You have bleeding problems.

◆ You are allergic to aspirin or other NSAIDs.

◆ You are taking other medications.

Pregnancy Safety in pregnancy not established. Discuss with your doctor.

Breast-feeding The drug passes into the breast milk and may affect the baby. Discuss with your doctor.

Infants and children Not recommended for children under 12 years.

Over 60 Reduced dose may be necessary. Increased likelihood of adverse effects.

Driving and hazardous work Avoid such activities until you have learned how ketoprofen affects you because the drug can cause dizziness and drowsiness.

Alcohol Avoid. Alcohol may increase the risk of stomach disorders with ketoprofen.

Surgery and general anaesthetics Ketoprofen may prolong bleeding. Discuss this with your doctor or dentist before having any surgery.

PROLONGED USE

There is an increased risk of bleeding from peptic ulcers and in the bowel with prolonged use of ketoprofen.

Lactulose

Brand names Duphalac, Lactugal, Laxose, Osmolax, Regulose
Used in the following combined preparations
None

QUICK REFERENCE
Drug group Laxative (p.43)
Overdose danger rating Low
Dependence rating Low
Prescription needed No
Available as generic Yes

GENERAL INFORMATION

Lactulose is an effective laxative that softens faeces by increasing the amount of water in the large intestine. It is used for the relief of constipation and faecal impaction, especially in the elderly. It is less likely than some of the other laxatives to disrupt normal bowel action.

Lactulose is also used for preventing and treating brain disturbance associated with liver failure, known as hepatic encephalopathy.

Because lactulose acts locally in the large intestine and is not absorbed into the body, it is safer than many other laxatives. However, the drug can cause stomach cramps and flatulence especially at the start of treatment.

INFORMATION FOR USERS

Follow instructions on the label. Call your doctor if symptoms worsen.
How taken Liquid, powder.
Frequency and timing of doses 2 x daily (chronic constipation); 3–4 x daily (liver failure).
Adult dosage range 15–30ml daily (chronic constipation); 90–150ml daily (liver failure).
Onset of effect 24–48 hours.
Duration of action 6–18 hours.
Diet advice It is important to maintain an adequate intake of fluid – up to 8 glasses of water daily.
Storage Keep in a closed container in a cool, dry place out of reach of children. Do not store after diluting.
Missed dose Take as soon as you remember. If your next dose is due within 3 hours, take a single dose now and skip the next.
Stopping the drug In the treatment of constipation, the drug can be safely stopped as soon as you no longer need it.

Exceeding the dose An occasional unintentional extra dose is unlikely to be a cause for concern. But if you notice any unusual symptoms, or if a large overdose has been taken, notify your doctor.

POSSIBLE ADVERSE EFFECTS

Adverse effects, which include belching and flatulence, nausea, abdominal distension, and stomach cramps, are rarely serious and often disappear when your body adjusts to the medicine. The occurrence of diarrhoea may indicate that the dosage of lactulose is too high.

INTERACTIONS

Mesalazine Lactulose may reduce the release of mesalazine at the site of action.

SPECIAL PRECAUTIONS

Be sure to consult your doctor or pharmacist before taking this drug if:
◆ You have severe abdominal pain.
◆ You suffer from lactose intolerance or galactosaemia.
◆ You are taking other medications.
Pregnancy No evidence of risk. Discuss with your doctor.
Breast-feeding No evidence of risk.
Infants and children Reduced dose necessary.
Over 60 No special problems.
Driving and hazardous work No known problems.
Alcohol No known problems.

PROLONGED USE

No problems expected.

Lamivudine

Brand names Epivir, Zeffix
Used in the following combined preparation
Combivir

QUICK REFERENCE
Drug group Drug for AIDS and immune deficiency (p.97)
Overdose danger rating Medium
Dependence rating Medium
Prescription needed Yes
Available as generic No

GENERAL INFORMATION

Lamivudine is an antiviral drug used in the treatment of HIV. It has also been used to treat hepatitis B virus infections. Lamivudine is a nucleoside reverse transcriptase inhibitor. When used to treat HIV, it is always prescribed with another drug to help prevent resistance from developing. The drug slows the progression of, but does not cure, the illness.

Often, when starting treatment, three drugs are used: two nucleoside reverse transcriptase inhibitors and a third from another class, such as ritonavir, a protease inhibitor. But these combinations may need to be changed during treatment if the patient's condition worsens.

Health workers and others who are occupationally exposed to HIV may be treated with these drugs to try to protect them from becoming HIV positive and developing AIDS.

INFORMATION FOR USERS

Your drug prescription is tailored for you. Do not alter dosage without checking with your doctor.

How taken Tablets, oral solution.
Frequency and timing of doses 2 x daily (HIV); once daily (Hepatitis B).
Adult dosage range HIV 300mg daily. Hepatitis B 100mg daily.
Onset of effect 1 hour.
Duration of action 12 hours.
Diet advice None.
Storage Keep in a closed container in a cool, dry place out of reach of children.
Missed dose Take as soon as you remember. If your next dose is due within 2 hours, take a single dose now and skip the next.
Stopping the drug Do not stop taking the drug without consulting your doctor because of the danger of drug resistance developing.
Exceeding the dose An occasional unintentional extra dose is unlikely to cause problems. But if you notice any unusual symptoms, or if a large overdose has been taken, notify your doctor.

POSSIBLE ADVERSE EFFECTS

Nausea, vomiting, diarrhoea, and abdominal pain are the most common adverse effects of lamivudine. A cough, headache, tingling, and a "pins and needles" sensation may also occur. If rash, hair loss, malaise, fever, jaundice, or sore throat occur, consult your doctor. If you experience severe abdominal pain, seek urgent medical advice.

INTERACTIONS

Trimethoprim and co-trimoxazole These drugs increase blood levels of lamivudine.

SPECIAL PRECAUTIONS

Be sure to tell your doctor if:
◆ You have liver or kidney problems.
◆ You have had a previous allergic reaction to lamivudine.
◆ You are taking other medications.
Pregnancy Safety not established. Discuss with your doctor.
Breast-feeding Safety not established. Discuss with your doctor.
Infants and children Safety not established under 3 months. Reduced dose necessary in older infants and children.
Over 60 Reduced dose may be necessary. Increased likelihood of adverse effects.
Driving and hazardous work No special problems.
Alcohol No special problems.

PROLONGED USE

White blood-cell production may be affected by lamivudine during long-term use.
Monitoring Regular blood counts are usually carried out.

Lamotrigine

Brand name Lamictal
Used in the following combined preparations
None

QUICK REFERENCE

Drug group Anticonvulsant drug (p.16)
Overdose danger rating Medium
Dependence rating Low
Prescription needed Yes
Available as generic No

GENERAL INFORMATION

Lamotrigine, introduced in 1993, is an anticonvulsant drug prescribed, either alone or in combination with other anticonvulsants, for the treatment of epilepsy. It acts by restoring the balance between excitatory and inhibitory neurotransmitters in the brain. The drug may be less sedating than older anticonvulsants, and there is no need for blood tests to determine its level in the blood.

Lamotrigine may cause a number of minor adverse effects (see below), most of which will respond to dosage adjustment. Unlike many of the older anticonvulsants, it does not interfere with the action of oral contraceptives.

INFORMATION FOR USERS
Your drug prescription is tailored for you. Do not alter dosage without checking with your doctor.
How taken Tablets, dispersible tablets.
Frequency and timing of doses 1–2 x daily.
Adult dosage range 100–500mg (100–200mg if given together with sodium valproate) daily (maintenance dose). Smaller doses are used at the start of treatment.
Onset of effect Approximately 5 days at a constant dose.
Duration of action Up to 24 hours.
Diet advice None.
Storage Keep in a closed container in a cool, dry place out of reach of children.
Missed dose Take as soon as you remember. If your next dose is due within 2 hours, take a single dose now and skip the next.
Stopping the drug Do not stop taking the drug without consulting your doctor, who will supervise a gradual reduction in dosage over a period of about two weeks. Abrupt cessation increases the risk of rebound fits.
Exceeding the dose An occasional unintentional extra dose is unlikely to be a cause for concern. Large overdoses may cause sedation, double vision, loss of muscular coordination, nausea, and vomiting. Contact your doctor immediately.

POSSIBLE ADVERSE EFFECTS
Serious adverse effects are rare. The most common side effects are rash, nausea, headache, tiredness, insomnia, blurred or double vision, dizziness, agitation, confusion, and poor muscle coordination. These will respond to a dose reduction, and a rash is less likely if the treatment is started at a low dose (25mg), increasing gradually over about 4 weeks. If sore throat, swelling around the face, flu-like symptoms, or persistent or unusual bruising occur, consult your doctor immediately.

INTERACTIONS
Sodium valproate increases and prolongs the effectiveness of lamotrigine; a reduced dose of lamotrigine will be used.
Carbamazepine may reduce lamotrigine blood levels, but lamotrigine may increase the side effects of carbamazepine.
Phenytoin and phenobarbital may decrease blood levels of lamotrigine so a higher dose of lamotrigine may be needed.

SPECIAL PRECAUTIONS
Be sure to tell your doctor if:
◆ You have long-term liver or kidney problems.
◆ You suffer from thalassaemia.
◆ You have heart disease.
◆ You are taking other medications.
Pregnancy Safety in pregnancy not established. Discuss with your doctor.
Breast-feeding Safety in breast-feeding not established. Discuss with your doctor.
Infants and children Not recommended under 2 years. Not recommended as a single therapy under 12 years. Doses may be relatively higher than adult doses due to increased metabolism.
Over 60s The dose may need to be reduced.
Driving and hazardous work Your underlying condition, as well as the possibility of sedation, dizziness, and visual disturbances while taking lamotrigine, may make such activities inadvisable. Discuss with your doctor.
Alcohol Alcohol may increase the adverse effects of this drug.

PROLONGED USE
No special problems.

Lansoprazole

Brand name Zoton
Used in the following combined preparations
None

QUICK REFERENCE
Drug group Anti-ulcer drug (p.41)
Overdose danger rating Low

Dependence rating Low
Prescription needed Yes
Available as generic No

GENERAL INFORMATION

Lansoprazole is an anti-ulcer drug that belongs to the group of drugs known as proton pump inhibitors (p.41). It is used to treat peptic ulcers, gastro-oesophageal reflux (in which the stomach acid rises into and irritates the oesophagus), and Zollinger-Ellison syndrome (in which large quantities of stomach acid are produced, leading to ulceration).

Lansoprazole may be used alone or, for peptic ulcers, with two antibiotics, as part of a seven-day regimen to eradicate *Helicobacter pylori* bacteria, which are the main cause of such ulcers.

INFORMATION FOR USERS

Your drug prescription is tailored for you. Do not alter dosage without checking with your doctor.
How taken Capsules, oral suspension.
Frequency and timing of doses 1–2 x daily in the morning.
Dosage range *Benign gastric ulcer* 30mg daily. NSAID-associated gastric ulcer 15–30mg daily. *Duodenal ulcer* 30mg daily; 15mg daily (maintenance dose). *Helicobacter. pylori-associated ulcer* 60mg daily.
Onset of effect 1–2 hours.
Duration of action 24 hours.
Diet advice No specific advice, although spicy foods and alcohol may exacerbate the condition.
Storage Keep in a closed container in a cool, dry place out of reach of children.
Missed dose Take as soon as you remember. If your next dose is due within 8 hours, take a single dose now and skip the next.
Stopping the drug Unless rash, itching, wheezing, or breathing difficulties occur (see below), do not stop taking the drug without consulting your doctor; symptoms may recur.
Exceeding the dose An occasional unintentional extra dose is unlikely to be a cause for concern. But if you notice any unusual symptoms, or if a large overdose has been taken, notify your doctor.

POSSIBLE ADVERSE EFFECTS

Common side effects include headache, fatigue or dizziness, indigestion, flatulence and abdominal pain, and diarrhoea or constipation. If you experience muscle or joint pain, excessive bruising, or swollen extremities, consult your doctor. Sore throat and breathlessness are rare but should be reported to your doctor at once. If you develop a rash, itching, wheezing, or breathing difficulties, stop taking the drug and consult your doctor urgently.

INTERACTIONS

Oral contraceptives, phenytoin, warfarin, theophylline Lansoprazole may reduce the effect of these drugs.
Antacids and sucralfate These drugs may reduce the absorption of, and should not be taken within an hour of, lansoprazole.

SPECIAL PRECAUTIONS

Be sure to tell your doctor if:
◆ You have liver problems.
◆ You are taking other medications.
Pregnancy Safety not established. Discuss with your doctor.
Breast-feeding Safety not established. Discuss with your doctor.
Infants and children Not recommended.
Over 60 No special problems.
Driving and hazardous work No special problems.
Alcohol Avoid. Alcohol may aggravate your condition and reduce the beneficial effects of lansoprazole.

PROLONGED USE

No problems expected.

Levodopa

Brand names None
Used in the following combined preparations Madopar, Sinemet

QUICK REFERENCE

Drug group Drug for parkinsonism (p.18)
Overdose danger rating Medium
Dependence rating Low
Prescription needed Yes
Available as generic Yes

GENERAL INFORMATION

The treatment of Parkinson's disease underwent dramatic change in the 1960s with the introduction of levodopa. Since the body can transform levodopa into dopamine, a chemical messenger in the brain the absence or shortage of which causes Parkinson's disease (see p.18), rapid improvements in control were obtained. These were a marked relief of symptoms but were not a cure for the disease.

However, it was found that, while levodopa was effective, it produced severe side effects, such as nausea, dizziness, and palpitations. Even when treatment was initiated gradually, it was difficult to balance the benefits against the adverse reactions.

Today the drug is combined with carbidopa or benserazide, which enhance its effects in the brain and help to reduce its side effects.

INFORMATION FOR USERS

Your drug prescription is tailored for you. Do not alter dosage without checking with your doctor.

How taken Tablets, capsules.
Frequency and timing of doses 3–6 x daily with food or milk.
Adult dosage range 125–500mg initially, increased until benefits and side effects are balanced.
Onset of effect Within 1 hour.
Duration of action 2–12 hours.
Diet advice None.
Storage Keep in a closed container in a cool, dry place out of reach of children. Protect from light.
Missed dose Take as soon as you remember. If your next dose is due within 2 hours, take a single dose now and skip the next.
Stopping the drug Unless palpitations occur, do not stop taking the drug without consulting your doctor; stopping the drug may lead to severe worsening of the underlying condition.
Exceeding the dose An occasional unintentional extra dose is unlikely to cause problems. Larger overdoses may cause vomiting or drowsiness. Notify your doctor.

POSSIBLE ADVERSE EFFECTS

Adverse effects are closely related to dosage levels. At the start of treatment, when dosage is usually low, unwanted effects are likely to be mild. These include digestive disturbances, abnormal movement, and nervousness or agitation. Dizziness, fainting, confusion, and vivid dreams may also occur and may increase in severity as the dosage is increased to boost the drug's beneficial effects. Darkening of the urine can be ignored; all other adverse effects should be discussed with your doctor. If you experience palpitations, stop taking the drug and seek urgent medical advice.

INTERACTIONS

Antidepressants Levodopa may interact with MAOIs to cause a dangerous rise in blood pressure. It may also interact with tricyclic antidepressants.
Iron This may reduce absorption of levodopa.
Antipsychotic drugs Some of these drugs may reduce the effect of levodopa.
Pyridoxine (vitamin B_6) Excessive intake of this vitamin may reduce the effect of levodopa.

SPECIAL PRECAUTIONS

Be sure to tell your doctor if:
◆ You have heart problems.
◆ You have long-term liver or kidney problems.
◆ You have a lung disorder, such as asthma or bronchitis.
◆ You have an overactive thyroid gland.
◆ You have had glaucoma.
◆ You have a peptic ulcer.
◆ You have diabetes.
◆ You have any serious mental illness.
◆ You have ever had malignant melanoma.
◆ You are taking other medications.
Pregnancy Unlikely to be required.
Breast-feeding Unlikely to be required.
Infants and children Not normally used.
Over 60 No special problems.
Driving and hazardous work Your underlying condition, and the possibility of the drug causing fainting and dizziness, may make such activities inadvisable. Discuss with your doctor.
Alcohol No known problems.

PROLONGED USE

Effectiveness usually declines in time, necessitating increased dosage or the addition of other drugs (see p.18). The adverse effects may become so severe that ultimately the drug must be stopped.

Levofloxacin

Brand name Tavanic
Used in the following combined preparations
None

QUICK REFERENCE
Drug group Antibacterial (p.64)
Overdose danger rating Medium
Dependence rating Low
Prescription needed Yes
Available as generic No

GENERAL INFORMATION

Levofloxacin is a quinolone antibacterial drug used for soft-tissue and respiratory and urinary tract infections that have not responded to other antibiotics.

The drug is usually prescribed as tablets, but it is administered by intravenous infusion to people with serious systemic infections or those who cannot take drugs by mouth.

Like other quinolones, levofloxacin may occasionally cause tendon inflammation and damage, especially in the elderly or in people taking corticosteroids. You should, therefore, stop taking the drug and report tendon pain or inflammation to your doctor immediately. The affected limb or limbs should be rested until the symptoms have subsided.

INFORMATION FOR USERS

Your drug prescription is tailored for you. Do not alter dosage without checking with your doctor.
How taken Tablets, injection.
Frequency and timing of doses 1 x 2 times daily for 7–14 days depending on infection (tablets).
Adult dosage range 250–1,000mg daily.
Onset of effect 1 hour.
Duration of action 12–24 hours.
Diet advice None.
Storage Keep in a closed container in a cool, dry place out of reach of children.
Missed dose Take as soon as you remember, then take your next dose when it is due.
Stopping the drug Unless severe adverse effects occur (see below), take the full course. Even if you feel better, the original infection may still be present, and symptoms may recur if treatment is stopped too soon.

Exceeding the dose An occasional unintentional extra dose is unlikely to cause problems. Larger overdoses may cause mental disturbances and fits. Notify your doctor.

POSSIBLE ADVERSE EFFECTS

Nausea and vomiting are the most common adverse effects of levofloxacin taken by mouth. Abdominal pain, diarrhoea, dizziness, headache, restlessness, drowsiness, itching, and rash, may also occur. Given by injection, the drug may cause palpitations and giddiness due to a fall in blood pressure. If jaundice, confusion, hallucinations, fever, rash, painful or inflamed tendons, itching, wheezing, or breathlessness occur, stop taking the drug and consult your doctor urgently.

INTERACTIONS

NSAIDs and theophylline There is an increased risk of convulsions when these drugs are taken with levofloxacin.

Anticoagulants The effect of these drugs may be increased by levofloxacin.

Antacids, adsorbents, sucralfate, iron and zinc These drugs may reduce the absorption of levofloxacin.

Ciclosporin There is an increased risk of kidney damage if ciclosporin is taken with levofloxacin.

SPECIAL PRECAUTIONS

Be sure to tell your doctor if:
◆ You have kidney problems.
◆ You suffer from epilepsy.
◆ You have glucose-6-phosphate dehydrogenase (G6PD) deficiency.
◆ You are taking aspirin or another NSAID.
◆ You have had a previous allergic reaction to a quinolone antibacterial.
◆ You have had a previous tendon problem with a quinolone.
◆ You are taking other medications.
Pregnancy Safety not established. Discuss with your doctor.
Breast-feeding Safety not established. Discuss with your doctor.
Infants and children Not recommended.
Over 60 No special problems, except that tendon damage is more likely over the age of 60.
Driving and hazardous work Avoid such activities until you have learned how levofloxacin

affects you because the drug can cause dizziness, drowsiness, visual disturbances, and hallucinations.

Alcohol Avoid. Alcohol may increase the sedative effects of levofloxacin.

PROLONGED USE
Not usually prescribed for long-term use.

Levonorgestrel

Brand names Microval, Norgeston
Used in the following combined preparations
Ciclo-progynova, Eugynon 30, Microgynon 30, Ovranette, and others

QUICK REFERENCE
Drug group Female sex hormone (p.86) and oral contraceptive (p.101)
Overdose danger rating Low
Dependence rating Low
Prescription needed Yes
Available as generic No

GENERAL INFORMATION
Levonorgestrel is a synthetic hormone similar to progesterone, a natural female sex hormone. The drug's primary use is as an ingredient in oral contraceptives. It performs this function by thickening the mucus at the neck of the uterus (cervix), thereby making it difficult for sperm to enter the uterus. Levonorgestrel is available both in combined oral contraceptives with an oestrogen drug and in progestogen- only preparations.

It is occasionally given alone or with an oestrogen for emergency, post-coital contraception. It is also given in combination with an oestrogen drug in hormone replacement therapy to treat menopausal symptoms.

Levonorgestrel rarely causes serious adverse effects. When it is used without an oestrogen, menstrual irregularities, especially mid-cycle, or "breakthrough", bleeding are common.

INFORMATION FOR USERS
Your drug prescription is tailored for you. Do not alter dosage without checking with your doctor.

How taken Tablets, implant, intrauterine device (IUD).

Frequency and timing of doses Once daily, at the same time each day.

Adult dosage range *Progestogen-only pills* 30 micrograms daily.

Onset of effect Levonorgestrel starts to act within 4 hours, but contraceptive protection may not be fully effective for 14 days, depending on which day of the cycle the tablets are started.

Duration of action 24 hours. Some effects may persist for up to 3 months after levonorgestrel is stopped.

Diet advice None.

Storage Keep in a closed container in a cool, dry place out of reach of children.

Missed dose If a tablet is delayed by 3 hours or more, regard it as a missed dose. See What to do if you miss a pill (p.104).

Stopping the drug The drug can be safely stopped as soon as contraceptive protection is no longer required. For treatment of menopausal symptoms, consult your doctor before stopping the drug.

Exceeding the dose An occasional unintentional extra dose is unlikely to be a cause for concern. But if you notice any unusual symptoms, or if a large overdose has been taken, notify your doctor.

POSSIBLE ADVERSE EFFECTS
Menstrual irregularities (blood spotting between menstrual periods or absence of menstruation) are the most common side effects of levonorgestrel alone. Fluid retention, leading to swollen feet or ankles, and weight gain may occur. Nausea, vomiting, and breast tenderness are also adverse effects. If you develop headache or depression, consult your doctor.

INTERACTIONS
General note The beneficial effects of many drugs, including bromocriptine, oral anticoagulants, anticonvulsants, and antihypertensive and antidiabetic drugs, may be affected by levonorgestrel. Many other drugs may affect the action of oral contraceptives, reducing contraceptive protection. These include anticonvulsants, antituberculous drugs, and antibiotics. Inform your doctor that you are taking this drug before taking additional prescribed medication.

SPECIAL PRECAUTIONS
Be sure to tell your doctor if:
◆ You have a liver problem.
◆ You have heart failure or high blood pressure.
◆ You have diabetes.
◆ You have unexplained abnormal vaginal bleeding.
◆ You have had blood clots or a stroke.
◆ You have ever had migraines or severe headaches.
◆ You are taking other medications.

Pregnancy Not prescribed. May cause abnormalities in the developing baby. Discuss with your doctor.

Breast-feeding The drug passes into the breast milk, but at normal doses adverse effects on the baby are unlikely. Discuss with your doctor.

Infants and children Not prescribed.

Over 60 Not prescribed.

Driving and hazardous work No known problems.

Alcohol No known problems.

PROLONGED USE
Problems are rare.

Lisinopril

Brand names Carace, Zestril
Used in the following combined preparations
Carace Plus, Zestoretic

QUICK REFERENCE
Drug group ACE inhibitor vasodilator (p.30)
Overdose danger rating Medium
Dependence rating Low
Prescription needed Yes
Available as generic No

GENERAL INFORMATION
Lisinopril belongs to the ACE (angiotensin converting enzyme) inhibitor group of drugs and is used to treat high blood pressure (p.34) and heart failure (in which the heart is unable to deal with its workload). It may also be given to patients following a heart attack and is sometimes used to prevent or delay kidney damage in patients with diabetes. It is also often given with a diuretic to increase its effect on high blood pressure and heart failure. Lisinopril works by relaxing the muscles in blood vessel walls, allowing the vessels to dilate (widen), which enables the blood to circulate more easily and helps to lower blood pressure. The drug is long acting and may be taken once daily. The first dose may cause a sudden drop in blood pressure, especially in patients taking a diuretic; for this reason, you should lie down for 2–3 hours afterwards.

A variety of minor side effects may occur with lisinopril; many people develop a persistent dry cough, while others experience taste disturbance, which a reduction in dose may help to minimize.

INFORMATION FOR USERS
Your drug prescription is tailored for you. Do not alter dosage without checking with your doctor.

How taken Tablets.
Frequency and timing of doses Once daily.
Adult dosage range *Hypertension* 2.5mg (starting dose) up to 40mg. *Heart failure/diabetic nephropathy* 2.5mg (starting dose) up to 20mg. *Prevention of further heart attacks* 2.5–5mg (starting dose) up to 10mg.
Onset of effect 1–2 hours; full beneficial effect may take several weeks.
Duration of action 12–24 hours.
Diet advice None.
Storage Keep in a closed container in a cool, dry place out of reach of children.
Missed dose Take as soon as you remember. If your next dose is due within 8 hours, take a single dose now and skip the next.
Stopping the drug Unless severe adverse effects occur (see below), do not stop taking the drug without consulting your doctor. Stopping the drug may lead to worsening of the underlying condition.
Exceeding the dose An occasional unintentional extra dose is unlikely to be a cause for concern. Larger overdoses may cause dizziness or fainting. Notify your doctor.

POSSIBLE ADVERSE EFFECTS
Dizziness on standing is likely to occur after the first dose. Nausea and headache are common but are usually mild and transient. A persistent dry cough is the most common

adverse effect, but this can be minimized by taking smaller, more frequent, doses; some people may have to stop taking the drug. Rash or itching may occur. If dizziness or fainting, runny nose or sore throat, confusion or mood changes, or chest pain or palpitations occur, consult your doctor. If you develop jaundice, swelling of the face, or breathing difficulties, stop taking the drug and seek urgent medical advice.

INTERACTIONS

Potassium supplements, potassium-sparing diuretics, and ciclosporin Taken with lisinopril, these drugs increase the risk of high blood potassium levels.

NSAIDs Some of these drugs may reduce the effect of lisinopril, and the risk of kidney damage is increased.

Vasodilators, diuretics, and other drugs for hypertension These drugs may increase the effect of lisinopril.

Lithium Blood levels of lithium may be increased by lisinopril.

Insulin and antidiabetic drugs Lisinopril may increase the effect of these drugs.

SPECIAL PRECAUTIONS

Be sure to tell your doctor if:
◆ You have suffered from severe allergies.
◆ You have long-term kidney problems.
◆ You have coronary artery disease.
◆ You peripheral vascular disease.
◆ You are on a low sodium diet.
◆ You are allergic to other ACE inhibitors.
◆ You are taking other medications.

Pregnancy Not prescribed. May cause defects in the developing baby.

Breast-feeding The drug passes into the breast milk, but at normal doses adverse effects on the baby are unlikely. Discuss with your doctor.

Infants and children Not usually prescribed.

Over 60 Reduced dose may be necessary.

Driving and hazardous work Avoid such activities until you have learned how lisinopril affects you because the drug can cause dizziness and fainting.

Alcohol Avoid excessive amounts. Alcohol may increase the blood-pressure lowering and adverse effects of this drug.

Surgery and general anaesthetics Notify your doctor or dentist that you are taking lisinopril.

PROLONGED USE

Rarely, prolonged use of lisinopril can lead to changes in blood count or kidney function.

Monitoring Periodic checks on potassium levels, white blood cell counts and urine are usually performed.

Lithium

Brand names Camcolit, Li-liquid, Liskonum, Litarex, Priadel

Used in the following combined preparation Efalith

QUICK REFERENCE

Drug group Antimanic drug (p.16)
Overdose danger rating High
Dependence rating Low
Prescription needed Yes
Available as generic No

GENERAL INFORMATION

Lithium, the lightest known metal, has been used since the 1940s in the form of various salts to treat a severe mental disturbance, manic depressive illness. Lithium decreases the intensity and frequency of the episodic swings from extreme excitement to deep depression that are characteristic of the disorder.

Although preferred for mania alone, it is also sometimes used to prevent and treat severe depression (see p.14). Treatment with lithium may be started in hospital for the more seriously ill. Careful monitoring is required because high blood levels of lithium can cause serious adverse effects. Since it may take two to three weeks for any benefit to become apparent, an antipsychotic drug (p.15) is often given with lithium until the lithium becomes effective.

INFORMATION FOR USERS

Your drug prescription is tailored for you. Do not alter dosage without checking with your doctor.

How taken Tablets, SR-tablets, liquid.

Frequency and timing of doses 1–2 x daily with meals. Always take the same brand of lithium to ensure a consistent effect; change of brand must be closely supervised.

Adult dosage range 0.25–2g daily. Dosage may vary according to individual response.

Onset of effect Some effects may be noticed in 3–5 days, but full benefits may not be felt for 3 weeks.

Duration of action 18–36 hours. Some effect may last for several days.

Diet advice Blood lithium levels are affected by the amount of sodium in the body; do not suddenly increase or reduce the amount of salt in your diet. Be sure to drink adequate volumes of fluids, especially in hot weather.

Storage Keep in a closed container in a cool, dry place out of reach of children.

Missed dose Take as soon as you remember. If your next dose is due within 4 hours, take a single dose now and skip the next.

Stopping the drug Unless severe adverse effects occur (see below), do not stop taking the drug without consulting your doctor; symptoms may recur.

OVERDOSE ACTION

Seek immediate medical advice in all cases. Take emergency action if convulsions or loss of consciousness occur.

POSSIBLE ADVERSE EFFECTS

Many of the following adverse effects may be signs of a high lithium level in the blood: tremor, muscle weakness, thirst and increased urine production, weight gain, nausea, vomiting, diarrhoea, drowsiness, lethargy, and blurred vision. Stop taking the drug and seek medical advice promptly if you notice any of these symptoms. Also stop taking the drug and consult your doctor urgently if you develop a rash.

INTERACTIONS

General note Many drugs interact with lithium. Do not take any over-the-counter or prescription drugs without consulting your doctor or pharmacist. Paracetamol should be used in preference to other analgesics for everyday pain relief.

SPECIAL PRECAUTIONS

Be sure to tell your doctor if:
◆ You have long-term liver or kidney problems.
◆ You have heart or circulation problems.

◆ You have an overactive thyroid gland. You have myasthenia gravis.
◆ You have Addison's disease.
◆ You are taking other medications.

Pregnancy Not usually prescribed. May cause defects in the unborn baby. Discuss with your doctor.

Breast-feeding The drug passes into the breast milk and may affect the baby. Discuss with your doctor.

Infants and children Not recommended.

Over 60 Reduced dose may be necessary. Increased likelihood of adverse effects.

Driving and hazardous work Avoid such activities until you have learned how lithium affects you because the drug can cause reduced alertness.

Alcohol Avoid. Alcohol may increase the sedative effects of this drug.

PROLONGED USE

Prolonged use may lead to kidney problems. Treatment for periods of longer than 5 years is not normally advised unless the benefits are significant and tests show no sign of reduced kidney function.

Monitoring Regular monitoring of blood levels of the drug and the composition of the blood is usually carried out. Kidney and thyroid function should also be monitored.

Lofepramine

Brand name Gamanil
Used in the following combined preparations None

QUICK REFERENCE

Drug group Tricyclic antidepressant drug (p.14)
Overdose danger rating Medium
Dependence rating Low
Prescription needed Yes
Available as generic Yes

GENERAL INFORMATION

Lofepramine belongs to the tricyclic antidepressant group of drugs. Used primarily in the long-term treatment of depression, the drug serves to elevate mood, improve appetite, increase physical activity, and restore interest in everyday activities.

Less sedating than some other tricyclics, lofepramine is particularly useful when the depression accompanied by lethargy.

The drug's main advantage is that it seems to have a weaker anticholinergic action and therefore milder side effects. In overdose, it is considered less harmful than older tricyclics.

INFORMATION FOR USERS
Your drug prescription is tailored for you. Do not alter dosage without checking with your doctor.
How taken Tablets.
Frequency and timing of doses 2–3 x daily.
Adult dosage range 140–210mg daily.
Onset of effect Can be felt within hours; full antidepressant effect may take 2–6 weeks.
Duration of action Antidepressant effect may last 6 weeks; adverse effects, only a few days.
Diet advice None.
Storage Keep in a closed container in a cool, dry place out of reach of children. Protect from light.
Missed dose Take as soon as you remember. If your next dose is due within 3 hours, take a single dose now and skip the next.
Stopping the drug Stopping abruptly can cause withdrawal symptoms and a recurrence of the original problem. Consult your doctor, who may supervise gradual dosage reduction.
Exceeding the dose An occasional unintentional extra dose is unlikely to cause problems. If you notice any unusual symptoms, or if a large overdose has been taken, notify your doctor.

POSSIBLE ADVERSE EFFECTS
The drug's possible adverse effects are mainly the result of its mild anticholinergic action; you may experience sweating or flushing, drowsiness, dry mouth, or blurred vision. Consult your doctor if constipation, dizziness, or difficulty in passing urine occur. If you experience palpitations, stop taking the drug and seek urgent medical attention.

INTERACTIONS
Sedatives All drugs that have sedative effects may intensify those of lofepramine.
Smoking may reduce lofepramine's effect .
MAOIs Serious interactions are possible. These drugs are only prescribed together under close medical supervision.

Antihypertensive drugs Lofepramine may reduce the effectiveness of some of these drugs.
Anti-arrhythmics and sotalol These drugs may increase the risk of abnormal heart rhythms.

SPECIAL PRECAUTIONS
Be sure to tell your doctor if:
◆ You have heart problems.
◆ You have had epileptic fits.
◆ You have long-term liver or kidney problems.
◆ You have glaucoma.
◆ You have an overactive thyroid gland.
◆ You have prostate trouble.
◆ You are taking other medications.
Pregnancy Safety in pregnancy not established. Discuss with your doctor.
Breast-feeding The drug passes into the breast milk and may affect the baby. Discuss with your doctor.
Infants and children Not recommended.
Over 60 Reduced dose may be necessary.
Driving and hazardous work Avoid such activities until you have learned how lofepramine affects you because the drug may cause blurred vision and reduced alertness.
Alcohol Avoid. Alcohol may increase the sedative effects of this drug.
Surgery and general anaesthetics Lofepramine may need to be stopped. Discuss this with your doctor or dentist before any surgery.

PROLONGED USE
No problems expected.

Loperamide

Brand names Arret, Diasorb, Diocalm Ultra, Imodium
Used in the following combined preparations
None

QUICK REFERENCE
Drug group Antidiarrhoeal drug (p.42)
Overdose danger rating Medium
Dependence rating Low
Prescription needed No
Available as generic Yes

GENERAL INFORMATION
Loperamide is an antidiarrhoeal drug available in either as capsule or liquid form. It

reduces the loss of water and salts from the bowel and slows bowel activity, resulting in the passage of firmer bowel movements at less frequent intervals.

A fast-acting drug, loperamide is widely prescribed for both sudden and recurrent bouts of diarrhoea. It is not generally recommended for diarrhoea caused by infection, however, because it may delay the expulsion of harmful substances from the bowel. The drug is often prescribed for people who have had a colostomy or an ileostomy, to reduce fluid loss from the stoma (outlet).

Adverse effects are rare and, unlike opium-based antidiarrhoeals, there is no risk of abuse. It can be purchased over the counter.

INFORMATION FOR USERS
Follow instructions on the label. Call your doctor if symptoms worsen.
How taken Capsules, liquid.
Frequency and timing of doses *Acute diarrhoea* A double dose at start of treatment, then a single dose after each loose faeces, up to maximum daily dose. *Chronic diarrhoea* 2 x daily.
Adult dosage range *Acute diarrhoea* 4mg (starting dose), then 2mg after each loose faeces (maximum 16mg daily). Use for up to 5 days only (3 days only for children between 4 and 8 years), then consult your doctor. *Chronic diarrhoea* 4–8mg daily.
Onset of effect Within 1–2 hours.
Duration of action 6–18 hours.
Diet advice Ensure adequate fluid, sugar, and salt intake during a diarrhoeal illness.
Storage Keep in a closed container in a cool, dry place out of reach of children.
Missed dose Do not take the missed dose. Take your next dose if needed.
Stopping the drug Can be safely stopped as soon as you no longer need it.
Exceeding the dose An occasional unintentional extra dose is unlikely to be a cause for concern. Large overdoses may cause constipation, vomiting, or drowsiness, and affect breathing. Notify your doctor.

POSSIBLE ADVERSE EFFECTS
Adverse effects are unusual, but dry mouth, drowsiness, or dizziness may occur. Some adverse effects are difficult to distinguish from the effects the drug is used to treat. If

constipation occurs, stop taking the drug. If symptoms such as bloating, abdominal pain, or fever persist or worsen during treatment with loperamide, consult your doctor. You may experience itching skin; if this develops into a rash, stop taking the drug.

INTERACTIONS
None.

SPECIAL PRECAUTIONS
Be sure to consult your doctor or pharmacist before taking this drug if:
◆ You have long-term liver or kidney problems.
◆ You have had recent abdominal surgery.
◆ You have an infection or blockage in the intestine, pseudomembranous colitis, or ulcerative colitis.
◆ You are taking other medications.
Pregnancy Safety in pregnancy not established. Discuss with your doctor.
Breast-feeding The drug passes into the breast milk and may affect the baby. Discuss with your doctor.
Infants and children Not to be given to infants and children under 4 years. Reduced dose necessary in older children.
Over 60 No special problems.
Driving and hazardous work No known problems.
Alcohol No known problems.

PROLONGED USE
Not usually taken for prolonged periods (except in medically diagnosed long-term gastrointestinal conditions), but special problems are not expected.

Loratadine

Brand name Clarityn
Used in the following combined preparations
None

QUICK REFERENCE
Drug group Antihistamine (p.56)
Overdose danger rating Low
Dependence rating Low
Prescription needed No
Available as generic No

GENERAL INFORMATION

Loratadine, a long-acting antihistamine drug, is used for the relief of symptoms associated with allergic rhinitis, such as sneezing, nasal discharge, and itching and burning of the eyes. Symptoms are normally relieved within an hour of oral administration. It is also used to treat allergic skin conditions such as chronic urticaria (itching). It has fewer sedative and anticholinergic effects than older antihistamines such as chlorphenamine. It is therefore less likely to cause drowsiness.

The drug should be discontinued about four days prior to skin testing for allergy, as it may decrease or prevent otherwise positive results.

INFORMATION FOR USERS

Follow instructions on the label. Call your doctor if symptoms worsen.

How taken Tablets, liquid.

Frequency and timing of doses Once daily.

Adult dosage range 10mg daily.

Onset of effect Usually within 1 hour.

Duration of action Up to 24 hours.

Diet advice None.

Storage Keep in a closed container in a cool, dry place out of reach of children.

Missed dose Take as soon as you remember. If your next dose is due within 6 hours, take a single dose now and skip the next.

Stopping the drug Can be safely stopped as soon as you no longer need it.

Exceeding the dose An occasional unintentional extra dose is unlikely to be a cause for concern. But if you notice any unusual symptoms, or if a large overdose has been taken, notify your doctor.

POSSIBLE ADVERSE EFFECTS

The incidence of adverse effects is low. Fatigue, nausea, and headache may occur. If you experience fainting or palpitations, stop taking the drug and consult your doctor.

INTERACTIONS

Cimetidine This drug may increase the effects of loratadine.

SPECIAL PRECAUTIONS

Be sure to consult your doctor or pharmacist before taking this drug if:
◆ You are taking other medications.

Pregnancy Safety in pregnancy not established. Discuss with your doctor.

Breast-feeding The drug passes into the breast milk, but effects on the baby are unlikely.

Infants and children Not recommended for children under 2 years. Reduced dose necessary for older children.

Over 60 No problems expected.

Driving and hazardous work Problems are unlikely.

Alcohol No known problems, but avoid excessive amounts.

PROLONGED USE

No problems expected.

Losartan

Brand name Cozaar

Used in the following combined preparation
Cozaar-Comp

QUICK REFERENCE

Drug group Vasodilator (p.30) and antihypertensive drug (p.34)

Overdose danger rating Medium

Dependence rating Low

Prescription needed Yes

Available as generic No

GENERAL INFORMATION

Losartan is a member of the group of vasodilator drugs called angiotensin-II blockers. Used to treat hypertension, the drug works by blocking the action of angiotensin-II, a naturally occurring substance that constricts blood vessels. This action causes the blood vessel walls to relax, thereby easing blood pressure.

Unlike ACE inhibitors, losartan does not cause a persistent dry cough, and its use is now being evaluated in conditions such as heart failure, for which ACE inhibitors are currently being used.

Losartan is prescribed with caution to people with stenosis (narrowing) of the arteries to the kidneys because the drug may make kidney function worse in people with this problem. It is important to notify your doctor if you know that you have this condition. Also, the initial dose causes a sudden drop in blood pressure. Adverse effects, which include diarrhoea, dizziness, and fatigue, are rare.

INFORMATION FOR USERS

Your drug prescription is tailored for you. Do not alter dosage without checking with your doctor.

How taken Tablets.

Frequency and timing of doses Once daily.

Adult dosage range 50–100mg. People over 75 years, and other groups especially sensitive to the drug's effects, may start on 25mg.

Onset of effect *Blood pressure* 1–2 weeks, with maximum effect in 3–6 weeks from start of treatment. *Other conditions* Within 1 hour.

Duration of action 12–24 hours.

Diet advice None.

Storage Keep in a closed container in a cool, dry place out of reach of children.

Missed dose Take as soon as you remember. If your next dose is due within 8 hours, take a single dose now and skip the next.

Stopping the drug Unless severe adverse effects occur (see below), do not stop taking the drug without consulting your doctor. Stopping the drug may lead to worsening of the underlying condition.

Exceeding the dose An occasional unintentional extra dose is unlikely to cause problems. Large overdoses may cause dizziness and fainting. Notify your doctor.

POSSIBLE ADVERSE EFFECTS

Adverse effects, of which dizziness and fatigue are the most common, are usually mild. Diarrhoea and migraine also occur, and some people experience taste disturbance. Dizziness, lightheadedness, or feeling faint may be signs of an excessive fall in blood pressure; consult your doctor. If you develop a blotchy rash, or you experience itching or wheezing, stop taking the drug immediately and consult your doctor urgently.

INTERACTIONS

Diuretics There is a risk of a sudden fall in blood pressure when these drugs are taken with losartan for the first time.

Potassium supplements, potassium-sparing diuretics, and ciclosporin Losartan increases the effect of these drugs, leading to raised levels of potassium in the blood.

Lithium Losartan may increase the levels and toxicity of lithium.

NSAIDs Certain NSAIDs may reduce the blood-pressure lowering effect of losartan.

SPECIAL PRECAUTIONS

Be sure to tell your doctor if:
◆ You have stenosis of the kidney arteries.
◆ You have liver or kidney problems. You have congestive heart failure.
◆ You have primary aldosteronism.
◆ You are taking other medications.

Pregnancy Not prescribed.

Breast-feeding Not prescribed. Safety not established.

Infants and children Not prescribed. Safety not established.

Over 60 Reduced dose may be necessary over 75 years.

Driving and hazardous work Do not undertake such activities until you have learned how losartan affects you because the drug can cause dizziness and fatigue.

Alcohol Avoid excessive amounts. Alcohol may raise blood pressure, reducing the effectiveness of losartan. Alcohol also causes blood vessels to dilate, increasing the likelihood of an excessive fall in blood pressure.

PROLONGED USE

No special problems.

Monitoring Blood pressure will be monitored during treatment with losartan, as with all antihypertensive drugs. Periodic checks on blood potassium levels and kidney function may also be performed.

Magnesium Hydroxide

Brand names Cream of Magnesia, Milk of Magnesia
Used in the following combined preparations
Carbellon, Maalox, Mucaine, Mucogel, and others

QUICK REFERENCE

Drug group Antacid (p.40) and laxative (p.43)
Overdose danger rating Low
Dependence rating Low
Prescription needed No
Available as generic Yes

GENERAL INFORMATION

Magnesium hydroxide, a fast-acting antacid given to neutralize stomach acid, is available in a number of over-the-counter preparations for indigestion and heartburn. It also prevents the pain of stomach and duodenal ulcers, gastritis, and reflux oesophagitis, but other drugs are normally used for these problems nowadays. It also acts as a laxative by drawing water into the intestine from the surrounding blood vessels to soften the faeces.

Magnesium hydroxide is not often used alone as an antacid because of its laxative effect. However, this effect is countered when the drug is used in combination with aluminium hydroxide, which can cause constipation.

INFORMATION FOR USERS

Follow instructions on the label. Call your doctor if symptoms worsen.

How taken Tablets, liquid, powder.
Frequency and timing of doses 4 x daily with water, preferably an hour after food.
Adult dosage range *Antacid* 1–2g per dose (tablets); 5–20ml per dose (liquid).
Laxative 5–20ml per dose (liquid).
Onset of effect Antacid within 15 minutes. Laxative 2–8 hours.
Duration of action 2–4 hours.
Diet advice None.
Storage Keep in a closed container in a cool, dry place out of reach of children.
Missed dose Take as soon as you remember.
Stopping the drug When used as an antacid, can be safely stopped as soon as you no longer need it. When given as ulcer treatment, follow your doctor's advice.
Exceeding the dose An occasional unintentional extra dose is unlikely to be a cause for

concern. But if you notice any unusual symptoms, or if a large overdose has been taken, notify your doctor.

POSSIBLE ADVERSE EFFECTS

Diarrhoea is the only common adverse effect of this drug. Dizziness and muscle weakness, due to absorption of excess magnesium in the body, may occur from prolonged heavy use of magnesium hydroxide in people with poor kidney function.

INTERACTIONS

General note Magnesium hydroxide interferes with the absorption of a wide range of drugs taken by mouth, including tetracycline antibiotics, iron supplements, diflunisal, phenytoin, and penicillamine.
Enteric-coated tablets As with other antacids, magnesium hydroxide may allow break-up of the enteric coating of tablets, sometimes leading to stomach irritation.

SPECIAL PRECAUTIONS

Be sure to consult your doctor or pharmacist before taking this drug if:
◆ You have a long-term kidney problem.
◆ You have a bowel disorder.
◆ You are taking other medications.
Pregnancy No evidence of risk.
Breast-feeding No evidence of risk.
Infants and children Not recommended under 1 year except on the advice of a doctor. Reduced dose necessary for older children.
Over 60 No special problems.
Driving and hazardous work No known problems.
Alcohol Avoid excessive alcohol as it irritates the stomach and may reduce the benefits of the drug.

PROLONGED USE

Magnesium hydroxide should not be used for prolonged periods without consulting your doctor. If you are over 40 years of age and are experiencing long-term indigestion or heartburn, your doctor will probably refer you to a specialist. Prolonged use of the drug in people with kidney damage may cause drowsiness, dizziness, and weakness, resulting from accumulation of magnesium in the body.

Malathion

Brand names Derbac M, Prioderm, Suleo-M
Used in the following combined preparations
None

QUICK REFERENCE

Drug group Drug to treat skin parasites (p.118)
Overdose danger rating Low (medium if swallowed)
Dependence rating Low
Prescription needed No
Available as generic No

GENERAL INFORMATION

Malathion is an insecticide used in the treatment of lice and mite infestations. It kills parasites by interfering with their nervous system function, causing paralysis and death.

Malathion is applied topically, either as shampoo or lotion: lotion being more convenient to use, requiring only a single application, and more effective because shampoo is diluted in use. However, lotions with a high alcohol content are unsuitable for small children or asthmatics, who may be affected by the solvent, or for treating crab lice in the genital area. Care should be taken to avoid contact of the drug with the eyes or broken skin.

If resistance occurs during treatment, your pharmacist will recommend an alternative.

INFORMATION FOR USERS

Follow instructions on the label. Call your doctor if symptoms worsen.
How taken Lotion, shampoo.
Frequency and timing of doses *Scabies* Once only (lotion). *Lice* 3 applications 3 days apart (shampoo); 2 doses, 7 days apart (lotion).
Adult dosage range As directed. Family members and close contacts should also be treated.
Onset of effect *Lotion* leave on for 12 hours (lice), or 24 hours (scabies), before washing off. *Shampoo* leave on for 5 minutes, rinse off, repeat, then use fine-toothed comb.
Duration of action Until washed off.
Diet advice None.
Storage Keep in closed container in a cool, dry place out of reach of children. Protect from light.
Missed dose If a repeat application of the shampoo is missed, it should be carried out as soon as is practicable.

Stopping the drug Should be applied as a single application or short course of treatment.
Exceeding the dose An extra application is unlikely to cause problems. Take emergency action if the insecticide has been swallowed.

POSSIBLE ADVERSE EFFECTS

Used correctly, malathion preparations are unlikely to produce adverse effects, other than skin irritation, although the alcoholic fumes given off by some lotions may cause wheezing in asthmatics.

INTERACTIONS

None.

SPECIAL PRECAUTIONS

Be sure to consult your doctor or pharmacist before using this drug if:
◆ You have asthma.
Pregnancy No evidence of risk. It is unlikely that enough malathion would be absorbed after occasional application to affect the developing fetus.
Breast-feeding No evidence of risk. It is unlikely that enough malathion would be absorbed after occasional application to affect the baby.
Infants and children No special problems.
Over 60 No special problems.
Driving and hazardous work No special problems.
Alcohol No special problems.

PROLONGED USE

Malathion is intended for intermittent use only. The lotions should not be used more than once a week for three weeks at a time.

Mebeverine

Brand names Colofac, Equilon, Fomac
Used in the following combined preparation
Fybogel-Mebeverine

QUICK REFERENCE

Drug group Drug for irritable bowel syndrome (p.43)
Overdose danger rating Low
Dependence rating Low
Prescription needed No (some preparations)
Available as generic Yes

GENERAL INFORMATION

Mebeverine is an antispasmodic drug used to relieve painful spasms of the intestine (colic), such as those that occur as a result of irritable bowel syndrome and other intestinal disorders such as diverticular disease. It has a direct relaxing effect on the muscle in the bowel wall and may also have an anticholinergic action, which reduces the transmission of nerve signals to the smooth muscle of the bowel wall, thereby preventing spasm. Mebeverine does not have serious side effects.

In addition to being available in both tablet and liquid form, mebeverine is also produced in a combined form with ispaghula husk to provide roughage in an easily assimilable formulation. Both the drug itself and the combined form are commonly used to improve symptoms in the control of irritable bowel syndrome.

INFORMATION FOR USERS

Follow instructions on the label. Call your doctor if symptoms worsen.
How taken Tablets, SR-capsules, liquid.
Frequency and timing of doses 3 x daily, 20 minutes before meals.
Adult dosage range 405–450mg daily.
Onset of effect 30–60 minutes.
Duration of action 6–8 hours.
Diet advice None.
Storage Keep in a closed container in a dry place at room temperature, out of reach of children. Protect from light.
Missed dose Take as soon as you remember, then return to your normal dosing schedule.
Stopping the drug The drug can be safely stopped as soon as you no longer need it.
Exceeding the dose An occasional unintentional extra dose is unlikely to be a cause for concern. Larger overdoses will probably cause constipation, and may cause central nervous system excitability.

POSSIBLE ADVERSE EFFECTS

Constipation may occur. Confusion and agitation are unusual complications; and if they occur, stop taking the drug and consult your doctor.

INTERACTIONS

None.

SPECIAL PRECAUTIONS

Be sure to consult your doctor or pharmacist before taking this drug if:
◆ You have cystic fibrosis.
◆ You have porphyria.
Pregnancy Safety in pregnancy not established. Discuss with your doctor.
Breast-feeding Safety in breast-feeding not established. Discuss with your doctor.
Infants and children Not used in in infants and children under 10 years.
Over 60 No special problems.
Driving and hazardous work No special problems.
Alcohol No special problems.

PROLONGED USE

No problems expected.

Medroxyprogesterone

Brand names Depo-Provera, Farlutal, Provera
Used in the following combined preparations
Improvera, Premique, Tridestra

QUICK REFERENCE

Drug group Female sex hormone (p.86)
Overdose danger rating Low
Dependence rating Low
Prescription needed Yes
Available as generic No

GENERAL INFORMATION

Medroxyprogesterone is a progestogen, a synthetic female sex hormone similar to the natural hormone progesterone. It is used to treat a range of menstrual disorders such as mid-cycle bleeding and amenorrhoea (absent periods).

The drug is also often used to treat endometriosis, in which there is abnormal growth of the uterine-lining tissue in the pelvic cavity.

Depot injections of the drug are used as a contraceptive. However, since they may cause serious side effects, such as persistent bleeding from the uterus, amenorrhoea, and delayed return of fertility, their use remains controversial, and they are recommended only under special circumstances in Britain.

Medroxyprogesterone may be used to treat some types of cancer, such as cancer of the breast, uterus, or prostate.

INFORMATION FOR USERS

Your drug prescription is tailored for you. Do not alter dosage without checking with your doctor.

How taken Tablets, depot injection.

Frequency and timing of doses 1–3 x daily with plenty of water (by mouth); tablets may need to be taken at certain times during your cycle; follow the instructions you have been given. Every 3 months (depot injection).

Adult dosage range *Menstrual disorders* 2.5–10mg daily. *Endometriosis* 30mg daily. *Cancer* 100–1,500mg daily. *Contraception* 150mg.

Onset of effect 1–2 months (cancer); 1–2 weeks (other conditions).

Duration of action 1–2 days (by mouth); up to some months (depot injection).

Diet advice None.

Storage Keep in a closed container in a cool, dry place out of reach of children.

Missed dose Take as soon as you remember. If your next dose is due within 3 hours, take a single dose now and skip the next.

Stopping the drug Unless itching, rash, or acne occur, do not stop taking the drug without consulting your doctor; symptoms may recur.

Exceeding the dose An occasional unintentional extra dose is unlikely to be a cause for concern. But if you notice any unusual symptoms, or if a large overdose has been taken, notify your doctor.

POSSIBLE ADVERSE EFFECTS

Medroxyprogesterone rarely causes serious adverse effects. Fluid retention may lead to weight gain, swollen feet or ankles, and breast tenderness. Nausea, fatigue, depression, and irregular menstruation may also occur. If you develop itching, a rash, or acne, stop taking the drug and consult your doctor.

INTERACTIONS

Antibacterials These drugs may reduce the effect of medroxyprogesterone.

Antivirals Nevirapine may reduced the contraceptive effect of medroxyprogesterone.

Ciclosporin Blood levels of ciclosporin may be raised by medroxyprogesterone.

SPECIAL PRECAUTIONS

Be sure to tell your doctor if:
◆ You have high blood pressure.
◆ You have diabetes.
◆ You have had blood clots or a stroke.
◆ You have long-term liver or kidney problems.
◆ You are taking other medications.

Pregnancy Not prescribed. May cause abnormalities in the unborn baby. Discuss with your doctor.

Breast-feeding The drug passes into the breast milk, but at normal doses adverse effects on the baby are unlikely. Discuss with your doctor.

Infants and children Not usually prescribed.

Over 60 No special problems.

Driving and hazardous work No known problems.

Alcohol No known problems.

PROLONGED USE

Long-term use of this drug may slightly increase the risk of blood clots in the leg veins. Irregular menstrual bleeding or spotting between periods may also occur during long-term use.

Monitoring Periodic checks on blood pressure and annual cervical smear tests are usually required.

Mefenamic Acid

Brand names Dysman, Ponstan

Used in the following combined preparations None

QUICK REFERENCE

Drug group Non-steroidal anti-inflammatory drug (p.48)

Overdose danger rating Medium

Dependence rating Low

Prescription needed Yes

Available as generic Yes

GENERAL INFORMATION

Mefenamic acid, introduced in 1963, is a non-steroidal anti-inflammatory drug (NSAID). Like other NSAIDs, it relieves pain and inflammation. The drug is an effective analgesic, and is used to treat headache, toothache, and menstrual pains (dysmenorrhoea), as well as to reduce excessive menstrual bleeding (menorrhagia). Mefenamic acid is also prescribed for long-term relief of pain and stiffness in rheumatoid arthritis and osteoarthritis.

The most common side effects of mefenamic acid are gastrointestinal: abdominal pain, nausea and vomiting, and indigestion. Other, more serious effects include kidney problems, blood disorders, and peptic ulcers, which may occasionally bleed.

INFORMATION FOR USERS

Your drug prescription is tailored for you. Do not alter dosage without checking with your doctor.

How taken Tablets, capsules, liquid.
Frequency and timing of doses 3 x daily with food.
Adult dosage range 1,500mg daily.
Onset of effect 1–2 hours.
Duration of action Up to 6 hours.
Diet advice None.
Storage Keep in a closed container in a cool, dry place out of reach of children.
Missed dose Take as soon as you remember. If your next dose is due within 2 hours, take a single dose now and skip the next.
Stopping the drug Can be safely stopped as soon as you no longer need it.
Exceeding the dose An occasional unintentional extra dose is unlikely to be a cause for concern. Large overdoses may cause poor co-ordination, muscle twitching, or fits. Notify your doctor.

POSSIBLE ADVERSE EFFECTS

Gastrointestinal disturbances such as indigestion and nausea are the most common side effects of mefenamic acid. Drowsiness and dizziness may also occur. The drug should be stopped if diarrhoea or a rash occur, and not used thereafter. If blood-stained vomit, black bowel movements, wheezing, or breathlessness occur, stop taking the drug and consult your doctor without delay.

INTERACTIONS

General note Mefenamic acid interacts with a wide range of drugs to increase the risk of bleeding and/or peptic ulcers. These drugs include other NSAIDs such as aspirin, oral anticoagulant drugs, and corticosteroids.

Antihypertensive drugs and diuretics The beneficial effects of these drugs may be reduced by mefenamic acid.
Lithium Mefenamic acid may raise blood levels of lithium.
Oral antidiabetic drugs Mefenamic acid may increase the blood glucose-lowering effect of these drugs.
ACE inhibitors Mefenamic acid reduces the effectiveness of these drugs, and the chance of experiencing adverse effects from mefenamic acid are increased.

SPECIAL PRECAUTIONS

Be sure to tell your doctor if:
◆ You have liver or kidney problems.
◆ You have had a peptic ulcer, oesophagitis, or acid indigestion.
◆ You have inflammatory bowel disease.
◆ You have asthma.
◆ You have high blood pressure.
◆ You are allergic to aspirin.
◆ You have porphyria.
◆ You are taking other medications.
Pregnancy Not usually prescribed. May cause defects in the unborn baby and, taken in late pregnancy, may affect the baby's cardiovascular system. Discuss with your doctor.
Breast-feeding The drug passes into the breast milk, but at normal doses adverse effects on the baby are unlikely. Discuss with your doctor.
Infants and children Reduced dose necessary.
Over 60 Increased likelihood of adverse effects.
Driving and hazardous work Avoid such activities until you have learned how mefenamic acid affects you because the drug can cause drowsiness and dizziness.
Alcohol Avoid excessive intake. Alcohol may increase the risk of stomach irritation with mefenamic acid.
Surgery and general anaesthetics Mefenamic acid may prolong bleeding. Discuss the possibility of stopping treatment with your doctor or dentist before any surgery.

PROLONGED USE

Prolonged use increases the risk of bleeding from peptic ulcers and in the bowel. Rarely, the drug may affect the liver and blood. Blood tests may be carried out during prolonged use.

Mefloquine

Brand name Lariam
Used in the following combined preparations
None

QUICK REFERENCE

Drug group Antimalarial drug (p.73)
Overdose danger rating High
Dependence rating Low
Prescription needed Yes
Available as generic No

GENERAL INFORMATION

Mefloquine is used for the prevention and treatment of malaria and is recommended for use in areas where malaria is resistant to other drugs (e.g., China, Southeast Asia, South America, and Central and Southern Africa).

However, the drug's use is limited by the fact that in some patients it can cause serious side effects that include depression, suicidal tendencies, anxiety, panic, confusion, hallucinations, paranoid delusions, and convulsions.

For most people, the benefits of the use of mefloquine outweigh the risks, although this should be discussed with your doctor.

INFORMATION FOR USERS

Your drug prescription is tailored for you. Do not alter dosage without checking with your doctor.
How taken Tablets.
Frequency and timing of doses *Prevention* Once weekly. *Treatment* Up to 3 x daily, every 6–8 hours.
Adult dosage range *Prevention* 1 tablet once weekly starting 1–3 weeks before departure and continuing until 4 weeks after leaving the malarial area. *Treatment* Initial dose 3 tablets (750mg) followed by further doses according to body weight.
Onset of effect 2–3 days.
Duration of action Over 1 week. Low levels of the drug may persist for several months.
Diet advice None.
Storage Keep in a cool, dry place out of reach of children.
Missed dose Take as soon as you remember. If your next dose is due within 48 hours (if taken once weekly for prevention), take a single dose now and skip the next.

Stopping the drug Unless serious adverse effects occur (see below), do not stop taking the drug without consulting your doctor about alternative treatment.

OVERDOSE ACTION

Seek immediate medical advice in all cases. Take emergency action if dizziness, palpitations, collapse, or loss of consciousness occur.

POSSIBLE ADVERSE EFFECTS

Mefloquine commonly causes dizziness, vertigo, nausea, vomiting, abdominal pain, and headache. Rarely, serious adverse effects on the nervous system can occur, including anxiety or panic attacks, depression, hallucinations, and paranoid delusions. If any of these, hearing problems, or palpitations occur, stop taking the drug and consult your doctor.

INTERACTIONS

Anticonvulsants Mefloquine may decrease the effect of these drugs.
Other antimalarials Mefloquine may increase the risk of adverse effects with these drugs.
General note Mefloquine may increase the effects on the heart of drugs such as beta blockers, calcium channel blockers, and digitalis drugs.

SPECIAL PRECAUTIONS

Be sure to tell your doctor if:
◆ You have long-term liver or kidney problems.
◆ You have had epileptic fits.
◆ You have had depression or other psychiatric illness.
◆ You have had a previous allergic reaction to mefloquine or quinine.
◆ You have heart problems.
◆ You are taking other medications.
Pregnancy Not prescribed. Pregnancy must be avoided during and for 3 months after mefloquine use.
Breast-feeding Not prescribed. The drug passes into the breast milk.
Infants and children Not used in infants under 3 months old. Reduced dose necessary in older children.
Over 60 Careful monitoring is necessary if liver or kidney problems or heart disease are present.

Driving and hazardous work Avoid such activities when taking mefloquine for prevention until you know how the drug affects you. Also avoid during treatment and for 3 weeks afterwards as the drug can cause dizziness or disturb balance.
Alcohol Keep consumption low.

PROLONGED USE
May be taken for prevention of malaria for up to one year.

Megestrol

Brand name Megace
Used in the following combined preparations
None

QUICK REFERENCE
Drug group Female sex hormone (p.86) and anticancer drug (p.94)
Overdose danger rating Low
Dependence rating Low
Prescription needed Yes
Available as generic No

GENERAL INFORMATION
Megestrol is a progestogen (a synthetic female sex hormone similar to the natural hormone progesterone). It is used in the treatment of certain types of advanced cancer affecting the breast and uterus that are sensitive to hormone treatment. Megestrol is often prescribed when the tumour cannot be removed by surgery, when the disease has recurred after surgery, or when treatment with other anticancer drugs or radiotherapy have failed.

Successful treatment with the drug reduces the size of the tumour and may also cause secondary growths to disappear. Improvement usually occurs within two months of starting treatment. Because megestrol does not eradicate the cancer completely, the drug may need to be continued indefinitely.

INFORMATION FOR USERS
Your drug prescription is tailored for you. Do not alter dosage without checking with your doctor.
How taken Tablets.
Frequency and timing of doses 1–4 x daily.

Adult dosage range *Breast cancer* 160mg daily. *Cancer of the uterus* 40–320mg daily.
Onset of effect Within 2 months.
Duration of action 1–2 days.
Diet advice None.
Storage Keep in a closed container in a cool, dry place out of reach of children.
Missed dose Take as soon as you remember.
Stopping the drug Unless a rash occurs, do not stop taking the drug without consulting your doctor. Stopping the drug may lead to worsening of your underlying condition.
Exceeding the dose An occasional unintentional extra dose is unlikely to be a cause for concern. But if you notice any unusual symptoms, or if a large overdose has been taken, notify your doctor.

POSSIBLE ADVERSE EFFECTS
Adverse effects are rare with meloxicam, but it may cause weight gain due to fluid retention (leading to swollen feet or ankles) or increased appetite and food intake. Other adverse effects include nausea, headache, and hair loss. If you develop a rash, stop taking the drug and consult your doctor .

INTERACTIONS
None known.

SPECIAL PRECAUTIONS
Be sure to tell your doctor if:
◆ You have long-term liver or kidney problems.
◆ You have had thrombosis.
◆ You have high blood pressure.
◆ You have heart problems.
◆ You are taking other medications.
Pregnancy Not usually prescribed.
Breast-feeding Breast-feeding is usually discontinued. Discuss with your doctor.
Infants and children Not usually required.
Over 60 No special problems.
Driving and hazardous work No known problems.
Alcohol No known problems.

PROLONGED USE
Long-term use of this drug may increase the risk of blood clots in the leg veins.
Monitoring Periodic checks on blood pressure may be performed.

Meloxicam

Brand name Mobic
Used in the following combined preparations
None

QUICK REFERENCE

Drug group Nonsteroidal anti-inflammatory drug (p.48)
Overdose danger rating Medium
Dependence rating Low
Prescription needed Yes
Available as generic No

GENERAL INFORMATION

Meloxicam is a member of the non-steroidal anti-inflammatory (NSAID) group of drugs. It reduces pain, stiffness, and inflammation and is used to relieve the symptoms of rheumatoid arthritis, ankylosing spondylitis, and acute episodes of osteoarthritis. It does not cure the underlying condition, however.

Meloxicam has less effect on the stomach, so it is less likely than many other NSAIDs to cause gastrointestinal bleeding, ulceration, and perforation. Elderly people, being more sensitive to the drug's effects, are usually prescribed only half the normal adult dose.

INFORMATION FOR USERS

Your drug prescription is tailored for you. Do not alter dosage without checking with your doctor.
How taken Tablets, suppositories.
Frequency and timing of doses Once daily.
Adult dosage range 7.5–15mg.
Onset of effect 1 hour.
Duration of action 24 hours.
Diet advice None.
Storage Keep in a closed container in a cool, dry place out of reach of children.
Missed dose Take as soon as you remember. If your next dose is due within 8 hours, take a single dose now and skip the next.
Stopping the drug The drug can be safely stopped as soon as you no longer need it (short term). Unless severe adverse effects occur (see below), do not stop taking the drug without consulting your doctor (long term).
Exceeding the dose An occasional unintentional extra dose is unlikely to cause problems.

Large overdoses can cause stomach and intestinal pain and damage. Notify your doctor.

POSSIBLE ADVERSE EFFECTS

Gastrointestinal disturbances, which may include abdominal pain, indigestion, diarrhoea, or constipation, are common adverse effects. Headache, lightheadedness or drowsiness, rash, or itching may also occur. If you experience palpitations, vertigo, ringing in the ears, or a persistent sore throat, consult your doctor. If black or bloodstained faeces or wheezing occur, stop taking the drug and report them your doctor without delay.

INTERACTIONS

Anticoagulants, other NSAIDs, oxpentifylline Taken with meloxicam, these drugs increase the risk of gastrointestinal bleeding.
Ciclosporin There is an increased risk of kidney damage when meloxicam is taken with ciclosporin.
Methotrexate Meloxicam may increase the risk of toxicity with this drug.
Lithium Meloxicam may increase the effects and risk of toxicity with lithium.
Antibacterials Meloxicam may increase the risk of convulsions with quinolones.

SPECIAL PRECAUTIONS

Be sure to tell your doctor if:
◆ You have asthma.
◆ You are allergic to aspirin or other NSAIDs.
◆ You have had a peptic ulcer, oesophagitis, or acid indigestion.
◆ You have liver or kidney problems.
◆ You have a bleeding disorder, proctitis, or haemorrhoids.
◆ You are taking other medications.
Pregnancy Safety not established. May affect the developing foetus. Discuss with your doctor.
Breast-feeding Safety not established. Discuss with your doctor.
Infants and children Not recommended.
Over 60 Reduced doses necessary. Increased likelihood of adverse effects.
Driving and hazardous work Avoid such activities until you have learned how meloxicam affects you because the drug can cause vertigo and drowsiness.

Alcohol Keep consumption low. Alcohol may increase the risk of stomach irritation with meloxicam.

PROLONGED USE
No special problems.
Monitoring Periodic tests on kidney function may be performed.

Mercaptopurine

Brand name Puri-Nethol
Used in the following combined preparations
None

QUICK REFERENCE
Drug group Anticancer drug (p.94)
Overdose danger rating Medium
Dependence rating Low
Prescription needed Yes
Available as generic No

GENERAL INFORMATION
Mercaptopurine, an anticancer drug, is widely used to prevent the recurrence of certain forms of leukaemia. Used with other anticancer drugs, mercaptopurine is also given to leukaemia victims who have not responded to other treatments.

Nausea and vomiting, mouth ulcers, and loss of appetite are the drug's most common side effects. Such symptoms tend to be milder than those of other cytotoxic drugs, and often disappear as the body adjusts to the drug. More seriously, mercaptopurine can interfere with blood cell production, resulting in blood clotting disorders and anaemia, and can also cause liver damage. The likelihood of infections is also increased.

INFORMATION FOR USERS
Your drug prescription is tailored for you. Do not alter dosage without checking with your doctor.
How taken Tablets.
Frequency and timing of doses Once daily.
Dosage range Dosage is determined individually according to body weight and response.
Onset of effect 1–2 weeks.
Duration of action Side effects may persist for several weeks after stopping treatment.

Diet advice None.
Storage Keep in a closed container in a cool, dry place out of reach of children. Protect from light.
Missed dose If your next dose is due within 6 hours, take a single dose now and skip the next. Tell your doctor that you missed a dose.
Stopping the drug Do not stop taking the drug without consulting your doctor; stopping the drug may lead to worsening of your underlying condition.
Exceeding the dose An occasional unintentional extra dose is unlikely to cause problems. Large overdoses may cause nausea and vomiting. Notify your doctor.

POSSIBLE ADVERSE EFFECTS
The most common adverse effects are nausea and vomiting and loss of appetite. Any other problems should be reported to your doctor urgently. Some people develop mouth ulcers, and infections are more likely. Jaundice may also occur but is reversible on stopping the drug. Because mercaptopurine interferes with the production of blood cells, it may cause anaemia and blood clotting disorders; and black faeces and bloodstained vomit may therefore occur due to bleeding in the intestine.

INTERACTIONS
Allopurinol This drug increases blood levels of mercaptopurine.
Warfarin The effects of warfarin may be decreased by mercaptopurine.

SPECIAL PRECAUTIONS
Be sure to tell your doctor if:
◆ You have long-term liver or kidney problems.
◆ You suffer from gout.
◆ You have recently had any infection.
◆ You have porphyria.
◆ You are taking other medications.
Pregnancy Not usually prescribed. Discuss with your doctor.
Breast-feeding Not advised. The drug passes into the breast milk and may affect the baby adversely. Discuss with your doctor.
Infants and children Reduced dose necessary.
Over 60 Reduced dose may be necessary. Increased risk of adverse effects.

Driving and hazardous work No known problems.

Alcohol Avoid. Alcohol may increase the adverse effects of this drug.

PROLONGED USE

Prolonged use of this drug may reduce bone marrow activity, leading to a reduction of all types of blood cells.

Monitoring Regular blood checks and tests on liver function are required.

Mesalazine

Brand names Asacol, Pentasa, Salofalk
Used in the following combined preparations
None

QUICK REFERENCE

Drug group Drug for inflammatory bowel disease (p.44)
Overdose danger rating Low
Dependence rating Low
Prescription needed Yes
Available as generic No

GENERAL INFORMATION

Mesalazine is prescribed for patients with ulcerative colitis and is sometimes used for Crohn's disease, which affects the large intestine. The drug is given to relieve symptoms in an acute attack and is also taken as a preventative measure. When mesalazine is used to treat severe cases, it is often taken with other drugs such as corticosteroids.

When taken in tablet form, the active component of the drug is released in the large intestine, where its local effect relieves the inflamed mucosa. Enemas and suppositories are also available and are particularly useful when the disease affects the rectum and lower colon.

This drug produces fewer side effects than some older treatments, such as sulfasalazine. People who cannot tolerate sulfasalazine may be able to take mesalazine without problems.

INFORMATION FOR USERS

Your drug prescription is tailored for you. Do not alter dosage without checking with your doctor.

How taken Tablets, suppositories, enema (aerosol).

Frequency and timing of doses 3 x daily, swallowed whole and not chewed (tablets); 3 x daily (suppositories); once daily at bedtime (enema).

Adult dosage range 1.5–2.4g daily (acute attack); 750mg–2.4g daily (maintenance dose).

Onset of effect Adverse effects may be noticed within a few days, but full beneficial effects may not be felt for a couple of weeks.

Duration of action Up to 12 hours.

Diet advice Your doctor may advise you, taking account of the condition affecting you.

Storage Keep in a closed container in a cool, dry place out of reach of children. Protect from light. Keep aerosol container out of direct sunlight.

Missed dose Take as soon as you remember. If your next dose is due within 2 hours, take a single dose now and skip the next.

Stopping the drug Unless severe adverse effects occur (see below), do not stop taking the drug without consulting your doctor; symptoms may recur.

Exceeding the dose An occasional unintentional extra dose is unlikely to be a cause for concern. But if you notice any unusual symptoms, or if a large overdose has been taken, notify your doctor.

POSSIBLE ADVERSE EFFECTS

The common side effects of mesalazine are on the gastrointestinal tract; nausea, abdominal pain, or diarrhoea may occur. Other problems are uncommon. However, unexplained bleeding, bruising, sore throat, fever, wheezing, or malaise should be reported to your doctor. If worsening of colitis, or a rash, occur, stop taking the drug and report them to your doctor without delay.

INTERACTIONS

Lactulose The release of mesalazine at its site of action may be reduced by lactulose.

SPECIAL PRECAUTIONS

Be sure to tell your doctor if:
◆ You have long-term liver or kidney problems.
◆ You are allergic to aspirin.
◆ You are taking other medications.

Pregnancy Negligible amounts of the drug cross the placenta. However, safety in pregnancy is not established. Discuss with your doctor.

Breast-feeding Negligible amounts of the drug pass into the breast milk. However, safety is not established. Discuss with your doctor.

Infants and children Not recommended under 15 years.

Over 60 Dosage reduction not normally necessary unless there is kidney impairment.

Driving and hazardous work No special problems.

Alcohol No special problems.

PROLONGED USE

No problems expected.

Metformin

Brand names Glucamet, Glucophage, Orabet
Used in the following combined preparations
None

QUICK REFERENCE

Drug group Antidiabetic drug (p.80)
Overdose danger rating High
Dependence rating Low
Prescription needed Yes
Available as generic Yes

GENERAL INFORMATION

Metformin is an antidiabetic drug used to treat adult (maturity-onset or Type 2) diabetes in which some insulin-secreting cells are still active in the pancreas. It is usually prescribed for patients who are overweight.

Metformin lowers blood glucose by reducing the absorption of glucose from the digestive tract into the bloodstream, by reducing the glucose production by cells in the liver and kidneys, and by increasing the sensitivity of cells to insulin so that they take up glucose more effectively from the blood.

The drug is given in conjunction with a special diabetic diet that limits sugar and fat intake. It is often given with another antidiabetic drug that stimulates insulin secretion by the pancreas, or with insulin for treatment of maturity-onset diabetes, especially to overweight patients.

INFORMATION FOR USERS

Your drug prescription is tailored for you. Do not alter dosage without checking with your doctor.

How taken Tablets.
Frequency and timing of doses 2–3 x daily with food.
Adult dosage range 1.5–3g daily.
Onset of effect Within 2 hours. It may take 2 weeks to achieve control of diabetes.
Duration of action 8–12 hours.
Diet advice For the drug to be fully effective, an individualized low-fat, low-sugar diet must be maintained. Follow your doctor's advice.
Storage Keep in a closed container in a cool, dry place out of reach of children.
Missed dose Take as soon as you remember. If your next dose is due within 2 hours, take a single dose now and skip the next.
Stopping the drug Do not stop taking the drug without consulting your doctor; stopping the drug may lead to worsening of the underlying condition.

OVERDOSE ACTION

Seek immediate medical advice in all cases. Take emergency action if fits or loss of consciousness occur .

POSSIBLE ADVERSE EFFECTS

Minor gastrointestinal symptoms such as nausea, vomiting, and loss of appetite are often helped by taking the drug with food. Diarrhoea usually settles after a few days of continued treatment. Dizziness, confusion, weakness, sweating, or rash are uncommon and should be discussed with your doctor.

INTERACTIONS

General note A number of drugs, including corticosteroids, oestrogens, and diuretics, reduce metformin's effects. Others, notably MAOIs and beta blockers, increase its effects.
Warfarin Metformin may increase the effect of this anticoagulant. The dosage of warfarin may need to be adjusted accordingly.

SPECIAL PRECAUTIONS

Be sure to tell your doctor if:
◆ You have long-term liver or kidney problems.
◆ You have heart failure.

◆ You are a heavy drinker.
◆ You are taking other medications.
Pregnancy Not usually prescribed. Insulin is usually substituted because it provides better diabetic control during pregnancy. Discuss with your doctor.
Breast-feeding Safety not established. Discuss with your doctor.
Infants and children Not recommended.
Over 60 Reduced dose may be necessary. Increased likelihood of adverse effects.
Driving and hazardous work Usually no problems. Avoid such activities if you have warning signs of low blood glucose.
Alcohol Avoid excessive amounts. Alcohol increases the risk of low blood glucose and can cause coma by increasing the blood's acidity.
Surgery and general anaesthetics The response to this drug may be reduced. Notify your doctor that you are diabetic before any surgery; insulin treatment may need to be substituted.

PROLONGED USE
Prolonged treatment with metformin can deplete reserves of vitamin B_{12}, and this may cause anaemia.
Monitoring Regular checks on kidney function and on levels of sugar in the urine and/or blood are usually required. Vitamin B_{12} levels may also be checked annually.

Methadone

Brand names Methadose, Metharose, Methex, Physeptone
Used in the following combined preparations
None

QUICK REFERENCE
Drug group Opioid analgesic (p.9)
Overdose danger rating High
Dependence rating High
Prescription needed Yes
Available as generic Yes

GENERAL INFORMATION
Methadone is a synthetic drug belonging to the opioid analgesic group. It is used in the control of severe pain and as a cough suppressant, but it is more widely used to replace morphine or heroin in the treatment

of dependence. In this situation, methadone can be given once daily to prevent withdrawal symptoms. In some cases, dosage can be reduced until the drug is no longer needed.
Tolerance to methadone is marked. Although the initial dose for a person not used to taking opioids is very low, the dose needed by someone who regularly takes the drug could be fatal for a non-user.

INFORMATION FOR USERS
Your drug prescription is tailored for you. Do not alter dosage without checking with your doctor.
How taken Tablets, liquid, injection.
Frequency and timing of doses *Pain* 3–4 x daily; 2 x daily (prolonged use). *Cough* 4–6 x daily (starting dose); 2 x daily (prolonged use). *Opioid addiction* Once daily.
Adult dosage range *Pain* 5–10mg per dose initially, adjusted according to response. *Cough* 1–2mg per dose. *Opioid addiction* 10–20mg (starting dose); 40–60mg daily (maintenance dose).
Onset of effect 15–60 minutes.
Duration of action 36–48 hours.
Diet advice None.
Storage Keep in a closed container in a cool, dry place out of reach of children. Protect injections and liquids from light.
Missed dose Take as soon as you remember and return to your normal dosing schedule as soon as possible. If you missed the dose because it caused you to vomit, or if you cannot swallow, consult your doctor.
Stopping the drug If the reason for taking the drug no longer exists, it can be safely stopped. Discuss with your doctor.

OVERDOSE ACTION
Seek immediate medical advice in all cases. Take emergency action if symptoms such as slow or irregular breathing, severe drowsiness, or loss of consciousness occur.

POSSIBLE ADVERSE EFFECTS
Drowsiness and nausea are the most common side effects, but these diminish as the body adapts. Other adverse effects include constipation, dizziness, and confusion. If you experience loss of consciousness or slow, difficult breathing, seek immediate medical advice.

INTERACTIONS

Phenytoin, carbamazepine, and ritonavir These drugs may reduce the effects of methadone.

MAOIs Taken with methadone, these drugs may produce a rise or fall in blood pressure.

Sedatives The effects of all drugs that have a sedative effect on the central nervous system are likely to be increased by methadone.

SPECIAL PRECAUTIONS

Be sure to tell your doctor if:
◆ You have heart or circulatory problems.
◆ You have liver or kidney problems.
◆ You have lung problems such as asthma or bronchitis.
◆ You have thyroid disease.
◆ You have a history of epileptic fits.
◆ You are an alcoholic.
◆ You are taking other medications.

Pregnancy Not prescribed in late pregnancy if possible. May cause breathing difficulties in the newborn baby. Discuss with your doctor.

Breast-feeding Safety not established. The drug passes into breast milk and may affect the baby adversely. Discuss with your doctor.

Infants and children Not recommended.

Over 60 Not recommended.

Driving and hazardous work Your underlying condition may make such activities inadvisable. Discuss with your doctor.

Alcohol Avoid. Alcohol increases the sedative effects of the drug and may depress breathing.

PROLONGED USE

Treatment is always closely monitored. If the drug is being taken long term, the dose must be carefully reduced before the drug is stopped.

Methotrexate

Brand name Maxtrex
Used in the following combined preparations
None

QUICK REFERENCE

Drug group Anticancer drug (p.94), antirheumatic drug (p.50), and drug for psoriasis, (p.120)
Overdose danger rating Medium
Dependence rating Low
Prescription needed Yes
Available as generic Yes

GENERAL INFORMATION

Methotrexate is an anticancer drug used, together with other anticancer drugs, in the treatment of leukaemia, lymphomas, and solid cancers such as those of the breast, bone, lung, bladder, head, and neck. It is also used for severe uncontrolled psoriasis until less potent drugs can be re-introduced. It is also prescribed for people with severe acute rheumatoid arthritis that has not responded to other treatment. Once the condition is under control, the dose is reduced to a minimum.

As with most anticancer drugs, methotrexate affects both healthy and cancerous cells, so that its usefulness is limited by its adverse effects and toxicity. When given in high doses, it is usually given with folinic acid to prevent the destruction of bone marrow cells that occurs when high doses are used.

Methotrexate has been reported to reduce the IQ of children. It may also reduce fertility by depressing sperm and egg development.

INFORMATION FOR USERS

Your drug prescription is tailored for you. Do not alter dosage without checking with your doctor.

How taken Tablets, injection.

Frequency and timing of doses Daily or every 2 days, for 4–5 doses, repeating at weekly intervals (some short chemotherapy courses only); once weekly (other conditions).

Adult dosage range *Cancer* Determined individually according to nature of condition, body weight, and response. *Rheumatoid arthritis* 7.5–20mg weekly. *Psoriasis* 10-25mg weekly.

Onset of effect 30–60 minutes.

Duration of action 10–15 hours.

Diet advice None.

Storage Keep in a closed container in a cool, dry place out of reach of children. Wash your hands after handling the tablets.

Missed dose Take as soon as you remember and consult your doctor.

Stopping the drug Unless sore throat, fever, or rash occur, do not stop taking the drug without consulting your doctor. Stopping the drug may lead to worsening of the underlying condition.

Exceeding the dose Tell your doctor if you accidentally take an extra tablet. Large overdoses damage the bone marrow and cause nausea and abdominal pain. Notify your doctor immediately.

POSSIBLE ADVERSE EFFECTS
Nausea and vomiting may occur within a few hours. Diarrhoea and mouth ulcers are also common side effects but should be mentioned to your doctor; you should also mention jaundice, mood changes, and confusion. Dry cough or chest pain may also occur. If you develop a sore throat, fever, or rash, stop taking the drug and consult your doctor.

INTERACTIONS
General Note Many drugs, including NSAIDs, diuretics, ciclosporin, phenytoin, and probenecid, may increase blood levels and toxicity of methotrexate.
Co-trimoxazole, trimethoprim, and nitrous oxide (including Entonox©) These drugs may enhance the effects of methotrexate.

SPECIAL PRECAUTIONS
Be sure to tell your doctor if:
◆ You have liver or kidney problems.
◆ You have porphyria.
◆ You have a problem with alcohol abuse.
◆ You have a peptic or other digestive-tract ulcer.
◆ You are taking other medications.
Pregnancy Not prescribed. Methotrexate may cause birth defects in the unborn baby.
Breast-feeding Not advised. The drug passes into the breast milk and may affect the baby adversely.
Infants and children For cancer treatment only. Reduced dose necessary.
Over 60 Reduced dose necessary. Increased likelihood of adverse effects.
Driving and hazardous work No special problems.
Alcohol Avoid. Alcohol may increase the adverse effects of methotrexate.

PROLONGED USE
Long-term treatment may be needed for rheumatoid arthritis. Once the condition is controlled, the drug is reduced as much as possible to the lowest effective dose.
Monitoring Full blood counts and kidney and liver function tests will be performed before treatment starts and at intervals during treatment. Blood concentrations of methotrexate may also be measured periodically.

Methylcellulose

Brand name Celevac
Used in the following combined preparations None

QUICK REFERENCE
Drug group Laxative (p.43) and antidiarrhoeal drug (p.42)
Overdose danger rating Low
Dependence rating Low
Prescription needed No
Available as generic No

GENERAL INFORMATION
Methylcellulose is a laxative used in the treatment of constipation, diverticular disease, and irritable bowel syndrome. Taken by mouth, it is not absorbed into the bloodstream but remains in the intestine, absorbing up to 25 times its volume of water, softening faeces and increasing their volume. It is also used to reduce frequency and increase firmness of faeces in chronic diarrhoea, and to control consistency of faeces after colostomies and ileostomies.
   The drug is also used with appropriate dieting in some cases of obesity. The bulking agent swells to give a feeling of fullness, encouraging adherence to a reducing diet.is found in contact lens irrigation solutions and in various lotions, creams, ointments, and pastes.

INFORMATION FOR USERS
Follow instructions on the label. Call your doctor if symptoms worsen.
How taken Tablets, eye drops
Frequency and timing of doses 1–4 x daily. Unless otherwise instructed, take with a full glass of water. Use eye drops as directed.
Adult dosage range 1.5–6g daily.
Onset of effect Within 24 hours.
Duration of action Up to 3 days.
Diet advice If taken as a laxative, drink plenty of fluids, at least 6–8 glasses daily.
Storage Keep in a closed container in a cool, dry place out of reach of children.
Missed dose Take as soon as you remember. Take the next dose as scheduled.

Stopping the drug Can be safely stopped as soon as you no longer need it.

Exceeding the dose An occasional unintentional extra dose is unlikely to be a cause for concern. But if you notice any unusual symptoms, or if a large overdose has been taken, notify your doctor.

POSSIBLE ADVERSE EFFECTS

When taken by mouth, the drug may cause bloating and excess wind. Insufficient fluid intake may cause blockage of the oesophagus (gullet) or intestine. Consult your doctor if you experience severe abdominal pain or if you have no bowel movement for 2 days after taking methylcellulose. When taken as eye drops, no adverse effects are expected.

INTERACTIONS

None.

SPECIAL PRECAUTIONS

Be sure to consult your doctor or pharmacist before taking this drug if:
◆ You have severe constipation and/or abdominal pain.
◆ You have unexplained rectal bleeding.
◆ You have difficulty in swallowing.
◆ You vomit readily.
◆ You are taking other medications.

Pregnancy No evidence of risk to developing baby.

Breast-feeding No evidence of risk.

Infants and children Reduced dose necessary.

Over 60 No special problems.

Driving and hazardous work No known problems.

Alcohol No known problems.

PROLONGED USE

No problems expected.

Methyldopa

Brand name Aldomet
Used in the following combined preparations
None

QUICK REFERENCE

Drug group Antihypertensive drug (p.34)
Overdose danger rating Medium

Dependence rating Low
Prescription needed Yes
Available as generic Yes

GENERAL INFORMATION

Introduced in the 1960s, methyldopa was, for many years, one of the most widely prescribed antihypertensive drugs for the treatment of high blood pressure. In recent years, its use has declined as newer drugs with fewer side effects have been introduced. It is effective in treating people for whom other, newer drugs are ineffective and for patients who have taken it for many years without experiencing side effects such as drowsiness, which can be a problems for others.

Because it does not reduce blood flow to the kidneys, methyldopa is sometimes used for patients with kidney disorders

Because methyldopa does not affect unborn babies, it is often prescribed to women who experience high blood pressure during late pregnancy.

INFORMATION FOR USERS

Your drug prescription is tailored for you. Do not alter dosage without checking with your doctor.

How taken Tablets, injection.

Frequency and timing of doses 2–4 x daily.

Dosage range _Adults_ 500mg–3g daily.
Children Reduced dose necessary.

Onset of effect 3–6 hours. Full effect begins in 2–3 days.

Duration of action 6–12 hours. Some effect may last for 1–2 days after stopping the drug.

Diet advice None.

Storage Keep in a closed container in a cool, dry place out of reach of children. Protect from light.

Missed dose Take as soon as you remember. If your next dose is due within 2 hours, take a single dose now and skip the next.

Stopping the drug Unless jaundice or rash occur, do not stop taking the drug without consulting your doctor, who will gradually reduce your dose. Stopping suddenly may lead to an increase in blood pressure.

Exceeding the dose An occasional unintentional extra dose is unlikely to cause problems. Large overdoses may cause drowsiness or palpitations. Notify your doctor.

POSSIBLE ADVERSE EFFECTS

Most adverse effects, such as drowsiness, head-aches, and stuffy nose, are uncommon and diminish in time. Depression and fever may also occur. The fluid retention that occurs during treatment is counteracted by taking a diuretic. If you develop a rash or jaundice, stop taking the drug and consult your doctor.

INTERACTIONS

Lithium Methyldopa may raise blood lithium levels, causing lithium toxicity.

Tricyclics These drugs may reduce the effects of methyldopa.

Levodopa The effects of methyldopa may be enhanced by levodopa.

SPECIAL PRECAUTIONS

Be sure to tell your doctor if:
◆ You have long-term liver or kidney problems.
◆ You have anaemia.
◆ You have angina.
◆ You suffer from depression.
◆ You are taking other medications.

Pregnancy No evidence of risk.

Breast-feeding The drug passes into the breast milk, but at normal doses adverse effects on the baby are unlikely. Discuss with your doctor.

Infants and children Reduced dose necessary.

Over 60 Reduced dose necessary.

Driving and hazardous work Avoid such activities until you have learned how methyldopa affects you because the drug can cause drowsiness.

Alcohol Avoid. Alcohol may increase the hypotensive and sedative effects of this drug.

Surgery and general anaesthetics Discuss with your doctor or dentist before any surgery.

PROLONGED USE

Liver and blood problems may occur rarely.

Monitoring Periodic checks on blood and urine are usually required.

Metoclopramide

Brand names Gastrobid, Gastroflux, Gastromax, Maxolon, Parmid, Primperan
Used in the following combined preparations
Migravess, Paramax

QUICK REFERENCE

Drug group Gastrointestinal motility regulator and anti-emetic drug (p.21)
Overdose danger rating Medium
Dependence rating Low
Prescription needed Yes
Available as generic Yes

GENERAL INFORMATION

Metoclopramide has a direct action on the gastrointestinal tract. It is used for conditions in which there is a need to encourage normal propulsion of food through the stomach and intestine.

The drug has powerful anti-emetic properties and its most common use is in the prevention and treatment of nausea and vomiting. It is particularly effective for the relief of the nausea that sometimes accompanies migraines, and the nausea caused by treatment with anticancer drugs. It is also given to alleviate symptoms of hiatus hernia caused by acid reflux into the oesophagus.

One of the drug's side effects, muscle spasm of the face and neck, is more likely to occur in children and young adults under 20 years. Other side effects are not usually troublesome.

INFORMATION FOR USERS

Your drug prescription is tailored for you. Do not alter dosage without checking with your doctor.

How taken Tablets, SR-tablets/capsules, liquid, injection.

Frequency and timing of doses Usually 3 x daily; 1–2 x daily (SR-preparations).

Adult dosage range Usually 15–30mg daily; may be higher for nausea caused by anti-cancer drugs.

Onset of effect Within 1 hour.

Duration of action 6–8 hours.

Diet advice Fatty and spicy foods and alcohol are best avoided if nausea is a problem.

Storage Keep in a closed container in a cool, dry place out of reach of children.

Missed dose Take as soon as you remember. If your next dose is due within 3 hours, take a single dose now and skip the next.

Stopping the drug Can be safely stopped as soon as you no longer need it.

Exceeding the dose An occasional unintentional extra dose is unlikely to be a cause for concern. Large overdoses may cause drowsiness and muscle spasms. Notify your doctor.

POSSIBLE ADVERSE EFFECTS

The main adverse effects are drowsiness or restlessness and, even less commonly, uncontrolled muscle spasm. Other symptoms rarely occur.

INTERACTIONS

Sedatives The sedative properties of metoclopramide are increased by all drugs that have a sedative effect on the central nervous system. Such drugs include anti-anxiety and sleeping drugs, antihistamines, antidepressants, opioid analgesics, and antipsychotics.

Phenothiazines Metoclopramide increases likelihood of adverse effects from these drugs.

Lithium Metoclopramide increases the risk of central nervous system side effects.

SPECIAL PRECAUTIONS

Be sure to tell your doctor if:
◆ You have long-term liver or kidney problems.
◆ You have acute porphyria.
◆ You are taking other medications.

Pregnancy Safety in pregnancy not established. Discuss with your doctor.

Breast-feeding The drug passes into the breast milk but at normal doses adverse effects on the baby are unlikely. Discuss with your doctor.

Infants and children Reduced dose necessary.

Over 60 Reduced dose may be necessary.

Driving and hazardous work Avoid such activities until you have learned how metoclopramide affects you because the drug can cause drowsiness.

Alcohol Avoid. Alcohol may oppose the drug's beneficial effects and increase its sedative effect.

PROLONGED USE

Not normally used long term, except under specialist supervision for certain gastrointestinal disorders.

Metoprolol

Brand names Betaloc, Betaloc SA, Lopresor, Lopresor SR, Mepranix
Used in the following combined preparations
Co-Betaloc, Co-Betaloc SA

QUICK REFERENCE

Drug group Beta-blocker (p.28)
Overdose danger rating High
Dependence rating Low
Prescription needed Yes
Available as generic Yes

GENERAL INFORMATION

Metoprolol is a member of the beta-blocker group of drugs. It is used to prevent the heart from beating too quickly in conditions such as angina, hypertension (high blood pressure), arrhythmias (abnormal heart rhythms), heart failure, and hyperthyroidism (overactive thyroid gland). Metoprolol is also used to prevent migraine attacks and to protect the heart from further damage following a heart attack.

Because metoprolol is cardioselective (see p.28), it is less likely to provoke breathing difficulties than other, non-cardioselective, beta blockers. Metoprolol should not be used by people with asthma, however, but the drug can be used with caution by people with bronchitis.

INFORMATION FOR USERS

Your drug prescription is tailored for you. Do not alter dosage without checking with your doctor.

How taken Tablets, SR-tablets, injection.

Frequency and timing of doses 1–2 x daily (hypertension); 2–3 x daily (angina/arrhythmias; 4 x daily for 2 days, then 2 x daily (heart attack prevention); 2 x daily (migraine prevention); 4 x daily (hyperthyroidism).

Adult dosage range 100–300mg daily.

Onset of effect 1–2 hours.

Duration of action 3–7 hours.

Diet advice None.

Storage Keep in a closed container in a cool, dry place out of reach of children.

Missed dose Take as soon as you remember. If your next dose is due within 2 hours, take a single dose now and skip the next.

Stopping the drug Do not stop taking the drug without consulting your doctor. Stopping suddenly may lead to worsening of the underlying condition.

OVERDOSE ACTION

Seek immediate medical advice in all cases.

Take emergency action if breathing difficulties, collapse, or loss of consciousness occur.

POSSIBLE ADVERSE EFFECTS

Like all beta blockers, metoprolol is associated with nightmares and cold fingers and toes. Fatigue, dizziness, headache, nausea, vomiting, and abdominal pain may also occur. Other common adverse effects include breathing difficulties and slow heart beat, which may lead to fainting.

INTERACTIONS

Verapamil This drug should not be taken with metoprolol because it may seriously slow or stop the heart beat and lower the blood pressure.

Decongestants Taken with metoprolol, these drugs may increase blood pressure and heart rate with metoprolol.

Ergotamine Taken with metoprolol, this drug increases the constriction of blood vessels in the extremities.

NSAIDs These drugs may oppose the blood-pressure lowering effects of metoprolol.

SPECIAL PRECAUTIONS

Be sure to tell your doctor if:
◆ You have liver or kidney problems.
◆ You have asthma, bronchitis, or emphysema.
◆ You have heart failure.
◆ You have diabetes.
◆ You have hyperthyroidism.
◆ You have phaeochromocytoma.
◆ You have poor circulation in the legs.
◆ You are taking other medications.

Pregnancy Not usually prescribed. May affect the baby. Discuss with your doctor.

Breast-feeding The drug passes into the breast milk, but at normal doses adverse effects on the baby are unlikely. Discuss with your doctor.

Infants and children Not recommended.

Over 60 There may be an increased risk of adverse effects.

Driving and hazardous work Avoid such activities until you have learned how metoprolol affects you because the drug can cause fatigue, dizziness, and drowsiness.

Alcohol No special problems.

PROLONGED USE

No special problems.

Metronidazole

Brand names Anabact, Elyzol, Flagyl, Metrogel, Metrolyl, Metrotop, Metrozol, Rozex, Vaginyl, Zadstat
Used in the following combined preparations
Flagyl Compak

QUICK REFERENCE

Drug group Antibacterial (p.64) and antiprotozoal drug (p.71)
Overdose danger rating Low
Dependence rating Low
Prescription needed Yes
Available as generic Yes

GENERAL INFORMATION

Metronidazole is prescribed to fight both protozoal, and a variety of bacterial, infections.

Metronidazole is widely used in the treatment of trichomonas infection of the vagina. Because the organism responsible for this disorder is sexually transmitted and may not cause any symptoms, a simultaneous course of treatment is usually advised for the sexual partner.

Certain infections of the abdomen, pelvis, and gums also respond well to metronidazole. The drug is used to treat *helicobacter pylori* infection of the stomach as well as septicaemia and infected leg ulcers and pressure sores. The drug may be given to prevent or treat infections after surgery; and because, in high doses, it can penetrate the brain, it is prescribed to treat abscesses occurring there.

Metronidazole is also prescribed for the treatment of amoebic dysentery and giardiasis, a rare protozoal infection.

Metronidazole may be applied topically in the form of a gel to treat some forms of acne, rosacea, infected tumours, and gum disease.

INFORMATION FOR USERS

Your drug prescription is tailored for you. Do not alter dosage without checking with your doctor.

How taken Tablets, liquid, injection, suppositories, gel.

Frequency and timing of doses 3 x daily for 5–10 days, depending on the condition being treated. Sometimes a single large dose is prescribed. Tablets should be taken after meals and swallowed whole with plenty of water.

Adult dosage range 600–1,200mg daily (by mouth); 3g daily (suppositories); 1.5g daily (injection).
Onset of effect The drug starts to work within an hour or so, but beneficial effects may not be felt for 1–2 days.
Duration of action 6–12 hours.
Diet advice None.
Storage Keep in a closed container in a cool, dry place out of reach of children. Protect from light.
Missed dose Take as soon as you remember. If your next dose is due within 2 hours, take a single dose now and skip the next.
Stopping the drug Take the full course. Even if you feel better the infection may still be present and symptoms may recur if treatment is stopped too soon.
Exceeding the dose An occasional unintentional extra dose is unlikely to be a cause for concern. But if you notice unusual symptoms, especially numbness or tingling, or if a large overdose has been taken, notify your doctor.

POSSIBLE ADVERSE EFFECTS
Minor gastrointestinal disturbances, such as dry mouth, metallic taste, nausea, and loss of appetite, are common but tend to diminish with time. The drug may cause a darkening of the urine, which is of no concern. Headache and dizziness may also occur. More serious adverse effects on the nervous system, causing numbness or tingling, are extremely rare.

INTERACTIONS
Oral anticoagulants Metronidazole may increase the effect of oral anticoagulants.
Lithium Metronidazole increases the risk of adverse effects on the kidneys.
Phenytoin Metronidazole may increase the effects of phenytoin.
Cimetidine This drug may increase the levels of metronidazole in the body.
Phenobarbital This drug may reduce the effects of metronidazole.

SPECIAL PRECAUTIONS
Be sure to tell your doctor if:
◆ You have long-term liver problems.
◆ You have a blood disorder.

◆ You have a disorder of the central nervous system, such as epilepsy.
◆ You are taking other medications.
Pregnancy Safety in pregnancy not established. Discuss with your doctor
Breast-feeding The drug passes into the breast milk, but at normal doses adverse effects on the baby are unlikely. However, metronidazole may give the milk a bitter taste. Discuss with your doctor.
Infants and children Reduced dose necessary.
Over 60 No special problems.
Driving and hazardous work Avoid such activities until you have learned how metronidazole affects you because the drug can cause dizziness and drowsiness.
Alcohol Avoid. Taken with metronidazole, alcohol may cause flushing, nausea, vomiting, abdominal pain, and headache.

PROLONGED USE
Not usually prescribed for longer than 10 days. Prolonged treatment may cause temporary loss of sensation in the hands and feet, and may also reduce production of white blood cells.

Miconazole
Brand names Daktarin, Dumicoat, Femeron, Gyno-Daktarin
Used in the following combined preparation Daktacort

QUICK REFERENCE
Drug group Antifungal drug (p.74)
Overdose danger rating Low
Dependence rating Low
Prescription needed No
Available as generic Yes

GENERAL INFORMATION
Miconazole is an antifungal drug used to treat candida (yeast) infections of the mouth, candida and bacterial infections of the vagina, and other fungal skin infections. Once given intravenously to treat systemic fungal infections, it has now been superseded for this use by newer drugs.

The drug is available for the treatment of oral infections in the form of a gel and antifungal denture paint. Cream, dusting powder, or ointment are used to treat skin infections, and several vaginal preparations are available.

Side effects usually only occur with oral preparations because miconazole is absorbed in only very small quantities following topical or vaginal application.

The pessaries, vaginal capsules, and vaginal cream damage latex condoms and diaphragms.

INFORMATION FOR USERS
Follow instructions on the label. Call your doctor if symptoms worsen.

How taken Pessaries, vaginal cream, vaginal capsules, cream, ointment, gel, dusting powder, dental lacquer.

Frequency and timing of doses 4 x daily after food (oral gel); once a week for 3 weeks (dental lacquer); 1–2 x daily (vaginal/skin preparations).

Adult dosage range *Vaginal infections* 1 x 5g applicatorful (cream); 1 x 100mg pessary; 1 x 1.2g vaginal capsule. *Oral/skin infections* As directed.

Onset of effect 2–3 days.

Duration of action Up to 12 hours.

Diet advice None.

Storage Keep in a closed container in a cool, dry place out of reach of children.

Missed dose No cause for concern, but apply the missed dose or application as soon as you remember.

Stopping the drug Unless wheezing or rash occur, apply the full course. Even if you feel better, the original infection may still be present and may recur if treatment is stopped too soon.

Exceeding the dose An occasional unintentional extra dose is unlikely to cause problems. But if you notice any unusual symptoms or if a large amount has been swallowed, notify your doctor.

POSSIBLE ADVERSE EFFECTS
Apart from local irritation, adverse effects are rare with miconazole and usually only occur with oral use. Nausea and vomiting may occur. If wheezing or a blotchy rash occur, stop taking the drug and seek urgent medical attention.

INTERACTIONS
Oral anticoagulants, ciclosporin, phenytoin, and antidiabetics Miconazole oral gel may increase the effects and toxicity of these drugs.

SPECIAL PRECAUTIONS
Be sure to consult your doctor or pharmacist before taking this drug if:
◆ You have porphyria.
◆ You are taking other medications.
Pregnancy Safety not established. Discuss with your doctor.
Breast-feeding Safety not established. Discuss with your doctor.
Infants and children Reduced dose necessary (oral gel).
Over 60 No special problems.
Driving and hazardous work No special problems.
Alcohol No special problems.

PROLONGED USE
No problems expected. Miconazole is not usually prescribed long term.

Minocycline

Brand names Aknemin, Blemix, Cyclomin, Dentomycin, Minocin MR
Used in the following combined preparations None

QUICK REFERENCE
Drug group Tetracycline antibiotic (p.60)
Overdose danger rating Low
Dependence rating Low
Prescription needed Yes
Available as generic No

GENERAL INFORMATION
Minocycline is a member of the tetracycline group of antibiotics but has a substantially longer duration of action than tetracycline itself. The drug is most commonly used to treat acne.

Minocycline may be given to treat pneumonia or to prevent infection in people suffering from chronic bronchitis. The drug is also used for the treatment of gonorrhea and non-gonococcal urethritis and may be used to treat other sexually transmitted diseases.

Minocycline is also used to treat chronic gum disease in adults.

The most frequent side effects of minocycline are nausea, vomiting, and diarrhoea. The drug also interferes with the functioning of the balance mechanism in the inner ear, with resultant nausea, dizziness, and unsteadiness, but these symptoms generally disappear after the drug is stopped. Minocycline is not prescribed for people with poor kidney function.

INFORMATION FOR USERS

Your drug prescription is tailored for you. Do not alter dosage without checking with your doctor.

How taken Tablets, capsules, gel.
Frequency and timing of doses 1–2 x daily.
Dosage range *Adults* 100–200mg daily. *Children* Reduced dose according to age and weight.
Onset of effect 4–12 hours.
Duration of action Up to 24 hours.
Diet advice Milk products may impair absorption of minocycline; avoid from 1 hour before, to 2 hours after, dosage.
Storage Keep in a closed container in a cool, dry, well-secured place out of reach of children.
Missed dose Take as soon as you remember. If your next dose is due within 4 hours, take a single dose now and skip the next.
Stopping the drug Unless you experience severe adverse effects (see below), use the full course. Even if you feel better, the original infection may still be present and symptoms may recur if treatment is stopped too soon.
Exceeding the dose An occasional unintentional extra dose is unlikely to be a cause for concern. But if you notice any unusual symptoms, or if a large overdose has been taken, notify your doctor.

POSSIBLE ADVERSE EFFECTS

Minocycline may occasionally cause nausea, vomiting, or diarrhoea. Other less common adverse effects are rash and increased sensitivity of the skin to sunlight. If you experience dizziness, loss of balance (vertigo), headaches, or blurred vision, stop taking the drug and consult your doctor urgently.

INTERACTIONS

Oral anticoagulants Minocycline may increase the anticoagulant action of these drugs.
Penicillin antibiotics Minocycline interferes with the antibacterial action of these drugs.
Oral contraceptive drugs Minocycline can reduce the effectiveness of oral contraceptive drugs.
Iron This mineral may interfere with the absorption of minocycline and may reduce its effectiveness.
Antacids and milk These interfere with the absorption of minocycline and may reduce its effectiveness. Doses should be separated by 1–2 hours.

SPECIAL PRECAUTIONS

Be sure to tell your doctor if:
◆ You have liver or kidney problems.
◆ You have previously suffered an allergic reaction to a tetracycline antibiotic.
◆ You are taking other medications.
Pregnancy Not prescribed. May damage the teeth and bones of the developing baby, as well as the mother's liver. Discuss with your doctor.
Breast-feeding The drug passes into the breast milk and may lead to discoloration of the baby's teeth. Discuss with your doctor.
Infants and children Not recommended under 13 years. Reduced dose necessary in older children.
Over 60 No special problems.
Driving and hazardous work Avoid such activities until you have learned how minocycline affects you because the drug can cause dizziness and drowsiness.
Alcohol No known problems.
How to take your tablets To prevent retention of the drug in the oesophagus, a small amount of water should be taken before, and a full glass of water taken after, each dose of minocycline. Take this medication while sitting or standing and do not lie down immediately afterwards.

PROLONGED USE

Prolonged use of minocycline may occasionally cause skin darkening and discoloration of the teeth.
Monitoring Regular blood tests should be carried out to assess liver function.

Minoxidil

Brand names Loniten, Regaine
Used in the following combined preparations
None

QUICK REFERENCE

Drug group Antihypertensive drug (p.34) and treatment for hair loss (p.123)
Overdose danger rating Medium
Dependence rating Low
Prescription needed Yes (except for scalp lotions)
Available as generic No

GENERAL INFORMATION

Minoxidil is a vasodilator drug (see p.30) that works by relaxing the muscles of artery walls and dilating blood vessels. It is effective in controlling dangerously high blood pressure that is rising very rapidly. Because minoxidil is stronger acting than many other antihypertensive drugs, it is particularly useful for people whose blood pressure is not controlled by other treatment.

Because the drug can cause fluid retention and increased heart rate, it is usually prescribed with a diuretic and a beta blocker to increase effectiveness and counteract its side effects. Unlike many other antihypertensives, minoxidil rarely causes dizziness and fainting. Its major drawback is that, if taken for more than two months, it increases hair growth, especially on the face. This can be controlled by shaving or depilatories, but the abnormal growth can be distressing. This effect is put to use, however, to treat baldness in men and women, and for this purpose minoxidil is applied locally as a solution.

INFORMATION FOR USERS

Your drug prescription is tailored for you. Do not alter dosage without checking with your doctor.
How taken Tablets, topical solution.
Frequency and timing of doses 1 x 2 times daily.
Adult dosage range 5mg daily initially, increasing gradually to maximum 50mg daily.
Onset of effect Blood pressure Within 1 hour (tablets). Hair growth Up to 1 year (solution).
Duration of action Up to 24 hours. Some effect may last for 2–5 days after drug is stopped.
Diet advice None.

Storage Keep in a closed container in a cool, dry place out of reach of children.
Missed dose Take as soon as you remember (tablets). If your next dose is due within 5 hours, take a single dose now and skip the next.
Stopping the drug Unless palpitations occur, do not stop taking the drug without consulting your doctor; stopping the drug may lead to worsening of the underlying condition.
Exceeding the dose An occasional unintentional extra dose is unlikely to cause problems. Large overdoses may cause nausea, vomiting, palpitations, or dizziness. Notify your doctor.

POSSIBLE ADVERSE EFFECTS

Side effects are very rare with the lotion. Fluid retention is common when the drug is taken by mouth and may lead to increased body weight; diuretics are often prescribed to control this adverse effect. Increased hair growth may occur. Nausea, breast tenderness, dizziness or lightheadedness, and rash are also recognized side effects. If palpitations develop, stop taking the drug and call your doctor immediately.

INTERACTIONS

Antidepressant drugs The hypotensive effects of minoxidil may be enhanced by antidepressant drugs.
Oestrogens and progestogens (including those in some contraceptive pills) may reduce the effects of minoxidil.

SPECIAL PRECAUTIONS

Be sure to tell your doctor if:
◆ You have a long-term kidney problem.
◆ You have heart problems.
◆ You retain fluid.
◆ You are taking other medications.
Pregnancy Safety in pregnancy not established. Discuss with your doctor.
Breast-feeding The drug passes into the breast milk, but at normal doses adverse effects on the baby are unlikely. Discuss with your doctor.
Infants and children Reduced dose necessary.
Over 60 Reduced dose may be necessary.
Driving and hazardous work Avoid such activities until you have learned how minoxidil affects you because the drug can cause dizziness and lightheadedness.
Alcohol Avoid. Alcohol may further reduce blood pressure.

Surgery and general anaesthetics Minoxidil may need to be stopped before you have a general anaesthetic. Discuss this with your doctor or dentist before any surgery.

PROLONGED USE
Prolonged use of this drug may lead to swelling of the ankles and increased hair growth.

Misoprostol

Brand name Cytotec
Used in the following combined preparations
Arthrotec, Condrotec, Napratec

QUICK REFERENCE
Drug group Anti-ulcer drug (p.41)
Overdose danger rating Low
Dependence rating Low
Prescription needed Yes
Available as generic No

GENERAL INFORMATION
Misoprostol reduces the amount of acid secreted in the stomach and promotes healing of gastric and duodenal ulcers. The drug is related to naturally occurring chemicals called prostaglandins. Gastric and duodenal ulcers may be caused by aspirin (p.138) and NSAIDs (p.48) that block certain prostaglandins; misoprostol can be used to prevent or cure these ulcers. The ulcers usually heal after a few weeks of misoprostol treatment. In some cases, misoprostol is given during treatment with these drugs as a preventative; and combined preparations are available that reduce the likelihood of ulcers occurring.

The most likely adverse effects are diarrhoea and abdominal pain, which, if severe, may necessitate stopping treatment. Diarrhoea can be made worse by antacids containing magnesium; these should therefore be avoided.

INFORMATION FOR USERS
Your drug prescription is tailored for you. Do not alter dosage without checking with your doctor.
How taken Tablets.
Frequency and timing of doses 2–4 x daily.
Adult dosage range 400–800 micrograms daily.
Onset of effect Within 24 hours.

Duration of action Up to 24 hours; some effects may be longer lasting.
Diet advice None.
Storage Keep in a closed container in a cool, dry place out of reach of children.
Missed dose Take as soon as you remember. If your next dose is due within 3 hours, take a single dose now and skip the next.
Stopping the drug Unless a rash occurs, do not stop taking the drug without consulting your doctor; symptoms may recur.
Exceeding the dose An occasional unintentional extra dose is unlikely to be a cause for concern. But if you notice any unusual symptoms, or if a large overdose has been taken, notify your doctor.

POSSIBLE ADVERSE EFFECTS
Adverse effects on the gastrointestinal tract, such as diarrhoea and nausea or vomiting, may occur. These can be reduced by spreading the doses out during the day. Taking the drug with food may be recommended. Bleeding between periods and abdominal pain may occur. If you develop a rash, stop taking the drug and consult your doctor.

INTERACTIONS
Magnesium-containing antacids These may increase the severity of any diarrhoea caused by misoprostol.

SPECIAL PRECAUTIONS
Be sure to tell your doctor if:
◆ You are, or intend to become, pregnant.
◆ You have had a stroke.
◆ You have heart or circulation problems.
◆ You have high blood pressure.
◆ You have bowel problems.
◆ You are taking other medications.
Pregnancy Misoprostol should not be taken during pregnancy since it can cause the uterus to contract before the baby is due.
Breast-feeding Safety not established. Discuss with your doctor.
Infants and children Not recommended.
Over 60 No special problems.
Driving and hazardous work No problems expected.
Alcohol No problems expected, but excessive amounts may undermine the desired effect of the drug.

PROLONGED USE
No problems expected.

Mometasone

Brand names Elocon, Nasonex
Used in the following combined preparations
None

QUICK REFERENCE
Drug group Corticosteroid (p.78)
Overdose danger rating Low
Dependence rating Low
Prescription needed Yes
Available as generic No

GENERAL INFORMATION
Mometasone is a corticosteroid drug used in the form of a nasal spray to relieve the symptoms of allergic rhinitis. The drug is also used topically for the treatment of severe inflammatory skin disorders and in conditions such as eczema that have not responded to other corticosteroids (see Topical corticosteroids, p.116).

Serious adverse effects are rare if mometasone is used for short periods or in small amounts. However, prolonged or excessive topical use of the drug may cause local side effects such as thin skin with enlarged capillaries, and systemic side effects such as weak bones, muscle weakness, and peptic ulcers. Because corticosteroids can affect growth, children using the nasal spray for prolonged periods may need to have their growth (height) monitored.

INFORMATION FOR USERS
Your drug prescription is tailored for you. Do not alter dosage without checking with your doctor.
How taken Cream, ointment, scalp lotion, nasal spray.
Frequency and timing of doses Once daily.
Dosage range Nasal spray 100 micrograms (2 puffs) into each nostril. Topical preparations As directed, applied thinly.
Onset of effect 12 hours. Full beneficial effect after 48 hours.
Duration of action 24 hours.
Diet advice None.

Storage Keep in a cool, dry place out of reach of children.
Missed dose Take as soon as you remember. If your next dose/application is due within 8 hours, take a single dose or apply the usual amount now and skip the next.
Stopping the drug Do not stop taking the drug without consulting your doctor; symptoms may recur.
Exceeding the dose An occasional unintentional extra dose/ application may not be a cause for concern, but if you notice unusual symptoms, notify your doctor.

POSSIBLE ADVERSE EFFECTS
Irritation of, and sometimes bleeding from, the nose are the most common side effects of mometasone treatment. In the skin, loss of colour, thinning, and increased size of capillaries may occur. Acne or dermatitis may develop around the mouth. Sore throat, weight gain, and mood changes are also recognized adverse effects. Discuss all unwanted effects with your doctor.

INTERACTIONS
None.

SPECIAL PRECAUTIONS
Be sure to tell your doctor if:
◆ You have a cold sore, measles, or chickenpox.
◆ You have any other nasal or skin infection.
◆ You have rosacea or acne.
Avoid exposure to chickenpox, measles, or shingles while using mometasone.
Pregnancy Safety not established. Discuss with your doctor.
Breast-feeding No evidence of risk. Discuss with your doctor.
Infants and children Only used for very short courses in children.
Over 60 No special problems.
Driving and hazardous work No special problems.
Alcohol No special problems.

PROLONGED USE
Not advisable. Prolonged use of topical preparations of this drug can cause permanent skin changes and should be avoided whenever possible.

Montelukast

Brand name Singulair
Used in the following combined preparations
None

QUICK REFERENCE

Drug group Anti-allergy drug (p.58)
Overdose danger rating Low
Dependence rating Low
Prescription needed Yes
Available as generic No

GENERAL INFORMATION

Montelukast belongs to the leukotriene receptor antagonist (blocker) group of anti-allergy drugs and is used in the prevention of asthma attacks. It is thought that chemicals called leukotrienes released in the lungs play a part in causing asthma. Montelukast works by blocking the receptors for these leukotrienes.

The drug is given as additional medication when combined treatment with corticosteroids and bronchodilators does not give adequate control. It is usually given as tablets, and a chewable form is available for children.

The drug is not a bronchodilator, and cannot be used to treat an acute asthma attack.

INFORMATION FOR USERS

Your drug prescription is tailored for you. Do not alter dosage without checking with your doctor.
How taken Tablets, chewable tablets.
Frequency and timing of doses Once daily at bedtime.
Adult dosage range 10mg.
Onset of effect 2 hours.
Duration of action 24 hours.
Diet advice None.
Storage Keep in a closed container in a cool, dry place out of reach of children. Protect from light.
Missed dose Take as soon as you remember. If your next dose is due within 8 hours, take a single dose now and skip the next.
Stopping the drug Do not stop taking the drug without consulting your doctor, symptoms may recur.
Exceeding the dose An occasional unintentional extra dose is unlikely to be a cause for concern. But if you notice any unusual symptoms, or if a large overdose has been taken, notify your doctor.

POSSIBLE ADVERSE EFFECTS

Severe adverse effects are rare with montelukast. There seems to be an increase in the incidence of chest infections among people taking this drug.

INTERACTIONS

None.

SPECIAL PRECAUTIONS

Be sure to tell your doctor if:
◆ You have phenylketonuria.
◆ You are taking other medications.
Pregnancy Safety not established. Discuss with your doctor.
Breast-feeding Safety not established. Discuss with your doctor.
Infants and children Safety not established under 6 years. Reduced dose necessary.
Over 60 No special problems.
Driving and hazardous work Avoid such activities until you have learned how montelukast affects you because the drug can cause dizziness.
Alcohol No special problems.

PROLONGED USE

No special problems.

Morphine/Diamorphine

Brand names Diagesil, MST Continus, MXL, Oramorph, Oramorph SR, Sevredol
Used in the following combined preparations
Cyclimorph, Omnopon

QUICK REFERENCE

Drug group Opioid analgesic (p.9)
Overdose danger rating High
Dependence rating High
Prescription needed Yes
Available as generic Yes

GENERAL INFORMATION

In use since the 19th century, morphine and diamorphine belong to a group of drugs called the opioid analgesics (see p.11). These drugs are derived from opium, which is obtained from the unripe seed capsules of the opium poppy.

The drugs are used to relieve severe pain that can be caused by heart attack, injury, surgery, or chronic diseases such as cancer. They are also sometimes given as premedication before surgery.

The painkilling effect of the drugs wears off quickly, in contrast to some other opioid analgesics, and morphine may be given in a special slow-release (long-acting) form to relieve continuous severe pain.

These drugs are habit-forming, and dependence and addiction can occur. However, patients who take them for pain relief over brief periods of time do not become dependent and are able to stop taking them without difficulty. Long-term use for painful conditions does not lead to dependence, but constipation can be a problem.

INFORMATION FOR USERS

Your drug prescription is tailored for you. Do not alter your dosage without checking with your doctor.

How taken Tablets, SR-tablets, capsules, SR-capsules, liquid, SR-granules, injection, suppositories.

Frequency and timing of doses Every 4 hours; every 12–24 hours (SR-preparations).

Adult dosage range
5–25mg per dose; however, some patients may need 75mg or more per dose. Doses vary considerably for each individual.

Onset of effect Within 1 hour; within 4 hours (SR-preparations).

Duration of action 4 hours; up to 24 hours (SR-tablets).

Diet advice None.

Storage Keep in a closed container in a cool, dry place out of reach of children.

Missed dose Take as soon as you remember. Return to your normal dosing schedule as soon as possible.

Stopping the drug If the reason for taking morphine and diamorphine no longer exists, you may stop taking the drugs and notify your doctor.

OVERDOSE ACTION

Seek immediate medical advice in all cases. Take emergency action if symptoms such as slow or irregular breathing, severe drowsiness, or loss of consciousness occur.

POSSIBLE ADVERSE EFFECTS

Nausea, vomiting, and constipation are common, especially with high doses of the drugs. Anti-nausea drugs or laxatives may be needed to counteract these symptoms. Drowsiness, dizziness, and confusion may occur. Slow or irregular breathing may be a sign of overdosage; stop taking the drugs and seek urgent medical attention.

INTERACTIONS

Sedatives Morphine and diamorphine increase the sedative effects of other sedating drugs including antidepressants, antipsychotics, sleeping drugs, and antihistamines.

MAOIs These drugs may produce a severe rise in blood pressure when taken with morphine and diamorphine.

SPECIAL PRECAUTIONS

Be sure to tell your doctor if:

◆ You have long-term liver or kidney problems.

◆ You have heart or circulatory problems.

◆ You have a lung disorder such as asthma or bronchitis.

◆ You have thyroid disease. You have a history of epileptic fits. You are taking other medications.

Pregnancy Not usually prescribed. May cause breathing difficulties in the newborn baby. Discuss with your doctor.

Breast-feeding The drug passes into the breast milk, but at low doses adverse effects on the baby are unlikely. Discuss with your doctor.

Infants and children Reduced dose necessary.

Over 60 Reduced dose may be necessary. Increased likelihood of adverse effects.

Driving and hazardous work People having morphine treatment are unlikely to be well enough to undertake such activities.

Alcohol Avoid. Alcohol may increase the sedative effects of these drugs.

PROLONGED USE

The effects of these drugs usually become weaker during prolonged use as the body adapts. Dependence may occur if they are taken for extended periods.

Moxonidine

Brand name Physiotens
Used in the following combined preparations
None

QUICK REFERENCE

Drug group Antihypertensive drug (p.34)
Overdose danger rating Medium
Dependence rating Low
Prescription needed Yes
Available as generic No

GENERAL INFORMATION

Moxonidine is a new antihypertensive drug that is related to clonidine but is more selective and may therefore have fewer side effects. It works by stimulating receptors within the central nervous system, reducing the signals that constrict the blood vessels. Moxonidine also reduces resistance to blood flow in the peripheral blood vessels. It also seems to have actions on the kidneys that result in more sodium and water being excreted.

The drug is less likely than clonidine to cause dry mouth, and, unlike clonidine, has no effect on blood fat levels or glucose. However, other side effects, such as headache and dizziness, may still occur.

INFORMATION FOR USERS

Your drug prescription is tailored for you. Do not alter dosage without checking with your doctor.
How taken Tablets.
Frequency and timing of doses
Once daily in the morning (initially); 1–2 x daily.
Adult dosage range 200 micrograms daily initially; increasing after 3 weeks to 400 micrograms daily, if necessary; increasing again after a further 3 weeks to maximum of 600 micrograms daily in 2 divided doses if necessary.
Onset of effect 30–180 minutes.
Duration of action 12 hours.
Diet advice None.
Storage Keep in a closed container in a cool, dry place out of reach of children.
Missed dose Take as soon as you remember. If your next dose is due within 4 hours, take a single dose now and skip the next.

Stopping the drug Do not stop taking the drug without consulting your doctor, who will supervise a gradual reduction in dosage over a period of 2 weeks.
Exceeding the dose An occasional unintentional extra dose is unlikely to cause problems. Large overdoses may cause drowsiness and a fall in blood pressure.

POSSIBLE ADVERSE EFFECTS

Side effects that appear at the start of treatment with moxonidine often decrease in frequency and intensity during the course of treatment. The commonest of these are dry mouth, headache, and weakness or fatigue. Dizziness, drowsiness, nausea, and sleep disturbance are less common.

INTERACTIONS

Other antihypertensives, thymoxamine and muscle relaxants These drugs may increase the blood-pressure lowering effect of moxonidine.
Sedatives and hypnotics The effect of these drugs may be increased by moxonidine.

SPECIAL PRECAUTIONS

Be sure to tell your doctor if:
◆ You have liver or kidney problems.
◆ You have heart problems.
◆ You have a history of angioedema.
◆ You have Raynaud's syndrome.
◆ You have epilepsy.
◆ You suffer from depression.
◆ You have Parkinson's disease.
◆ You have glaucoma.
◆ You are taking other medications.
Pregnancy Safety not established. Discuss with your doctor.
Breast-feeding Safety in breast-feeding not established. Discuss with your doctor.
Infants and children Not recommended.
Over 60 No special problems.
Driving and hazardous work Avoid such activities until you have learned how moxonidine affects you because the drug can cause drowsiness and dizziness.
Alcohol Avoid excessive amounts. Alcohol may increase the sedative effects of this drug.

PROLONGED USE

No special problems.

Naftidrofuryl

Brand names Praxilene, Stimlor
Used in the following combined preparations
None

QUICK REFERENCE
Drug group Vasodilator (p.30)
Overdose danger rating Medium
Dependence rating Low
Prescription needed Yes
Available as generic Yes

GENERAL INFORMATION

Naftidrofuryl is a vasodilator drug used in the treatment of peripheral circulatory disorders such as Raynaud's syndrome or intermittent claudication (cramplike pain). Most of these conditions are caused by blockage of blood vessels due to spasms or sclerosis (hardening) of the vessel walls.

The drug may improve symptoms and mobility in these conditions, but it is not known if it has any influence on their progress. Lifestyle changes such as giving up smoking and taking exercise (and keeping warm in the case of Raynaud's) are often helpful.

Naftidrofuryl has also been tried for night cramps and circulatory disorders in the brain.

INFORMATION FOR USERS

Your drug prescription is tailored for you. Do not alter dosage without checking with your doctor.
How taken Capsules.
Frequency and timing of doses 3 x daily.
Adult dosage range 300–600mg daily.
Onset of effect 1 hour.
Duration of action 8 hours.
Diet advice None.
Storage Keep in a closed container in a cool, dry place out of reach of children.
Missed dose Take when you remember. If your next dose is due within 2 hours, take a single dose now and skip the next.
Stopping the drug Unless you experience severe adverse effects, do not stop taking the drug without consulting your doctor; symptoms may recur.
Exceeding the dose An occasional unintentional extra dose is unlikely to cause problems. Large overdoses may cause

heart problems and convulsions. Notify your doctor immediately.

POSSIBLE ADVERSE EFFECTS

Naftidrofuryl is generally well tolerated, but nausea commonly occurs. Stop taking the drug and consult your doctor urgently if you experience rare side effects such as a rash, chest pain, jaundice, or convulsions.

INTERACTIONS
None.

SPECIAL PRECAUTIONS

Be sure to tell your doctor if:
◆ You have liver or kidney problems.
◆ You are taking other medications.
Pregnancy Safety not established. Discuss with your doctor.
Breast-feeding Safety not established. Discuss with your doctor.
Infants and children Not recommended.
Over 60 No special problems.
Driving and hazardous work No special problems.
Alcohol No special problems.

PROLONGED USE

Treatment should be reviewed after 3 months to see if the condition is improving, or if the drug should be stopped.

Naproxen

Brand names Arthrosin, Arthroxen, Laraflex, Naprosyn, Nycopren, Prosaid, Synflex, Timpron, Valrox
Used in the following combined preparations
Condrotec, Napratec

QUICK REFERENCE
Drug group Non-steroidal anti-inflammatory drug (p.48) and drug for gout (p.51)
Overdose danger rating Medium
Dependence rating Low
Prescription needed Yes
Available as generic Yes

GENERAL INFORMATION

Naproxen, one of the non-steroidal anti-inflammatory drugs (NSAIDs), is used to reduce pain, stiffness, and inflammation.

The drug relieves the symptoms of adult and juvenile rheumatoid arthritis, ankylosing spondylitis, and osteoarthritis, although it does not cure the underlying disease.

Naproxen is also used to treat acute attacks of gout, and may sometimes be prescribed for the relief of migraine and pain following orthopaedic surgery, dental treatment, strains, and sprains. It is also effective for treating painful menstrual cramps.

Gastrointestinal side effects are fairly common, and there is an increased risk of bleeding. However, it may be safer than aspirin, and in long-term use it needs to be taken only twice daily.

INFORMATION FOR USERS
Your drug prescription is tailored for you. Do not alter dosage without checking with your doctor.

How taken Tablets, liquid, granules, suppositories.

Frequency and timing of doses Every 6–8 hours as required (general pain relief); 1–2 x daily (muscular pain and arthritis); every 8 hours (gout). All doses should be taken with food.

Adult dosage range *Mild to moderate pain, menstrual cramps* 500mg (starting dose), then 250mg every 6–8 hours as required. *Muscular pain and arthritis* 500–1,250mg daily. Gout 750mg (starting dose), then 250mg every 8 hours until attack has subsided.

Onset of effect Pain relief begins within 1 hour. Full anti-inflammatory effect may take 2 weeks.

Duration of action Up to 12 hours.

Diet advice None.

Storage Keep in a closed container in a cool, dry place out of reach of children. Protect from light.

Missed dose Take as soon as you remember. If your next dose is due within 4 hours, take a single dose now and skip the next.

Stopping the drug When taken for short-term pain relief, naproxen can be safely stopped as soon as you no longer need it. Seek medical advice before stopping long-term treatment unless serious adverse effects occur (see below).

Exceeding the dose An occasional unintentional extra dose is unlikely to be a cause for concern. But if you notice any unusual symptoms, or if a large overdose has been taken, notify your doctor.

POSSIBLE ADVERSE EFFECTS
Most adverse effects are not serious and may diminish with time. Stomach irritation is common and may lead to dyspepsia or abdominal pain. Discuss headache, inability to concentrate, ringing in the ears, and swollen feet or ankles with your doctor. Stop taking the drug and notify your doctor immediately if rash or itching, wheezing or breathlessness, or black or bloodstained bowel movements occur.

INTERACTIONS
General note Naproxen interacts with a wide range of drugs to increase the risk of bleeding and/or peptic ulcers. It may also alter the blood levels of lithium.

Antihypertensive drugs and diuretics The beneficial effects of these drugs may be reduced by naproxen.

SPECIAL PRECAUTIONS
Be sure to tell your doctor if:
◆ You have long-term liver or kidney problems.
◆ You have heart problems.
◆ You have a bleeding disorder.
◆ You have high blood pressure.
◆ You have had a peptic ulcer, oesophagitis, or acid indigestion.
◆ You are allergic to aspirin.
◆ You suffer from asthma. You are taking other medications.

Pregnancy Not usually prescribed. When taken in the last three months of pregnancy, may increase the risk of adverse effects on the baby's heart and may prolong labour. Discuss with your doctor.

Breast-feeding The drug passes into the breast milk, but at normal doses adverse effects on the baby are unlikely. Discuss with your doctor.

Infants and children Prescribed only to treat juvenile arthritis. Reduced dose necessary.

Over 60 Reduced dose may be necessary. Increased likelihood of adverse effects.

Driving and hazardous work Avoid such activities until you have learned how naproxen affects you because the drug may reduce your ability to concentrate.

Alcohol Keep consumption low. Alcohol may increase the risk of stomach irritation with naproxen.

Surgery and general anaesthetics Naproxen may prolong bleeding. Discuss with your doctor or dentist before surgery.

PROLONGED USE

There is an increased risk of bleeding from peptic ulcers and in the bowel when naproxen is used long term.

Nicorandil

Brand name Ikorel
Used in the following combined preparations
None

QUICK REFERENCE

Drug group Anti-angina drug (p.33)
Overdose danger rating Medium
Dependence rating Low
Prescription needed Yes
Available as generic No

GENERAL INFORMATION

Nicorandil, introduced in 1994 for the treatment of angina pectoris, is the first of a new group of drugs known as the potassium channel openers.

The symptoms of angina result from the failure of narrowed coronary blood vessels to deliver sufficient oxygen to the heart. Like the older drugs for angina, nicorandil acts by widening blood vessels, but it dilates them by a different mechanism and is notable because it widens both veins and arteries. As a result of this widening of the vessels, more oxygen-carrying blood reaches the heart muscle and, at the same time, the heart's work load is reduced since the resistance against which it has to pump is decreased.

Because nicorandil is a new drug, its precise role in the treatment of angina is still unclear, and it is currently used mostly for treating angina that is resistant to older drugs.

INFORMATION FOR USERS

Your drug prescription is tailored for you. Do not alter dosage without checking with your doctor.

How taken Tablets.
Frequency and timing of doses 2 x daily.
Adult dosage range 10–60mg daily.
Onset of effect Within 1 hour.
Duration of action Approximately 12 hours.
Diet advice None.
Storage Keep in a closed container in a cool, dry place out of reach of children.
Missed dose Take as soon as you remember. If your next dose is due within 4 hours, take a single dose now and skip the next.
Stopping the drug Unless you experience palpitations, do not stop taking the drug without consulting your doctor; stopping the drug may lead to worsening of the underlying condition.
Exceeding the dose An occasional unintentional extra dose is unlikely to cause problems. Large overdoses may cause unusual dizziness and dangerously low blood pressure. Notify your doctor.

POSSIBLE ADVERSE EFFECTS

Adverse effects, such as headache, flushing, nausea, and dizziness, are generally minor and usually wear off with continued treatment, but may necessitate a dose reduction in some cases. Stop taking the drug and consult your doctor urgently if you experience palpitations.

INTERACTIONS

Tricyclic antidepressant drugs may increase the effects of nicorandil on blood pressure, resulting in dizziness.

Antihypertensive drugs Nicorandil may increase the effects of these drugs.

SPECIAL PRECAUTIONS

Be sure to tell your doctor if:
◆ You are taking other medications.
Pregnancy Safety in pregnancy not established. Discuss with your doctor.
Breast-feeding Safety not established. Discuss with your doctor.
Infants and children Not recommended.
Over 60 No special problems.
Driving and hazardous work Avoid such activities until you have learned how nicorandil affects you because the drug can cause dizziness as a result of lowered blood pressure.
Alcohol Avoid until you are accustomed to the effect of nicorandil. Alcohol may further

reduce blood pressure, causing dizziness or other symptoms.

PROLONGED USE
No problems expected.

Nicotine

Brand names Boots Nicotine Gum, Boots NRT Patch, Nicorette, Nicotinell, NiQuitin CQ
Used in the following combined preparations
None

QUICK REFERENCE
Overdose danger rating Medium
Dependence rating Low
Prescription needed No
Available as generic No

GENERAL INFORMATION
Smoking is a difficult habit to stop due to the addiction to nicotine and the psychological attachment to cigarettes or a pipe. Taking nicotine in a different form can help the smoker deal with the two aspects of the habit separately.

Nicotine is available as chewing gum, nasal spray, and skin patches for the relief of withdrawal symptoms on giving up smoking.

The patches should be applied every 24 hours to unbroken, dry, and non-hairy skin on the trunk or the upper arm. Replacement patches should be placed on a different area, and the same area of application avoided for several days. The strength of the patch is gradually reduced, and abstinence is generally achieved within three months.

The chewing gum or nasal spray are used when the urge to smoke occurs. The gum is chewed slowly for up to 30 minutes, by which time all available nicotine has been released.

INFORMATION FOR USERS
Follow instructions on the label. Call your doctor if symptoms worsen.
How taken Skin patch, nasal spray, chewing gum.
Frequency and timing of doses Every 24 hours, removing the patch after 16 hours (patches); when the urge to smoke is felt (gum or spray).

Adult dosage range Will depend on your previous smoking habits. 7–22mg per day (patches); 1 x 2mg piece to 15 x 4mg pieces per day (gum); up to 64 x 0.5mg puffs (spray).
Onset of effect A few hours (patches); within minutes (gum and spray).
Duration of action Up to 24 hours (patches); 30 minutes (gum and spray).
Diet advice None.
Storage Keep in a cool, dry place out of reach of children.
Missed dose Change your patch as soon as you remember, and keep the new patch on for the required amount of time before removing it.
Stopping the drug The dose of nicotine is normally reduced gradually.
Exceeding the dose Application of several nicotine patches at the same time could result in serious overdosage. Seek immediate medical help. Overdosage with the gum or spray can occur only if many pieces are chewed simultaneously or if the spray is used more than 4 times an hour. Seek immediate medical help.

POSSIBLE ADVERSE EFFECTS
Any skin reaction to nicotine patches will usually disappear in a couple of days. The chewing gum and nasal spray may cause local irritation of the throat or nose and increased salivation. Other recognized side effects of the drug include headache, dizziness, nausea, flu-like symptoms, indigestion, and insomnia.

INTERACTIONS
General note Nicotine patches, chewing gum, and nasal spray should not be used with other nicotine-containing products, including cigarettes. Stopping smoking may increase the blood levels of some drugs (such as warfarin and theophylline/aminophylline). Discuss with your doctor or pharmacist.

SPECIAL PRECAUTIONS
Be sure to consult your doctor or pharmacist before taking this drug if:
◆ You have long-term liver or kidney problems.
◆ You have diabetes mellitus.

◆ You have thyroid disease.
◆ You have circulation problems.
◆ You have heart problems.
◆ You have a peptic ulcer.
◆ You have phaeochromocytoma.
◆ You have any skin disorders.
◆ You are taking other medications.

Pregnancy Nicotine should not be used (in any form) during pregnancy.

Breast-feeding Nicotine should not be used (in any form) while breast-feeding.

Infants and children Nicotine products should not be administered to children.

Over 60 No special problems.

Driving and hazardous work Usually no problems.

Alcohol No special problems.

PROLONGED USE
Nicotine should not normally be used for more than three months.

Nifedipine

Brand names Adalat, Adipine, Angiopine, Cardilate MR, Coracten, Nifelease, Tensipine MR, and others
Used in the following combined preparations
Beta-Adalat, Tenif

QUICK REFERENCE
Drug group Anti-angina drug (p.33) and antihypertensive drug (p.34)
Overdose danger rating Medium
Dependence rating Low
Prescription needed Yes
Available as generic Yes

GENERAL INFORMATION
Nifedipine belongs to the group of drugs known as calcium channel blockers (p.33), which interfere with conduction of signals in the muscles of the heart and blood vessels.

Nifedipine is given for the treatment of angina, as a regular medication to help prevent attacks. The drug can be used safely by asthmatics, unlike some other anti-angina drugs (such as beta blockers).

Nifedipine is also widely used to reduce high blood pressure and is often helpful in improving circulation to the limbs in disorders such as Raynaud's disease.

In common with other drugs of its class, it may cause blood pressure to fall too low, and may occasionally cause disturbances of heart rhythm. In rare cases, angina worsens as a result of taking nifedipine, and another drug must be substituted.

INFORMATION FOR USERS
Your drug prescription is tailored for you. Do not alter dosage without checking with your doctor.

How taken Tablets, capsules, SR-tablets, SR-capsules.

Frequency and timing of doses 3 x daily; 1–2 x daily (SR-preparations). For angina attacks, a capsule may be bitten and the liquid kept in the mouth or swallowed.

Adult dosage range 15–90mg daily.

Onset of effect 30–60 minutes. When capsules are bitten effects may be felt within minutes.

Duration of action 6–24 hours.

Diet advice Nifedipine should not be taken with grapefruit juice.

Storage Keep in a closed container in a cool, dry place out of reach of children. Protect from light.

Missed dose Take as soon as you remember, or when needed. If your next dose is due within 3 hours, take a single dose now and skip the next.

Stopping the drug Unless your angina worsens, do not stop taking the drug without consulting your doctor; symptoms may recur.

Exceeding the dose An occasional unintentional extra dose is unlikely to cause problems. Large overdoses may cause dizziness. Notify your doctor.

POSSIBLE ADVERSE EFFECTS
Nifedipine can cause a variety of minor adverse effects. These include headache, flushing, ankle swelling, and frequency in passing urine. Dizziness or lightheadedness, especially on rising, may be caused by an excessive reduction in blood pressure. Patients with angina may notice an increase in the severity or frequency of attacks after starting nifedipine treatment. Stop taking the drug and consult your doctor urgently. Sometimes an adjustment in dosage or a change of drug may be necessary.

INTERACTIONS

Antihypertensive and anti-angina drugs Nifedipine may increase the effects of these drugs.

Phenytoin Nifedipine may increase the effects of phenytoin.

Digoxin Nifedipine may increase the effects and toxicity of digoxin.

Rifampicin This drug may decrease the effects of nifedipine.

Grapefruit juice This may block the breakdown of nifedipine, increasing its effects.

SPECIAL PRECAUTIONS

Be sure to tell your doctor if:

◆ You have liver or kidney problems.

◆ You have heart failure.

◆ You have had a recent heart attack.

◆ You have aortic stenosis.

◆ You have diabetes.

◆ You are taking other medications.

Pregnancy Not usually prescribed. The drug may cause abnormalities in the developing fetus and delay labour. Discuss with your doctor.

Breast-feeding The drug passes into the breast milk and may affect the baby. Discuss with your doctor.

Infants and children Not recommended.

Over 60 Reduced dose may be necessary. Increased likelihood of adverse effects.

Driving and hazardous work Avoid such activities until you have learned how nifedipine affects you because the drug can cause dizziness as a result of lowered blood pressure.

Alcohol Keep consumption low. Alcohol may further reduce blood pressure, causing dizziness or other symptoms.

PROLONGED USE

No problems expected.

Norethisterone

Brand names Micronor, Noriday, Noristerat, Primolut N, Utovlan, and others

Used in the following combined preparations
Brevinor, Loestrin, Norinyl, Synphase, TriNovum, and others

QUICK REFERENCE

Drug group Female sex hormone (p.86)

Overdose danger rating Low
Dependence rating Low
Prescription needed Yes
Available as generic No

GENERAL INFORMATION

Norethisterone is a progestogen, a synthetic hormone similar to a natural female sex hormone, progesterone. It has a wide variety of uses including the postponement of menstruation and the treatment of menstrual disorders such as endometriosis (p.101). When used for these disorders, it is only taken on certain days during the menstrual cycle. It is also prescribed in the treatment of certain types of breast cancer.

One of the major uses for norethisterone is as an ingredient of oral contraceptive preparations, either on its own or with an oestrogen drug. The drug is also available in an injectable contraceptive preparation, which is used in special circumstances.

Adverse effects from this drug are rare, but contraceptive preparations containing this drug may cause "breakthrough" bleeding (see p.103).

INFORMATION FOR USERS

Your drug prescription is tailored for you. Do not alter dosage without checking with your doctor.

How taken Tablets, injection.

Frequency and timing of doses 1–3 x daily (tablets); once every 8 weeks (injection).

Adult dosage range 10–15mg daily (menstrual disorders); 15mg daily (postponement of menstruation); 350 micrograms daily (progestogen-only contraceptives); 30–60mg daily (cancer).

Onset of effect The drug starts to act within a few hours.

Duration of action 24 hours.

Diet advice None.

Storage Keep in a closed container in a cool, dry place out of reach of children. Protect from light.

Missed dose Take as soon as you remember. If you are taking the drug for contraception, see What to do if you miss a pill (p.104).

Stopping the drug The drug can be safely stopped as soon as contraceptive protection is no longer required. If it is prescribed for

an underlying disorder, do not stop taking the drug without consulting your doctor.
Exceeding the dose An occasional unintentional extra dose is unlikely to be a cause for concern. But if you notice any unusual symptoms, or if a large overdose has been taken, notify your doctor.

POSSIBLE ADVERSE EFFECTS

Adverse effects are rarely troublesome with norethisterone and are generally typical of drugs of this type. They include breakthrough bleeding, swollen feet or ankles, weight gain, headache, and depression. Prolonged treatment may cause jaundice due to liver damage. Stop taking the drug and notify your doctor immediately.

INTERACTIONS

General note Norethisterone may interfere with the beneficial effects of many drugs, including oral anticoagulants, anticonvulsants, antihypertensives, and antidiabetic drugs. Many other drugs may reduce the contraceptive effect of norethisterone-containing pills. These include anticonvulsants, antituberculous drugs, and antibiotics. Be sure to inform your doctor that you are taking norethisterone before taking additional prescribed medication.
Ciclosporin Levels of ciclosporin may be raised by norethisterone.

SPECIAL PRECAUTIONS

Be sure to tell your doctor if:
◆ You have liver or kidney problems.
◆ You have diabetes.
◆ You have had epileptic fits.
◆ You suffer from migraines.
◆ You have acute porphyria.
◆ You have heart or circulatory problems.
◆ You are taking other medications.
Pregnancy Not usually prescribed. May cause defects in the baby. Discuss with your doctor.
Breast-feeding The drug passes into the breast milk, but at normal doses adverse effects on the baby are unlikely. Discuss with your doctor.
Infants and children Not prescribed.
Over 60 Not usually prescribed.
Driving and hazardous work No special problems.
Alcohol No special problems.

PROLONGED USE

Prolonged use may in rare cases cause liver damage.
Monitoring Blood tests to check liver function may be carried out.

Nystatin

Brand names Nystamont, Nystan
Used in the following combined preparations Dermovate-NN, Nystaform, Timodine, Tinaderm-M, and others

QUICK REFERENCE

Drug group Antifungal drug (p.74)
Overdose danger rating Low
Dependence rating Low
Prescription needed Yes
Available as generic Yes

GENERAL INFORMATION

Nystatin is an antifungal drug named after the New York State Institute of Health, where it was developed in the early 1950s.

Nystatin has been used effectively against candidiasis (thrush), an infection caused by the *Candida* yeast. Available in a variety of dosage forms, it is used for infections of the skin, mouth, throat, intestinal tract, oesophagus, and vagina. Because it is poorly absorbed into the bloodstream from the digestive tract, the drug is of little use against systemic infections. Nystatin is not given by injection.

Nystatin rarely causes adverse effects and can be used during pregnancy to treat vaginal candidiasis.

INFORMATION FOR USERS

Your drug prescription is tailored for you. Do not alter dosage without checking with your doctor.
How taken Tablets, pastilles, liquid, pessaries, cream, ointment, gel.
Frequency and timing of doses *Mouth or throat infections* 4 x daily; liquid should be held in the mouth for several minutes before being swallowed. *Intestinal infections* 4 x daily. *Skin infections* 2–4 x daily. *Vaginal infections* Once daily for 2 weeks.
Adult dosage range 2–4 million units daily (by mouth); 100,000–200,000 units at night

(pessaries); 1–2 applicatorfuls (vaginal cream); as directed (skin preparations).

Onset of effect Full beneficial effect may not be felt for 7–14 days.

Duration of action Up to 6 hours.

Diet advice None.

Storage Keep in a closed container in a cool, dry place out of reach of children. Protect from light.

Missed dose Take as soon as you remember. Take your next dose as usual.

Stopping the drug Take the full course. Even if the affected area seems to be cured, the original infection may still be present, and symptoms may recur if treatment is stopped too soon.

Exceeding the dose An occasional unintentional extra dose is unlikely to be a cause for concern. But if you notice any unusual symptoms, or if a large overdose has been taken, notify your doctor.

POSSIBLE ADVERSE EFFECTS

Adverse effects are uncommon and are usually mild and transient. Nausea and vomiting may occur when high doses of the drug are taken by mouth. If you develop diarrhoea or a rash, consult your doctor.

INTERACTIONS

None.

SPECIAL PRECAUTIONS

Be sure to tell your doctor if:
◆ You are taking other medications.

Pregnancy No evidence of risk to developing fetus.

Breast-feeding No evidence of risk.

Infants and children Reduced dose necessary.

Over 60 No special problems.

Driving and hazardous work No known problems.

Alcohol No known problems.

PROLONGED USE

No problems expected. Nystatin is usually given as a course of treatment until the infection is cured.

Olanzapine

Brand name Zyprexa
Used in the following combined preparations
None

QUICK REFERENCE
Drug group Antipsychotic drug (p.15)
Overdose danger rating Medium
Dependence rating Low
Prescription needed Yes
Available as generic No

GENERAL INFORMATION

Olanzapine is a benzodiazepine antipsychotic drug that is prescribed for the treatment of schizophrenia. The drug works by blocking several different receptors in the brain, including dopamine, histamine, and serotonin receptors.

Olanzapine is effective in maintaining control of the condition in people who have responded to initial treatment. It can be used to treat both "positive" symptoms (delusions, hallucinations, and thought disorders) and "negative" symptoms (blunted affect, emotional and social withdrawal).

Olanzapine stays in the body longer in women, non-smokers, and the elderly than in younger men and smokers. As a result, women, non-smokers, and older people may need a lower starting dose and lower maintenance doses.

INFORMATION FOR USERS

Your drug prescription is tailored for you. Do not alter dosage without checking with your doctor.
How taken Tablets.
Frequency and timing of doses Once daily.
Adult dosage range 10mg daily (starting dose), then 5–20mg daily. Doses greater than 15mg are prescribed only after clinical re-assessment.
Onset of effect 4–8 hours.
Duration of action 30–38 hours, but longer in women than in men, and longer in the elderly.
Diet advice None.
Storage Keep in a closed container in a cool, dry place out of reach of children. Protect from light.

Missed dose Take as soon as you remember. If your next dose is due within 8 hours take a single dose now and skip the next.
Stopping the drug Do not stop taking the drug without consulting your doctor; symptoms may recur.
Exceeding the dose An occasional unintentional extra dose is unlikely to cause problems. Large overdoses may cause unusual drowsiness, depressed breathing, and low blood pressure. Notify your doctor.

POSSIBLE ADVERSE EFFECTS
Unusual drowsiness and weight gain are the most common adverse effects of olanzapine treatment. Consult your doctor if you experience dizziness or fainting, tremor, or a persistent sore throat.

INTERACTIONS
Sedatives All drugs that have a sedative effect on the central nervous system may increase the sedative effects of olanzapine.
Anticonvulsants Olanzapine opposes the effect of these drugs. Carbamazepine decreases the effect of olanzapine.
Anti-arrhythmics There is an increased risk of arrhythmias when certain of these drugs are used with olanzapine.

SPECIAL PRECAUTIONS
Be sure to tell your doctor if:
◆ You have an enlarged prostate.
◆ You have glaucoma.
◆ You are taking other medications.
Pregnancy Safety not established. Discuss with your doctor.
Breast-feeding Safety not established. Discuss with your doctor.
Infants and children Not recommended.
Over 60 Reduced dose necessary.
Driving and hazardous work Avoid. Olanzapine can cause unusual drowsiness.
Alcohol Avoid. Alcohol increases the sedative effects of this drug.

PROLONGED USE
Prolonged use of olanzapine may, in rare cases, cause *tardive dyskinesia*, in which there are involuntary movements of the tongue and face.

Omeprazole

Brand name Losec
Used in the following combined preparations
None

QUICK REFERENCE

Drug group Anti-ulcer drug (p.41)
Overdose danger rating Low
Dependence rating Low
Prescription needed Yes
Available as generic No

GENERAL INFORMATION

Omeprazole, an anti-ulcer drug, was introduced in 1989 and is used to treat stomach and duodenal ulcers as well as reflux oesophagitis, a condition in which acid from the stomach rises into the oesophagus. It reduces (by about 70 per cent) the amount of acid produced by the stomach and works in a different way to some of the other anti-ulcer drugs that reduce acid secretion.

Treatment is usually given for four to eight weeks, depending on the problem being treated. Omeprazole may also be given with antibiotics to eradicate the *Helicobacter pylori* bacteria that cause many gastric ulcers. Reflux oesophagitis may be treated for four to twelve weeks.

Omeprazole causes few serious side effects. However, because the drug may affect the actions of enzymes in the liver, where many drugs are broken down, it may increase the effects of ciclosporin, warfarin, and phenytoin, and these drugs require more careful monitoring when they are being used with omeprazole.

INFORMATION FOR USERS

Your drug prescription is tailored for you. Do not alter dosage without checking with your doctor.
How taken Capsules.
Frequency and timing of doses 1–2 x daily.
Adult dosage range 10–40mg daily and sometimes up to 120mg daily.
Onset of effect 2–5 hours.
Duration of action 24 hours.
Diet advice None, although spicy foods and alcohol may exacerbate the underlying condition.

Storage Keep in a closed container in a cool, dry place out of reach of children. Omeprazole is very sensitive to moisture. It must not be transferred to another container and must be used within 3 months of opening.
Missed dose Take as soon as you remember. If your next dose is due within 8 hours, take a single dose now and skip the next.
Stopping the drug Unless a rash occurs, do not stop taking the drug without consulting your doctor; symptoms may recur.
Exceeding the dose An occasional unintentional extra dose is unlikely to be a cause for concern. But if you notice any unusual symptoms, or if a large overdose has been taken, notify your doctor.

POSSIBLE ADVERSE EFFECTS

Adverse effects such as headache and diarrhoea are usually mild, and often diminish with continued use of the drug. Less commonly, rash, nausea and constipation may occur. If you develop a rash, stop taking the drug and notify your doctor.

INTERACTIONS

Warfarin The effects of warfarin may be increased by omeprazole.
Phenytoin The effects of phenytoin may be increased by omeprazole.
Ciclosporin Blood levels of ciclosporin are raised by omeprazole.

SPECIAL PRECAUTIONS

Be sure to tell your doctor if:
◆ You have a long-term liver problem.
◆ You are taking other medications.
Pregnancy Safety in pregnancy not established. Discuss with your doctor.
Breast-feeding The drug may pass into the breast milk. Safety in breast-feeding not established. Discuss with your doctor.
Infants and children Not recommended.
Over 60 No special problems.
Driving and hazardous work No special problems.
Alcohol Avoid. Alcohol may aggravate your underlying condition and reduce the beneficial effects of this drug.

PROLONGED USE

No problems expected.

Ondansetron

Brand name Zofran
Used in the following combined preparations
None

QUICK REFERENCE

Drug group Anti-emetic (p.21)
Overdose danger rating Low
Dependence rating Low
Prescription needed Yes
Available as generic No

GENERAL INFORMATION

Ondansetron, an anti-emetic, is used especially for treating the nausea and vomiting
associated with radiotherapy and anticancer
drugs such as cisplatin. It may also be given
for nausea and vomiting following surgery.

Its dose and frequency depend on the
anti-cancer drug. In most cases, you will receive a dose, either by mouth or injection, before infusion of the anti-cancer agent, then
tablets for up to five days after the treatment
has finished. The activity of ondansetron
against the delayed nausea and vomiting that
occur several days after chemotherapy is much
less than its activity against the symptoms
that occur soon after anticancer treatment.

To enhance the drug's effectiveness, it is
usually taken with other drugs, such as dexamethasone. Serious adverse effects are unlikely.

INFORMATION FOR USERS

Your drug prescription is tailored for you.
Do not alter dosage without checking with
your doctor.
How taken Tablets, injection.
Frequency and timing of doses Normally 2 x
daily but the frequency will depend on the
reason for which it is being used.
Adult dosage range 4–32mg daily depending
on the reason for which it is being used.
Onset of effect Within 1 hour.
Duration of action Approximately 12 hours.
Diet advice None.
Storage Keep in a closed container in a cool,
dry place out of reach of children. Protect
from light.
Missed dose Take as soon as you remember. If
your next dose is due within 2 hours, take a
single dose now and skip the next.

Stopping the drug Can be safely stopped as
soon as you no longer need it.
Exceeding the dose An occasional unintentional extra dose is unlikely to be a cause for
concern. But if you notice any unusual
symptoms, or if a large overdose has been
taken, notify your doctor.

POSSIBLE ADVERSE EFFECTS

Ondansetron is considered to be safe and is
generally well tolerated. It does not cause
sedation and movement disorders – adverse
effects of some of the other anti-emetics.
Constipation, headache, and a warm feeling
in the head or stomach sometimes occur.

INTERACTIONS

None

SPECIAL PRECAUTIONS

Be sure to tell your doctor if:
◆ You have a long-term liver problem.
◆ You are taking other medications.
Pregnancy Safety in pregnancy not estab-
lished. Discuss with your doctor.
Breast-feeding The drug passes into the
breast milk. Discuss with your doctor.
Infants and children Reduced dose necessary.
Over 60 No special problems.
Driving and hazardous work No problems
expected.
Alcohol No known problems.

PROLONGED USE

Not generally prescribed long term.

Orlistat

Brand name Xenical
Used in the following combined preparations
None

QUICK REFERENCE

Overdose danger rating Low
Dependence rating Low
Prescription needed Yes
Available as generic No

GENERAL INFORMATION

Orlistat blocks the action of stomach and
pancreatic enzymes (lipases) that digest fats,

so that the fats are not absorbed into the body but pass through to be excreted in the faeces. As a result, the body must burn stored fat to provide energy, which gradually reduces fat stores and produces weight loss. The drug's effectiveness varies from person to person.

Because orlistat works by making the faeces oily, flatulence can occur. The drug's effect may be partly due to people reducing their fat intake to avoid the unpleasant side effects.

As fat absorption is greatly reduced, there is a danger that fat soluble vitamins might be lost to the body. Vitamin supplements may be prescribed to compensate for this. The vitamins should be taken at a different time from the orlistat; bedtime might be best, or at least 2 hours apart from any orlistat dose.

INFORMATION FOR USERS
Your drug prescription is tailored for you. Do not alter dosage without checking with your doctor.

How taken Capsules.
Frequency and timing of doses Just before, during, or up to 1 hour after each main meal (up to 3 x daily). If a meal is omitted or contains no fat, do not take the dose of orlistat.
Adult dosage range 120–360mg daily.
Onset of effect 30 minutes; excretion of excess faecal fat begins about 24–48 hours after the first dose.
Duration of action The drug is not absorbed from the gut and can continue to work as it passes through the intestines. Faeces return to normal 48–72 hours after treatment is stopped.
Diet advice Eat a balanced diet that does not contain quite enough calories, and that provides about 30 percent of the calories as fat. Eat lots of fruit and vegetables. The intake of fat, carbohydrate, and protein should be distributed over the three main meals.
Storage Keep in a closed container in a cool dry place. Keep out of reach of children.
Missed dose No cause for concern. Take the next dose with the next meal.
Stopping the drug The drug can be safely stopped as soon as it is no longer needed, but notify your doctor.

POSSIBLE ADVERSE EFFECTS
Most side effects depend on how much fat is eaten and the dose of orlistat. They include

liquid, oily stools, faecal urgency, abdominal or rectal pain, headache, nausea, flatulence, menstrual irregularities, anxiety, and fatigue.

INTERACTIONS
Acarbose, metformin, and fibrates increase the effects of orlistat.

SPECIAL PRECAUTIONS
Be sure to tell your doctor if:
◆ You have diabetes.
◆ You have chronic malabsorption syndrome.
◆ You have gallbladder or liver problems.
◆ You are taking lipid-lowering drugs.
◆ You are taking other medications.
Pregnancy Safety not established. Discuss with your doctor.
Breast-feeding Safety not established. Discuss with your doctor.
Infants and children Not prescribed.
Over 60 No known problems.
Driving and hazardous work No special problems.
Alcohol No special problems.

PROLONGED USE
Treatment should be stopped after 12 weeks if you have not lost 5 percent of your body weight since starting treatment. If you have, the drug may be continued for a maximum of 2 years until target weight is approached.

Orphenadrine

Brand names Biorphen, Disipal
Used in the following combined preparations None

QUICK REFERENCE
Drug group Anticholinergic muscle relaxant (p.52) and drug for parkinsonism (p.18)
Overdose danger rating High
Dependence rating Low
Prescription needed Yes
Available as generic Yes

GENERAL INFORMATION
Orphenadrine is an anticholinergic drug that is prescribed to treat all forms of Parkinson's disease. Although less effective than other drugs used in the treatment of this disorder,

it is often preferred because its adverse effects tend to be less severe. Orphenadrine is particularly valuable for relieving the muscle rigidity that often occurs with Parkinson's disease; it is less helpful for improving slowing of movement that also commonly occur.

The drug possesses significant muscle-relaxant properties. It produces this effect by blocking nerve pathways responsible for muscle rigidity and spasm. Consequently, it is prescribed for the relief of muscle spasm caused by muscle injury, prolapsed ("slipped") disc, and whiplash injuries.

INFORMATION FOR USERS

Your drug prescription is tailored for you. Do not alter dosage without checking with your doctor.

How taken Tablets, liquid, injection.
Frequency and timing of doses 2–3 x daily.
Adult dosage range 150–400mg daily.
Onset of effect Within 60 minutes (by mouth); within 5 minutes (by injection).
Duration of action 8–12 hours.
Diet advice None.
Storage Keep in a closed container in a cool, dry place out of reach of children. Protect from light.
Missed dose Take as soon as you remember. If your next dose is due within 2 hours, take a single dose now and skip the next.
Stopping the drug Unless rash, itching or palpitations occur, do not stop taking the drug without consulting your doctor; symptoms may recur.

OVERDOSE ACTION

Seek immediate medical advice in all cases. Take emergency action if palpitations, fits, or loss of consciousness occur.

POSSIBLE ADVERSE EFFECTS

The drug's adverse effects are similar to those of other anticholinergic drugs. The more common symptoms, such as dry mouth and blurred vision, can often be overcome by an adjustment in dosage. Other anticholinergic symptoms include difficulty in passing urine, constipation, dizziness, and confusion or agitation. If any of these, a rash, itching, or palpitations occur, stop taking the drug and consult your doctor.

INTERACTIONS

Anticholinergics These drugs are likely to increase orphenadrine's anticholinergic effects.
Dextropropoxyphene/co-proxamol Confusion, anxiety, and tremors may occur if these drugs are taken with orphenadrine.
Sedatives All drugs that have a sedative effect on the central nervous system are likely to increase the effects of orphenadrine.

SPECIAL PRECAUTIONS

Be sure to tell your doctor if:
◆ You have long-term liver or kidney problems.
◆ You have heart problems.
◆ You have had glaucoma.
◆ You have difficulty in passing urine.
◆ You have myasthenia gravis.
◆ You are taking other medications.
Pregnancy Safety in pregnancy not established. Discuss with your doctor.
Breast-feeding The drug passes into the breast milk, but at normal doses adverse effects on the baby are unlikely. Discuss with your doctor.
Infants and children Not usually prescribed.
Over 60 Increased likelihood of adverse effects. Reduced dose may therefore be necessary.
Driving and hazardous work Avoid such activities until you have learned how orphenadrine affects you because the drug can cause dizziness, lightheadedness, and blurred vision.
Alcohol Avoid. Alcohol may increase the sedative effects of this drug.

PROLONGED USE

No problems expected. Effectiveness in treating Parkinson's disease may diminish with time.

Oxybutynin

Brand names Contimin, Cystrin, Ditropan
Used in the following combined preparations None

QUICK REFERENCE

Drug group Drug for urinary disorders (p.108)
Overdose danger rating Medium
Dependence rating Low
Prescription needed Yes
Available as generic Yes

GENERAL INFORMATION

Oxybutynin is an anticholinergic and anti-spasmodic drug used to treat urinary incontinence and frequency in adults and bedwetting in children. It works by reducing bladder contraction, allowing the bladder to hold more urine. It stops bladder spasms and delays the desire to empty the bladder. The drug also has some local anaesthetic effect.

The drug's usefulness is, to some extent, limited by its side effects, especially in children and the elderly. It can aggravate conditions such as an enlarged prostate or coronary heart disease in the elderly. Children are more susceptible to effects on the central nervous system (CNS), such as restlessness, disorientation, hallucinations, and convulsions.

INFORMATION FOR USERS

Your drug prescription is tailored for you. Do not alter dosage without checking with your doctor.

How taken Tablets, liquid.
Frequency and timing of doses 2–4 x daily.
Adult dosage range 10–20mg daily.
Onset of effect 1 hour.
Duration of action Up to 10 hours.
Diet advice None.
Storage Keep in a closed container in a cool, dry place out of reach of children. Protect liquid from light.
Missed dose Take as soon as you remember. If your next dose is due within 2 hours, take a single dose now and skip the next.
Stopping the drug Do not stop taking the drug without consulting your doctor; symptoms may recur.
Exceeding the dose An occasional unintentional extra dose is unlikely to cause problems. Larger overdoses may cause restlessness or psychotic behaviour, a fall in blood pressure, breathing difficulties, paralysis, or coma. Notify your doctor immediately.

POSSIBLE ADVERSE EFFECTS

Dosage adjustment is necessary in children and the elderly to minimize adverse effects. The drug can also precipitate glaucoma. Dry mouth, constipation, nausea, facial flushing, dry skin, and difficulty in passing urine may occur. Consult your doctor if headache, confusion, rash, eye pain, or blurred vision occur.

INTERACTIONS

General note If oxybutynin is taken with other drugs that have anticholinergic effects, the risk of accumulated side effects is increased.

SPECIAL PRECAUTIONS

Be sure to tell your doctor if:
◆ You have liver or kidney problems.
◆ You have hyperthyroidism.
◆ You have heart problems.
◆ You have an enlarged prostate.
◆ You have porphyria.
◆ You have hiatus hernia.
◆ You have ulcerative colitis.
◆ You have glaucoma.
◆ You have myasthenia gravis.
◆ You are taking other medications.
Pregnancy Safety not established. May harm the unborn baby. Discuss with your doctor.
Breast-feeding Safety not established. Discuss with your doctor.
Infants and children Not recommended under 5 years. Reduced dose necessary in older children.
Over 60 Reduced dose necessary.
Driving and hazardous work Avoid such activities until you have learned how oxybutynin affects you because the drug can cause drowsiness, disorientation, and blurred vision.
Alcohol Avoid excessive amounts. Alcohol increases the sedative effects of oxybutynin.

PROLONGED USE

No special problems.

Paracetamol

Brand names Alvedon, Calpol, Disprol, Hedex, Panadol, Panaleve, and many others
Used in the following combined preparations
Anadin Extra, Migraleve, Panadeine, Paradote, Tylex, and others

QUICK REFERENCE

Drug group Non-opioid analgesic (p.9)
Overdose danger rating High
Dependence rating Low
Prescription needed No
Available as generic Yes

GENERAL INFORMATION

Although paracetamol has been known since the early 1900s, it was not widely used as an analgesic until the 1950s. One of a group of drugs known as the non-opioid analgesics, it is kept in the home to relieve occasional bouts of mild pain and to reduce fever. It is suitable for children as well as adults.

One of the primary advantages of paracetamol is that it does not cause stomach upset or bleeding problems. This makes it particularly useful for people who suffer from peptic ulcers or those who cannot tolerate aspirin. It is also safe for occasional use by those being treated with anticoagulants.

Although safe when used as directed, paracetamol is dangerous when taken in overdose, and it is capable of causing serious damage to the liver and kidneys. Large doses may also be toxic if you regularly drink even moderate amounts of alcohol.

INFORMATION FOR USERS

Follow instructions on the label. Call your doctor if symptoms worsen.
How taken Tablets, capsules, liquid, suppositories.
Frequency and timing of doses Every 4–6 hours as necessary, but not more than 4 doses per 24 hours in children.
Dosage range *Adults* 500mg–1g per dose up to 4g daily. *Children* 60–120mg per dose (3 months–1 year); 120–250mg per dose (1–5 years); 250–500mg per dose (6–12 years).
Onset of effect Within 15–60 minutes.
Duration of action Up to 6 hours.
Diet advice None.

Storage Keep in a closed container in a cool, dry place out of reach of children.
Missed dose Take as soon as you remember if required to relieve pain. Otherwise do not take the missed dose, and take a further dose only when you are in pain.
Stopping the drug Can be safely stopped as soon as you no longer need it.

OVERDOSE ACTION

Seek immediate medical advice in all cases. Take emergency action if nausea, vomiting, or stomach pain occur.

POSSIBLE ADVERSE EFFECTS

Paracetamol has rarely been found to produce any side effects when taken as recommended, although nausea may occur. If you develop a rash, stop taking the drug and notify your doctor.

INTERACTIONS

Anticoagulants such as warfarin may need dosage adjustment if paracetamol is taken regularly in high doses.
Cholestyramine reduces the absorption of paracetamol and may reduce its effectiveness.

SPECIAL PRECAUTIONS

Be sure to consult your doctor or pharmacist before using this drug if:
◆ You have long-term liver or kidney problems.
◆ You are taking other medications.
Pregnancy No evidence of risk with occasional use.
Breast-feeding No evidence of risk.
Infants and children Infants under 3 months on doctor's advice only. Reduced dose necessary up to 12 years.
Over 60 No special problems.
Driving and hazardous work No special problems.
Alcohol Prolonged heavy intake in combination with excess paracetamol may substantially increase the risk of injury to the liver.

PROLONGED USE

You should not normally take this drug for longer than 48 hours except on the advice of your doctor. However, there is no evidence of harm from long-term use.

Paroxetine

Brand name Seroxat
Used in the following combined preparations
None

QUICK REFERENCE
Drug group Antidepressant drug (p.14)
Overdose danger rating Medium
Dependence rating Low
Prescription needed Yes
Available as generic No

GENERAL INFORMATION
Paroxetine is one of the group of drugs
known as selective serotonin re-uptake inhibitors (SSRIs). It is used for mild to moderate
depression and helps to control the anxiety
often accompanying depression. It is also used
for panic and obsessive-compulsive disorders.

Unlike older tricyclics, paroxetine and other
SSRIs are less likely to cause anticholinergic
side effects such as dry mouth, blurred vision,
and difficulty in passing urine. They are also
much less dangerous if taken in overdose.

The most common adverse effects include
nausea, drowsiness, sweating, tremor, weakness, insomnia, and sexual dysfunction.

INFORMATION FOR USERS
Your drug prescription is tailored for you.
Do not alter dosage without checking with
your doctor.
How taken Tablets.
Frequency and timing of doses Once daily, in
the morning.
Dosage range 20–60mg daily.
Onset of effect The onset of therapeutic
response usually occurs within 7–14 days of
starting treatment, but full antidepressant
effect may not be felt for 3–4 weeks.
Duration of action Up to 24 hours.
Diet advice None.
Storage Keep in a closed container in a cool,
dry place out of reach of children.
Missed dose Take as soon as you remember.
Stopping the drug Unless rash or joint pains
occur, do not stop taking the drug without
consulting your doctor. Stopping abruptly
can cause withdrawal symptoms.
Exceeding the dose An occasional unintentional extra dose is unlikely to be a cause for

concern. Large doses may cause unusual
drowsiness. Notify your doctor immediately.

POSSIBLE ADVERSE EFFECTS
The most common adverse effects are nausea, drowsiness, sweating, tremor, weakness,
insomnia, and sexual dysfunction (lack of
orgasm, male ejaculation problems). Less
commonly, nervousness, anxiety, agitation,
worsening appetite, and weight loss may
occur. Convulsions are a rare complication.
If you develop a blotchy or irritating rash or
joint pains, stop taking the drug and consult
your doctor immediately.

INTERACTIONS
General note Any drug that affects the breakdown of others in the liver may alter blood
levels of paroxetine or vice versa.
Anticoagulants Paroxetine may increase the
effects of these drugs.
Sedatives All sedatives are likely to increase
the sedative effects of paroxetine.
Tricyclic antidepressants Paroxetine may increase the toxicity of these drugs.
MAOIs Paroxetine should not be taken during
or within 14 days of MAOI treatment because serious reactions may occur.

SPECIAL PRECAUTIONS
Be sure to tell your doctor if:
◆ You have long-term liver or kidney prob-
lems.
◆ You have a heart problem.
◆ You have a history, or family history, of fits.
◆ You are taking other medications.
Pregnancy Safety in pregnancy not estab-
lished. Discuss with your doctor.
Breast-feeding The drug passes into the breast
milk. Discuss with your doctor.
Infants and children Not recommended under
18 years.
Over 60 No special problems.
Driving and hazardous work Avoid such activ-
ities until you have learned how paroxetine
affects you because the drug can cause
drowsiness.
Alcohol Avoid. Alcohol may increase the
sedative effects of this drug.

PROLONGED USE
No problems expected. However, mild

withdrawal symptoms may occur if paroxetine treatment is not stopped gradually.

Permethrin

Brand name Lyclear
Used in the following combined preparations
None

QUICK REFERENCE
Drug group Drug to treat skin parasites (p.118)
Overdose danger rating Low
Dependence rating Low
Prescription needed No
Available as generic No

GENERAL INFORMATION
Permethrin is an insecticide related to the natural substance, pyrethrum, which is obtained from the flower of the same name. The drug is used to treat head lice and scabies infestations. It works by interfering with the nervous system function of the parasites, causing paralysis and death. Permethrin has the advantage of being less toxic than some other types of insecticide.

Permethrin is used topically as liquid for head lice and cream for scabies infestations. In children, the entire body surface, including the face, scalp, neck, and ears, is covered; adults are treated from the neck downwards.

For both head lice and scabies, all family members should be treated at the same time, to prevent recontamination, and the process repeated after a week.

There are signs that the parasites are developing resistance to permethrin. If it does not work for you, your pharmacist should be able to suggest an alternative treatment.

INFORMATION FOR USERS
Follow instructions on the label. Call your doctor if symptoms worsen.
How taken Cream, topical liquid.
Frequency and timing of doses Once only, repeating after 7 days. Avoid contact with eyes and broken or infected skin.
Adult dosage range As directed.
Onset of effect Liquid should be rinsed off after 10 minutes (head lice); cream should be washed off after 8–12 hours (scabies).

Duration of action Until washed off.
Diet advice None.
Storage Keep in a closed container in a cool, dry place out of reach of children. Protect from light.
Missed dose Timing of second application is not rigid; use as soon as you remember.
Stopping the drug Not applicable.
Exceeding the dose An occasional extra application is unlikely to cause problems. If accidentally swallowed, take emergency action.

POSSIBLE ADVERSE EFFECTS
In general, permethrin is well tolerated on the skin, although mild skin irritation is common. The skin may be reddened or stinging, and occasionally a rash may occur.

INTERACTIONS
None.

SPECIAL PRECAUTIONS
Be sure to consult your doctor or pharmacist before taking this drug if:
◆ You are taking other medications.
Pregnancy Safety not established. Discuss with your doctor.
Breast-feeding Safety not established. Discuss with your doctor.
Infants and children No special problems.
Over 60 No special problems.
Driving and hazardous work No special problems.
Alcohol No special problems.

PROLONGED USE
Permethrin is intended for intermittent use only and should not be used long term.

Phenobarbital

Brand name Gardenal
Used in the following combined preparations
None

QUICK REFERENCE
Drug group Barbiturate anticonvulsant drug (p.16)
Overdose danger rating High
Dependence rating High
Prescription needed Yes
Available as generic Yes

GENERAL INFORMATION

Phenobarbital, introduced more than 70 years ago, belongs to the group of drugs known as barbiturates. It is used mainly in the treatment of epilepsy but is now being superseded by newer drugs. It was also used as a sleeping drug and sedative before the development of safer drugs.

In the treatment of epilepsy, the drug is usually given together with another anticonvulsant drug such as phenytoin.

The main disadvantage of the drug is that it often causes unwanted sedation. However, tolerance develops within a week or two, and most patients have no problem in long-term use. In children and the elderly, it may occasionally cause excessive excitement.

Because of their sedative effects, phenobarbital and other barbiturates are sometimes abused.

INFORMATION FOR USERS

Your drug prescription is tailored for you. Do not alter dosage without checking with your doctor.

How taken Tablets, liquid, injection.
Frequency and timing of doses 1–3 x daily.
Dosage range Adults 60–180mg daily.
Onset of effect 30–60 minutes (by mouth).
Duration of action 24–48 hours (some effect may persist for up to 6 days).
Diet advice None.
Storage Keep in a closed container in a cool, dry place out of reach of children.
Missed dose Take as soon as you remember. If you take once daily and the next dose is due within 10 hours, take a single dose now and skip the next. If you take 2–3 times daily and the next dose is due within 2 hours, take a single dose now and skip the next.
Stopping the drug Unless rash or swelling occur, do not stop taking the drug without consulting your doctor. He or she may supervise a gradual reduction in dosage because abrupt cessation may cause fits or lead to restlessness, trembling, and insomnia.

OVERDOSE ACTION

Seek immediate medical advice in all cases. Take emergency action if unsteadiness, severe weakness, confusion, or loss of consciousness occur.

POSSIBLE ADVERSE EFFECTS

Most adverse effects of phenobarbital are the result of its sedative effect. These include drowsiness, clumsiness or unsteadiness, dizziness, fainting, and confusion, which can sometimes be minimized by a medically supervised reduction of dosage. If a rash or localized swellings occur, stop taking the drug and call your doctor urgently.

INTERACTIONS

Corticosteroids Phenobarbital may reduce the effect of corticosteroid drugs.
Antipsychotics and antidepressants may reduce the anticonvulsant effect of phenobarbital.
Anticoagulants The effect of these drugs may be reduced when they are taken with phenobarbital.
Oral contraceptives Phenobarbital may reduce the effectiveness of oral contraceptives. Discuss with your doctor.
Sedatives All drugs that have a sedative effect on the central nervous system are likely to increase the sedative properties of phenobarbital.

SPECIAL PRECAUTIONS

Be sure to tell your doctor if:
◆ You have long-term liver or kidney problems.
◆ You have heart problems.
◆ You have poor circulation.
◆ You have porphyria.
◆ You have breathing problems.
◆ You are taking other medications.
Pregnancy The drug may affect the fetus and increase the tendency of bleeding in newborn babies. Discuss with your doctor.
Breast-feeding The drug passes into the breast milk and could cause drowsiness in the baby. Discuss with your doctor.
Infants and children Reduced dose necessary.
Over 60 Increased likelihood of confusion. Reduced dose may therefore be necessary.
Driving and hazardous work Your underlying condition, in addition to the possibility of reduced alertness while taking phenobarbital, may make such activities inadvisable. Discuss with your doctor.
Alcohol Never drink while under treatment with phenobarbital. Alcohol may interact dangerously with this drug.

PROLONGED USE

After starting the drug, its sedative effect can build up, causing excessive drowsiness and lethargy. However, tolerance may develop, reducing these effects. Withdrawal symptoms may occur if the drug is stopped suddenly.

Monitoring Blood samples may be taken periodically to test blood levels of the drug.

Phenoxymethylpenicillin

Brand names Apsin, Tenkicin
Used in the following combined preparations
None

QUICK REFERENCE

Drug group Penicillin antibiotic (p.60)
Overdose danger rating Low
Dependence rating Low
Prescription needed Yes
Available as generic Yes

GENERAL INFORMATION

Phenoxymethylpenicillin, also known as Penicillin V, is a synthetic penicillin-type antibiotic prescribed for a wide range of infections.

Various commonly occurring respiratory tract infections, such as some types of tonsillitis and pharyngitis, as well as ear infections, often respond well to this drug. It is also effective for the treatment of the gum disease, Vincent's gingivitis.

Phenoxymethylpenicillin is also used to treat less common infections caused by the Streptococcus bacterium, such as scarlet fever and erysipelas (a skin infection). It is also prescribed long term to prevent recurrence of rheumatic fever, a rare but potentially serious condition. It is also used long term to prevent infections following removal of the spleen or in sickle cell disease.

As with other penicillins, the most serious adverse effect that may rarely occur is an allergic reaction that may cause collapse, wheezing, and a rash in susceptible people.

INFORMATION FOR USERS

Your drug prescription is tailored for you. Do not alter dosage without checking with your doctor.
How taken Tablets, liquid.

Frequency and timing of doses 2–4 x daily, at least 30 minutes before food.
Dosage range Adults 2–3g daily. Children Reduced dose according to age.
Onset of effect 1–2 days.
Duration of action Up to 12 hours.
Diet advice None.
Storage Keep in a closed container in a cool, dry place out of reach of children.
Missed dose Take as soon as you remember. If your next dose is due within 2 hours, take a single dose now and skip the next.
Stopping the drug Take the full course. Only stop if rash, itching, wheezing, or breathing difficulties occur. Even if you feel better, the original infection may still be present and may recur if treatment is stopped too soon.
Exceeding the dose An occasional unintentional extra dose is unlikely to be a cause for concern. But if you notice any unusual symptoms, or if a large overdose has been taken, notify your doctor.

POSSIBLE ADVERSE EFFECTS

Most people experience no serious adverse effects. However, nausea, vomiting, and diarrhoea may occur. The drug may also provoke an allergic reaction in susceptible people. Stop taking the drug and call your doctor urgently if you experience rash, itching, wheezing, or breathing difficulties.

INTERACTIONS

Oral contraceptives Phenoxymethylpenicillin may reduce the contraceptive effect of these drugs. Discuss with your doctor.
Probenecid increases the level of phenoxymethylpenicillin in the blood.

SPECIAL PRECAUTIONS

Be sure to tell your doctor if:
◆ You have a long-term kidney problem.
◆ You have had a previous allergic reaction to a penicillin or cephalosporin antibiotic.
◆ You have an allergic disorder such as asthma or urticaria.
◆ You are taking other medications.
Pregnancy No evidence of risk.
Breast-feeding The drug passes into the breast milk, but at normal doses adverse effects on the baby are unlikely. Discuss with your doctor.
Infants and children Reduced dose necessary.

Over 60 No special problems.
Driving and hazardous work No known problems.
Alcohol No known problems.

PROLONGED USE
Prolonged use may increase the risk of *Candida* infections and diarrhoea.

Phenylpropanolamine

Used in the following combined preparations
Contac 400, Day Nurse Capsules, Dimotapp, Eskornade, Mucron, Sinutab, Triogesic, Triominic, Vicks Coldcare, and others.

QUICK REFERENCE
Drug group Decongestant (p.24)
Overdose danger rating High
Dependence rating Low
Prescription needed No
Available as generic No

GENERAL INFORMATION
Phenylpropanolamine belongs to the sympathomimetic group of drugs. It is used as a decongestant in many over-the-counter cold relief preparations. By reducing inflammation and swelling of blood vessels in the lining of the nose, the drug relieves the nasal congestion in head colds, hay fever, and sinusitis.

Phenylpropanolamine mimics some of the actions of the sympathetic nervous system (see Autonomic nervous system, p.8), and as a consequence it can produce undesirable stimulant side effects. It may raise the heart rate and severely elevate blood pressure and can also cause palpitations and wakefulness.

INFORMATION FOR USERS
Follow instructions on the label. Call your doctor if symptoms worsen.
How taken Tablets, SR-tablets, capsules, liquid.
Frequency and timing of doses 3–4 x daily; 2 x daily (SR-tablets).
Dosage range 75–100mg daily.
Onset of effect Within 30 minutes.
Duration of action 4–6 hours. Up to 12 hours (SR-tablets).
Diet advice None.

Storage Keep in a closed container in a cool, dry place out of reach of children. Protect from light.
Missed dose Take as soon as you remember if needed. If you take the medication twice daily, and your next dose is due within 12 hours, take a single dose now and skip the next. If you take it 3–4 times daily and your next dose is due within 2 hours, take a single dose now and skip the next.
Stopping the drug Can be safely stopped as soon as you no longer need it.

OVERDOSE ACTION
Seek immediate medical advice in all cases. Take emergency action if delirium, convulsions, or loss of consciousness occur.

POSSIBLE ADVERSE EFFECTS
High doses may be associated with anxiety, nausea, dizziness, and, rarely, with a marked rise in blood pressure, causing palpitations, headache, and breathlessness. If these signs of a rise in blood pressure occur, or if you develop a rash, stop taking the drug and call your doctor urgently.

INTERACTIONS
Other sympathomimetics These increase the risk of adverse effects with the drug.
Beta blockers A severe rise in blood pressure can occur if beta blockers are taken with phenylpropanolamine.
Tricyclic antidepressants and digoxin There is an increased risk of abnormal heart rhythms if these drugs are taken with phenylpropanolamine.
MAOIs These dangerously increase the risk of high blood pressure with phenylpropanolamine. It should not be taken during or within 14 days of MAOI treatment.

SPECIAL PRECAUTIONS
Be sure to consult your doctor or pharmacist before taking this drug if:
◆ You have high blood pressure.
◆ You have heart problems.
◆ You have had glaucoma.
◆ You have an overactive thyroid gland.
◆ You have diabetes.
◆ You have urinary difficulties.
◆ You are taking other medications.

Pregnancy Safety in pregnancy not established. Discuss with your doctor.
Breast-feeding The drug passes into the breast milk and may affect the baby. Discuss with your doctor.
Infants and children Not recommended under 8 years.
Over 60 Reduced dose may be necessary. Increased likelihood of adverse effects.
Driving and hazardous work Do not undertake such activities until you know how phenyl-propanolamine affects you because the drug can cause dizziness.
Alcohol No known problems.

PROLONGED USE
The drug should not be taken long term without medical supervision because it may raise the blood pressure, straining the heart.

Phenytoin/Fosphenytoin

Brand names Epanutin, Pentran
Used in the following combined preparations
None

QUICK REFERENCE
Drug group Anticonvulsant drug (p.16)
Overdose danger rating Medium
Dependence rating Low
Prescription needed Yes
Available as generic Yes

GENERAL INFORMATION
Phenytoin decreases the likelihood of convulsions by reducing abnormal electrical discharges within the brain. Introduced in the 1930s, it is prescribed for the treatment of epilepsy, including grand mal and temporal lobe epilepsy. Fosphenytoin is a new type of phenytoin given by injection for severe fits.

Over the years, various other uses have been found for phenytoin. It has been given for migraine, trigeminal neuralgia, and the correction of certain abnormal heart rhythms.

Some adverse effects (such as overgrowth of the gums) are more pronounced in children, so the drug is prescribed for children only when other drugs are unsuitable. is also avoided, if possible, in young women as it can affect the developing fetus.

INFORMATION FOR USERS
Your drug prescription is tailored for you. Do not alter dosage without checking with your doctor.
How taken Tablets, capsules, liquid, injection.
Frequency and timing of doses 1–3 x daily with food or plenty of water.
Dosage range Adults 200–500mg daily. Children According to age and weight.
Onset of effect Full anticonvulsant effect may not be felt for 7–10 days.
Duration of action 24 hours.
Diet advice Folic acid and vitamin D deficiency may occasionally occur while taking this drug. Make sure you eat a balanced diet containing fresh, green vegetables.
Storage Keep in a tightly closed container in a cool, dry place out of reach of children.
Missed dose Take as soon as you remember.
Stopping the drug Do not stop taking the drug without consulting your doctor; symptoms may recur.
Exceeding the dose An occasional, unintentional extra dose is unlikely to cause problems. However, if you notice unusual drowsiness, slurred speech, or confusion, notify your doctor.

POSSIBLE ADVERSE EFFECTS
Phenytoin has a number of adverse effects, many of which appear only after prolonged use. Dizziness or headache, confusion, nausea, and insomnia are common. If they become severe, your doctor may prescribe a different anticonvulsant. Long-term effects include increased body hair, overgrowth of gums, and a rash. Consult your doctor if you develop a fever, sore throat, or mouth ulcers.

INTERACTIONS
General note Many drugs may interact with phenytoin, causing either an increase or a reduction in the phenytoin blood level. The dosage of phenytoin may need to be adjusted. Consult your doctor.
Ciclosporin Blood levels of ciclosporin may be reduced with phenytoin.
Antidepressants/antipsychotics These drug may reduce the effect of phenytoin.
Warfarin The anticoagulant effect of this drug may be altered. An adjustment in its dosage may be necessary.

Oral contraceptives Phenytoin may reduce their effectiveness.

SPECIAL PRECAUTIONS
Be sure to tell your doctor if:
◆ You have long-term liver or kidney problems.
◆ You have diabetes.
◆ You have porphyria.
◆ You are taking other medications.

Pregnancy May be associated with malformation and a tendency to bleeding in newborn babies. Folic acid supplements should be taken by the mother. Discuss with your doctor.

Breast-feeding The drug passes into the breast milk, but at normal doses adverse effects on the baby are unlikely. Discuss with your doctor.

Infants and children Reduced dose necessary. Increased likelihood of overgrowth of the gums and excessive growth of body hair.

Over 60 Reduced dose may be necessary.

Driving and hazardous work Your underlying condition, as well as the effects of phenytoin, may make such activities inadvisable. Discuss with your doctor.

Alcohol Avoid. Alcohol increases the sedative effects of this drug.

PROLONGED USE
There is a slight risk that blood abnormalities may occur. Prolonged use may also lead to adverse effects on skin, gums, and bones. It may also disrupt control of diabetes.

Monitoring Periodic blood tests may be performed to monitor levels of the drug in the body and composition of the blood cells and blood chemistry.

Pilocarpine

Brand names Minims Pilocarpine, Ocusert Pilo, Salagen, Sno Pilo
Used in the following combined preparation
Isopto Carpine

QUICK REFERENCE
Drug group Miotic drug for glaucoma (p.110)
Overdose danger rating Medium
Dependence rating Low
Prescription needed Yes
Available as generic Yes

GENERAL INFORMATION
Pilocarpine, in use since 1875, is a miotic drug used to treat chronic glaucoma and, less often, severe glaucoma prior to surgery.

It is prescribed most frequently as eye drops. These are quick-acting but have to be re-applied every four to eight hours in chronic glaucoma. A slow-release formulation inserted once a week under the eyelid (Ocusert) may be more convenient for long-term use.

Pilocarpine, like similar drugs, frequently causes blurred vision; and excessive spasm of the eye muscles may cause headaches, particularly at the start of treatment. However, serious adverse effects are rare.

The tablets are used to treat dry mouth following radiotherapy to the head and neck.

INFORMATION FOR USERS
Your drug prescription is tailored for you. Do not alter dosage without checking with your doctor.

How taken Tablets, eye drops, SR-inserts (Ocuserts).

Frequency and timing of doses *Eye drops* 3–6 x daily (chronic glaucoma). In acute glaucoma, pilocarpine is given at 5-minute intervals until the condition is controlled. *Ocusert* Once every 7 days at bedtime. *Tablets* 3 x daily after food with plenty of water.

Dosage range According to formulation and condition. In general, 1–2 eye drops are used per application. *Tablets* 15–30 mg daily.

Onset of effect 15–30 minutes.

Duration of action 4–8 weeks for maximum effect (tablets); 3–8 hours (eye drops); about 7 days (Ocuserts).

Diet advice None.

Storage Keep in a closed container in a cool, dry place out of reach of children (tablets/ eye drops). Discard eye drops 1 month after opening.

Missed dose Use as soon as you remember. If not remembered until 2 hours before your next dose, skip the missed dose and take the next dose now.

Stopping the drug Do not stop taking the drug without consulting your doctor; symptoms may recur.

Exceeding the dose An occasional unintentional extra application is unlikely to cause problems. Excessive use may cause facial flushing, an increase in the flow of saliva, and sweating. If accidentally swallowed, seek medical attention immediately.

POSSIBLE ADVERSE EFFECTS
Alterations in vision, such as blurred vision or poor night vision, are common. Ocuserts may cause irritation if they move out of position. Brow ache and eye pain are common at the start of treatment but usually wear off after a few days. Twitching eyelids, and red, watery eyes may also occur.

INTERACTIONS
General note A wide range of drugs (including aminoglycoside antibiotics, clindamycin, colistin, chloroquine, quinine, quinidine, lithium, and procainamide) may block the effect of pilocarpine.
Beta blockers These drugs may reduce the effects of pilocarpine.
Calcium channel blockers These drugs may increase pilocarpine's systemic effects.

SPECIAL PRECAUTIONS
Be sure to tell your doctor if:
◆ You have asthma.
◆ You have inflamed eyes.
◆ You wear contact lenses.
◆ You have heart, liver, or gastrointestinal problems.
◆ You are taking other medications.
Pregnancy No evidence of risk at the doses used for chronic glaucoma.
Breast-feeding The drug passes into the breast milk, but at normal doses adverse effects on the baby are unlikely. Discuss with your doctor.
Infants and children Not usually prescribed.
Over 60 Reduced night vision is particularly noticeable.
Driving and hazardous work Avoid such activities, especially in poor light, until you have learned how pilocarpine affects you because the drug may cause short sight and poor night vision.
Alcohol No known problems.

PROLONGED USE
The effect of the drug may occasionally wear off with prolonged use as the body adapts, but may be restored by changing temporarily to another antiglaucoma drug.

Piroxicam

Brand names Feldene, Flamatrol, Kentene, Larapram, Piroflam, Pirozip
Used in the following combined preparations
None

QUICK REFERENCE
Drug group Non-steroidal anti-inflammatory drug (p.48) and drug for gout (p.51)
Overdose danger rating Medium
Dependence rating Low
Prescription needed Yes
Available as generic Yes

GENERAL INFORMATION
Piroxicam, introduced in 1980, is a non-steroidal anti-inflammatory drug (NSAID). Like other drugs in this group, it reduces pain, stiffness, and inflammation. Blood levels of the drug remain high for many hours after a dose. Therefore, it needs to be taken only once daily.

Piroxicam is used to treat osteoarthritis, rheumatoid arthritis, acute attacks of gout, and ankylosing spondylitis. The drug relieves the symptoms of arthritis, but it does not cure the disease. Piroxicam is sometimes prescribed in conjunction with slow-acting drugs in the treatment of rheumatoid arthritis to relieve pain and inflammation while the slow-acting drugs take effect. Piroxicam may also be given for pain relief after sports injuries, to treat conditions such as tendinitis and bursitis, and following minor surgery.

As with all NSAIDs, there is a risk of stomach ulcers occurring.

INFORMATION FOR USERS
Your drug prescription is tailored for you. Do not alter dosage without checking with your doctor.
How taken Tablets, dispersible tablets, capsules, injection, suppositories, gel.
Frequency and timing of doses 1–3 x daily with food or plenty of water.
Adult dosage range 10–40mg daily.
Onset of effect Pain relief begins in 3–4 hours. Used for arthritis, the full anti-inflammatory effect develops over 2–4 weeks. Used for gout, this effect develops over 4–5 days.

Duration of action Up to 2 days. Some effect may last for 7–10 days after treatment has been stopped.

Diet advice None.

Storage Keep in a closed container in a cool, dry place out of reach of children. Protect from light.

Missed dose Take as soon as you remember. If your next dose is due within 4 hours, take a single dose now and skip the next.

Stopping the drug When taken for short-term pain relief, the drug can be safely stopped as soon as you no longer need it. Unless serious adverse effects occur (see below), seek medical advice before stopping long-term treatment of arthritis .

Exceeding the dose An occasional unintentional extra dose is unlikely to be a cause for concern. Large overdoses may cause nausea and vomiting. Notify your doctor.

POSSIBLE ADVERSE EFFECTS

Dizziness, headache and gastrointestinal side effects, such as nausea and indigestion, are not generally serious. Discuss symptoms such as abdominal pain and swollen feet or ankles with your doctor. If you develop a rash, or if you experience wheezing or breathlessness, bruising, or bleeding or black bowel movements, stop taking piroxicam and call your doctor immediately.

INTERACTIONS

General note Piroxicam interacts with many drugs, including other NSAIDs, corticosteroids, and oral anticoagulant drugs, to increase the risk of bleeding and/or peptic ulcers.

Lithium Piroxicam may raise blood levels of lithium.

Antihypertensive drugs and diuretics The beneficial effects of these drugs may be reduced by piroxicam.

Ciprofloxacin, norfloxacin, and ofloxacin Piroxicam may increase the risk of convulsions when taken with these drugs.

SPECIAL PRECAUTIONS

Be sure to tell your doctor if:
◆ You have liver or kidney problems.
◆ You have heart problems or high blood pressure

◆ You have had a peptic ulcer, oesophagitis, or acid indigestion.
◆ You have porphyria.
◆ You have asthma.
◆ You are allergic to aspirin.
◆ You are taking other medications.

Pregnancy Not usually prescribed. When taken in the last three months of pregnancy, the drug increase the risk of adverse effects on the baby's heart and may prolong labour. Discuss with your doctor.

Breast-feeding The drug passes into the breast milk but at normal doses adverse effects are unlikely. Discuss with your doctor.

Infants and children Not recommended under 6 years. Reduced dose necessary.

Over 60 Reduced dose may be necessary. Increased likelihood of adverse effects.

Driving and hazardous work Avoid such activities until you have learned how piroxicam affects you because the drug can cause dizziness.

Alcohol Avoid. Alcohol may increase the risk of stomach disorders with piroxicam.

Surgery and general anaesthetics Piroxicam may prolong bleeding. Discuss with your doctor or dentist before any surgery.

PROLONGED USE

There is an increased risk of bleeding from peptic ulcers and in the bowel.

Monitoring Periodic blood counts and liver function tests may be performed.

Pizotifen

Brand name Sanomigran
Used in the following combined preparations
None

QUICK REFERENCE

Drug group Drug for migraine (p.20)
Overdose danger rating Medium
Dependence rating Low
Prescription needed Yes
Available as generic No

GENERAL INFORMATION

Pizotifen is an antihistamine drug with a chemical structure similar to that of the tricyclic antidepressants (p.14); it also has similar anticholinergic effects. This drug is prescribed for the prevention of migraine headaches in people who suffer frequent, disabling attacks. The drug is thought to work by blocking the chemicals (histamine and serotonin) that act on blood vessels in the brain.

Pizotifen has also been prescribed to relieve the symptoms of carcinoid syndrome, a disorder in which excess production of serotonin causes attacks of flushing and diarrhoea.

The main disadvantage of prolonged use of pizotifen is that it stimulates the appetite and, as a result, often causes weight gain. It is usually prescribed only for people in whom other measures for migraine prevention – for example, avoidance of stress and foods that trigger attacks – have failed.

The sweetener used in the liquid medicine may affect blood sugar levels.

INFORMATION FOR USERS

Your drug prescription is tailored for you. Do not alter dosage without checking with your doctor.

How taken Tablets, liquid.

Frequency and timing of doses Once a day (at night) or 3 x daily.

Adult dosage range 1.5–4.5mg daily. Maximum single dose 3mg.

Onset of effect Full beneficial effects may not be felt for several days.

Duration of action Effects of this drug may last for several weeks.

Diet advice Migraine sufferers may be advised to avoid foods that trigger headaches in their case.

Storage Keep in a closed container in a cool, dry place out of reach of children. Protect from light.

Missed dose Take as soon as you remember. If your next dose is due within 4 hours, take a single dose now and skip the next.

Stopping the drug Do not stop taking the drug without consulting your doctor; symptoms may recur.

Exceeding the dose An occasional unintentional extra dose is unlikely to cause problems. Large overdoses may cause drowsiness, nausea, palpitations, and fits. Notify your doctor.

POSSIBLE ADVERSE EFFECTS

Drowsiness is a common adverse effect of pizotifen treatment that can often be minimized by starting treatment with a low dose that is gradually increased. Increased appetite may lead to weight gain. Other adverse effects include nausea, dry mouth, dizziness, blurred vision, and muscle pains. If you begin to become depressed, be sure to consult your doctor.

INTERACTIONS

Anticholinergic drugs The weak anticholinergic effects of pizotifen may be increased by other anticholinergic drugs, including tricyclic antidepressants.

MAOIs A dangerous rise in blood pressure may occur if pizotifen is taken with these drugs.

Sedatives All drugs that have a sedative effect on the central nervous system are likely to increase the sedative properties of pizotifen. These include sleeping drugs, anti-anxiety drugs, opioid analgesic drugs, and antihistamines.

SPECIAL PRECAUTIONS

Be sure to tell your doctor if:
◆ You have a long-term kidney problem.
◆ You have glaucoma.
◆ You have prostate trouble.
◆ You are taking other medications.

Pregnancy Safety in pregnancy not established. Discuss with your doctor.

Breast-feeding The drug passes into the breast milk, but at normal doses adverse effects on the baby are unlikely. Discuss with your doctor.

Infants and children Reduced dose usually necessary.

Over 60 No special problems.

Driving and hazardous work Avoid such activities until you have learned how pizotifen affects you because the drug can cause drowsiness.

Alcohol Avoid. Alcohol may increase the sedative effects of this drug.

PROLONGED USE

Pizotifen often causes weight gain during long-term use. Treatment is usually reviewed every 6 months.

Pravastatin

Brand name Lipostat
Used in the following combined preparations
None

QUICK REFERENCE

Drug group Lipid-lowering drug (p.35)
Overdose danger rating Medium
Dependence rating Low
Prescription needed Yes
Available as generic No

GENERAL INFORMATION

Pravastatin belongs to the statin group of lipid-lowering drugs. It is prescribed for people with hypercholesterolaemia (high levels of cholesterol in the blood) who have not responded to other treatments, such as a special diet, and who are at risk of developing heart disease. The drug works by blocking the action of an enzyme that is needed for the manufacture of cholesterol, mainly in the liver. As a result, blood levels of cholesterol are lowered, which can help to prevent heart disease.

Rarely, statins can cause muscle pain, inflammation, and damage. This seems to be more likely if another kind of lipid-lowering drug called a fibrate is given with the statin.

INFORMATION FOR USERS

Your drug prescription is tailored for you. Do not alter dosage without checking with your doctor.
How taken Tablets.
Frequency and timing of doses Once daily at night.
Adult dosage range 10–40mg daily, changed after intervals of at least 4 weeks.
Onset of effect Within 2 weeks. Full beneficial effect may be felt within 4 weeks.
Duration of action 24 hours.
Diet advice A low fat diet is usually recommended.
Storage Keep in a closed container in a cool, dry place out of reach of children. Protect from light.
Missed dose Take as soon as you remember. If your next dose is due within 8 hours, do not take the missed dose, but take the next dose as usual.

Stopping the drug Do not stop taking the drug without consulting your doctor; stopping may lead to worsening of the underlying condition.
Exceeding the dose An occasional unintentional extra dose is unlikely to cause problems. Large overdoses may cause liver problems. Notify your doctor.

POSSIBLE ADVERSE EFFECTS

Most adverse effects such as headache, nausea, and fatigue are mild and usually disappear with time. Report symptoms such as jaundice, abdominal pain, rash, and muscle pain or weakness to your doctor urgently.

INTERACTIONS

Anticoagulants Pravastatin may increase the effect of these drugs.
Antifungal drugs Taken with pravastatin, itraconazole, ketoconazole, and possibly other antifungal drugs, may increase the risk of muscle damage.
Orlistat This drug increases blood levels and toxicity of pravastatin.
Other lipid-lowering drugs (fibrates) Taken with pravastatin, these drugs may increase the risk of muscle damage.
Ciclosporin and other immunosuppressant drugs There is an increased risk of muscle damage if pravastatin is taken with these drugs. They are not usually prescribed together.

SPECIAL PRECAUTIONS

Be sure to tell your doctor if:
◆ You have had liver problems.
◆ You are taking other medications.
Pregnancy Not usually prescribed. Safety not established. Discuss with your doctor.
Breast-feeding Safety not established. Discuss with your doctor.
Infants and children Not recommended.
Over 60 No special problems.
Driving and hazardous work No special problems.
Alcohol Avoid excessive amounts. Alcohol may increase the risk of developing liver problems with this drug.

PROLONGED USE

Long-term use of pravastatin can affect liver function.

Monitoring Regular blood tests to check liver and muscle function are usually required.

Prednisolone

Brand names Deltacortril, Deltastab, Minims prednisolone, Precortisyl, Predenema, Predfoam, Pred Forte, Predsol, and others
Used in the following combined preparations Predsol-N, Scheriproct

QUICK REFERENCE
Drug group Corticosteroid (p.78)
Overdose danger rating Low
Dependence rating Low
Prescription needed Yes
Available as generic Yes

GENERAL INFORMATION
Prednisolone, a powerful corticosteroid, is used for a wide range of conditions, including some skin diseases, rheumatic disorders, allergic states, and certain blood disorders. It is used in the form of eye drops to reduce inflammation in conjunctivitis or iritis and may be given as an enema to treat inflammatory bowel disease. The drug can also be injected into joints to relieve rheumatoid and other forms of arthritis. Prednisolone is also prescribed with fludrocortisone for pituitary or adrenal gland disorders.

Low doses taken short term either by mouth or topically rarely cause serious side effects. However, long-term treatment with large doses can cause fluid retention, indigestion, diabetes, hypertension, and acne. Enteric-coated tablets reduce the drug's local effects on the stomach but not the systemic effects.

INFORMATION FOR USERS
Your drug prescription is tailored for you. Do not alter dosage without checking with your doctor.
How taken Tablets, injection, suppositories, enema, foam, eye and ear drops.
Frequency and timing of doses 1–2 x daily or on alternate days with food (tablets/injection); 2–4 x daily, more frequently initially (eye/ear drops).
Adult dosage range Considerable variation. Follow your doctor's instructions.

Onset of effect 2–4 days.
Duration of action 12–72 hours.
Diet advice A low-sodium/high-potassium diet is recommended when the oral or injected form of prednisolone is prescribed for extended periods. Follow your doctor's advice.
Storage Keep in a closed container in a cool, dry place out of reach of children. Protect from light.
Missed dose Take as soon as you remember. If your next dose is due within 6 hours, take a single dose now and skip the next.
Stopping the drug Do not stop taking the drug without consulting your doctor. Abrupt cessation of long-term treatment by mouth or injection may be dangerous.
Exceeding the dose An occasional unintentional extra dose is unlikely to be a cause for concern. But if you notice any unusual symptoms, or if a large overdose has been taken, notify your doctor.

POSSIBLE ADVERSE EFFECTS
Indigestion, acne, weight gain, muscle weakness, and mood changes or depression are among the wide range of adverse effects of prednisolone taken by mouth and should be reported to your doctor. If you have black or bloodstained bowel movements, call your doctor urgently. This adverse effect only occurs when high doses are taken by mouth or injection or for long periods. If you are taking prednisolone by mouth, avoid close personal contact with chickenpox or herpes zoster (shingles), and seek urgent medical attention if exposed.

INTERACTIONS
Anticonvulsant drugs Carbamazepine, phenytoin, and phenobarbital can reduce the effects of prednisolone.
Anticoagulant drugs Prednisolone may affect the response to these drugs.
Diuretics Prednisolone may increase the adverse effects of these drugs.
Antihypertensive and antidiabetic drugs and insulin Prednisolone may reduce the effects of these drugs.
Vaccines Serious reactions can occur when vaccinations are given with this drug. Discuss with your doctor.

SPECIAL PRECAUTIONS

Be sure to tell your doctor if:
◆ You have had a peptic ulcer.
◆ You have glaucoma.
◆ You have had tuberculosis.
◆ You suffer from depression.
◆ You have any infection.
◆ You have diabetes.
◆ You have osteoporosis.
◆ You are taking other medications.
Avoid exposure to chickenpox, shingles, or measles if you are on systemic treatment.

Pregnancy No evidence of risk with drops or joint injections. Taken as tablets in low doses, harm to the fetus is unlikely. Discuss with your doctor.

Breast-feeding No evidence of risk with drops or injections. Taken by mouth, it passes into the breast milk, but at low doses adverse effects on the baby are unlikely. Discuss with your doctor.

Infants and children Only given when essential. Reduced dose may be necessary.

Over 60 Reduced dose may be necessary. Increased likelihood of adverse effects.

Driving and hazardous work No known problems.

Alcohol Keep consumption low. Alcohol may increase the risk of peptic ulcers with prednisolone taken by mouth or injection.

PROLONGED USE

Prolonged systemic use can lead to adverse effects such as diabetes, glaucoma, cataracts, and osteoporosis, and may retard growth in children. Dosages are usually tailored to minimize these. People on long-term treatment are advised to carry a treatment card.

Primidone

Brand name Mysoline
Used in the following combined preparations
None

QUICK REFERENCE

Drug group Anticonvulsant (p.16)
Overdose danger rating High
Dependence rating Medium
Prescription needed Yes
Available as generic No

GENERAL INFORMATION

Introduced in the 1950s, primidone is in the anticonvulsant group of drugs. It is chemically related to the barbiturates (see Sleeping drugs, p.11) and is partially converted to phenobarbital in the body. Largely superseded by newer anticonvulsant drugs, primidone is still used mainly for its effect in suppressing epileptic fits. However, the drug is also prescribed to treat people who suffer from certain types of tremor.

Although this drug may be prescribed on its own, it is more frequently taken with another anticonvulsant. Its major adverse effects are due to its sedative action on the central nervous system.

INFORMATION FOR USERS

Your drug prescription is tailored for you. Do not alter dosage without checking with your doctor.

How taken Tablets, liquid.

Frequency and timing of doses 1–3 x daily, usually 2 x daily.

Adult dosage range Initially 125mg, increased gradually to a maximum of 1.5g daily (1g daily in children).

Onset of effect Within 1 hour.

Duration of action Up to 24 hours.

Diet advice None.

Storage Keep in a closed container in a cool, dry place out of reach of children.

Missed dose Take as soon as you remember. If you normally take once daily, and your next dose is due within 8 hours, take a single dose now and skip the next. If you normally take 2–3 times daily, and your next dose is due within 2 hours, take a single dose now and skip the next.

Stopping the drug Do not stop taking the drug without consulting your doctor; symptoms may recur and withdrawal reactions can result.

OVERDOSE ACTION

Seek immediate medical advice in all cases. Take emergency action if loss of consciousness occurs.

POSSIBLE ADVERSE EFFECTS

Most people experience very few adverse effects with this drug, but when blood levels become too high, the adverse effects are common and the dose may need to be reduced. These effects include drowsiness, clumsiness, unsteadiness, dizziness, light-headedness, nausea, and headache. If you develop a rash, notify your doctor.

INTERACTIONS

Sedatives All drugs that have a sedative effect are likely to increase the sedative properties of primidone. Such drugs include sleeping drugs, antihistamines, opioid analgesics, antipsychotic drugs, and antidepressant drugs.

Anticoagulants Primidone may reduce the effect of anticoagulant drugs.

Oral contraceptives Primidone may reduce the effectiveness of oral contraceptives. An alternative form of contraception may be necessary. Discuss with your doctor.

Corticosteroids Primidone may reduce the effect of some of these drugs.

SPECIAL PRECAUTIONS

Be sure to tell your doctor if:
◆ You have long-term liver or kidney problems.
◆ You have heart problems.
◆ You have poor circulation.
◆ You have a lung disorder such as asthma or bronchitis.
◆ You have porphyria.
◆ You are taking other medications.

Pregnancy Not usually prescribed. May cause abnormalities in the fetus. Discuss with your doctor.

Breast-feeding The drug passes into the breast milk and may affect the baby. Discuss with your doctor.

Infants and children Reduced dose necessary, depending on weight.

Over 60 Reduced dose may be necessary.

Driving and hazardous work Your underlying condition, as well as the possibility of reduced alertness while taking primidone, may make such activities inadvisable. Discuss with your doctor.

Alcohol Avoid. Alcohol may dangerously increase the sedative effects of this drug.

PROLONGED USE

Continued use may sometimes lead to dependence. In rare cases, joint pain may occur.

Monitoring Regular blood tests may be performed to measure blood levels and to check the blood cells.

Prochlorperazine

Brand names Buccastem, Prozière, Stemetil
Used in the following combined preparations
None

QUICK REFERENCE

Drug group Phenothiazine antipsychotic drug (p.15) and anti-emetic (p.21)
Overdose danger rating Medium
Dependence rating Low
Prescription needed Yes
Available as generic Yes

GENERAL INFORMATION

Prochlorperazine was introduced in the late 1950s and belongs to a group of drugs called the phenothiazines, which act on the central nervous system.

In small doses, prochlorperazine controls nausea and vomiting, especially when they occur as side effects of medical treatment by drugs or radiation, or of anaesthesia. It is also used to treat the nausea that occurs with inner-ear disorders (e.g., vertigo). In large doses, the drug is used as an antipsychotic to tranquillize, reduce aggressiveness, and suppress abnormal behaviour (see p.21). It thus minimizes and controls the abnormal behaviour of schizophrenia, mania, and other mental disorders. It does not cure any of these diseases but helps to relieve symptoms.

INFORMATION FOR USERS

Your drug prescription is tailored for you. Do not alter the dosage without checking with your doctor.

How taken Tablets, capsules, SR-capsules, liquid, powder, injection, suppositories.

Frequency and timing of doses 2–3 x daily (tablets); 2–3 x daily (suppositories); 1–2 x daily (SR-capsules); 2–3 x daily (injection).

Adult dosage range *Nausea and vomiting* 20mg initially, then 5–10mg per dose (tablets); 5–25mg per dose (suppositories); 10–15mg per dose (SR-capsules). *Mental illness* 15–40mg daily. Larger doses may be given.

Onset of effect Within 60 minutes (by mouth or suppository); 10–20 minutes (by injection).
Duration of action 3–6 hours (up to 12 hours SR-preparations).
Diet advice None.
Storage Keep in a closed container in a cool, dry place out of reach of children. Protect from light.
Missed dose Take as soon as you remember. If your next dose is due within 2 hours, take a single dose now and skip the next.
Stopping the drug Can be safely stopped as soon as it is no longer needed for nausea or vomiting. When used for mental illness, do not stop taking the drug without consulting your doctor; symptoms may recur.
Exceeding the dose An occasional unintentional extra dose is unlikely to be a cause for concern. Large overdoses may cause unusual drowsiness and may affect the heart. Notify your doctor.

POSSIBLE ADVERSE EFFECTS

The drug has a strong anticholinergic effect, which can cause minor symptoms, such as drowsiness, lethargy, dry mouth, and dizziness, that often become less marked with time. The most significant adverse effect with high doses is parkinsonism, caused by changes in the balance of brain chemicals. Discuss this and rash, jaundice, fever, and stiffness of the neck, jaws, or tongue urgently with your doctor.

INTERACTIONS

Sedatives All drugs with a sedative effect are likely to increase the sedative effects of prochlorperazine.
Drugs for parkinsonism Prochlorperazine may block the beneficial effect of these.
Anticholinergic drugs Prochlorperazine may increase the side effects of these drugs.

SPECIAL PRECAUTIONS

Be sure to tell your doctor if:
◆ You have heart problems.
◆ You have liver or kidney problems.
◆ You have had epileptic fits.
◆ You have Parkinson's disease.
◆ You have an underactive thyroid gland.
◆ You have prostate problems.
◆ You have glaucoma.
◆ You are taking other medications.

Pregnancy Safety in pregnancy not established. Discuss with your doctor.
Breast-feeding The drug passes into the breast milk and may affect the baby. Discuss with your doctor.
Infants and children Not recommended in infants weighing less than 10kg and young children. Reduced dose necessary in older children due to increased risk of adverse effects.
Over 60 Reduced dose may be necessary. Increased likelihood of adverse effects.
Driving and hazardous work Avoid such activities until you have learned how prochlorperazine affects you because the drug can cause drowsiness and reduced alertness.
Alcohol Avoid. Alcohol may increase and prolong the sedative effects of this drug.

PROLONGED USE

Use of this drug for more than a few months may lead to the development of involuntary, potentially irreversible, eye, mouth, and tongue, movements (tardive dyskinesia). Occasionally, jaundice may occur.
Monitoring Periodic blood tests may be performed.

Procyclidine

Brand names Arpicolin, Kemadrin
Used in the following combined preparations
None

QUICK REFERENCE

Drug group Anticholinergic drug for parkinsonism (p.18)
Overdose danger rating High
Dependence rating Low
Prescription needed Yes
Available as generic Yes

GENERAL INFORMATION

Introduced in the 1950s, procyclidine is an anticholinergic drug that is used to treat Parkinson's disease. It is especially helpful in the early stages of the disorder for treating muscle rigidity. It also helps to reduce muscle tremor and excess salivation. However, the drug has less effect on the shuffling gait and slowness of muscular movement that characterize Parkinson's disease.

Procyclidine is also often used to treat parkinsonism resulting from treatment with antipsychotics.

The drug may cause various minor adverse effects (see below), but these are rarely serious enough to warrant stopping treatment.

INFORMATION FOR USERS
Your drug prescription is tailored for you. Do not alter dosage without checking with your doctor.

How taken Tablets, liquid, injection.
Frequency and timing of doses 2–3 x daily.
Adult dosage range 7.5–30mg daily, exceptionally up to 60mg daily. Dosage is determined individually in order to find the best balance between effective relief of symptoms and the occurrence of adverse effects.
Onset of effect Within 30 minutes.
Duration of action 8–12 hours.
Diet advice None.
Storage Keep in a closed container in a cool, dry place out of reach of children.
Missed dose Take as soon as you remember. If your next dose is due within 2 hours, take a single dose now and skip the next.
Stopping the drug Do not stop taking the drug without consulting your doctor; symptoms may recur.

OVERDOSE ACTION
Seek immediate medical advice in all cases. Take emergency action if palpitations, fits, or unconsciousness occur.

POSSIBLE ADVERSE EFFECTS
The possible adverse effects are mainly the result of the drug's anticholinergic action. Some more common symptoms, such as dry mouth, constipation, and blurred vision, may be overcome by dosage adjustment. Nausea and vomiting, nervousness, confusion, drowsiness, and rash have occasionally been reported. If you experience difficulty in passing urine, notify your doctor. If palpitations occur, seek immediate medical attention.

INTERACTIONS
Anticholinergics and antihistamines These drugs may increase procyclidine's adverse effects .
Antidepressants These drugs may increase the adverse effects of procyclidine.

Glyceryl trinitrate This may be less effective in the relief of heart pain, since dry mouth may prevent its dissolution under the tongue.

SPECIAL PRECAUTIONS
Be sure to tell your doctor if:
◆ You have long-term liver or kidney problems.
◆ You suffer from or have a family history of glaucoma.
◆ You have high blood pressure.
◆ You suffer from constipation.
◆ You have prostate trouble.
◆ You are taking other medications.
Pregnancy Safety in pregnancy not established. Discuss with your doctor.
Breast-feeding The drug passes into the breast milk and may affect the baby. Discuss with your doctor.
Infants and children Not recommended.
Over 60 Reduced dose may be necessary.
Driving and hazardous work Avoid such activities until you have learned how procyclidine affects you because the drug can cause drowsiness, blurred vision, and mild confusion.
Alcohol Avoid. Alcohol may increase the sedative effect of this drug.

PROLONGED USE
Prolonged use of this drug may provoke the onset of glaucoma.
Monitoring Periodic eye examinations are usually advised.

Proguanil
Brand name Paludrine
Used in the following combined preparations
None

QUICK REFERENCE
Drug group Antimalarial drug (p.73)
Overdose danger rating Medium
Dependence rating Low
Prescription needed No
Available as generic No

GENERAL INFORMATION
An antimalarial drug in use for over 30 years, proguanil is given to prevent malaria from developing in people visiting parts of the

world where it is prevalent. Treatment must be started one week before travel and continued for four weeks after you return. In some parts of the world the parasite is resistant to proguanil, so another drug such as chloroquine may also be needed to ensure adequate protection. Always seek expert advice on malaria prevention well ahead of travelling. To be effective, the drug must be taken regularly. Consult your doctor at once if you become ill within three months of returning.

Adverse effects with proguanil are rare and usually subside with continued treatment.

Preventative drug treatment should be combined with personal protection against being bitten, such as keeping well covered and using mosquito nets and repellents.

INFORMATION FOR USERS
Follow instructions on the label.
How taken Tablets.
Frequency and timing of doses Once daily with water after food.
Adult dosage range 200mg (2 tablets) daily.
Onset of effect After 24 hours.
Duration of action 24–48 hours.
Diet advice None.
Storage Keep in a closed container in a cool, dry place out of reach of children.
Missed dose Take as soon as you remember. If your next dose is due at this time, take both doses together.
Stopping the drug Do not stop taking the drug for 4 weeks after leaving a malaria-infected area, otherwise there is a risk that you may develop the disease.
Exceeding the dose An occasional unintentional extra dose is unlikely to cause problems. Large overdoses may cause abdominal pain and vomiting. Notify your doctor.

POSSIBLE ADVERSE EFFECTS
Adverse effects are rare. Stomach irritation is the most common problem and may cause indigestion, nausea, vomiting, and abdominal pain, but these usually settle as the treatment continues. Mouth ulcers and hair loss are also recognized adverse effects.

INTERACTIONS
Warfarin The effects of warfarin may be enhanced by proguanil.

Antacids The absorption of proguanil may be reduced by antacids.

SPECIAL PRECAUTIONS
Be sure to tell your doctor if:
◆ You have a long-term kidney problem.
◆ You are taking other medications.
Pregnancy Safety in pregnancy not established, but benefits are generally considered to outweigh risks. Folic acid supplements must be taken. Discuss with your doctor.
Breast-feeding The drug passes into the breast milk, but at normal doses adverse effects on the baby are unlikely. Breast-feeding while taking proguanil will not protect the baby from malaria. Discuss with your doctor.
Infants and children Reduced dose necessary.
Over 60 No known problems.
Driving and hazardous work No known problems.
Alcohol No special problems.

PROLONGED USE
No known problems.

Promazine
Brand name Sparine
Used in the following combined preparations
None

QUICK REFERENCE
Drug group Anti-anxiety drug (p.13)
Overdose danger rating Medium
Dependence rating Low
Prescription needed Yes
Available as generic Yes

GENERAL INFORMATION
Promazine, introduced in the late 1950s, is a member of the group of drugs called phenothiazines, which act on the brain to regulate abnormal behaviour (see Antipsychotics, p.15).

The main use of promazine is to calm agitated and restless behaviour. The drug is also given as a sedative for the short-term treatment of severe anxiety, especially in the elderly and during terminal illness.

In theory, promazine may cause unpleasant side effects, in particular parkinsonism (abnormal movements and shaking of the arms and legs). In practice, however, the drug is rarely used for long enough to produce these problems.

INFORMATION FOR USERS

Your drug prescription is tailored for you. Do not alter dosage without checking with your doctor.

How taken Tablets, liquid, injection.
Frequency and timing of doses 4 x daily.
Adult dosage range 100–800mg daily (tablets).
Onset of effect 30 minutes–1 hour.
Duration of action 4–6 hours.
Diet advice None.
Storage Keep in a closed container in a cool, dry place out of reach of children. Protect from light.
Missed dose Take as soon as you remember. If your next dose is due within 2 hours, take a single dose now and skip the next.
Stopping the drug Do not stop taking the drug without consulting your doctor; symptoms may recur.
Exceeding the dose An occasional unintentional extra dose is unlikely to be a cause for concern. Large overdoses may cause drowsiness, dizziness, unsteadiness, fits, and coma. Notify your doctor.

POSSIBLE ADVERSE EFFECTS

The more common adverse effects of promazine, such as drowsiness, dry mouth, constipation, and blurred vision, may be helped by adjustment of dosage. Promazine may affect the body's ability to regulate body temperature (especially in the elderly). The most significant adverse effect with high doses is parkinsonism, caused by changes in the balance of brain chemicals. Discuss this with your doctor.

INTERACTIONS

Sedatives All drugs that have a sedative effect are likely to increase the sedative properties of promazine.
Anticonvulsants Promazine may reduce the effectiveness of anticonvulsants.
Drugs for parkinsonism The effectiveness of these drugs may be reduced by promazine.
Antiemetics There is an increased risk of parkinsonism if antiemetic drugs such as metoclopramide are taken with promazine.

SPECIAL PRECAUTIONS

Be sure to tell your doctor if:
◆ You have heart problems.
◆ You have long-term liver or kidney problems.
◆ You have myasthenia gravis or phaeochromocytoma.
◆ You have had epileptic fits.
◆ You have breathing problems.
◆ You have prostate problems.
◆ You have glaucoma.
◆ You have Parkinson's disease.
◆ You are diabetic.
◆ You are taking other medications.
Pregnancy Safety in early pregnancy not established. The drug is sometimes injected during labour. Discuss with your doctor.
Breast-feeding The drug passes into the breast milk, but at normal doses adverse effects on the baby are unlikely. Discuss with your doctor.
Infants and children Not recommended.
Over 60 Reduced dose may be necessary. Increased likelihood of adverse effects.
Driving and hazardous work Avoid such activities until you have learned how promazine affects you because the drug can cause drowsiness and reduced alertness.
Alcohol Avoid. Alcohol may increase the sedative effect of this drug.

PROLONGED USE

Use of this drug for more than a few months may be associated with jaundice and abnormal movements. Sometimes a reduction in dose may be recommended.
Monitoring Periodic blood tests and eye examinations may be performed.

Promethazine

Brand names Avomine, Phenergan, Sominex
Used in the following combined preparations
Medised, Night Nurse, Pamergan P100, Phensedyl Plus, Tixylix Night-time

QUICK REFERENCE
Drug group Antihistamine (p.56) and anti-emetic (p.21)
Overdose danger rating Medium
Dependence rating Low
Prescription needed No
Available as generic No

GENERAL INFORMATION

Promethazine is one of a class of drugs known as the phenothiazines, which were developed in the 1950s for their beneficial effect on abnormal behaviour arising from mental illnesses (see Antipsychotics, p.15). Promethazine was found, however, to have effects more like the antihistamines used to treat allergies (see p.56) and some types of nausea and vomiting (see Anti-emetics, p.21). The drug is widely used to reduce itching in a variety of skin conditions including urticaria (hives), chickenpox, and eczema. It can also relieve the nausea and vomiting caused by inner ear disturbances such as Ménière's disease and motion sickness. Because of its sedative effect, promethazine is sometimes used for short periods as a sleeping medicine, and is also given as premedication before surgery.

Promethazine is used in combined preparations together with opioid cough suppressants for the relief of coughs and nasal congestion, and it is given at night for its sedative effect.

INFORMATION FOR USERS

Follow instructions on the label. Call your doctor if symptoms worsen.

How taken Tablets, liquid, injection.

Frequency and timing of doses *Allergic symptoms* 1–3 x daily or as a single dose at night. *Motion sickness* Bedtime on night before travelling, repeating following morning if necessary, then every 6–8 hours as necessary. *Nausea and vomiting* Every 4–6 hours as necessary.

Dosage range (promethazine hydrochloride) *Adults* 20–75mg per dose.
Children Reduced dose according to age.

Onset of effect Within 1 hour. If dose is taken after nausea has started, the onset of effect is delayed.

Duration of action 8–16 hours.

Diet advice None.

Storage Keep in a closed container in a cool, dry place out of reach of children. Protect from light.

Missed dose No cause for concern, but take as soon as you remember. Adjust the timing of your next dose accordingly.

Stopping the drug Can be safely stopped as soon as symptoms disappear.

Exceeding the dose An occasional unintentional extra dose is unlikely to cause problems. Large overdoses may cause drowsiness or agitation, fits, unsteadiness, and coma. Notify your doctor.

POSSIBLE ADVERSE EFFECTS

Promethazine usually causes only minor anticholinergic effects, including drowsiness, lethargy, dry mouth, and blurred vision. If you develop a rash on light-exposed areas of skin, stop taking the drug and consult your doctor.

INTERACTIONS

MAOIs These drugs may cause a severe reaction if taken with promethazine. Avoid taking promethazine if MAOIs have been taken in the last 14 days.

Sedatives All drugs that have a sedative effect are likely to increase the sedative properties of promethazine. Such drugs include other antihistamines, sleeping drugs, and antipsychotics.

SPECIAL PRECAUTIONS

Be sure to consult your doctor or pharmacist before taking this drug if:
◆ You have liver or kidney problems.
◆ You have had epileptic fits.
◆ You have heart disease.
◆ You have glaucoma.
◆ You suffer from asthma.
◆ You have Parkinson's disease.
◆ You have urinary difficulties.
◆ You are taking other medications.

Pregnancy Safety in pregnancy not established. Discuss with your doctor.

Breast-feeding The drug passes into the breast milk, but at normal doses adverse effects on the baby are unlikely. Discuss with your doctor.

Infants and children Not recommended for infants under two years. Reduced dose necessary for older children.

Over 60 No special problems.

Driving and hazardous work Avoid such activities until you have learned how promethazine affects you because the drug can cause drowsiness.

Alcohol Avoid. Alcohol may increase the sedative effects of this drug.

Sunlight Avoid exposure to strong sunlight.

PROLONGED USE
Prolonged use is rarely necessary. The drug may sometimes cause abnormal movements of the face and limbs (parkinsonism), but this normally disappears on stopping the drug.

Propranolol

Brand names Angilol, Apsolol, Berkolol, Beta-Prograne, Cardinol, Inderal, Inderal-LA, Propanix, and others
Used in the following combined preparations
Inderetic, Inderex

QUICK REFERENCE
Drug group Beta blocker (p.28) and anti-anxiety drug (p.13)
Overdose danger rating High
Dependence rating Low
Prescription needed Yes
Available as generic Yes

GENERAL INFORMATION
Propranolol, introduced in 1965, was the first widely available beta blocker in the UK. It is most often used to treat hypertension, angina, and abnormal heart rhythms but is also helpful in controlling the fast heart rate and other symptoms of an overactive thyroid gland. It also helps to reduce the palpitations, sweating, and tremor of severe anxiety and is also used to prevent migraine headaches.

Propranolol is not prescribed to people with asthma because it can cause breathing difficulties. The drug can be useful for diabetics who are at high risk of heart disease, but, like all beta blockers, it may affect the body's response to low blood sugar.

INFORMATION FOR USERS
Your drug prescription is tailored for you. Do not alter dosage without checking with your doctor.
How taken Tablets, SR-capsules, liquid, injection.
Frequency and timing of doses 2–4 x daily. Once daily (SR-capsules).
Adult dosage range *Abnormal heart rhythms* 30–160mg daily. *Angina* 80–240mg daily.

Hypertension 160–320mg daily. *Migraine prevention and anxiety* 40–160mg daily.
Onset of effect 1–2 hours (tablets); after 4 hours (SR-capsules). In hypertension and migraine, it may be several weeks before full benefits of this drug are felt.
Duration of action 6–12 hours (tablets); 24–30 hours (SR-capsules).
Diet advice None.
Storage Keep in a closed container in a cool, dry place out of reach of children. Protect from light.
Missed dose Take as soon as you remember. If your next dose is due within 2 hours (tablets) or 12 hours (SR-capsules), take a single dose now and skip the next.
Stopping the drug Do not stop taking the drug without consulting your doctor. Abrupt cessation may lead to worsening of the underlying condition.

OVERDOSE ACTION
Seek immediate medical advice in all cases. Take emergency action if breathing difficulties, collapse, or loss of consciousness occur.

POSSIBLE ADVERSE EFFECTS
Cold hands and feet, dry eyes, aching muscles, and nightmares or vivid dreams are adverse effects that are common to most beta blockers. Symptoms such as fatigue and nausea are usually temporary and diminish with long-term use. Fainting may be a sign that the drug has slowed the heart beat excessively and should be reported to your doctor promptly. You should also report any shortness of breath or wheezing.

INTERACTIONS
Antihypertensives Propranolol may enhance the blood pressure lowering effect.
Diltiazem and verapamil Combining either of these drugs with propranolol may have adverse effects on heart function.
Cimetidine and hydralazine These drugs may increase the effects of propranolol.
NSAIDs (e.g., indomethacin) These may reduce the antihypertensive effect of propranolol.

SPECIAL PRECAUTIONS
Be sure to tell your doctor if:
◆ You have long-term liver or kidney problems.

◆ You have a breathing disorder such as asthma, bronchitis, or emphysema.
◆ You have heart failure.
◆ You have diabetes.
◆ You have poor circulation in the legs.
◆ You are taking other medications.

Pregnancy May affect the baby. Discuss with your doctor.

Breast-feeding The drug passes into the breast milk, but at normal doses adverse effects on the baby are unlikely. Discuss with your doctor.

Infants and children Reduced dose necessary.

Over 60 Increased risk of adverse effects.

Driving and hazardous work No special problems.

Alcohol No special problems.

Surgery and general anaesthetics Propranolol may need to be stopped before you have a general anaesthetic. Discuss this with your doctor or dentist before any surgery.

PROLONGED USE
No problems expected.

Propylthiouracil

Brand names None
Used in the following combined preparations None

QUICK REFERENCE
Drug group Antithyroid drug (p.82)
Overdose danger rating Medium
Dependence rating Low
Prescription needed Yes
Available as generic Yes

GENERAL INFORMATION
Propylthiouracil is an antithyroid drug used to manage an overactive thyroid gland (hyperthyroidism). In some people, particularly those with Graves' disease (the most common form of the disorder), drug treatment alone may bring on a remission. Propylthiouracil may also be prescribed for long-term treatment of the disease in people who may be at special risk from surgery, such as children and pregnant women.

The drug is also used to restore the normal functioning of the thyroid gland before its partial removal by surgery. It is sometimes given with thyroxine in order to prevent the development of hypothyroidism (low thyroid hormone levels). Propylthiouracil is preferred to other antithyroid drugs when treatment is essential during pregnancy.

The most important adverse effect that sometimes occurs is a reduction in white blood cells, leading to the risk of infection. If you develop a sore throat or mouth ulceration, see your doctor immediately; this might be a sign that your blood is being affected.

INFORMATION FOR USERS
Your drug prescription is tailored for you. Do not alter dosage without consulting your doctor.

How taken Tablets.

Frequency and timing of doses 1–3 x daily.

Dosage range Initially 300–600mg daily. Dose can usually be reduced to 50–150mg daily.

Onset of effect 10–20 days. Full beneficial effects may not be felt for 6–10 weeks.

Duration of action 24–36 hours.

Diet advice Your doctor may advise you to avoid foods that are high in iodine.

Storage Keep in a closed container in a cool, dry place out of reach of children. Protect from light.

Missed dose Take as soon as you remember. If your next dose is due within 3 hours, take a single dose now and skip the next.

Stopping the drug Do not stop taking the drug without consulting your doctor; stopping the drug may lead to a recurrence of hyperthyroidism.

Exceeding the dose An occasional unintentional extra dose is unlikely to cause problems. Large overdoses may cause nausea, vomiting, and headache. Notify your doctor.

POSSIBLE ADVERSE EFFECTS
Serious side effects are rare with this drug. Rashes and itching are fairly common. Nausea, vomiting, headache, and joint pain may also occur. Sore throat or fever may indicate adverse effects on the blood. If these or jaundice occur, inform your doctor immediately.

INTERACTIONS
Anticoagulants Propylthiouracil may increase the effects of these drugs, making an adjustment in dosage necessary.

SPECIAL PRECAUTIONS

Be sure to tell your doctor if:
◆ You have long-term liver or kidney problems.
◆ You are taking other medications.

Pregnancy Prescribed with caution. Risk of goitre and hypothyroidism (thyroid hormone deficiency) in the newborn baby if too high a dose is used. Discuss with your doctor.
Breast-feeding The drug passes into the breast milk and may affect the baby. Discuss with your doctor.
Infants and children Reduced dose necessary.
Over 60 No special problems.
Driving and hazardous work No problems expected.
Alcohol No known problems.

PROLONGED USE

High doses over a prolonged period may reduce the number of white blood cells.
Monitoring Periodic tests of thyroid function are usually required, and blood cell counts may also be carried out.

Pyridostigmine

Brand name Mestinon
Used in the following combined preparations
None

QUICK REFERENCE

Drug group Drug for myasthenia gravis (p.53)
Overdose danger rating High
Dependence rating Low
Prescription needed Yes
Available as generic No

GENERAL INFORMATION

Pyridostigmine is used to treat a rare autoimmune condition involving faulty transmission of nerve impulses to the muscles, known as myasthenia gravis (p.53). It improves muscle strength by prolonging nerve signals but does not cure the disease. In severe cases, the drug may be given with corticosteroids or other drugs. It may also be given to reverse temporary paralysis of the bowel and urinary retention following operations.

Side effects, including abdominal cramps, nausea, and diarrhoea, usually disappear as a result of reducing dosage of pyridostigmine.

INFORMATION FOR USERS

Your drug prescription is tailored for you. Do not alter dosage without checking with your doctor.
How taken Tablets.
Frequency and timing of doses Every 3–4 hours initially. Thereafter, according to the needs of the individual.
Dosage range *Adults* 150mg–1.2g daily (by mouth) according to response and side effects. *Children* Reduced dose necessary according to age and weight.
Onset of effect 30–60 minutes.
Duration of action 3–6 hours.
Diet advice None.
Storage Keep in a closed container in a cool, dry place out of reach of children. Protect from light.
Missed dose Take as soon as you remember. If your next dose is due within 2 hours, take a single dose now and skip the next.
Stopping the drug Do not stop taking the drug without consulting your doctor; symptoms may recur.

OVERDOSE ACTION

Seek immediate medical advice in all cases. You may experience severe abdominal cramps, vomiting, weakness, and tremor. Take emergency action if wheezing, unusually slow heart beat, fits, or loss of consciousness occur.

POSSIBLE ADVERSE EFFECTS

Adverse effects are usually dose-related and can be avoided by adjusting the dose. These effects include nausea, vomiting, increased salivation, abdominal cramps, diarrhoea, watering eyes, small pupils, sweating, and headache. In rare cases hypersensitivity may occur, leading to an allergic rash.

INTERACTIONS

General note Drugs that suppress the transmission of nerve signals may oppose the effect of pyridostigmine; they include aminoglycoside antibiotics, digoxin, procainamide, quinidine, lithium, and chloroquine.
Propranolol This beta blocker antagonizes the effect of pyridostigmine.

SPECIAL PRECAUTIONS

Be sure to tell your doctor if:

◆ You have a long-term kidney problem.
◆ You have heart problems.
◆ You have had epileptic fits.
◆ You have asthma.
◆ You have difficulty in passing urine.
◆ You have a peptic ulcer.
◆ You have Parkinson's disease.
◆ You are taking other medications.

Pregnancy No evidence of risk to the developing fetus in the first 6 months. Large doses near the time of delivery may cause premature labour and temporary muscle weakness in the baby. Discuss with your doctor.

Breast-feeding No evidence of risk, but the baby should be monitored for signs of muscle weakness.

Infants and children Reduced dose necessary, calculated according to age and weight.

Over 60 Reduced dose is usually given. Increased likelihood of adverse effects.

Driving and hazardous work Your underlying condition may make such activities inadvisable. Discuss with your doctor.

Alcohol No special problems.

Surgery and general anaesthetics Pyridostigmine interacts with some anaesthetic agents. Discuss your treatment with your doctor, dentist, and anaesthetist before any surgery.

PROLONGED USE

No problems expected.

Pyrimethamine

Brand name Daraprim
Used in the following combined preparations
Fansidar, Maloprim

QUICK REFERENCE

Drug group Antimalarial drug (p.73)
Overdose danger rating Medium
Dependence rating Low
Prescription needed Yes
Available as generic No

GENERAL INFORMATION

Pyrimethamine is an antimalarial drug now reserved for use against types of malaria resistant to other drugs. Since the malaria parasites can readily develop resistance to pyrimethamine, the drug is now usually given combined with the antibacterial drug sulfadoxine (Fansidar) or dapsone (Maloprim). The activity of these combinations greatly exceeds that of either drug alone. Fansidar is used to suppress the symptoms of malaria during treatment with quinine. Maloprim is now used with chloroquine only to protect against malaria in areas with a high risk of chloroquine-resistant malaria.

Pyrimethamine and sulfadiazine are given together to treat toxoplasmosis in immuno-compromised patients.

Because blood disorders can arise during prolonged use, blood counts are monitored regularly and vitamin supplements are given.

INFORMATION FOR USERS

Your drug prescription is tailored for you. Do not alter dosage without checking with your doctor.

How taken Tablets.

Frequency and timing of doses *Prevention of malaria* Once weekly starting 1 week before travel and continuing for at least 4 weeks after leaving malarial area.

Dosage range *Adults* 25mg per dose (prevention of malaria).
Children Reduced dose necessary according to age.

Onset of effect 24 hours.

Duration of action Up to 1 week.

Diet advice None.

Storage Keep in a closed container in a cool, dry place out of reach of children. Protect from light.

Missed dose Take as soon as you remember. If your next dose is due within 24 hours, take a single dose now and alter the dosing day so that your next dose is one week later.

Stopping the drug Do not stop taking the drug until 4 weeks after leaving a malaria-infected area, otherwise there is a risk that you may develop the disease.

Exceeding the dose An occasional unintentional extra dose is unlikely to cause problems. Large overdoses may cause trembling, breathing difficulty, fits, and blood disorders. Notify your doctor.

POSSIBLE ADVERSE EFFECTS

Side effects of pyrimethamine, such as indigestion and insomnia, occur only rarely with the low doses that are given for the prevention of malaria. Unusual tiredness, weakness, bleeding, bruising, and sore throat may be signs of a blood disorder. Notify your doctor promptly if these occur. Breathing difficulties, rash, or signs of chest infection should also be reported to your doctor.

INTERACTIONS

General note Drugs that suppress the bone marrow or cause folic acid deficiency may increase the risk of serious blood disorders when taken with pyrimethamine. Such drugs include anticancer and antirheumatic drugs, phenylbutazone, sulfasalazine, co-trimoxazole, trimethoprim, and phenytoin.

SPECIAL PRECAUTIONS

Be sure to tell your doctor if:
◆ You have long-term liver or kidney problems.
◆ You have had epileptic fits.
◆ You have anaemia.
◆ You are allergic to sulphonamides.
◆ You have glucose-6-phosphate dehydrogenase (G6PD) deficiency.
◆ You are taking other medications.
Pregnancy Pyrimethamine may cause folic acid deficiency in the unborn fetus. Pregnant women receiving this drug should take a folic acid supplement. Discuss with your doctor.
Breast-feeding The drug passes into the breast milk, but at normal doses adverse effects on the baby are unlikely. Discuss with your doctor.
Infants and children Reduced dose necessary.
Over 60 No special problems.
Driving and hazardous work No special problems.
Alcohol No known problems.

PROLONGED USE

Prolonged use of this drug may cause folic acid deficiency, leading to serious blood disorders. Supplements of folic acid may be recommended (in the form of folinic acid).
Monitoring Regular blood cell counts are required during high-dose or long-term treatment.

Quetiapine

Brand name Seroquel
Used in the following combined preparations
None

QUICK REFERENCE

Drug group Antipsychotic drug (p.15)
Overdose danger rating Medium
Dependence rating Low
Prescription needed Yes
Available as generic No

GENERAL INFORMATION

Quetiapine is an antipsychotic drug that is prescribed for the treatment of schizophrenia. It can be used to treat "positive" symptoms (thought disorders, delusions, and hallucinations) and "negative" symptoms (blunted affect and emotional and social withdrawal). Quetiapine may be more effective when it is used to treat positive symptoms, however.

Unlike the similar drug olanzapine, quetiapine stays in the body for the same length of time in both men and women. Elderly people excrete the drug up to 50 percent more slowly than the usual adult rate. They therefore require much lower doses in order to avoid adverse effects.

Parkinsonism is a common adverse effect of this and many other antipsychotic drugs.

INFORMATION FOR USERS

Your drug prescription is tailored for you. Do not alter dosage without checking with your doctor.
How taken Tablets.
Frequency and timing of doses 2 x daily.
Adult dosage range 50mg daily (day 1), 100mg daily (day 2), 200mg daily (day 3), 300mg daily (day 4), then changing according to response. Usual range is 300-450mg daily, maximum 750mg daily.
Onset of effect 1 hour.
Duration of action Up to 12 hours.
Diet advice None.
Storage Keep in a closed container in a cool, dry place out of reach of children.
Missed dose Take as soon as you remember. If your next dose is due within 4 hours take a single dose now and skip the next.

Stopping the drug Do not stop taking the drug without consulting your doctor; symptoms may recur.
Exceeding the dose
An occasional unintentional extra dose is unlikely to cause problems. Large overdoses may cause unusual drowsiness, palpitations, and low blood pressure. Notify your doctor.

POSSIBLE ADVERSE EFFECTS

Unusual drowsiness and weight gain are common adverse effects of quetiapine. Digestive upset and parkinsonism are less common. If persistent sore throat, dizziness or fainting, or palpitations occur, consult your doctor.

INTERACTIONS

Sedatives All drugs that have a sedative effect on the central nervous system are likely to increase the sedative properties of quetiapine.
Anticonvulsants Quetiapine opposes the effect of these drugs. Phenytoin decreases the effect of quetiapine.

SPECIAL PRECAUTIONS

Be sure to tell your doctor if:
◆ You have epilepsy.
◆ You have Parkinson's disease.
◆ You have liver or kidney problems.
◆ You have heart problems.
◆ You have blood problems.
◆ You are taking other medications.
Pregnancy Safety not established. Discuss with your doctor.
Breast-feeding Safety not established. Discuss with your doctor.
Infants and children Not recommended.
Over 60 Reduced doses necessary. The elderly eliminate quetiapine much more slowly than younger adults.
Driving and hazardous work Avoid. Quetiapine can cause drowsiness.
Alcohol Avoid. Alcohol increases the sedative effects of this drug.

PROLONGED USE

Prolonged use of quetiapine has been reported to produce tardive dyskinesia (in which there are involuntary movements of the tongue and face).

Quinine

Brand names None
Used in the following combined preparations
None

QUICK REFERENCE

Drug group Antimalarial drug (p.73) and muscle relaxant (p.52)
Overdose danger rating High
Dependence rating Low
Prescription needed Yes
Available as generic Yes

GENERAL INFORMATION

Quinine, which is obtained from the bark of the cinchona tree, was introduced in the last century and is the earliest antimalarial drug. Quinine often causes side effects, but it is still given for malaria that is resistant to safer treatments. Owing to resistance of the malaria parasite to chloroquine and some of the more modern antimalarials, quinine remains the mainstay of treatment but is not used as a preventative.

At the high doses used to treat malaria, quinine may cause a group of symptoms known as cinchonism. These include ringing in the ears, headaches, nausea, hearing loss, and blurred vision. In rare cases, quinine may cause bleeding into the skin due to reduced blood platelets.

In many countries quinine is often used, in small doses, to prevent painful night-time leg cramps.

INFORMATION FOR USERS

Your drug prescription is tailored for you. Do not alter dosage without checking with your doctor.
How taken Tablets, injection.
Frequency and timing of doses *Malaria* Every 8 hours. *Muscle cramps* Once daily at bedtime.
Adult dosage range 1.8g daily (malaria); 200–300mg daily (cramps).
Onset of effect 1–2 days (malaria); 2–3 hours (cramps).
Duration of action Up to 24 hours.
Diet advice None.
Storage Keep in a closed container in a cool, dry place out of reach of children. Protect from light.

Missed dose Take as soon as you remember. If your next dose is due within 4 hours, skip the missed one and return to your normal dosing schedule thereafter.
Stopping the drug If prescribed for malaria, take the full course. Even if you feel better, the original infection may still be present and may recur if treatment is stopped too soon. If taken for muscle cramps, the drug can safely be stopped as soon as you no longer need it.

OVERDOSE ACTION

Seek immediate medical advice in all cases. Take emergency action if breathing problems, fits, or loss of consciousness occur.

POSSIBLE ADVERSE EFFECTS

Adverse effects are unlikely with quinine at low doses. At antimalarial doses, headache and blurred vision are more common; and dizziness, ringing in the ears, and temporary deafness may occur. Quinine may also cause nausea and diarrhoea. Report any rash to your doctor.

INTERACTIONS

Cimetidine This drug increases the blood levels of quinine.
Digoxin Quinine increases the blood levels of digoxin, and so the dose of digoxin should be reduced. Discuss with your doctor.

SPECIAL PRECAUTIONS

Be sure to consult your doctor if:
◆ You have a long-term kidney problem.
◆ You have tinnitus (ringing in the ears).
◆ You have optic neuritis.
◆ You have myasthenia gravis.
◆ You have glucose-6-phosphate dehydrogenase (G6PD) deficiency.
◆ You have heart problems.
◆ You are taking other medications.
Pregnancy Not usually prescribed. May cause defects in the unborn baby. Discuss with your doctor.
Breast-feeding The drug passes into the breast milk, but at normal doses adverse effects on the baby are unlikely. Discuss with your doctor.
Infants and children Reduced dose necessary.
Over 60 No special problems.

Driving and hazardous work Avoid these activities until you know how quinine affects you because the drug's side effects may distract you.
Alcohol No known problems.

PROLONGED USE
No problems expected with low doses used to control night-time leg cramps.

Raloxifene

Brand name Evista
Used in the following combined preparations
None

QUICK REFERENCE

Drug group Drug for bone disorders (p.54)
Overdose danger rating Low
Dependence rating Low
Prescription needed Yes
Available as generic No

GENERAL INFORMATION

Raloxifene is a non-steroidal anti-oestrogen drug (oestrogen is a naturally occurring female sex hormone, see p.86) that is related to clomifene (p.177) and tamoxifen (p.375). Raloxifene is prescribed to prevent vertebral fractures in postmenopausal women who are at increased risk of osteoporosis. There is some evidence that the drug would also be useful for preventing fractures of the hip, but its use in the prevention of other bone fractures is uncertain.

Raloxifene has no beneficial effect on other menopausal problems such as hot flushes. The drug is not prescribed to women who might become pregnant because it may harm the unborn baby, and it is not prescribed to men.

There is an increased risk of a deep vein thrombosis (blood clot developing in a vein in the leg), but the risk is similar to that due to HRT (see p.87). However, because of this risk, raloxifene is usually stopped if the woman taking it becomes immobile or bedbound, when clots are more likely to form. Treatment is restarted when full activity is resumed.

INFORMATION FOR USERS

Your drug prescription is tailored for you. Do not alter dosage without checking with your doctor.
How taken Tablets.
Frequency and timing of doses Once daily.
Adult dosage range 60mg daily.
Onset of effect 1–4 hours.
Duration of action 24–48 hours.
Diet advice Calcium supplements are recommended if dietary calcium is low.

Storage Keep in a closed container in a cool, dry place out of reach of children. Protect from light.
Missed dose Take as soon as you remember. If your next dose is due within 8 hours, take a single dose now and skip the next.
Stopping the drug Do not stop taking the drug without consulting your doctor except under specified conditions such as immobility, which increases the risk of deep-vein thrombosis.
Exceeding the dose An occasional unintentional extra dose is unlikely to be a cause for concern. But if you notice any unusual symptoms, or if a large overdose has been taken, notify your doctor.

POSSIBLE ADVERSE EFFECTS

Raloxifene may cause hot flushes, leg cramps, and swollen feet or ankles. Pain, tenderness, or swelling in the leg indicate the possibility of a deep vein thrombosis. If any of these adverse effects occur, seek urgent medical attention.

INTERACTIONS

Anticoagulants Raloxifene reduces the effect of warfarin and acenocoumarol (nicoumalone).
Colestyramine This drug reduces the absorption of raloxifene by the body.

SPECIAL PRECAUTIONS

Be sure to tell your doctor if:
◆ You have had a blood clot in a vein.
◆ You have uterine bleeding.
◆ You have liver or kidney problems.
◆ You are taking other medications.
Pregnancy Not prescribed to premenopausal women.
Breast-feeding Not prescribed to premenopausal women.
Infants and children Not prescribed.
Over 60 No special problems.
Driving and hazardous work No special problems.
Alcohol No special problems.

PROLONGED USE

No special problems. Raloxifene is normally used long term.

Ramipril

Brand name Tritace
Used in the following combined preparations
None

QUICK REFERENCE

Drug group ACE inhibitor vasodilator (p.30)
Overdose danger rating Medium
Dependence rating Low
Prescription needed Yes
Available as generic No

GENERAL INFORMATION

Ramipril belongs to the ACE (angiotensin converting enzyme) inhibitor group of drugs and is used to treat high blood pressure (p.34) and heart failure (in which the heart is unable to deal with its workload). It may also be given to patients following a heart attack and is sometimes used to prevent or delay kidney damage in patients with diabetes. It is also often given with a diuretic to increase its effect on high blood pressure and heart failure. Ramipril works by relaxing the muscles in blood vessel walls, allowing the vessels to dilate (widen), which enables the blood to circulate more easily and helps to lower blood pressure. The drug is long acting and is taken once or twice daily. The first dose may cause a sudden drop in blood pressure, especially in patients taking a diuretic. For this reason, you should lie down for 2–3 hours afterwards.

A variety of minor side effects may occur with ramipril; many people develop a persistent dry cough, while others experience taste disturbance, which a reduction in dose may help to minimize.

INFORMATION FOR USERS

Your drug prescription is tailored for you. Do not alter dosage without checking with your doctor.
How taken Capsules.
Frequency and timing of doses With water, with or after food. *High blood pressure* Usually once daily. *Heart failure* after a heart attack 2 x daily.
Adult dosage range *High blood pressure* 1.25–10mg daily. *Heart failure* after heart attack 5–10mg daily.

Onset of effect Within 2 hours.
Duration of action Up to 24 hours.
Diet advice You may be advised to lower your salt intake to help control your blood pressure.
Storage Keep in a closed container in a cool, dry place out of reach of children.
Missed dose Take as soon as you remember. If your next dose is due within 6 hours, take a single dose now and skip the next. Subsequently, continue with your usual routine.
Stopping the drug Unless severe adverse effects occur (see below), do not stop taking the drug without consulting your doctor. Treatment of hypertension and heart failure is normally lifelong, it may be necessary to substitute alternative therapy.
Exceeding the dose If you notice any unusual symptoms or if a large overdose has been taken, notify your doctor.

POSSIBLE ADVERSE EFFECTS

Dizziness on standing is likely to occur after the first dose. Nausea and headache are common but are usually mild and transient. A persistent dry cough is the most common adverse effect, but this can be minimized by taking smaller, more frequent, doses; some people may have to stop taking the drug. Rash or itching may occur. If dizziness or fainting, runny nose or sore throat, confusion or mood changes, or chest pain or palpitations occur, consult your doctor. If you develop jaundice, swelling of the face, or breathing difficulties, stop taking the drug and consult your doctor urgently.

INTERACTIONS

NSAIDs (e.g., ibuprofen) may reduce the antihypertensive effect of ramipril and increase the risk of kidney damage.
Ciclosporin This drug increases the risk of high potassium levels.
Potassium supplements and potassium-sparing diuretics These may cause excess levels of potassium in the body.
Lithium Like other ACE inhibitors, ramipril may cause raised blood lithium levels and toxicity.

SPECIAL PRECAUTIONS

◆ You have suffered from severe allergies.
◆ You have long-term kidney problems.

◆ You have coronary artery disease.
◆ You peripheral vascular disease.
◆ You are on a low sodium diet
◆ You are allergic to other ACE inhibitors.
◆ You are taking other medications.

Pregnancy Not prescribed. May cause defects in the developing baby.

Breast-feeding The drug passes into the breast milk, but at normal doses adverse effects on the baby are unlikely. Discuss with your doctor.

Infants and children Not usually prescribed.

Over 60 Reduced dose may be necessary.

Driving and hazardous work Avoid such activities until you have learned how ramipril affects you because the drug can cause dizziness and fainting.

Alcohol Avoid excessive amounts. Alcohol may increase the blood-pressure lowering and adverse effects of this drug.

Surgery and general anaesthetics Notify your doctor or dentist that you are taking ramipril.

PROLONGED USE
No problems expected.

Ranitidine

Brand name Zantac
Used in the following combined preparations
None

QUICK REFERENCE
Drug group Anti-ulcer drug (p.41)
Overdose danger rating Low
Dependence rating Low
Prescription needed No (tablets in limited quantities); Yes (other preparations)
Available as generic Yes

GENERAL INFORMATION
Ranitidine is prescribed in the treatment of stomach and duodenal ulcers. In combination with antibiotics, the drug is used for ulcers caused by *Helicobacter pylori* infection. It is also used to protect against duodenal (but not stomach) ulcers in people taking NSAIDs (p.48), who may be prone to ulcers. This drug reduces the discomfort and ulceration of reflux oesophagitis, and may prevent stress ulceration and gastric bleeding in

severely ill patients. Ranitidine reduces the amount of stomach acid produced, allowing ulcers to heal. It is usually given in courses lasting four to eight weeks, with further courses if symptoms recur.

Ranitidine does not affect the actions of enzymes in the liver, where many drugs are broken down. Consequently, unlike the similar drug cimetidine, ranitidine does not increase blood levels of other drugs such as anticoagulants and anti-convulsants, which might reduce their effectiveness.

Most people experience no serious effects during ranitidine treatment. As it promotes healing of the stomach lining, there is a risk that ranitidine may mask stomach cancer, delaying diagnosis. It is therefore usually prescribed only when the possibility of stomach cancer has been ruled out.

INFORMATION FOR USERS
Your drug prescription is tailored for you. Do not alter dosage without checking with your doctor.

How taken Tablets, capsules, oral liquid, injection.

Frequency and timing of doses Once daily at bedtime or 2–3 x daily.

Adult dosage range 150mg–6g daily, depending on the condition being treated. Usual dose is 150mg twice daily.

Onset of effect Within 1 hour.

Duration of action 12 hours.

Diet advice None.

Storage Keep in a closed container in a cool, dry place out of reach of children. Protect from light.

Missed dose Take as soon as you remember. If your next dose is due within 3 hours, take a single dose now and skip the next.

Stopping the drug Do not stop taking the drug without consulting your doctor; symptoms may recur.

Exceeding the dose An occasional unintentional extra dose is unlikely to be a cause for concern. But if you notice any unusual symptoms, or if a large overdose has been taken, notify your doctor.

POSSIBLE ADVERSE EFFECTS
Adverse effects, which include headache, dizziness, nausea, vomiting, constipation and

diarrhoea, are uncommon and are usually related to dosage level and almost always disappear when treatment finishes.

INTERACTIONS

Ketoconazole Ranitidine may reduce absorption of ketoconazole. Ranitidine should be taken at least 2 hours after ketoconazole.

Sucralfate High doses (2g) of sucralfate may reduce the absorption of ranitidine. Sucralfate should be taken at least 2 hours after ranitidine.

SPECIAL PRECAUTIONS

Be sure to tell your doctor if:
◆ You have long-term liver or kidney problems.
◆ You are taking other medications.
Pregnancy Safety in pregnancy not established. Discuss with your doctor.
Breast-feeding The drug passes into the breast milk and may affect the baby. Discuss with your doctor.
Infants and children Reduced dose necessary.
Over 60 No special problems.
Driving and hazardous work No known problems. Dizziness can occur in a very small proportion of patients.
Alcohol Avoid. Alcohol may aggravate your underlying condition and reduce the beneficial effects of this drug.

PROLONGED USE

No problems expected.

Repaglinide

Brand name NovoNorm
Used in the following combined preparations
None

QUICK REFERENCE

Drug group Oral antidiabetic drug (p.80)
Overdose danger rating Medium
Dependence rating Low
Prescription needed Yes
Available as generic No

GENERAL INFORMATION

Repaglinide is a drug used to treat non-insulin dependent diabetes that cannot be adequately controlled by diet and exercise alone. It acts in a similar manner to sulphonylurea drugs by stimulating the release of insulin from the pancreas. Therefore, some of the pancreatic cells need to be functioning in order for it to be effective.

Repaglinide is quick acting, but its effects last for only about four hours. The drug is sometimes given with metformin if that drug is not providing adequate diabetic control.

Repaglinide is best taken just before a meal in order for the insulin that is released to cope with the food. If a meal is likely to be missed, the dose of repaglinide should not be taken. If a tablet has been taken and a meal is not forthcoming, some carbohydrate (as specified by your doctor or dietitian) should be eaten as soon as possible.

INFORMATION FOR USERS

Your drug prescription is tailored for you. Do not alter dosage without checking with your doctor.
How taken Tablets.
Frequency and timing of doses 1–4 x daily (up to 30 minutes before a meal, and up to 4 meals a day). If you are going to miss a meal, do not take the tablet.
Adult dosage range 500 micrograms (starting dose), increased at intervals of 1–2 weeks according to response; 4–16mg daily (maintenance dose).
Onset of effect 30 minutes.
Duration of action 4 hours.
Diet advice Follow the diet advised by your doctor or dietitian.
Storage Keep in a closed container in a cool, dry place out of reach of children.
Missed dose Do not take tablets between meals. Discuss with your doctor.
Stopping the drug Do not stop taking the drug without consulting your doctor.
Exceeding the dose An overdose will cause hypoglycaemia with dizziness, sweating, trembling, confusion, and headache. Notify your doctor.

POSSIBLE ADVERSE EFFECTS

Intestinal problems, such as nausea, vomiting, abdominal pain, and diarrhoea or constipation, are common at the start of treatment with repaglinide. However, such adverse effects tend to become less trouble-some as treatment continues. If rash or itching occur, consult your doctor.

INTERACTIONS
MaOls, beta-blockers, ACE inhibitors, and NSAIds These drugs may increase the effect of repaglinide.
Oral contraceptives, thiazide diuretics, corticosteroids, danazol, thyroid hormones and sympathomimetics These drugs may decrease the effect of repaglinide.

SPECIAL PRECAUTIONS
Be sure to tell your doctor if:
◆ You have liver or kidney problems.
◆ You are taking other medications.
Pregnancy Safety not established. Discuss with your doctor.
Breast-feeding Safety not established. Discuss with your doctor.
Infants and children Not recommended.
Over 60 No special problems, but safety not established over 75 years.
Driving and hazardous work Avoid if low blood sugar without warning signs is likely.
Alcohol Avoid. Alcohol may upset diabetic control and may increase and prolong the effects of repaglinide.

PROLONGED USE
Repaglinide is usually prescribed indefinitely. No special problems.

Rifampicin

Brand names Rifadin, Rimactane
Used in the following combined preparations
Rifater, Rifinah, Rimactazid

QUICK REFERENCE
Drug group Antituberculous drug (p.65)
Overdose danger rating Medium
Dependence rating Low
Prescription needed Yes
Available as generic Yes

GENERAL INFORMATION
Rifampicin is an antibacterial drug that is highly effective in the treatment of tuberculosis. Taken by mouth, the drug is well absorbed in the intestine and widely distributed throughout the body, including the brain. As a result, rifampicin is particularly useful in the treatment of tuberculous meningitis. In order to prevent recurrent disease in later life, a course of treatment may last up to a year.

Rifampicin is also used to treat leprosy and other serious infections, including Legionnaires' disease and infections of the bone (osteomyelitis). Additionally, it is given to anyone in close contact with meningococcal meningitis in order to prevent infection. Rifampicin is always prescribed with antibiotics or other antituberculous drugs because of rapid resistance in some bacteria.

A harmless red-orange coloration may be imparted to the urine, saliva, and tears, and soft contact lenses may become permanently stained.

INFORMATION FOR USERS
Your drug prescription is tailored for you. Do not alter dosage without checking with your doctor.
How taken Tablets, capsules, liquid, injection.
Frequency and timing of doses 1 x daily, 30 minutes before breakfast (leprosy, tuberculosis) or once a month (leprosy); 2 x daily (prevention of meningococcal meningitis); 2–4 x daily, 30 minutes before or 2 hours after meals (other serious infections).
Adult dosage range According to weight; usually 450–600mg daily (tuberculosis, leprosy) or 600mg once a month (leprosy); 600mg–1.2g daily (other serious infections); 1.2g daily for 2 days (meningococcal meningitis).
Onset of effect Over several days.
Duration of action Up to 24 hours.
Diet advice None.
Storage Keep in a closed container in a cool, dry place out of reach of children. Protect from light.
Missed dose Take as soon as you remember. If your next dose is due within 6 hours, take a single dose now, then return to normal dosing schedule.
Stopping the drug Take the full course. Even if you feel better, the original infection may still be present and symptoms may recur if treatment is stopped too soon. In rare cases

stopping the drug suddenly after high-dose treatment can lead to a severe flu-like illness. **Exceeding the dose** An occasional unintentional extra dose is unlikely to cause problems. Large overdoses may cause liver damage, nausea, vomiting, and lethargy. Notify your doctor immediately.

POSSIBLE ADVERSE EFFECTS

A harmless red-orange discoloration of body fluids normally occurs. Serious adverse effects are rare. They include nausea, vomiting, diarrhoea, muscle cramps or aches, and Jaundice, which usually improves during treatment but should be reported to your doctor. You should consult your doctor promptly if you have a flu-like illness or you develop a rash or itching. Headache and breathing difficulties may occur after stopping high-dose treatment.

INTERACTIONS

General note Rifampicin may reduce the effectiveness of a wide variety of drugs, such as oral contraceptives (in which case alternative contraceptive methods may be necessary), phenytoin, corticosteroids, oral antidiabetics, disopyramide, and oral anticoagulants. Dosage adjustment of these drugs may be necessary at the start or end of treatment with rifampicin. Consult your doctor or pharmacist for advice.

SPECIAL PRECAUTIONS

Be sure to tell your doctor if:
◆ You have a long-term liver problem.
◆ You wear contact lenses.
◆ You are taking other medications.
Pregnancy Safety in pregnancy not established. Discuss with your doctor.
Breast-feeding The drug passes into the breast milk, but at normal doses adverse effects on the baby are unlikely. Discuss with your doctor.
Infants and children Reduced dose necessary.
Over 60 Reduced dose may be necessary. Increased risk of adverse effects.
Driving and hazardous work No problems expected.
Alcohol Avoid excessive amounts. Heavy alcohol consumption may increase the risk of liver damage.

PROLONGED USE

Prolonged use of rifampicin may cause liver damage.
Monitoring Periodic blood tests may be performed to monitor liver function.

Risperidone

Brand names Risperdal
Used in the following combined preparations
None

QUICK REFERENCE

Drug group Antipsychotic drug (p.15)
Overdose danger rating Medium
Dependence rating Low
Prescription needed Yes
Available as generic No

GENERAL INFORMATION

Risperidone is used to treat patients with acute psychiatric disorders and long-term psychotic illness such as schizophrenia. Although it does not cure the underlying disorder, the drug helps to alleviate the distressing symptoms. It is effective for relieving both "positive" symptoms (for example, hallucinations, thought disturbances, and hostility) and "negative" symptoms (for example, emotional and social withdrawal). The drug may also help with various other symptoms that are often associated with schizophrenia, such as depression and anxiety. Risperidone has less of a sedative effect and is also less likely to cause movement disorders as a side effect than some other antipsychotics.

INFORMATION FOR USERS

Your drug prescription is tailored for you. Do not alter dosage without checking with your doctor.
How taken Tablets.
Frequency and timing of doses 1–2 x daily.
Adult dosage range 2mg daily (starting dose) increasing to 6–10mg, sometimes up to 16mg, daily (maintenance dose).
Onset of effect Within 2–3 days, but it may take up to 4 weeks for the maximum effect to be seen.
Duration of action Approximately 2 days.

Diet advice None.

Storage Keep in a closed container in a cool, dry place out of reach of children. Protect from light.

Missed dose Take as soon as you remember. If your next dose is due within 3 hours, take a single dose now and skip the next.

Stopping the drug Unless severe adverse effects occur (see below), do not stop taking the drug without consulting your doctor; symptoms may recur.

Exceeding the dose An occasional unintentional extra dose is unlikely to cause problems. If larger doses have been taken, notify your doctor.

POSSIBLE ADVERSE EFFECTS

Risperidone is generally well tolerated and there is low incidence of movement disorders. It is less sedating than some of the other antipsychotics, but adverse effects include insomnia, anxiety, agitation, headache, drowsiness, difficulty in concentrating, and dizziness. Weight gain, rash and excessive thirst may also occur; consult your doctor. If you develop a high fever or rigid muscles, stop taking the drug and consult your doctor urgently.

INTERACTIONS

Drugs for parkinsonism Risperidone may reduce the effect of these drugs.

Carbamazepine This drug reduces the effects of risperidone.

Sedatives All drugs that have a sedative effect on the central nervous system are likely to increase any sedative effect of risperidone.

SPECIAL PRECAUTIONS

Be sure to tell your doctor if:
◆ You have liver or kidney problems.
◆ You have heart or circulation problems.
◆ You have had epileptic fits.
◆ You have Parkinson's disease.
◆ You are taking other medications.

Pregnancy Safety in pregnancy not established. Discuss with your doctor.

Breast-feeding The drug probably passes into breast milk. Discuss with your doctor.

Infants and children Not recommended under 15 years.

Over 60 Reduced dose necessary.

Driving and hazardous work Avoid such activities until you have learned how risperidone affects you because the drug may cause difficulty in concentration and slowed reactions.

Alcohol Avoid excessive amounts. Alcohol may increase the sedative effects of this drug.

Surgery and general anaesthetics Risperidone treatment may need to be stopped before you have a general anaesthetic. Discuss this with your doctor or dentist before any operation.

PROLONGED USE

Permanent movement disorders (tardive dyskinesia) may occur but are less likely than with many other antipsychotics.

Rivastigmine

Brand names Exelon
Used in the following combined preparations None

QUICK REFERENCE

Drug group Drug for dementia (p.19)
Overdose danger rating Medium
Dependence rating Low
Prescription needed Yes
Available as generic No

GENERAL INFORMATION

Rivastigmine is an anticholinesterase drug (an inhibitor of the enzyme acetylcholinesterase). The enzyme usually breaks down the neurotransmitter acetylcholine from the blood, thus limiting its effects. Blocking the enzyme increases and prolongs the effect of acetylcholine. Rivastigmine has been found to improve the symptoms of dementia due to Alzheimer's disease and slows the rate of deterioration in around half of the patients treated. The drug has no effect on dementia due to other causes. It is usual to assess anyone being treated with rivastigmine after about three months to decide whether the drug is helping and whether it is worth continuing treatment. As the disease progresses, the benefit obtained may diminish.

Side effects may include agitation, confusion and depression, which could be thought due to Alzheimer's disease. Weight loss should be watched for.

INFORMATION FOR USERS

Your drug prescription is tailored for you. Do not alter dosage without checking with your doctor.

How taken Capsules.

Frequency and timing of doses 2 x daily.

Adult dosage range 3mg daily (starting dose); 6–12mg daily (maintenance dose).

Onset of effect 30–60 minutes.

Duration of action 9–12 hours.

Diet advice None.

Storage Keep in a closed container in a cool, dry place out of reach of children.

Missed dose Take as soon as you remember. If your next dose is due within 4 hours, take a single dose now and skip the next. A carer should be overseeing the taking of tablets.

Stopping the drug Do not stop taking the drug without consulting your doctor; symptoms may recur.

Exceeding the dose An occasional unintentional extra dose is unlikely to be a problem. Large overdoses may cause nausea, vomiting and diarrhoea. Notify your doctor.

POSSIBLE ADVERSE EFFECTS

Adverse effects include mental changes, such as agitation, confusion, depression, drowsiness, and dizziness, and intestinal problems such as reduced appetite, nausea, abdominal pain and weight loss. Though common, these effects are usually quite mild. Weakness, trembling, sweating, malaise, headache, and insomnia may also occur. If you experience difficulty in passing urine, consult your doctor. If convulsions occur, seek urgent medical attention.

INTERACTIONS

Aminoglycoside antibiotics, clindamycin, and colistin These antibiotics block the effect of rivastigmine.

Antimalarials and anti-arrhythmics Certain drugs from these groups may block the effects of rivastigmine.

Muscle relaxants used in surgery Rivastigmine may increase the effects of some muscle relaxants, but it may also block the effects of some others.

SPECIAL PRECAUTIONS

Be sure to tell your doctor if:

♦ You have a heart problem.

♦ You have liver or kidney problems.

♦ You have asthma or respiratory problems.

♦ You have had a peptic ulcer.

♦ You are taking an NSAID regularly.

♦ You are taking other medications.

Pregnancy Not usually prescribed. Safety not established.

Breast-feeding Not usually prescribed. Safety not established.

Infants and children Not usually prescribed.

Over 60 No special problems.

Driving and hazardous work Your underlying condition may make such activities inadvisable. Discuss with your doctor.

Alcohol Avoid. Alcohol increases the sedative effects of rivastigmine.

Surgery and general anaesthetics Treatment with rivastigmine may need to be stopped before you have a general anaesthetic. Discuss this with your doctor or dentist before any operation.

PROLONGED USE

May be continued for as long as there is benefit. Stopping the drug leads to a gradual loss of the improvements.

Monitoring Periodic checks may be carried out to test whether the drug is still providing some benefit.

Salbutamol

Brand name Aerolin, Airomir, Asmasal, Asmaven, Maxivent, Salamol, Salbulin, Ventodisks, Ventolin, Volmax

Used in the following combined preparations
Aerocrom, Combivent, Ventide

QUICK REFERENCE

Drug group Bronchodilator (p.23) and drug used in premature labour (p.106)
Overdose danger rating Low
Dependence rating Low
Prescription needed Yes
Available as generic Yes

GENERAL INFORMATION

Salbutamol is a sympathomimetic broncho-dilator that relaxes the muscle surrounding the bronchioles (airways in the lungs).

It is used to relieve symptoms of asthma and may help some people with chronic bronchitis, and emphysema. Although it can be taken by mouth, inhalation is considered more effective because the drug is delivered directly to the bronchioles, thus giving rapid relief, allowing smaller doses, and causing fewer side effects. Inhaled corticosteroids are commonly also given with salbutamol.

Compared with some similar drugs, salbu-tamol has little stimulant effect on the heart rate and blood pressure, making it safer for people with heart problems or high blood pressure. Because it relaxes the muscles of the uterus, it is also used to prevent pre-mature labour.

The most common side effect of salbuta-mol is fine tremor of the hands, which may interfere with precise manual work. Anxiety, tension, and restlessness may also occur.

INFORMATION FOR USERS

Your drug prescription is tailored for you. Do not alter dosage without checking with your doctor.
How taken Tablets, SR-tablets, liquid, injec-tion, inhaler, powder for inhalation.
Frequency and timing of doses 1–2 inhalations 3–4 x daily (inhaler); 3–4 x daily (tablets/liquid); 2 x daily (SR-tablets).
Dosage range 400–800 micrograms daily (inhaler); 8–32mg daily (by mouth).

Onset of effect Within 5–15 minutes (inha-ler); within 30–60 minutes (by mouth).
Duration of action Up to 6 hours (inhaler); up to 8 hours (by mouth).
Diet advice None.
Storage Keep in a closed container in a cool, dry place out of reach of children. Protect from light. Do not puncture or burn inhalers.
Missed dose Take as soon as you remember if needed. If your next dose is due within 2 hours, take a single dose now and skip the next.
Stopping the drug Do not stop taking the drug without consulting your doctor; symp-toms may recur.
Exceeding the dose An occasional uninten-tional extra dose is unlikely to be a cause for concern. But if you notice any unusual symptoms, or if a large overdose has been taken, notify your doctor.

POSSIBLE ADVERSE EFFECTS

Muscle tremor, which particularly affects the hands, anxiety, and restlessness are the most common adverse effects. Muscle cramps and headache may also occur. If palpitations occur, consult your doctor urgently.

INTERACTIONS

Theophylline There is a risk of low potassium levels in blood occurring if this drug is taken with salbutamol.
MAOIs These drugs can interact with salbu-tamol to produce a dangerous rise in blood pressure.
Other sympathomimetics These drugs may increase the effects of salbutamol, thereby also increasing the risk of adverse effects.
Beta blockers These may oppose the action of salbutamol and should not be taken with it; but salbutamol may be given to relieve the airways when beta blockers cause wheezing.

SPECIAL PRECAUTIONS

Be sure to tell your doctor if:
◆ You have heart problems.
◆ You have high blood pressure.
◆ You have an overactive thyroid gland.
◆ You have diabetes.
◆ You are taking other medications.
Pregnancy No evidence of risk when used to treat asthma, or to treat or prevent prema-ture labour. Discuss with your doctor.

Breast-feeding The drug passes into the breast milk, but at normal doses adverse effects on the baby are unlikely. Discuss with your doctor.
Infants and children Reduced dose necessary.
Over 60 Reduced dose may be necessary. Increased likelihood of adverse effects.
Driving and hazardous work Avoid such activities until you have learned how salbutamol affects you because the drug can cause tremors.
Alcohol No known problems.

PROLONGED USE

No problems expected, but contact your doctor if you need to use your inhaler more than usual; this may be a result of worsening asthma that requires urgent medical attention.

Salmeterol

Brand name Serevent
Used in the following combined preparation
Seretide

QUICK REFERENCE

Drug group Bronchodilator (p.23)
Overdose danger rating Low
Dependence rating Low
Prescription needed Yes
Available as generic No

GENERAL INFORMATION

Salmeterol is a sympathomimetic bronchodilator used to treat conditions, such as asthma and bronchospasm, in which the airways become constricted. Its advantage over salbutamol (p.361) is that it is longer acting.

Salmeterol relaxes the muscle surrounding the airways in the lungs but, because of its slow onset of effect, it is not used to relieve the immediate symptoms of asthma. It is prescribed to prevent attacks, however, and can be helpful in controlling night-time asthma.

Taken by inhalation, salmeterol is delivered directly to the airways. This allows smaller doses to be taken and reduces the risk of adverse effects.

INFORMATION FOR USERS

Your drug prescription is tailored for you. Do not alter dosage without checking with your doctor.

How taken Inhaler, powder for inhalation.
Frequency and timing of doses 2 x daily.
Adult dosage range 100–200 micrograms daily.
Onset of effect 10–20 minutes.
Duration of action 12 hours.
Diet advice None.
Storage Keep in a cool, dry place out of reach of children.
Missed dose Take as soon as you remember. If your next dose is due within 4 hours, take a single dose now and skip the next.
Stopping the drug Unless wheezing and breathlessness occur, do not stop taking the drug without consulting your doctor; symptoms may recur.
Exceeding the dose An occasional unintentional extra dose is unlikely to be a cause for concern. But if you notice any unusual symptoms, or if a large overdose has been taken, notify your doctor.

POSSIBLE ADVERSE EFFECTS

Side effects are usually mild. The most common is tremor, but headache and palpitations may also occur; consult your doctor. If wheezing and breathlessness (paradoxical bronchospasm) occur, stop taking the drug and notify your doctor immediately.

INTERACTIONS

Corticosteroids, theophylline, and diuretics The risk of low blood potassium levels is increased when high doses of salmeterol are taken with these drugs.

SPECIAL PRECAUTIONS

Be sure to tell your doctor if:
◆ You have heart problems.
◆ You have high blood pressure.
◆ You have an overactive thyroid.
◆ You have diabetes.
◆ You are taking other medications.
Pregnancy No evidence of risk when used to treat asthma. Discuss with your doctor.
Breast-feeding No known problems.
Infants and children Reduced dose necessary. Not recommended under 4 years.
Over 60 No special problems.
Driving and hazardous work No special problems.
Alcohol No known problems.

PROLONGED USE

Salmeterol is intended to be used long term. The main problem comes from using combinations of anti-asthma drugs, leading to low blood potassium levels.

Sildenafil

Brand name Viagra
Used in the following combined preparations
None

QUICK REFERENCE

Drug group Drug for impotence (p.105)
Overdose danger rating Medium
Dependence rating Low
Prescription needed Yes
Available as generic No

GENERAL INFORMATION

Sildenafil is a new type of drug used to treat impotence. It does not cause an erection directly, but it produces a chemical change that prevents the muscle walls of the blood-filled chambers in the penis from relaxing.

Sildenafil does not need to be taken regularly; it is only used to produce an erection and only needs to be taken before sexual activity is undertaken.

Because it is a vasodilator, sildenafil can cause a small fall in blood pressure while it is active, and it may increase the effect of antihypertensive drugs. The drug is not usually prescribed with nitrates (see p.30) because it greatly increases their effects.

INFORMATION FOR USERS

Your drug prescription is tailored for you. Do not alter dosage without checking with your doctor.
How taken Tablets.
Frequency and timing of doses Maximum once daily, 1 hour before sexual activity.
Adult dosage range 25–100mg.
Onset of effect 30 minutes.
Duration of action 4 hours.
Diet advice None, but sildenafil takes longer to work after food, especially a high fat meal. It is absorbed faster on an empty stomach.
Storage Keep in a closed container in a cool, dry place out of reach of children.

Missed dose Take the next dose when you need to. Do not use more than one dose in a 24-hour period.
Stopping the drug Can be safely stopped as soon as you no longer need it.
Exceeding the dose An occasional unintentional extra dose is unlikely to cause problems. Large overdoses may cause headache, dizziness, flushing, altered vision, and nasal congestion. Notify your doctor.

POSSIBLE ADVERSE EFFECTS

Most adverse effects of sildenafil are common and short lived. These include headache, flushing, dizziness, indigestion, nasal congestion, and a bluish colour to vision. However, if priapism (a prolonged, painful erection) occurs, discontinue the drug and consult your doctor. Sildenafil has been reported to cause muscle aches when taken more frequently than recommended. It is not certain that this effect is due to the drug.

INTERACTIONS

Nitrates The effects of these drugs are greatly increased by sildenafil, and they are therefore not prescribed with it.
Cimetidine, erythromycin, and ketoconazole (oral) These drugs increase the blood levels and toxicity of sildenafil.
Antihypertensives Sildenafil may enhance the blood-pressure lowering effect of these drugs.
Other drugs for impotence Safety not established. Not recommended.

SPECIAL PRECAUTIONS

Be sure to tell your doctor if:
◆ You have heart problems.
◆ You have had a stroke or heart attack.
◆ You have sickle cell anaemia.
◆ You have multiple myeloma.
◆ You have leukaemia.
◆ You have liver or kidney problems.
◆ You have an inherited eye problem.
◆ You have an abnormality of the penis.
◆ You are taking a nitrate drug.
◆ You are taking other medications.
Pregnancy Not prescribed.
Breast-feeding Not prescribed.
Infants and children Not prescribed under 18 years.
Over 60 Reduced dose may be necessary.

Driving and hazardous work Avoid such activities until you have learned how sildenafil affects you because the drug can cause dizziness.
Alcohol No special problems.

PROLONGED USE
No problems expected.

Simvastatin

Brand name Zocor
Used in the following combined preparations
None

QUICK REFERENCE
Drug group Lipid-lowering drug (p.35)
Overdose danger rating Medium
Dependence rating Low
Prescription needed Yes
Available as generic No

GENERAL INFORMATION
Introduced in 1989, simvastatin is a lipid-lowering drug that blocks the action of an enzyme that enables cholesterol to be manufactured in the liver, and as a result the blood levels of cholesterol are lowered. The drug is prescribed for people with hypercholesterolaemia (high levels of cholesterol in the blood) who have not responded to other forms of therapy, such as a special diet, and who are at risk of developing heart disease. It is also sometimes prescribed for people who have had a heart attack, to reduce the risk of a further attack. Studies are currently being carried out on simvastatin because it may a have a beneficial effect on bone strength and mental function.

Side effects are usually mild and often wear off with time. In the body, simvastatin is found mainly in the liver, and it may raise the levels of various liver enzymes. This effect does not usually indicate serious liver damage.

INFORMATION FOR USERS
Your drug prescription is tailored for you. Do not alter dosage without checking with your doctor.
How taken Tablets.

Frequency and timing of doses Once daily at night.
Adult dosage range 10–40mg daily.
Onset of effect Within 2 weeks; full beneficial effects may not be felt for 4–6 weeks.
Duration of action Up to 24 hours.
Diet advice A low-fat diet is usually recommended.
Storage Keep in a closed container in a cool, dry place out of reach of children. Protect from light.
Missed dose Take as soon as you remember. If your next dose is due within 8 hours, do not take the missed dose, but take the next dose on schedule.
Stopping the drug Unless a rash occurs, do not stop taking the drug without consulting your doctor. Stopping the drug has no effect in the short term but may eventually lead to worsening of the underlying condition.
Exceeding the dose An occasional unintentional extra dose is unlikely to cause problems. Large overdoses may cause liver problems. Notify your doctor.

POSSIBLE ADVERSE EFFECTS
Adverse effects are usually mild and do not last long. The most common are those affecting the gastrointestinal system, such as nausea, flatulence, abdominal pain, and constipation or diarrhoea. Headaches may also occur. If you develop a rash, stop taking the drug and consult your doctor. Simvastatin may very rarely cause muscle problems; any muscle pain or weakness should be reported to your doctor at once.

INTERACTIONS
Anticoagulants Simvastatin may increase the effect of anticoagulants. The dose may need to be adjusted, and prothrombin time should be monitored regularly.
Ciclosporin and other immunosuppressant drugs Simvastatin and these drugs are not usually prescribed together because of the risk of muscle toxicity.
Other lipid-lowering drugs Taken with simvastatin, these drugs may increase the risk of muscle toxicity.
Itraconazole, ketoconazole, erythromycin Taken with simvastatin, these drugs may increase the risk of muscle toxicity.

SPECIAL PRECAUTIONS
Be sure to tell your doctor if:
◆ You have liver or kidney problems.
◆ You have eye or vision problems.
◆ You have muscle weakness.
◆ You have a thyroid disorder.
◆ You have had problems with alcohol abuse.
◆ You have porphyria.
◆ You have angina.
◆ You have high blood pressure.
◆ You are taking other medications.
Pregnancy Not usually prescribed. Safety in pregnancy not established. Discuss with your doctor.
Breast-feeding Safety not established. Discuss with your doctor.
Infants and children Not recommended.
Over 60 No special problems.
Driving and hazardous work No special problems.
Alcohol Avoid excessive amounts. Alcohol may increase the risk of developing liver problems with this drug.

PROLONGED USE
Prolonged treatment can adversely affect liver function.
Monitoring Regular blood tests to assess liver function and muscle strength are recommended.

Sodium Bicarbonate
Used in the following combined preparations
Alka-Seltzer, Bismag, Bisodol, Carbalax, Dioralyte, Gastrocote, Gaviscon, Mictral, Roter, and many others

QUICK REFERENCE
Drug group Antacid (p.40)
Overdose danger rating Medium
Dependence rating Low
Prescription needed No
Available as generic Yes

GENERAL INFORMATION
Sodium bicarbonate is available without prescription for the relief of occasional episodes of indigestion and heartburn, either alone or in multi-ingredient preparations. The drug may also relieve the discomfort caused by peptic ulcers. However, sodium bicarbonate is now seldom recommended by doctors because other drugs are safer and more effective.

Because sodium bicarbonate also reduces the acidity of the urine, relieving painful urination, it is sometimes recommended for cystitis. It should be avoided by people with heart failure and a history of kidney disease, however. It is sometimes given by injection to reduce the acidity of the blood and body tissues in metabolic acidosis, a potentially fatal condition that may occur in life-threatening illnesses or following cardiac arrest. Ear drops containing sodium bicarbonate are sometimes used for the softening, prior to the removal of, ear wax.

INFORMATION FOR USERS
Follow instructions on the label. Call your doctor if symptoms worsen.
How taken Tablets, capsules, liquid, powder (dissolved in water), injection, ear drops.
Frequency and timing of doses *Indigestion* As required (by mouth).
Adult dosage range Dependent on the condition being treated. As an antacid: 1–5g per dose.
Onset of effect Within 15 minutes as an antacid.
Duration of action 30–60 minutes as an antacid.
Diet advice None.
Storage Keep in a closed container in a cool, dry place out of reach of children.
Missed dose No cause for concern.
Stopping the drug When taken for indigestion, sodium bicarbonate can be safely stopped. When taken for other disorders, consult your doctor.
Exceeding the dose An occasional unintentional extra dose is unlikely to cause problems. Large overdoses may cause unusual weakness, dizziness, or headache. Notify your doctor.

POSSIBLE ADVERSE EFFECTS
Belching and stomach pain may arise from the carbon dioxide produced as sodium bicarbonate neutralizes stomach acid, and can be caused by a single dose. Other effects, such as muscle cramps, weakness, vomiting,

shortness of breath, and swollen ankles, result from the long-term regular use of sodium bicarbonate.

INTERACTIONS

General note Sodium bicarbonate interferes with the absorption or excretion of a wide range of drugs taken by mouth. Consult your doctor if you are taking oral anticoagulants, tetracycline antibiotics, phenothiazine antipsychotics, oral iron preparations, or lithium, and wish to take more than an occasional dose of sodium bicarbonate.

Diuretics The beneficial effects of these drugs may be reduced by sodium bicarbonate.

Corticosteroids Large doses of sodium bicarbonate may hasten potassium loss, and increase fluid retention and high blood pressure.

SPECIAL PRECAUTIONS

Be sure to consult your doctor or pharmacist before taking this drug if:
◆ You have long-term liver or kidney problems.
◆ You have heart problems.
◆ You have high blood pressure.
◆ You have severe abdominal pain or vomiting.
◆ You are on a low-sodium diet.
◆ You are taking other medications.

Pregnancy No evidence of risk, but it is not likely to help morning sickness, and can encourage fluid retention.

Breast-feeding No evidence of risk.

Infants and children Not recommended under 6 years except on the advice of a doctor. Reduced dose necessary.

Over 60 Reduced dose may be necessary.

Driving and hazardous work No special problems.

Alcohol Avoid excessive amounts. Alcohol irritates the stomach and may counter the beneficial effects of this drug.

PROLONGED USE

Severe weakness, fatigue, and muscle cramps may occur when this drug is taken regularly for extended periods. It should not be used daily for longer than 2 weeks without consulting your doctor.

Monitoring Blood and urine tests may be performed during prolonged use.

Sodium Cromoglicate

Brand names Cromogen, Intal, Nalcrom, Opticrom, Rynacrom

Used in the following combined preparations
Aerocrom, Intal Compound, Rynacrom Compound

QUICK REFERENCE

Drug group Anti-allergy drug (p.58)
Overdose danger rating Low
Dependence rating Low
Prescription needed No (some preparations)
Available as generic No

GENERAL INFORMATION

Sodium cromoglicate, introduced in the 1970s, is used primarily to prevent asthma and allergic conditions.

When taken by inhaler as a powder (Spinhaler) or spray, it is commonly used to reduce the frequency and severity of asthma attacks, and is also effective in helping to prevent attacks induced by exercise or cold air. The drug has a slow onset of action, and it may take up to six weeks to produce its full anti-asthmatic effect. It is not effective for the relief of an asthma attack, and aside from its use in asthma prevention, it is also given as eye drops to prevent allergic conjunctivitis. Taken as a nasal spray, the drug is used to prevent allergic rhinitis (hay fever). It is also given, as capsules, for food allergy.

Side effects are mild. Coughing and wheezing occurring on inhalation of the drug may be prevented by using a sympathomimetic bronchodilator (p.23) first. Hoarseness and throat irritation can be avoided by rinsing the mouth with water after inhalation.

INFORMATION FOR USERS

Follow instructions on the label. Call your doctor if symptoms worsen.

How taken Capsules, eye ointment, inhaler (various types), eye and nose drops, nasal spray.

Frequency and timing of doses *Capsules* 4 x daily before meals, swallowed whole or dissolved in water. *Inhaler, nasal preparations* 4–6 x daily. *Eye preparations* 4 x daily (drops); 2–3 x daily (eye ointment).

Dosage range 800mg daily (capsules); as directed (inhaler); apply to each nostril as directed (nasal preparations); 1–2 drops in each eye per dose (eye drops).

Onset of effect Varies with dosage, form, and condition treated. Eye conditions and allergic rhinitis may respond after a few days' treatment with drops, while asthma and chronic allergic rhinitis may take take 2–6 weeks to show improvement.

Duration of action 4–6 hours. Some effect persists for several days after treatment is stopped.

Diet advice You may be advised to avoid certain foods (Capsules). Follow your doctor's advice.

Storage Keep in a closed container in a cool, dry place out of reach of children. Protect from light.

Missed dose Take as soon as you remember. If your next dose is due within 2 hours, take a single dose now and skip the next.

Stopping the drug Do not stop taking the drug without consulting your doctor; symptoms may recur.

Exceeding the dose An occasional unintentional extra dose is unlikely to be a cause for concern. But if you notice any unusual symptoms, or if a large overdose has been taken, notify your doctor.

POSSIBLE ADVERSE EFFECTS

Coughing and hoarseness are common with inhalation of sodium cromoglicate. Nasal spray may cause sneezing. These symptoms usually diminish with continued use.

INTERACTIONS

None.

SPECIAL PRECAUTIONS

Be sure to consult your doctor or pharmacist before taking this drug if:
◆ You are taking other medications.

Pregnancy No evidence of risk.
Breast-feeding No evidence of risk.
Infants and children Reduced dose necessary.
Over 60 No special problems.
Driving and hazardous work No known problems.
Alcohol No known problems.

PROLONGED USE

No problems expected.

Sodium Valproate

Brand names Convulex (valproic acid), Epilim, Orlept
Used in the following combined preparations
None

QUICK REFERENCE
Drug group Anticonvulsant drug (p.16)
Overdose danger rating Medium
Dependency rating Low
Prescription needed Yes
Available as generic Yes

GENERAL INFORMATION

Sodium valproate is an anticonvulsant often used for the treatment of a variety of types of epilepsy. Its action is similar to that of other anticonvulsants; it reduces electrical discharges in the brain, preventing their excessive build-up, which can lead to epileptic fits.

Beneficial in long-term treatment, this drug does not have a sedative effect. This makes it particularly suitable for children who suffer either from atonic epilepsy (the sudden relaxing of the muscles throughout the body) or absence seizures (during which the person appears to be daydreaming).

INFORMATION FOR USERS

Your drug prescription is tailored for you. Do not alter dosage without checking with your doctor.

How taken Tablets, capsules, liquid, injection.
Frequency and timing of doses 1–2 x daily.
Dosage range 600mg–2.5g daily, adjusted as necessary.
Onset of effect Within 60 minutes.
Duration of action 12 hours or more.
Diet advice None.
Storage Keep in a tightly closed container in a cool, dry place out of reach of children. Protect from light.
Missed dose Take as soon as you remember. If your next dose is due within 2 hours, take a single dose now and skip the next.
Stopping the drug Do not stop taking the drug without consulting your doctor; symptoms may recur.
Exceeding the dose An occasional unintentional extra dose is unlikely to cause problems. Large overdoses may lead to coma. Notify your doctor.

POSSIBLE ADVERSE EFFECTS

Apart from nausea and indigestion, adverse effects are uncommon. Temporary hair loss and weight gain may occur. More serious adverse effects such as liver failure or platelet and bleeding abnormalities are rare. If you experience vomiting, appetite loss, jaundice, a rash or abnormal bleeding or bruising, consult your doctor urgently. Menstrual periods may become irregular or cease.

INTERACTIONS

Other anticonvulsant drugs These drugs may reduce blood levels of sodium valproate.

Aspirin This drug may increase the effects of sodium valproate.

Antidepressants and antipsychotics These drugs may reduce sodium valproate's effectiveness.

Cholestyramine This drug may reduce the absorption of oral sodium valproate.

Antimalarials Chloroquine and mefloquine reduce reduce sodium valproate's effectiveness.

Cimetidine This drug may increase the effects of valproate.

Zidovudine When zidovudine and sodium valproate are taken together, the blood levels of zidovudine may increase, leading to increased adverse effects.

SPECIAL PRECAUTIONS

Be sure to tell your doctor if:
◆ You have long-term liver or kidney problems.
◆ You are taking other medications.

Pregnancy Not usually prescribed. May cause abnormalities in the unborn baby. Discuss with your doctor.

Breast-feeding The drug passes into the breast milk, but at normal doses adverse effects on the baby are unlikely. Discuss with your doctor.

Infants and children Reduced dose necessary.

Over 60 Reduced dose may be necessary.

Driving and hazardous work Your underlying condition may make such activities inadvisable. Discuss with your doctor.

Alcohol Avoid. Alcohol may increase the sedative effects of this drug.

PROLONGED USE

This drug may cause liver damage, which is more likely in the first 6 months of use.

Monitoring Periodic checks on blood levels of the drug are usually required. Blood tests of liver function and blood composition may also be carried out.

Sotalol

Brand names Beta-Cardone, Sotacor
Used in the following combined preparations
None

QUICK REFERENCE

Drug group beta blocker (p.28)
Overdose danger rating Medium
Dependence rating Low
Prescription needed Yes
Available as generic Yes

GENERAL INFORMATION

Sotalol is a non-cardioselective beta blocker used in the prevention and treatment of ventricular and supraventricular arrhythmias (see p.32). It has an additional anti-arrhythmic action to other beta blockers.

Sotalol is no longer prescribed for the other conditions that beta blockers are prescribed for. This is due to a serious side effect called 'torsades de pointes', a kind of ventricular arrhythmia that is serious enough to produce symptoms and, rarely, death. For this reason, anyone taking sotalol will be carefully monitored.

INFORMATION FOR USERS

Your drug prescription is tailored for you. Do not alter dosage without checking with your doctor.

How taken Tablets, injection.

Frequency and timing of doses 2 x daily (tablets); 6-hourly intervals when necessary (injections).

Adult dosage range 80mg daily initially, increased at 2–3-day intervals to 160–320mg daily. Higher doses of 480–640mg under specialist supervision.

Onset of effect 30–60 minutes.

Duration of action 12 hours.

Diet advice None.

Storage Keep in a closed container in a cool, dry place out of reach of children. Protect from light.

Missed dose Take as soon as you remember. If your next dose is due within 3 hours, take a single dose now and skip the next.

Stopping the drug Do not stop taking the drug without consulting your doctor, who will supervise a gradual reduction in dosage. Sudden withdrawal may lead to worsening of your condition.

Exceeding the dose An occasional unintentional extra dose is unlikely to be a cause for concern. Large overdoses may cause low blood pressure, slow heart rate, heart block, bronchospasm, and heart arrhythmias. Notify your doctor immediately.

POSSIBLE ADVERSE EFFECTS

Sotalol may cause lethargy, fatigue, dizziness, cold hands and feet, and nightmares or vivid dreams. A very fast heart rate with palpitations could be a symptom of torsades de pointes; if you experience this or suffer from dizzy spells or fainting, notify your doctor immediately. You should also consult your doctor if you develop shortness of breath or wheezing.

INTERACTIONS

Phenothiazines, antidepressants, vincamine, fenoxedil, and erythromycin (IV) These drugs increase the risk of torsades de pointes with sotalol.

Verapamil and diltiazem Combining these drugs with sotalol will have very adverse effects on heart function.

Anti-arrhythmics such as amiodarone, disopyramide, quinidine, lidocaine, procainamide Taking any of these drugs with sotalol may slow the heart rate and affect heart function.

Calcium channel blockers These may cause low blood pressure, slow heartbeats and heart failure if taken with sotalol.

Potassium-sparing diuretics, amphotericin, corticosteroids, and some laxatives These drugs may lower blood potassium levels, increasing the risk of torsades de pointes.

Sympathomimetics such as adrenaline, noradrenaline and dobutamine There is a risk of severe high blood pressure if these drugs are taken with sotalol.

SPECIAL PRECAUTIONS

Be sure to tell your doctor if:
◆ You have liver or kidney problems.

◆ You have a breathing disorder such as asthma, bronchitis, or emphysema.
◆ You have heart failure.
◆ You have diabetes.
◆ You have poor circulation in the legs.
◆ You are taking other medications.

Pregnancy Not usually prescribed. May affect the unborn baby. Discuss with your doctor.

Breast-feeding The drug passes into the breast milk and may affect the baby. Discuss with your doctor.

Infants and children Not prescribed.

Over 60 Reduced dose may be necessary.

Driving and hazardous work No problems expected.

Alcohol No special problems.

PROLONGED USE

Sotalol may be taken indefinitely for prevention of ventricular arrhythmias.

Monitoring Periodic blood tests are usually performed to monitor levels of potassium and magnesium. The electrocardiogram is usually monitored for signs of development of torsades de pointes.

Streptokinase

Brand names Kabikinase, Streptase
Used in the following combined preparation
Varidase

QUICK REFERENCE

Drug group Thrombolytic drug (p.38)
Overdose danger rating Medium
Dependence rating Low
Prescription needed Yes
Available as generic No

GENERAL INFORMATION

Streptokinase, an enzyme produced by the streptococcus bacteria, is used in hospitals to dissolve the fibrin (see p.36) of blood clots, especially those in the arteries of the heart and lungs. It is also used on the clots formed in shunts during kidney dialysis.

Administered into a vein in the early stages of a heart attack to dissolve a clot in the coronary arteries (thrombosis), streptokinase can reduce the amount of damage to heart muscle. A fast-acting drug, it is is most effective in dissolving any newly formed clots, and it is often released at the site of the clot via a catheter inserted into an artery. Because excessive bleeding is a common side effect, treatment is closely supervised.

Streptokinase is also used to treat wounds and ulcers in combination with another enzyme called streptodornase. For this use, powder is applied locally.

Streptokinase is a protein and can cause allergic reactions. Antihistamines may be given at the start of treatment to reduce this risk.

INFORMATION FOR USERS

The drug is only given under medical super-vision and is not for self-administration.

How taken Powder, injection.

Frequency and timing of doses By a single injection or continuously over a period of 24–72 hours. *Powder* 1–2 x daily.

Dosage range Dosage is determined individ-ually by the patient's condition and response.

Onset of effect As soon as streptokinase reaches the blood clot, it begins to dissolve within minutes. Most of the clot will be dissolved within a few hours.

Duration of action Effect disappears within a few minutes of stopping the drug.

Diet advice None.

Storage Not applicable. This drug is not normally kept in the home.

Missed dose Not applicable. This drug is given only in hospital under close medical supervision.

Stopping the drug The drug is usually given for up to 3 days.

Exceeding the dose Overdosage is unlikely since treatment is carefully monitored.

POSSIBLE ADVERSE EFFECTS

Streptokinase is given under strict super-vision and all adverse effects are closely monitored so that they can be quickly dealt with. Excessive bleeding is the most impor-tant adverse effect. Nausea or vomiting, rash or itching, fever, wheezing, and abnormal heart rhythms may also occur.

INTERACTIONS

Anticoagulants There is an increased risk of bleeding when these drugs are taken at the same time as streptokinase.

Antiplatelet drugs The risk of bleeding is inc-reased if these are given with streptokinase.

SPECIAL PRECAUTIONS

Streptokinase is prescribed only under close medical supervision, usually only in life-threatening circumstances.

Pregnancy Not usually prescribed. If used during the first 18 weeks of pregnancy there is a risk that the placenta may separate from the wall of the uterus.

Breast-feeding No evidence of risk.

Infants and children Reduced dose necessary.

Over 60 Increased likelihood of bleeding into the brain.

Driving and hazardous work Not applicable.

Alcohol Not applicable.

PROLONGED USE

Streptokinase is never used long term.

Further instructions Once you have had a dose, you will be given a card which you must keep with you at all times and present to any doc-tor in case further treatment is required. A second course of treatment would not nor-mally be given within 6 months of the first.

Sucralfate

Brand name Antepsin
Used in the following combined preparations
None

QUICK REFERENCE

Drug group Ulcer-healing drug (p.41)
Overdose danger rating Low
Dependence rating Low
Prescription needed Yes
Available as generic No

GENERAL INFORMATION

Sucralfate, a drug that is partly derived from aluminium, is prescribed to treat gast-ric and duodenal ulcers. The drug does not neutralize stomach acid, but it forms a pro-tective barrier over the ulcer that protects it from attack by digestive juices, giving it time to heal.

If antacids are necessary during treatment to relieve pain, they should be taken at least half an hour before or after taking sucralfate.

SULFASALAZINE

Apart from constipation, sucralfate does not have many common adverse effects. However, the safety of the drug for long-term use has not yet been confirmed. Therefore, courses of more than 12 weeks are not recommended.

INFORMATION FOR USERS
Your drug prescription is tailored for you. Do not alter dosage without checking with your doctor.
How taken Tablets, liquid.
Frequency and timing of doses 2–4 x daily, 1 hour before each meal and at bedtime, at least 2 hours after food. The tablets may be dispersed in a little water before swallowing. Occasionally, up to 6 x daily.
Dosage range 4–8g daily.
Onset of effect Some improvement may be noted after one or two doses, but it takes a few weeks for an ulcer to heal.
Duration of action Up to 5 hours.
Diet advice Your doctor will advise if supplements are needed.
Storage Keep in a closed container in a cool, dry place out of reach of children.
Missed dose Do not make up the dose you missed. Take your next dose on your original schedule.
Stopping the drug Do not stop taking the drug without consulting your doctor; symptoms may recur.
Exceeding the dose An occasional unintentional extra dose is unlikely to be a cause for concern. But if you notice any unusual symptoms, or if a large overdose has been taken, notify your doctor.

POSSIBLE ADVERSE EFFECTS
Most people do not experience any adverse effects while they are taking sucralfate. The most common is constipation, which will diminish as your body adjusts to the drug. Some people may experience indigestion, nausea, diarrhoea, a dry mouth, dizziness, insomnia, and a rash or itching.

INTERACTIONS
Antacids and other indigestion remedies These reduce the effectiveness of sucralfate and should be taken more than 30 minutes before or after sucralfate.

Phenytoin The effect of this drug may be reduced if it is taken with sucralfate.
Warfarin The effects of warfarin may be reduced if it is taken with sucralfate.
Tetracyclines, ciprofloxacin, norfloxacin, and ofloxacin Sucralfate may reduce the effect of these antibiotics.
Digoxin The effects of this drug may be reduced.
Thyroxine The effects of this drug may be reduced.

SPECIAL PRECAUTIONS
Be sure to tell your doctor if:
◆ You have a long-term kidney problem.
◆ You are taking other medications.
Pregnancy Safety in pregnancy not established. Discuss with your doctor.
Breast-feeding No evidence of risk.
Infants and children Not usually prescribed.
Over 60 No special problems.
Driving and hazardous work Usually no problems, but sucralfate may cause dizziness in some people.
Alcohol Avoid. Alcohol may counteract the beneficial effect of this drug.

PROLONGED USE
Not usually prescribed for periods longer than 12 weeks at a time. Prolonged use may lead to deficiency of vitamins A, D, E, and K.

Sulfasalazine
Brand name Salazopyrin
Used in the following combined preparations
None

QUICK REFERENCE
Drug group Drug for inflammatory bowel disease (p.44) and antirheumatic drug (p.50)
Overdose danger rating Low
Dependence rating Low
Prescription needed Yes
Available as a generic Yes

GENERAL INFORMATION
Sulfasalazine, chemically related to the sulphonamide antibacterial drugs, is used to treat two inflammatory disorders affecting the bowel. One is ulcerative colitis (which

371

mainly affects the large intestine); the other is Crohn's disease (which usually affects the small intestine). In recent years, sulfasalazine has also been found effective in the treatment of rheumatoid arthritis.

Adverse effects such as nausea, loss of appetite, and general discomfort are more likely when higher doses are taken. Side effects caused by stomach irritation may be avoided by changing to a specially coated tablet form of the drug. Allergic reactions such as fever and rash may be avoided or minimized by low initial doses of the drug, followed by gradual increases. Maintenance of adequate fluid intake is important while taking this drug. In rare cases among men, temporary sterility may occur.

INFORMATION FOR USERS

Your drug prescription is tailored for you. Do not alter dosage without checking with your doctor.

How taken Tablets, liquid, suppositories, enema.

Frequency and timing of doses 4 x daily after meals with a glass of water (tablets); 2 x daily (suppositories); once daily, usually at bedtime (enema).

Adult dosage range 4–8g daily (Crohn's disease/ulcerative colitis); 500mg–3g daily (rheumatoid arthritis).

Onset of effect Adverse effects may occur within a few days, but full beneficial effects may take 1–3 weeks, depending on the severity of the condition.

Duration of action Up to 24 hours.

Diet advice It is important to drink plenty of liquids (at least 1.5 litres a day) during treatment. Sulfasalazine may reduce the absorption of folic acid from the intestine, leading to a deficiency of this vitamin. Eat plenty of green vegetables.

Storage Keep in a closed container in a cool, dry place out of reach of children.

Missed dose Take as soon as you remember. If your next dose is due within 2 hours, take a single dose now and skip the next.

Stopping the drug Do not stop taking the drug without consulting your doctor; symptoms may recur.

Exceeding the dose An occasional unintentional extra dose is unlikely to be a cause for concern. But if you notice any unusual symptoms, or if a large overdose has been taken, notify your doctor.

POSSIBLE ADVERSE EFFECTS

Adverse effects, including headache, malaise, loss of appetite, joint pain, and ringing in the ears, are common with high doses, but may disappear with a reduction in the dose. Symptoms such as nausea and vomiting may be helped by taking the drug with food. Orange or yellow discoloration of the urine is no cause for alarm. If you develop a fever or rash, or you experience bleeding or abnormal bruising, consult your doctor urgently.

INTERACTIONS

General note 1 Sulfasalazine may increase the effects of a variety of drugs, including oral anticoagulants, oral antidiabetics, anticonvulsants, and methotrexate.

General note 2 Sulfasalazine reduces the absorption and effect of some drugs, including digoxin, folic acid, and iron.

SPECIAL PRECAUTIONS

Be sure to tell your doctor if:
◆ You have long-term liver or kidney problems.
◆ You have glucose-6-phosphate dehydrogenase (G6PD) deficiency.
◆ You have a blood disorder.
◆ You suffer from porphyria.
◆ You are allergic to sulphonamides or aspirin.
◆ You wear soft contact lenses.
◆ You are taking other medications.

Pregnancy No evidence of risk to developing fetus. Folic acid supplements may be required. Discuss with your doctor.

Breast-feeding The drug passes into the breast milk and may affect the baby. Discuss with your doctor.

Infants and children Not recommended under 2 years. Reduced dose necessary for older children, according to body weight.

Over 60 No special problems.

Driving and hazardous work No special problems.

Alcohol No known problems.

PROLONGED USE

Blood disorders may occur with prolonged

use of this drug. Maintenance dosage is usually continued indefinitely.

Monitoring Periodic tests of blood composition and liver function are usually required.

Sumatriptan

Brand name Imigran
Used in the following combined preparations
None

QUICK REFERENCE
Drug group Drug for migraine (p.20)
Overdose danger rating Medium
Dependence rating Low
Prescription needed Yes
Available as generic No

GENERAL INFORMATION
Sumatriptan is a highly effective drug for migraine, usually given to people who fail to respond to analgesics (such as aspirin and paracetamol). The drug is of considerable value in the treatment of acute migraine attacks, whether or not they are preceded by an aura, but is not meant to be taken regularly to prevent attacks. Sumatriptan is also used for the acute treatment of cluster headache (a form of migraine headache). It should be taken as soon as possible after the onset of the attack, although, unlike other drugs used in migraine, it will still be of benefit at whatever stage of the attack it is taken.

Sumatriptan relieves the symptoms of migraine by preventing the dilation of blood vessels in the brain, which causes the attack.

INFORMATION FOR USERS
Your drug prescription is tailored for you. Do not alter dosage without checking with your doctor.

How taken Tablets, injection, nasal spray.
Frequency and timing of doses Should be taken as soon as possible after the onset of an attack. However, it is equally effective at whatever stage it is taken. DO NOT take a second dose for the same attack. The tablets should be swallowed whole with water.

Adult dosage range Tablets 50–100mg per attack, up to maximum of 300mg in 24 hours if another attack occurs. Injection 6mg per attack, up to maximum of 12mg (two injections) in 24 hours if another attack occurs. Nasal spray 20mg per attack, up to maximum of 40mg (2 puffs) in 24 hours if another attack occurs.

Onset of effect 30 minutes (tablets); 10–15 minutes (injection).

Duration of action Tablets The maximum effect occurs after 2–4 hours. Injection The maximum effect occurs after 11/2–2 hours.

Diet advice None unless otherwise advised.

Storage Keep in a closed container in a cool, dry place out of reach of children. Protect from light.

Missed dose Not applicable, as it is taken only to treat a migraine attack.

Stopping the drug Taken only to treat a migraine attack.

Exceeding the dose An occasional unintentional extra tablet or injection is unlikely to cause problems. But if you notice any unusual symptoms, or if a large overdose has been taken, notify your doctor.

POSSIBLE ADVERSE EFFECTS
Adverse effects of sumatriptan include pain at the injection site; flushing; a hot, tingling feeling; dizziness; a feeling of heaviness or weakness; fatigue; and drowsiness. Many of the adverse effects will disappear after about 1 hour as your body becomes adjusted to the medicine. If the symptoms persist or are severe, contact your doctor. If you experience palpitations or chest pain, consult your doctor urgently.

INTERACTIONS
Antidepressants MAOIs and some other antidepressants, such as fluvoxamine, fluoxetine, paroxetine, and sertraline, increase the risk of adverse effects with sumatriptan.

Lithium Patients taking lithium should not take sumatriptan due to the high risk of adverse effects.

Ergotamine must be taken at least 6 hours after sumatriptan, and sumatriptan must be taken at least 24 hours after ergotamine.

SPECIAL PRECAUTIONS
Be sure to tell your doctor if:
◆ You have liver or kidney problems.
◆ You have heart problems.

◆ You have high blood pressure.
◆ You have had a heart attack.
◆ You have angina.
◆ You are allergic to some medicines.
◆ You are taking other medications.

Pregnancy Safety in pregnancy not established. Discuss with your doctor.

Breast-feeding Safety not established. Discuss with your doctor.

Infants and children Not recommended.

Over 60 Not recommended for patients over 65 years.

Driving and hazardous work It is inadvisable to undertake such activities once a migraine attack appears to be developing.

Alcohol No special problems, but some drinks may provoke migraine in some people.

Surgery and general anaesthetics Notify your doctor or dentist if you have used sumatriptan within 48 hours prior to surgery.

PROLONGED USE

Sumatriptan should not be used continuously to prevent migraine but only to treat migraine attacks.

Tamoxifen

Brand names Emblon, Fentamox, Nolvadex, Oestrifen, Tamofen
Used in the following combined preparations
None

QUICK REFERENCE

Drug group Anticancer drug (p.94)
Overdose danger rating Low
Dependence rating Low
Prescription needed Yes
Available as generic Yes

GENERAL INFORMATION

Tamoxifen is an anti-oestrogen drug (oestrogen is a naturally occurring female sex hormone, see p.86). It is used for two conditions: infertility and breast cancer. When given as treatment of certain types of infertility, tamoxifen is taken only on certain days of the menstrual cycle. Used as an anticancer drug for breast cancer, it works against oestrogens. By latching on to cells that recognize these hormones, it can slow the growth of the tumour and even shrink it. It can also be used to prevent the recurrence of a breast cancer that has been surgically removed.

As its effect is specific, tamoxifen has fewer adverse effects than most other drugs used for breast cancer.

INFORMATION FOR USERS

Your drug prescription is tailored for you. Do not alter dosage without checking with your doctor.
How taken Tablets.
Frequency and timing of doses 1–2 x daily.
Adult dosage range 20mg daily (breast cancer). 20–80mg daily (infertility).
Onset of effect Side effects may be felt within days, but beneficial effects may take 4–10 weeks.
Duration of action Effects may be felt for several weeks after stopping the drug.
Diet advice None.
Storage Keep in a closed container in a cool, dry place out of reach of children. Protect from light.
Missed dose Take as soon as you remember. If your next dose is due within 2 hours, take a single dose now and skip the next.

Stopping the drug Do not stop taking the drug without consulting your doctor; stopping the drug may lead to worsening of your underlying condition.
Exceeding the dose An occasional unintentional extra dose is unlikely to be a cause for concern. But if you notice any unusual symptoms, or if a large overdose has been taken, notify your doctor.

POSSIBLE ADVERSE EFFECTS

Adverse effects are rarely serious with tamoxifen and do not usually require treatment to be stopped. Nausea, vomiting, and hot flushes are the most common reactions. Ankle swelling may also occur. There is a small risk of endometrial cancer (cancer of the uterine lining) developing. You should therefore notify your doctor of any symptoms such as irregular vaginal bleeding or discharge as soon as possible. If you experience bone or tumour pain, develop a rash or itching, or experience blurred vision or headache, consult your doctor.

INTERACTIONS

Anticoagulants People treated with anticoagulants such as warfarin usually need a lower dose of the anticoagulant.

SPECIAL PRECAUTIONS

Be sure to tell your doctor if:
◆ You have cataracts or poor eyesight.
◆ You suffer from porphyria.
◆ You are taking other medications.
Pregnancy Not usually prescribed. May have effects on the developing baby. Discuss with your doctor.
Breast-feeding Not usually prescribed. Discuss with your doctor.
Infants and children Not prescribed.
Over 60 No special problems.
Driving and hazardous work No special problems.
Alcohol No known problems.

PROLONGED USE

There is a small increase in the risk of endometrial cancer with long-term treatment. This is far outweighed by the benefits of treatment, however.

There is a risk of damage to the eye with long-term, high-dose treatment.
Monitoring Eyesight may be tested periodically.

Tamsulosin

Brand name Flomax MR
Used in the following combined preparations
None

QUICK REFERENCE
Drug group Drug for urinary disorders (p.108)
Overdose danger rating Medium
Dependence rating Low
Prescription needed Yes
Available as generic No

GENERAL INFORMATION
Tamsulosin is a selective alpha-blocker drug used to treat urinary retention due to benign prostatic hypertrophy, or BPH (an enlarged prostate gland). The drug, as it passes through the prostate, relaxes the muscle in the wall of the urethra, thereby increasing urine flow.

To exclude other conditions with similar symptoms, your doctor will arrange for you to have a physical examination and a special blood test, which may be repeated at intervals during treatment.

Like other alpha-blockers, tamsulosin may lower blood pressure rapidly after the first dose. For this reason, the first dose should be taken at home so that, if dizziness or weakness occur, you can lie down until they have disappeared.

Tamsulosin is not used to treat hypertension (high blood pressure) because the dose used in the treatment of benign prostatic hypertrophy is low.

INFORMATION FOR USERS
Your drug prescription is tailored for you. Do not alter dosage without checking with your doctor.
How taken SR-capsules.
Frequency and timing of doses Once daily after breakfast.
Adult dosage range 400 micrograms.
Onset of effect 1–2 hours.
Duration of action 24 hours.

Diet advice None.
Storage Keep in a closed container in a cool, dry place out of reach of children.
Missed dose Taken as soon as you remember. If your next dose is due within 4 hours, take a single dose now and skip the next.
Stopping the drug Do not stop taking the drug without consulting your doctor; stopping tamsulosin suddenly may lead to a rise in blood pressure.
Exceeding the dose An occasional unintentional extra dose is unlikely to cause problems. Large overdoses may produce sedation, dizziness, low blood pressure and rapid pulse. Notify your doctor immediately.

POSSIBLE ADVERSE EFFECTS
Dizziness seems to be the most common adverse effect of treatment with tamsulosin, but this usually improves after the first few doses. Other adverse effects include headache, drowsiness, nausea, vomiting, diarrhoea, constipation, ejaculatory problems, and palpitations. If you develop a rash or itching, consult your doctor.

INTERACTIONS
Antidepressants, beta-blockers, calcium channel blockers, diuretics, and thymoxamine These drugs are likely to increase the blood-pressure lowering effect of tamsulosin.

SPECIAL PRECAUTIONS
Be sure to tell your doctor if:
◆ You have had low blood pressure.
◆ You have liver or kidney problems.
◆ You have heart failure.
◆ You have a history of depression.
◆ You are taking an MAOI drug.
◆ You are taking drugs for high blood pressure.
◆ You are taking other medications.
Pregnancy Not prescribed.
Breast-feeding Not prescribed.
Infants and children Not prescribed.
Over 60 No special problems.
Driving and hazardous work Avoid such activities until you have learned how tamsulosin because the drug can cause drowsiness and dizziness.
Alcohol Avoid excessive amounts. Alcohol can further lower blood pressure.

PROLONGED USE
No special problems.

Temazepam

Brand name None
Used in the following combined preparations
None

QUICK REFERENCE
Drug group Benzodiazepine sleeping drug (p.11)
Overdose danger rating Medium
Dependence rating High
Prescription needed Yes
Available as generic Yes

GENERAL INFORMATION
Temazepam belongs to a group of drugs known as the benzodiazepines. The actions and adverse effects of this group of drugs are described more fully under Anti-anxiety drugs (p.13).

Temazepam is used in the short-term treatment of insomnia. Because it is a short-acting drug compared with some other benzodiazepines, it is less likely to cause drowsiness and/or lightheadedness the following day. For this reason, the drug is not usually effective in preventing early wakening, but hangover is less common than with other benzodiazepines.

Like other benzodiazepines, the drug can be habit-forming if taken regularly over a long period. Its effects also grow weaker with time. For these reasons, treatment is usually only continued for a few days at a time.

INFORMATION FOR USERS
Your drug prescription is tailored for you. Do not alter dosage without checking with your doctor.
How taken Tablets, liquid.
Frequency and timing of doses Once daily, 30 minutes before bedtime.
Adult dosage range 10–60mg.
Onset of effect 15–40 minutes, or longer.
Duration of action 6–8 hours.
Diet advice None.
Storage Keep in a closed container in a cool, dry place out of reach of children. Protect from light.

Missed dose If you fall asleep without having taken a dose and wake some hours later, do not take the missed dose. If necessary, return to your normal dose schedule the following night.
Stopping the drug If you have been taking the drug continuously for less than 2 weeks, it can be safely stopped as soon as you no longer need it. If you have been taking the drug for longer, consult your doctor, who may supervise a gradual reduction in dosage. Stopping the drug abruptly may lead to withdrawal symptoms.
Exceeding the dose An occasional unintentional extra dose is unlikely to be a cause for concern. Large overdoses may cause unusual drowsiness. Notify your doctor.

POSSIBLE ADVERSE EFFECTS
The principal adverse effects of this drug are related to its sedative and tranquillizing properties. They include dizziness, unsteadiness, daytime drowsiness, vivid dreams, nightmares, headache, and confusion. These effects normally diminish after the first few days of treatment.

INTERACTIONS
Sedatives All drugs that have a sedative effect on the central nervous system are likely to increase the sedative properties of temazepam. Such drugs include other anti-anxiety and sleeping drugs, opioid analgesics, antidepressants, antihistamines, and antipsychotics.

SPECIAL PRECAUTIONS
Be sure to tell your doctor if:
◆ You have severe respiratory disease.
◆ You suffer from porphyria.
◆ You suffer from depression.
◆ You have liver or kidney problems.
◆ You have myasthenia gravis.
◆ You have had problems with alcohol or drug abuse.
◆ You are taking other medications.
Pregnancy Safety in pregnancy not established. Discuss with your doctor.
Breast-feeding The drug passes into the breast milk, but at normal doses adverse effects on the baby are unlikely. Discuss with your doctor.
Infants and children Not recommended.

Over 60 Reduced dose may be necessary. Increased likelihood of adverse effects.

Driving and hazardous work Avoid such activities until you have learned how temazepam affects you because the drug can cause reduced alertness and slowed reactions.

Alcohol Avoid. Alcohol may increase the sedative effect of this drug.

PROLONGED USE

Regular use of temazepam over several weeks can lead to a reduction in its effect as the body adapts. It may also be habit-forming when taken for extended periods. It should not normally be used for longer than 1–2 weeks.

Terbinafine

Brand name Lamisil
Used in the following combined preparations
None

QUICK REFERENCE

Drug group Antifungal drug (p.74)
Overdose danger rating Low
Dependence rating Low
Prescription needed Yes
Available as generic No

GENERAL INFORMATION

Terbinafine is an antifungal drug used to treat fungal infections of the skin and nails, particularly tinea (ringworm). It is also used as a cream for candida (yeast) infections.

Terbinafine has largely replaced older drugs such as griseofulvin because it is more easily absorbed and is therefore more effective.

Tinea infections are treated in two to six weeks, but treatment of nail infections may take up to 6 months.

Rare adverse effects of terbinafine treatment include jaundice and a severe rash, both of which should be reported to your doctor without delay.

INFORMATION FOR USERS

Your drug prescription is tailored for you. Do not alter dosage without checking with your doctor.

How taken Tablets, cream.

Frequency and timing of doses Once daily (tablets); 1–2 x daily (cream).

Adult dosage range *Tinea infection* 250mg (tablets). *Candida infection* As directed (cream).

Onset of effect 1 hour.

Duration of action 24 hours.

Diet advice None.

Storage Keep in a closed container in a cool, dry place out of reach of children. Protect from light.

Missed dose Take as soon as you remember. If your next dose is due within 4 hours, take a single dose now and skip the next.

Stopping the drug Take the full course. Even if you feel better, the original infection may still be present and may recur if treatment is stopped too soon.

Exceeding the dose An occasional unintentional extra dose is unlikely to be a cause for concern. But if you notice any unusual symptoms, or if a large overdose has been taken, notify your doctor.

POSSIBLE ADVERSE EFFECTS

Side effects are generally mild and transient and include nausea, indigestion, bloating, mild abdominal pain, diarrhoea, and headache. Some people may experience disturbance or loss of taste, dizziness, "pins and needles", and muscle or joint pain. If you develop jaundice or a severe rash, consult your doctor urgently.

INTERACTIONS

Oral contraceptives "Breakthrough" bleeding may occur when these are taken with terbinafine.

Rifampicin This drug may reduce the blood level and effect of terbinafine.

Cimetidine This drug may increase the blood level of terbinafine.

SPECIAL PRECAUTIONS

Be sure to tell your doctor if:
◆ You have liver or kidney problems.
◆ You are taking other medications.

Pregnancy Safety in pregnancy not established. Discuss with your doctor.

Breast-feeding The drug passes into the breast milk and may affect the baby adversely. Discuss with your doctor.

Infants and children Safety not established. Discuss with your doctor.

Over 60 No special problems.
Driving and hazardous work No known problems.
Alcohol No known problems.

PROLONGED USE
No special problems.

Terbutaline

Brand names Bricanyl, Monovent
Used in the following combined preparations
None

QUICK REFERENCE
Drug group Bronchodilator (p.23)
Overdose danger rating Low
Dependence rating Low
Prescription needed Yes
Available as generic No

GENERAL INFORMATION
Terbutaline is a sympathomimetic broncho-dilator that dilates the small airways in the lungs. It is used in the treatment and prevention of the bronchospasm occurring with asthma, chronic bronchitis, and emphysema. The drug may be given orally or by inhaler when rapid relief of breathlessness is required.

Muscle tremor, especially of the hands, is common with terbutaline and usually disappears on reduction of the dose or with continued use as the body adapts to the drug. In common with the other sympathomimetic drugs, it may produce nervousness and restlessness.

INFORMATION FOR USERS
Your drug prescription is tailored for you. Do not alter dosage without checking with your doctor.
How taken Tablets, liquid, injection, inhaler.
Frequency and timing of doses 3 x daily (tablets); as necessary (inhaler).
Dosage range *Adults* 7.5–15mg daily (tablets); up to 2mg daily (inhaler). *Children* Reduced dose according to age and weight.
Onset of effect Within a few minutes (inhaler); within 1–2 hours (tablets).
Duration of action 4–8 hours (tablets).
Diet advice None.

Storage Keep in a closed container in a cool, dry place out of reach of children. Protect from light. Do not puncture or burn aerosol containers.
Missed dose Do not take the missed dose. Take your next dose as usual.
Stopping the drug Do not stop taking the drug without consulting your doctor; symptoms may recur.
Exceeding the dose An occasional unintentional extra dose is unlikely to be a cause for concern. But if you notice any unusual symptoms, or if a large overdose has been taken, notify your doctor.

POSSIBLE ADVERSE EFFECTS
Possible adverse effects include tremor, nervousness, anxiety, restlessness, muscle cramps, and nausea. These may be reduced by adjustment of dosage. Palpitations and headache, resulting from stimulation of the heart and narrowing of the blood vessels, are rare. Nausea or vomiting and muscle cramps may also occur.

INTERACTIONS
Other sympathomimetics may add to the effects of terbutaline and vice versa, so increasing the risk of adverse effects.
MAOIs Terbutaline may interact with these drugs to cause a dangerous rise in blood pressure.
Beta blockers may reduce the beneficial effects of terbutaline.

SPECIAL PRECAUTIONS
Be sure to tell your doctor if:
◆ You have heart problems.
◆ You have high blood pressure.
◆ You have diabetes.
◆ You have an overactive thyroid.
◆ You are taking other medications.
Pregnancy Safety in early pregnancy not established, although problems are unlikely with inhaled terbutaline. It is given by injection in late pregnancy to prevent premature labour. Discuss with your doctor.
Breast-feeding No problems expected with inhaled terbutaline.
Infants and children Reduced dose necessary.
Over 60 Reduced dose may be necessary. Increased likelihood of adverse effects.

Driving and hazardous work No problems expected.
Alcohol No special problems.

PROLONGED USE
Prolonged use may result in tolerance to terbutaline's effects. However, failure to respond to the drug may be the result of worsening asthma, requiring prompt medical attention.

Testosterone

Brand names Andropatch, Primoteston Depot, Restandol, Sustanon, Virormone
Used in the following combined preparations
None

QUICK REFERENCE
Drug group Male sex hormone (p.85)
Overdose danger rating Low
Dependence rating Low
Prescription needed Yes
Available as generic Yes

GENERAL INFORMATION
Testosterone is a male sex hormone produced by the testes and, in small quantities, by the ovaries in women. The hormone encourages bone and muscle growth in both men and women and stimulates sexual development in men.

The drug is used to initiate puberty in adolescent males if it has been delayed through deficiency of the natural hormone. It may help to increase fertility in men suffering from either pituitary or testicular disorders. Rarely, testosterone is used to treat breast cancer.

Testosterone can interfere with growth or cause over-rapid sexual development in adolescents. High doses may cause deepening of the voice, excessive hair growth, or hair loss in women.

INFORMATION FOR USERS
Your drug prescription is tailored for you. Do not alter dosage without checking with your doctor.
How taken Capsules, injection, patch, implanted pellets.
Frequency and timing of doses 2 x daily (capsules); once every 3 weeks to 2 x weekly (injection) depending on condition being treated; every 6 months (implant); once daily (patch).
Dosage range Varies with method of administration and the condition being treated.
Onset of effect 2–3 days.
Duration of action 1–2 days (capsules and patch); 1–3 weeks (injection); approximately 6 months (implant).
Diet advice None.
Storage Keep in a closed container in a cool, dry place out of reach of children. Protect from light.
Missed dose No cause for concern, but take as soon as you remember. If your next dose (by mouth) is due within 3 hours, take a single dose now and skip the next.
Stopping the drug Do not stop taking the drug without consulting your doctor.
Exceeding the dose An occasional unintentional extra dose is unlikely to be a cause for concern. But if you notice unusual symptoms, or if a large overdose was taken, notify your doctor.

POSSIBLE ADVERSE EFFECTS
Most of the more serious adverse effects are likely to occur only with long-term treatment with testosterone, and may be helped by a reduction in dosage. Men may experience difficulty in passing urine and abnormal erection, while women may experience unusual hair growth, voice changes, and an enlarged clitoris. Fluid retention, leading to ankle swelling, may occur. If you develop jaundice, seek urgent medical advice.

INTERACTIONS
Anticoagulants Testosterone may increase the effect of these drugs. Dosage of anticoagulants may need to be adjusted accordingly.
Antidiabetic agents As testosterone may lower the blood sugar, dosage of antidiabetic drugs and insulin may need to be reduced.

SPECIAL PRECAUTIONS
Be sure to tell your doctor if:
◆ You have long-term liver or kidney problems.
◆ You have heart problems.
◆ You have prostate trouble.
◆ You have high blood pressure.
◆ You have epilepsy or migraine headaches.

◆ You have diabetes.
◆ You are taking other medications.
Pregnancy Not prescribed.
Breast-feeding Not prescribed.
Infants and children Not prescribed for infants and young children. Reduced dose necessary in adolescents.
Over 60 Rarely required. Increased risk of prostate problems in elderly men. Reduced dose may therefore be necessary.
Driving and hazardous work No special problems.
Alcohol No special problems.

PROLONGED USE
Prolonged use of this drug may lead to reduced growth in adolescents.
Monitoring Regular checks of the effects of testosterone treatment are required.

Tetracycline

Brand names Achromycin, Economycin, Tetrachel, Topicycline
Used in the following combined preparations
Deteclo, Mysteclin

QUICK REFERENCE
Drug group Tetracycline antibiotic (p.60)
Overdose danger rating Low
Dependence rating Low
Prescription needed Yes
Available as generic Yes

GENERAL INFORMATION
Tetracyclines were a very widely used group of antibiotics. However, the development of strains of bacteria resistant to these drugs has reduced their effectiveness in many types of infection. Tetracycline is still used for chest infections caused by chlamydia (for example, psittacosis) and mycoplasma microorganisms. It is also used in non-specific urethritis and a number of rarer conditions, such as Q fever, Rocky Mountain spotted fever, cholera, and brucellosis.

Acne improves following long-term treatment with tetracycline drugs either taken by mouth or applied to the skin as a solution.

Common side effects of this drug are nausea, vomiting, and diarrhoea. Rashes may also occur. Tetracycline may discolour developing teeth if it is taken by children or by the mother during pregnancy. It is not prescribed for people with poor kidney function as it can cause further deterioration.

INFORMATION FOR USERS
Your drug prescription is tailored for you. Do not alter your dosage without checking with your doctor.
How taken Tablets, capsules, ointment, eye/ear ointment.
Frequency and timing of doses *By mouth* 4 x daily, at least 1 hour before or 2 hours after meals. Long-term treatment of acne may require only a single dose daily.
Skin preparations 1–3 times daily as directed.
Adult dosage range *Infections* 1–2g daily.
Acne 250mg–1g daily.
Onset of effect 4–12 hours. Improvement in acne may not be noticed for up to 4 weeks.
Duration of action Up to 6 hours.
Diet advice Milk products should be avoided for 1 hour before and 2 hours after taking the drug, since they may impair its absorption.
Storage Keep in a closed container in a cool, dry place out of reach of children.
Missed dose Take as soon as you remember. If your next dose is due within 2 hours, take a single dose now and skip the next.
Stopping the drug Take the full course. Even if you feel better, the original infection may still be present and may recur if treatment is stopped too soon.
Exceeding the dose An occasional unintentional extra dose is unlikely to be a cause for concern. But if you notice any unusual symptoms, or if a large overdose has been taken, notify your doctor.

POSSIBLE ADVERSE EFFECTS
Adverse effects from skin preparations are rare. But taken mouth, the drug may cause nausea, vomiting, or diarrhoea. If you develop a rash, itching, headache or visual disturbances, consult your doctor urgently.

INTERACTIONS
Iron This may reduce the effectiveness of tetracycline.
Oral anticoagulants Tetracycline may increase the action of these drugs.

THEOPHYLLINE/AMINOPHYLLINE

Retinoids These may increase the adverse effects of tetracycline.

Oral contraceptives Tetracycline may reduce the effectiveness of oral contraceptives.

Antacids and milk These interfere with the absorption of tetracycline and may reduce its effectiveness. Doses should be separated by 1–2 hours.

SPECIAL PRECAUTIONS

Be sure to tell your doctor if:
◆ You have long-term liver or kidney problems.
◆ You have previously suffered an allergic reaction to a tetracycline antibiotic.
◆ You are taking other medications.

Pregnancy Not usually prescribed. May cause discoloured teeth and damage bones of the developing fetus. Discuss with your doctor.

Breast-feeding The drug passes into the breast milk and may damage developing bones and discolour the baby's teeth. Discuss with your doctor.

Infants and children Not recommended under 12 years. Reduced dose necessary in older children. May discolour developing teeth.

Over 60 No special problems.

Driving and hazardous work No known problems.

Alcohol No known problems.

Taking your tablets To prevent irritation to the oesophagus, each dose should be taken with a full glass of water while standing.

PROLONGED USE

No problems expected.

Theophylline/ Aminophylline

Brand names [theophylline] Lasma, Nuelin, Theo-Dur, Uniphyllin; [aminophylline] Amnivent, Phyllocontin
Used in the following combined preparations
[theophylline] Do-Do Tablets, Franol, Fanolyn

QUICK REFERENCE

Drug group Bronchodilator (p.23)
Overdose danger rating High
Dependence rating Low
Prescription needed No
Available as generic Yes

GENERAL INFORMATION

Theophylline (and aminophylline, which breaks down to theophylline in the body) is used to treat bronchospasm (constriction of the air passages) in patients suffering from asthma, bronchitis, and emphysema.

It is usually taken continuously as a preventative measure, but it is also used to treat acute attacks.

Slow-release formulations of the drugs are effective for up to 12 hours. These preparations may be prescribed twice daily, but they are also useful as a single dose taken at night to prevent night-time asthma and early morning wheezing.

Treatment with theophylline must be monitored because the effective dose is very close to the toxic dose. Some adverse effects, such as indigestion, nausea, headache, and agitation, can be controlled by regulating the dosage and checking blood levels of the drug.

INFORMATION FOR USERS

Your drug prescription is tailored for you. Do not alter dosage without checking with your doctor.

How taken Tablets, SR-tablets, SR-capsules, liquid, injection.

Frequency and timing of doses 3–4 x daily (tablets, liquid); every 12 or 24 hours (SR-tablets/SR-capsules). The drug should be taken at the same time each day in relation to meals.

Dosage range Adults 375–1,000mg daily, depending on which product is used.

Onset of effect Within 30 minutes (by mouth); within 90 minutes (SR-tablets/SR-capsules).

Duration of action Up to 8 hours (by mouth); 12–24 hours (SR-tablets/SR-capsules).

Diet advice None.

Storage Keep in a closed container in a cool, dry place out of reach of children.

Missed dose Take as soon as you remember. If your next dose is due within 2 hours, take half the dose now (short-acting preparations) or leave out the missed dose and take your next dose now (SR-preparations). Return to your normal dose schedule thereafter.

Stopping the drug Unless palpitations occur, do not stop taking the drug without consulting your doctor; stopping the drug may lead to worsening of the underlying condition.

OVERDOSE ACTION

Seek immediate medical advice in all cases. Take emergency action if chest pains, confusion, or loss of consciousness occur.

POSSIBLE ADVERSE EFFECTS

Most adverse effects of theophylline are related to dosage. These include effects related to the drug's action on the central nervous system, such as headache, agitation and insomnia. Nausea, vomiting, and diarrhoea may also occur. If you experience palpitations, stop taking the drug and seek urgent medical advice.

INTERACTIONS

General note Many drugs increase the effect of theophylline (e.g., erythromycin and cimetidine); others reduce its effect (e.g., carbamazepine, phenytoin, and rifampicin). Discuss with your doctor.

SPECIAL PRECAUTIONS

Be sure to consult your doctor or pharmacist before taking this drug if:
◆ You have a long-term liver problem.
◆ You have angina or irregular heart beat.
◆ You have epilepsy.
◆ You have stomach ulcers.
◆ You smoke.
◆ You are taking other medications.
Pregnancy Safety in pregnancy not established. Discuss with your doctor.
Breast-feeding The drug passes into the breast milk and may affect the baby. Discuss with your doctor.
Infants and children Reduced dose necessary according to age and weight.
Over 60 Reduced dose may be necessary.
Driving and hazardous work No known problems
Alcohol Avoid excess as this may alter levels of the drug and may increase gastrointestinal symptoms.

PROLONGED USE

No problems expected.
Monitoring Periodic checks on blood levels of this drug are usually required.

Thioridazine

Brand names Melleril, Rideril
Used in the following combined preparations
None

QUICK REFERENCE

Drug group Phenothiazine antipsychotic drug (p.15)
Overdose danger rating Medium
Dependence rating Low
Prescription needed Yes
Available as generic Yes

GENERAL INFORMATION

Thioridazine is a member of the phenothiazine antipsychotic group of drugs and was first used in 1959.

Once widely prescribed to treat a variety of psychiatric conditions, this tranquillizer is now used only as a second-line treatment because, in rare cases, it can affect the heart rhythm. Thioridazine is used in the treatment of schizophrenia in adults; its tranquillizing effect suppresses abnormal behaviour. The drug has a similar action to chlorpromazine, but it is less sedating and does not produce movement disorders to the same extent.

Side effects such as hypotension are dose-related and can be controlled by medically supervised adjustment of dosage. The main drawback to the use of this drug is that when given in high doses it can cause eye problems, particularly blurred vision. If large doses are required for long periods, another antipsychotic drug is usually substituted.

INFORMATION FOR USERS

Your drug prescription is tailored for you. Do not alter your dosage without checking with your doctor.
How taken Tablets, liquid.
Frequency and timing of doses 2–4 x daily.
Adult dosage range 50–300mg daily.
Onset of effect 2–3 hours.
Duration of action 4–10 hours. Some effects may last as long as 36 hours.
Diet advice None.
Storage Keep in a closed container in a cool, dry place out of reach of children.
Missed dose Take as soon as you remember. If your next dose is due within 3 hours, take a single dose now and skip the next.

Stopping the drug Unless dizziness and fainting or palpitations occur, do not stop taking the drug without consulting your doctor; symptoms may recur.

Exceeding the dose Tell your doctor if you accidentally exceed the dose. Large overdoses of thioridazine may cause unusual drowsiness, muscle rigidity, fainting, agitation, and palpitations. Notify your doctor.

POSSIBLE ADVERSE EFFECTS
Thioridazine has a strong anticholinergic effect (see Drugs that act on the parasympathetic nervous system, p.9), which can cause a range of minor symptoms that often diminish with time. The most significant adverse effect is a variety of eye problems, such as blurred vision. Drowsiness; dry mouth; stuffy nose; muscle stiffness or tremor; and a fast, irregular heartbeat also occur. Adverse effects can be controlled by medically supervised adjustment of dosage or a change of drug. If you experience dizziness and fainting or palpitations, stop taking the drug and consult your doctor.

INTERACTIONS
Sedatives All drugs that have a sedative effect are likely to increase the sedative properties of thioridazine.

Drugs used for parkinsonism Thioridazine may counter the beneficial effect of these drugs.

Anticholinergic drugs The side effects of these drugs may be increased by thioridazine.

SPECIAL PRECAUTIONS
Be sure to tell your doctor if:
◆ You have liver or kidney problems.
◆ You have heart or circulation problems.
◆ You have had epileptic fits.
◆ You have glaucoma.
◆ You have a heart condition.
◆ You have Parkinson's disease.
◆ You have myasthenia gravis.
◆ You have difficulty in passing urine.
◆ You have porphyria.
◆ You are taking other medications.

Pregnancy Safety in pregnancy not established. Discuss with your doctor.

Breast-feeding The drug passes into the breast milk and may affect the baby. Discuss with your doctor.

Infants and children Not prescribed.
Over 60 Reduced dose may be necessary. Increased likelihood of adverse effects.
Driving and hazardous work Avoid such activities until you have learned how thioridazine affects you because the drug may cause drowsiness and blurred vision.
Alcohol Avoid. Alcohol may increase the sedative effects of this drug.

PROLONGED USE
Use of thioridazine for more than a few months may lead to eye problems and abnormal movements of the face and limbs (tardive dyskinesia). Occasionally, jaundice may occur.
Monitoring Eye examinations should be carried out at intervals during long term use.

Thyroxine
Brand name Eltroxin
Used in the following combined preparations
None

QUICK REFERENCE
Drug group Thyroid hormone (p.82)
Overdose danger rating Medium
Dependence rating Low
Prescription needed Yes
Available as generic Yes

GENERAL INFORMATION
Thyroxine is the major hormone produced by the thyroid gland. Hypothyroidism (deficiency of the natural hormone) may sometimes lead to myxoedema, a condition characterized by slowing of body functions and facial puffiness. A synthetic preparation is used to replace the natural hormone when it is deficient.

Certain types of goitre (an enlarged thyroid gland) are helped by thyroxine, and it may be prescribed to prevent the development of goitre during treatment with antithyroid drugs. Thyroxine is also prescribed for some forms of thyroid cancer.

Adults who have thyroid deficiency are sensitive to thyroid hormones. Therefore treatment is introduced gradually and increased slowly in order to prevent adverse effects. Particular care is required in patients with heart problems such as angina.

INFORMATION FOR USERS
Your drug prescription is tailored for you. Do not alter dosage without checking with your doctor.
How taken Tablets.
Frequency and timing of doses Once daily.
Dosage range *Adults* 50–100 micrograms daily, increased at 3–4-week intervals as required. The maximum dose is 200 micrograms daily.
Onset of effect Within 48 hours. Full beneficial effects may not be felt for several weeks.
Duration of action 1–3 weeks.
Diet advice None.
Storage Keep in a closed container in a cool, dry place out of reach of children. Protect from light.
Missed dose Take as soon as you remember. If your next dose is due within 8 hours, take a single dose now and skip the next.
Stopping the drug Do not stop taking the drug without consulting your doctor; symptoms may recur.
Exceeding the dose An occasional unintentional extra dose is unlikely to cause problems. Large overdoses may cause palpitations during the next few days. Notify your doctor.

POSSIBLE ADVERSE EFFECTS
Adverse effects are rare and are usually due to overdosage causing thyroid overactivity. They include anxiety or agitation, diarrhoea, weight loss, sweating or flushing, and muscle cramps but diminish as the dose is lowered. Too low a dose may cause signs of thyroid underactivity. If you experience palpitations or chest pain, consult your doctor urgently.

INTERACTIONS
Oral anticoagulants Thyroxine may increase the effect of these drugs.
Cholestyramine This drug may reduce the absorption of thyroxine.
Sucralfate The absorption of thyroxine may be reduced by sucralfate.
Antidiabetics Doses of these drugs may need increasing once thyroxine treatment is started.

SPECIAL PRECAUTIONS
Be sure to tell your doctor if:

- You have high blood pressure.
- You have heart problems.
- You have diabetes.
- You are taking other medications.

Pregnancy No evidence of risk.
Breast-feeding The drug passes into the breast milk, but at normal doses adverse effects on the baby are unlikely. Discuss with your doctor.
Infants and children Dosage depends on age and weight.
Over 60 Reduced dose usually necessary.
Driving and hazardous work No known problems.
Alcohol No known problems.

PROLONGED USE
No special problems.
Monitoring Periodic tests of thyroid function are usually required.

Tibolone

Brand name Livial
Used in the following combined preparations
None

QUICK REFERENCE
Drug group Female sex hormone (p.86)
Overdose danger rating Low
Dependence rating Low
Prescription needed Yes
Available as generic No

GENERAL INFORMATION
Tibolone is used for treating symptoms of natural or surgical menopause, such as sweating, depressed mood, and decreased sex drive, and is particularly effective in controlling hot flushes. The drug is taken continuously and, unlike most of the other available hormone replacement therapies, the treatment does not require a cyclical course of progestogen to be taken as well. This is because the drug has both oestrogenic and progestogenic activity.

Incidence of side effects is low. The drug does not cause withdrawal bleeding in postmenopausal women but is not used long term to prevent postmenopausal osteoporosis.

INFORMATION FOR USERS
Your drug prescription is tailored for you.

Do not alter dosage without checking with your doctor.

How taken Tablets.

Frequency and timing of doses Daily, preferably at the same time each day. Swallow the tablets whole – do not chew.

Adult dosage range 2.5mg daily.

Onset of effect You may notice improvement of symptoms within a few weeks but the best results are obtained when the drug is taken for at least 3 months.

Duration of action A few days.

Diet advice None.

Storage Keep in a closed container in a cool, dry place out of reach of children. Protect from light.

Missed dose Take as soon as you remember.

Stopping the drug Do not stop taking the drug without consulting your doctor; symptoms may recur.

Exceeding the dose An occasional unintentional extra dose is unlikely to be a cause for concern. Several tablets are taken together may cause a stomach upset. Notify your doctor.

POSSIBLE ADVERSE EFFECTS

Tibolone is well tolerated and incidence of adverse effects is low. They include weight gain, ankle swelling, dizziness, acne, headache, stomach upset, and facial hair growth. If you experience jaundice, consult your doctor urgently. Vaginal bleeding is more likely if it is less than one year since the menopause, so the drug is not recommended if less than 12 months has passed since your last period.

INTERACTIONS

Some anticonvulsants Phenytoin, phenobarbitone, primidone, and carbamazepine can accelerate the metabolism of tibolone and so decrease its blood levels and effectiveness.

Rifampicin This can accelerate the metabolism of tibolone, decreasing its blood levels and effectiveness.

SPECIAL PRECAUTIONS

Be sure to tell your doctor if:

◆ You have long-term liver or kidney problems.

◆ You suffer from epilepsy or migraine.

◆ You have diabetes.

◆ You have a tumour.

◆ You have a history of cardiovascular or cerebrovascular disease.

◆ You have a high cholesterol level.

◆ You have vaginal bleeding.

◆ You have had a period in the last 12 months.

◆ You are taking other medications.

Pregnancy Not prescribed.

Breast-feeding Not prescribed.

Infants and children Not prescribed.

Over 60 No special problems.

Driving and hazardous work No problems expected.

Alcohol No known problems.

PROLONGED USE

Monitoring Periodic examination by your doctor is advised.

Timolol

Brand names Betim, Blocadren, Glau-opt, Timoptol
Used in the following combined preparations
Moducren, Prestim

QUICK REFERENCE

Drug group Beta blocker (p.28) and drug for glaucoma (p.110)
Overdose danger rating High
Dependence rating Low
Prescription needed Yes
Available as generic No

GENERAL INFORMATION

Timolol is a beta blocker drug that is prescribed to treat hypertension (high blood pressure) and angina (pain due to narrowing of the coronary arteries). It may be given after a heart attack to prevent further damage to the heart muscle. When used to treat hypertension, timolol may also be given with a diuretic. The drug is commonly administered as eye drops to people with certain types of glaucoma, and is occasionally given to prevent migraine.

Timolol can cause breathing difficulties, especially in people suffering from asthma, chronic bronchitis, or emphysema. This problem is more likely to occur in people taking the drug in tablet form, although it can also occur in those individuals using timolol eye drops. As with other beta blockers, timolol may mask the response of the body to low blood sugar and, for that reason, it is prescribed with caution to diabetics.

INFORMATION FOR USERS
Your drug prescription is tailored for you. Do not alter dosage without checking with your doctor.

How taken Tablets, eye drops.

Frequency and timing of doses 1–3 x daily.

Adult dosage range *By mouth* 10–60mg daily (hypertension); 10–45mg daily (angina); 10–20mg daily (after a heart attack); 10–20mg daily (migraine prevention).

Onset of effect Within 30 minutes (by mouth).

Duration of action Up to 24 hours.

Diet advice None.

Storage Keep in a closed container in a cool, dry place out of reach of children.

Missed dose Take as soon as you remember. If your next dose is due within 3 hours, take a single dose now and skip the next.

Stopping the drug Do not stop taking the drug without consulting your doctor; stopping the drug may lead to worsening of the underlying condition.

OVERDOSE ACTION
Seek immediate medical advice in all cases of overdose by mouth. Take emergency action if breathing difficulties, palpitations, or loss of consciousness occur.

POSSIBLE ADVERSE EFFECTS
Timolol taken by mouth can cause lethargy, fatigue, headache, nightmares, vivid dreams, and cold hands or feet. It may also occasionally provoke or worsen heart problems and asthma. If you experience breathlessness or wheezing, stop taking the drug and consult your doctor urgently. Fainting may be a sign that the drug has slowed the heartbeat excessively. Eye drops cause these problems only rarely; eye irritation, headache, or blurred vision is more likely.

INTERACTIONS
Sympathomimetics Present in many cough and cold remedies, these drugs can cause a dangerous rise in blood pressure when taken with timolol.

Salbutamol, salmeterol, and other beta agonists Because these drugs have opposing effects to beta blockers, their effects may be reduced by timolol.

SPECIAL PRECAUTIONS
Be sure to tell your doctor if:
◆ You have a lung disorder such as asthma, bronchitis, or emphysema.
◆ You have diabetes.
◆ You have myasthenia gravis.
◆ You have poor circulation.
◆ You have allergies.
◆ You are taking other medications.

Pregnancy Safety in pregnancy not established. Discuss with your doctor.

Breast-feeding The drug passes into the breast milk, but at normal doses adverse effects on the baby are unlikely. Discuss with your doctor.

Infants and children Not usually prescribed.

Over 60 Reduced dose may be necessary.

Driving and hazardous work Avoid such activities until you have learned how timolol affects you because the tablets may cause drowsiness and the eye drops may cause blurred vision.

Alcohol May enhance lowering of blood pressure; avoid excessive amounts.

Surgery and general anaesthetics Timolol by mouth may need to be stopped before you have a general anaesthetic. Discuss with your doctor or dentist before any surgery.

PROLONGED USE
No problems expected.

Tolbutamide

Brand name None
Used in the following combined preparations
None

QUICK REFERENCE
Drug group Antidiabetic drug (p.80)
Overdose danger rating High
Dependence rating Low
Prescription needed Yes
Available as generic Yes

GENERAL INFORMATION

Tolbutamide is an antidiabetic agent that lowers blood sugar by stimulating insulin secretion from the pancreas. Taken by mouth, it is used to treat adult (maturity-onset or Type 2) diabetes in which active insulin-secreting cells are still present. Where these are lacking, as in juvenile diabetes, the drug is ineffective.

Tolbutamide does not act in isolation, but is administered in conjunction with a special diabetic diet that limits the patient's carbohydrate intake.

Shorter-acting than many other oral antidiabetic drugs, tolbutamide may help in the initial control of diabetes. It may also be given to people with impaired kidney function because it is less likely to build up in the body and cause excessive lowering of blood sugar. As with other oral antidiabetic drugs, tolbutamide may need to be replaced with insulin during serious illnesses, injury, or surgery, when diabetic control is lost.

INFORMATION FOR USERS

Your drug prescription is tailored for you. Do not alter dosage without checking with your doctor.

How taken Tablets.

Frequency and timing of doses Taken with meals either once daily in the morning, or 2 x daily in the morning and evening.

Adult dosage range 500mg–2g daily.

Onset of effect Within 1 hour.

Duration of action 6–10 hours.

Diet advice A low-fat, low-carbohydrate diet must be maintained for the drug to be fully effective. Follow the advice of your doctor.

Storage Keep in a closed container in a cool, dry place out of reach of children. Protect from light.

Missed dose Take as soon as you remember. If your next dose is due within 2 hours, take a single dose now and skip the next.

Stopping the drug Do not stop taking the drug without consulting your doctor; stopping the drug may lead to worsening of the underlying condition.

OVERDOSE ACTION

Seek immediate medical advice in all cases. If faintness, confusion, or headache occur, eat something sugary. Take emergency action if fits or loss of consciousness occur.

POSSIBLE ADVERSE EFFECTS

Serious adverse effects are rare. Symptoms such as dizziness, sweating, weakness, and confusion may indicate low blood sugar levels. Headache and nausea or vomiting may also occur. If jaundice, a rash, or itching occur, consult your doctor immediately.

INTERACTIONS

General note A variety of drugs may oppose the effect of tolbutamide and may therefore raise blood sugar levels. Such drugs include corticosteroids, oestrogens, diuretics, and rifampicin. Other drugs increase the risk of low blood sugar. These include warfarin, sulphonamides, beta blockers, chloramphenicol, clofibrate, aspirin and other NSAIDs, and MAOIs.

SPECIAL PRECAUTIONS

Be sure to tell your doctor if:
◆ You have long-term liver or kidney problems.
◆ You are allergic to sulphonamides.
◆ You have thyroid problems.
◆ You are taking other medications.

Pregnancy Not usually prescribed. May cause birth defects if taken in the first 3 months of pregnancy. Discuss with your doctor.

Breast-feeding The drug passes into the breast milk and may affect the baby. Discuss with your doctor.

Infants and children Not prescribed.

Over 60 Reduced dose is usually necessary. Increased risk of low blood sugar.

Driving and hazardous work Usually no problem. Avoid these activities if you have warning signs of low blood sugar.

Alcohol Keep consumption low. Alcohol may upset diabetic control.

Surgery and general anaesthetics Notify your doctor that you are diabetic before any surgery; insulin treatment may need to be substituted.

PROLONGED USE

No problems expected.

Monitoring Regular monitoring of urine and/or blood sugar is required.

Tolterodine

Brand name Detrusitol
Used in the following combined preparations
None

QUICK REFERENCE

Drug group Drug for urinary disorders (p.108)
Overdose danger rating Medium
Dependence rating Low
Prescription needed Yes
Available as generic No

GENERAL INFORMATION

Tolterodine is an anticholinergic and anti-spasmodic drug similar to atropine (p.142). It is used to treat urinary frequency and incontinence in adults. It works by reducing contraction of the bladder, allowing it to expand and hold more. It also stops spasms and delays the desire to empty the bladder.

Tolterodine's usefulness is limited to some extent by its side effects, and dosage needs to be reduced in the elderly. Children are more susceptible than adults to its anticholinergic effects. The drug can also trigger glaucoma.

INFORMATION FOR USERS

Your drug prescription is tailored for you. Do not alter dosage without checking with your doctor.
How taken Tablets.
Frequency and timing of doses 2 x daily.
Dosage range 4mg daily, reduced to 2mg daily, if necessary, to minimize side effects.
Onset of effect 1 hour.
Duration of action 12 hours.
Diet advice None.
Storage Keep in a closed container in a cool, dry place out of reach of children.
Missed dose Take as soon as you remember. If your next dose is due within 2 hours, take a single dose now and skip the next.
Stopping the drug Do not stop taking the drug without consulting your doctor; symptoms may recur.
Exceeding the dose An occasional unintentional extra dose is unlikely to cause problems. Large overdoses may cause visual disturbances, urinary difficulties, hallucinations, convulsions, and breathing difficulties. Notify your doctor.

POSSIBLE ADVERSE EFFECTS

The most common side effects of tolterodine, such as dry mouth, digestive upset, constipation, dry eyes, or blurred vision are the result of the drug's anticholinergic action and may improve with time. Other adverse effects include headache, drowsiness, and nervousness. If you experience chest pain or confusion or have difficulty in passing urine, consult your doctor.

INTERACTIONS

General note All drugs that have an anti-cholinergic effect will have increased side effects when taken with tolterodine.
Domperidone and metoclopramide Tolterodine may decrease the effects of these drugs.
Erythromycin, clarithromycin, itraconazole, ketoconazole, and miconazole These drugs may increase blood levels of tolterodine.

SPECIAL PRECAUTIONS

Be sure to tell your doctor if:
◆ You have liver or kidney problems.
◆ You have thyroid problems.
◆ You have heart problems.
◆ You have porphyria.
◆ You have hiatus hernia.
◆ You have ulcerative colitis.
◆ You have glaucoma.
◆ You have myasthenia gravis.
◆ You are taking other medications.
Pregnancy Safety in pregnancy not established. May harm the unborn baby. Discuss with your doctor.
Breast-feeding Safety not established. Discuss with your doctor.
Infants and children Not recommended. Safety not established.
Over 60 Reduced dose may be necessary.
Driving and hazardous work Avoid such activities until you have learned how tolterodine affects you because the drug can cause drowsiness, disorientation, and blurred vision.
Alcohol No special problems.

PROLONGED USE

No special problems. Effectiveness of the drug, and continuing clinical need for it, are usually reviewed after 6 months.
Monitoring Periodic eye tests for glaucoma may be performed.

Tramadol

Brand names Tramake, Zamadol, Zydol
Used in the following combined preparations
None

QUICK REFERENCE

Drug group Analgesic (p.9)
Overdose danger rating High
Dependence rating Low
Prescription needed Yes
Available as generic Yes

GENERAL INFORMATION

Tramadol is a synthetic opioid analgesic chemically similar to natural opioids. It is used to prevent or treat moderately severe pain of injury, surgery, or cancer, for example.

The painkilling effect of tramadol wears off after about 4 hours, but the drug can be given in a slow-release (long -acting) form, which gives relief for up to 12 hours.

Tramadol can be habit-forming, and dependence may occur. But most people who take it for a short time do not become dependent and are able to stop taking it without difficulty. The drug is said to be less likely than the older opioids to cause breathing problems and constipation. Side effects include hallucinations and confusion.

INFORMATION FOR USERS

Your drug prescription is tailored for you. Do not alter dosage without checking with your doctor.

How taken Tablets, SR-tablets, capsules, SR-capsules, injection, sachets.
Frequency and timing of doses Up to 6 x daily.
Adult dosage range Up to 400mg daily (by mouth); 600mg daily (injection).
Onset of effect 30–60 minutes (by mouth); 15–30 minutes (injection).
Duration of action 4 hours.
Diet advice None.
Storage Keep in a closed container in a cool, dry place out of reach of children.
Missed dose Take as soon as you remember, and return to your normal schedule as soon as possible.
Stopping the drug If the reason for taking tramadol no longer exists, you may stop taking the drug and notify your doctor. If you

have been taking it for a long time, you may experience withdrawal effects.

OVERDOSE ACTION

Seek immediate medical advice in all cases. Take emergency action if breathing difficulties, severe drowsiness, or loss of consciousness occur.

POSSIBLE ADVERSE EFFECTS

Adverse effects such as tiredness and drowsiness seem more common than with some other opioids. Other effects include dry mouth, dizziness, headache, nausea, and vomiting. If you experience confusion or hallucinations, consult your doctor. If convulsions, wheezing, or breathlessness occur, stop taking the drug and seek urgent medical advice.

INTERACTIONS

Antidepressants Taken with tramadol, some of these may increase the risk of convulsions.
Carbamazepine This drug may reduce blood levels and effects of tramadol.
Sedatives All drugs that have a sedative effect are likely to increase the sedative effects of tramadol. Such drugs include antidepressants, antipsychotics, antihistamines, and sleeping drugs.

SPECIAL PRECAUTIONS

Be sure to tell your doctor if:
◆ You have had a head injury.
◆ You have liver or kidney problems.
◆ You have heart or circulatory problems.
◆ You have a lung disorder such as asthma or bronchitis.
◆ You have thyroid disease.
◆ You have a history of epileptic fits.
◆ You are taking other medications.
Pregnancy Safety not established. Discuss with your doctor.
Breast-feeding The drug passes into the breast milk and may make the baby drowsy. Discuss with your doctor.
Infants and children Not recommended under 12 years.
Over 60 Reduced dose may be necessary.
Driving and hazardous work Avoid. Tramadol can cause drowsiness.
Alcohol Avoid. Alcohol increases the sedative effects of tramadol.

PROLONGED USE
Dependence may occur if tramadol is taken for long periods.

Trazodone

Brand name Molipaxin
Used in the following combined preparations
None

QUICK REFERENCE
Drug group Antidepressant (p.14)
Overdose danger rating Medium
Dependence rating Low
Prescription needed Yes
Available as generic No

GENERAL INFORMATION
Trazodone is one of many drugs used to treat depression. It helps to elevate the patient's mood and restore interest in everyday activities. Because the drug has a strong sedative effect, it is particularly useful when the depression is accompanied by anxiety, insomnia, or both. Consequently, when taken at night trazodone helps to reduce the need for sleeping drugs.

Trazodone is less likely to cause side effects than tricyclics. It is also safer for people with heart problems, and is therefore commonly used to treat depression in elderly patients.

INFORMATION FOR USERS
Your drug prescription is tailored for you. Do not alter dosage without checking with your doctor.
How taken Tablets, capsules, liquid.
Frequency and timing of doses 1–3 x daily with food.
Adult dosage range 150mg daily (starting dose), increased to 200–300mg, occasionally up to 600mg, daily (maintenance dose).
Onset of effect Some benefits and adverse effects may appear within a few days of starting treatment, but full antidepressant effect may not be felt for 2–4 weeks.
Duration of action Adverse effects may last up to 24 hours after stopping the drug. Antidepressant effect may persist for up to 6 weeks on stopping prolonged treatment.
Diet advice None.

Storage Keep in a closed container in a cool, dry place out of reach of children. Protect from light.
Missed dose Take as soon as you remember. If your next dose is due within 3 hours, take a single dose now and skip the next.
Stopping the drug Unless a rash occurs, do not stop taking the drug without consulting your doctor; symptoms may recur.
Exceeding the dose An occasional unintentional extra dose is unlikely to cause problems. Large doses may cause unusual drowsiness. Notify your doctor.

POSSIBLE ADVERSE EFFECTS
Trazodone has fewer common adverse effects than some of the other antidepressants, mainly because it has a much weaker anticholinergic action; drowsiness is the most common. Other effects include constipation or diarrhoea, dry mouth, headache, and dizziness or fainting. Painful or prolonged erection is a rare problem. If this occurs, seek urgent medical advice. If you develop a rash, stop taking the drug and consult your doctor.

INTERACTIONS
Sedatives All drugs that have a sedative effect on the central nervous system are likely to increase the sedative properties of trazodone. Such drugs include sleeping drugs, antipsychotic drugs, antihistamines, and opioid analgesics.
Anticonvulsants Trazodone may reduce the effects of these drugs.
MAOIs Trazodone may cause serious adverse effects if given with these antidepressants.

SPECIAL PRECAUTIONS
Be sure to tell your doctor if:
◆ You have had epileptic fits.
◆ You have long-term liver or kidney problems.
◆ You have heart disease or are recovering from a recent heart attack.
◆ You are taking other medications.
Pregnancy Safety in pregnancy not established. Discuss with your doctor.
Breast-feeding The drug passes into the breast milk, but at normal doses adverse effects on the baby are unlikely. Discuss with your doctor.

Infants and children Not recommended.
Over 60 Reduced dose may be necessary. Increased likelihood of adverse effects.
Driving and hazardous work Avoid such activities until you have learned how trazodone affects you because the drug can cause drowsiness.
Alcohol Avoid. Alcohol may increase the sedative effects of this drug.

PROLONGED USE
No problems expected.

Triamterene

Brand name Dytac
Used in the following combined preparations
Dyazide (co-triamterzide), Dytide, Frusene, Kalspare, Triam-Co, TriamaxCo

QUICK REFERENCE
Drug group Potassium-sparing diuretic (p.30)
Overdose danger rating Low
Dependence rating Low
Prescription needed Yes
Available as generic No

GENERAL INFORMATION
Triamterene belongs to the class of drugs known as potassium-sparing diuretics. In combination with thiazide or loop diuretics, it is given for the treatment of hypertension and oedema (fluid retention). Triamterene, either on its own or, more commonly, with a thiazide diuretic, may be used to treat oedema as a complication of heart failure, nephrotic syndrome, or cirrhosis of the liver.

Triamterene is quick to act; its effect on urine flow is apparent within two hours and may last for 12 hours. For this reason, you should take the drug early in the day. As with other potassium-sparing diuretics, unusually high levels of potassium may build up in the blood if the kidneys are functioning abnormally. Therefore, triamterene is prescribed with caution to people with kidney failure.

INFORMATION FOR USERS
Your drug prescription is tailored for you. Do not alter dosage without checking with your doctor.

How taken Tablets.
Frequency and timing of doses 1–2 x daily after meals or on alternate days.
Adult dosage range 50–250mg daily.
Onset of effect Within 2 hours.
Duration of action 9–12 hours.
Diet advice Avoid foods that are high in potassium, such as dried fruit and salt substitutes.
Storage Keep in a closed container in a cool, dry place out of reach of children.
Missed dose Take as soon as you remember. However, if it is late in the day, do not take the missed dose, or you may need to get up at night to pass urine. Take the next scheduled dose as usual.
Stopping the drug Do not stop taking the drug without consulting your doctor; symptoms may recur.
Exceeding the dose An occasional unintentional extra dose is unlikely to be a cause for concern. But if you notice any unusual symptoms, or if a large overdose has been taken, notify your doctor.

POSSIBLE ADVERSE EFFECTS
Triamterene has few adverse effects; the main problem is the possibility of potassium being retained by the body, causing muscle weakness and numbness. Dry mouth, digestive disturbance, and headache may also occur. If you develop muscle weakness or a rash, consult your doctor. The drug may colour your urine blue, but this is not a cause for concern.

INTERACTIONS
Lithium Triamterene may increase the blood levels of lithium, leading to an increased risk of lithium toxicity.
NSAIDs may increase the risk of raised blood levels of potassium.
ACE inhibitors These drugs increase the risk of raised blood levels of potassium with triamterene.
Ciclosporin This drug may increase levels of potassium with triamterene.

SPECIAL PRECAUTIONS
Be sure to tell your doctor if:
◆ You have long-term liver or kidney problems.
◆ You have had kidney stones.

◆ You have gout.
◆ You are taking other medications.
Pregnancy Not usually prescribed. May cause a reduction in the blood supply to the developing fetus. Discuss with your doctor.
Breast-feeding The drug passes into breast milk and may affect the baby. It could also reduce your milk supply. Discuss with your doctor.
Infants and children Not usually prescribed. Reduced dose necessary.
Over 60 Increased likelihood of adverse effects. Reduced dose may therefore be necessary.
Driving and hazardous work No special problems.
Alcohol No known problems.

PROLONGED USE
Serious problems are unlikely, but levels of salts such as sodium and potassium may occasionally become abnormal during prolonged use.
Monitoring Blood tests may be performed to check on kidney function and levels of body salts.

Trimethoprim

Brand names Monotrim, Trimogal, Trimopan, Triprimix
Used in the following combined preparations Comixco, Co-trimoxazole, Fectrim, Septrin, and others

QUICK REFERENCE
Drug group Antibacterial drug (p.64)
Overdose danger rating Low
Dependence rating Low
Prescription needed Yes
Available as generic Yes

GENERAL INFORMATION
Trimethoprim is an antibacterial drug that became popular in the 1970s for prevention and treatment of infections of the urinary and respiratory tracts. The drug has been used for many years in combination with another antibacterial, sulfamethoxazole, in a preparation known as co-trimoxazole (see p.189). Trimethoprim has fewer adverse effects than co-trimoxazole, however, and is

equally effective in treating many conditions. The drug can also be given by injection to treat severe infections.
Although side effects of trimethoprim are not usually troublesome, tests to monitor blood composition are often advised when the drug is taken for prolonged periods.

INFORMATION FOR USERS
Your drug prescription is tailored for you. Do not alter dosage without checking with your doctor.
How taken Tablets, liquid, injection.
Frequency and timing of doses 1–2 x daily.
Adult dosage range 300–400mg daily (treatment); 100–200mg daily (prevention).
Onset of effect 1–4 hours.
Duration of action Up to 24 hours.
Diet advice None.
Storage Keep in a closed container in a cool, dry place out of reach of children. Protect from light.
Missed dose Take as soon as you remember.
Stopping the drug Unless severe adverse effects occur (see below), take the full course. Even if you feel better, the original infection may still be present and symptoms may recur if treatment is stopped too soon.
Exceeding the dose An occasional unintentional extra dose is unlikely to be a cause for concern. But if you notice any unusual symptoms, or if a large overdose has been taken, notify your doctor.

POSSIBLE ADVERSE EFFECTS
Taken on its own, trimethoprim rarely causes side effects other than nausea. However, additional adverse effects may occur when trimethoprim is taken in combination with sulfamethoxazole. If you develop a sore throat, itching, or a rash, stop taking the drug and consult your doctor immediately.

INTERACTIONS
Phenytoin Taken with trimethoprim, this drug may increase the risk of folic acid deficiency, which results in blood abnormalities.
Warfarin Trimethoprim may increase the anticoagulant effect of warfarin.
Ciclosporin Trimethoprim increases the risk of this drug causing kidney damage.

Antimalarials containing pyrimethamine Drugs such as fansidar or maloprim may increase the risk of folic acid deficiency, resulting in blood abnormalities, if they are taken with trimethoprim.

SPECIAL PRECAUTIONS

Be sure to tell your doctor if:
◆ You have long-term liver or kidney problems.
◆ You have a blood disorder.
◆ You have porphyria.
◆ You are taking other medications.

Pregnancy Safety in pregnancy not established. Discuss with your doctor.

Breast-feeding The drug passes into the breast milk, but at normal doses adverse effects on the baby are unlikely. Discuss with your doctor.

Infants and children Reduced dose necessary.

Over 60 Reduced dose may be necessary. Increased likelihood of adverse effects.

Driving and hazardous work No known problems.

Alcohol No known problems.

PROLONGED USE

Long-term use of this drug may lead to folate deficiency, which, in turn, may lead to blood abnormalities. Folate supplements may be prescribed.

Monitoring Periodic blood tests to monitor blood composition are usually advised.

Venlafaxine

Brand name Efexor
Used in the following combined preparations
None

QUICK REFERENCE

Drug group Antidepressant (p.14)
Overdose danger rating High
Dependence rating Low
Prescription needed Yes
Available as generic No

GENERAL INFORMATION

Venlafaxine is a new antidepressant with a chemical structure unlike the other groups of antidepressant. It combines the therapeutic properties of the selective serotonin reuptake inhibitors (SSRIs) and tricyclic antidepressants, without anticholinergic adverse effects.

As with other antidepressants, venlafaxine acts to elevate mood, control disturbed sleep patterns, and restore interest in everyday activities.

Nausea, dizziness, drowsiness or insomnia, and restlessness are common adverse effects. Weight loss may occur due to decreased appetite. The drug can elevate blood pressure, which should be monitored during the course of treatment.

INFORMATION FOR USERS

Your drug prescription is tailored for you. Do not alter dosage without checking with your doctor.
How taken Tablets.
Frequency and timing of doses 2–3 x daily (tablets); once daily (SR-tablets). The tablets should be taken with food.
Dosage range 75–150mg daily (outpatients); up to 375mg daily (severely depressed patients).
Onset of effect Can appear within days, although full antidepressant effect may not be felt for 2–4 weeks, or longer.
Duration of action About 8–12 hours; 24 hours for SR-tablets. Following prolonged treatment, antidepressant effects may persist for up to 6 weeks.
Diet advice None.
Storage Keep in the original container in a cool, dry place out of reach of children.

Missed dose Do not make up a missed dose; just take your next scheduled dose.
Stopping the drug Unless severe adverse effects occur (see below), do not stop taking the drug without consulting your doctor, who may supervise a gradual reduction in dosage.

OVERDOSE ACTION

Seek immediate medical advice in all cases. Take emergency action if fits, slow or irregular pulse, or loss of consciousness occur.

POSSIBLE ADVERSE EFFECTS

The most common adverse effects, some of which may wear off within a few days, are weakness, nausea, decreased appetite, restlessness, drowsiness, and dizziness. Restlessness may include anxiety, nervousness, tremor, insomnia, abnormal dreams, agitation, and confusion. If sexual dysfunction, itching, or a rash occur, stop taking the drug and consult your doctor.

INTERACTIONS

Sedatives All drugs with a sedative effect are likely to increase the sedative effects of venlafaxine.
Antihypertensive drugs Treatment with venlafaxine may reduce the effectiveness
MAOIs Venlafaxine may interact with MAOIs to produce a dangerous rise in blood pressure. At least 14 days should elapse between stopping them and starting venlafaxine.

SPECIAL PRECAUTIONS

Be sure to tell your doctor if:
◆ You have had an adverse reaction to any other antidepressants.
◆ You have long-term liver or kidney problems.
◆ You have a heart problem or elevated blood pressure.
◆ You have had epileptic fits.
◆ You have had problems with alcohol or drug misuse/abuse.
◆ You are taking other medications.
Pregnancy Safety in pregnancy not established. Discuss with your doctor.
Breast-feeding Not recommended. Discuss with your doctor.
Infants and children Not recommended under 18 years.

Over 60 Reduced dose may be necessary. Increased likelihood of adverse effects.

Driving and hazardous work Avoid such activities until you have learned how venlafaxine affects you because the drug can cause dizziness, drowsiness, and blurred vision.

Alcohol Avoid. Alcohol may increase the sedative effects of this drug.

PROLONGED USE
No problems expected.

Monitoring Blood pressure should be measured periodically.

Verapamil

Brand names Berkatens, Cordilox, Ethimil, Securon-SR, Univer, Verapress

Used in the following combined preparations None

QUICK REFERENCE
Drug group Anti-angina drug (p.33), anti-arrhythmic drug (p.32), and antihypertensive drug (p.34)

Overdose danger rating Medium

Dependence rating Low

Prescription needed Yes

Available as generic Yes

GENERAL INFORMATION
Verapamil belongs to the group of drugs known as calcium channel blockers, which interfere with the conduction of electrical signals in the muscles of the heart and blood vessels. It is used in the treatment of hypertension, abnormal heart rhythms, and angina. It reduces the frequency of angina attacks but does not work quickly enough to relieve pain during an attack. Verapamil increases the ability to tolerate physical exertion and, unlike some drugs, does not affect breathing, so it can be used safely by asthmatics.

Because of its effects on the heart, verapamil is also prescribed for certain types of abnormal heart rhythm, for which it can be given by injection or taken as tablets.

Verapamil is not generally prescribed for people with low blood pressure, slow heart beat, or heart failure, because it may worsen these conditions. The drug may also cause constipation.

INFORMATION FOR USERS
Your drug prescription is tailored for you. Do not alter dosage without checking with your doctor.

How taken Tablets, SR-tablets, SR-capsules, liquid, injection.

Frequency and timing of doses 2–3 x daily (tablets, liquid); 1–2 x daily (SR-tablets).

Adult dosage range 120–480mg daily.

Onset of effect 1–2 hours (tablets); 2–3 minutes (injection).

Duration of action 6–8 hours. During prolonged treatment some beneficial effects may last for up to 12 hours. SR-tablets act for 12–24 hours.

Diet advice Avoid grapefruit juice, which may increase blood levels of verapamil.

Storage Keep in a closed container in a cool, dry place out of reach of children.

Missed dose Take as soon as you remember. If your next dose is due within 3 hours (tablets, liquid) or 8 hours (SR-tablets, SR-capsules), take a single dose now and skip the next.

Stopping the drug Do not stop taking the drug without consulting your doctor; symptoms may recur.

Exceeding the dose An occasional unintentional extra dose is unlikely to be a cause for concern. Large overdoses may cause dizziness. Notify your doctor.

POSSIBLE ADVERSE EFFECTS
Verapamil has fewer adverse effects than other calcium channel blockers but can still cause a variety of minor symptoms, such as nausea, constipation, and headache. Other effects include ankle swelling, flushing, and dizziness. If you develop a rash, consult your doctor promptly.

INTERACTIONS
Beta blockers When verapamil is taken with these drugs, there is a slight risk of abnormal heart beat and heart failure.

Carbamazepine The effects of this drug may be enhanced by verapamil.

Ciclosporin The blood levels of this drug may be increased by verapamil and its dose may need to be reduced.

Antihypertensive drugs Blood pressure may be further lowered when these drugs are taken with verapamil.

Digoxin The effects of this drug may be increased if it is taken with verapamil. The dosage of digoxin may need to be reduced.

Grapefruit juice Grapefruit juice may increase the effects of verapamil and is best avoided.

SPECIAL PRECAUTIONS

Be sure to tell your doctor if:
◆ You have a long-term liver problem.
◆ You have porphyria.
◆ You are taking other medications.

Pregnancy Not usually prescribed. May inhibit labour if taken during later stages of pregnancy. Discuss with your doctor.

Breast-feeding The drug passes into the breast milk, but at normal doses adverse effects on the baby are unlikely. Discuss with your doctor.

Infants and children Reduced dose necessary.

Over 60 No special problems.

Driving and hazardous work Avoid such activities until you have learned how verapamil affects you because the drug can cause dizziness.

Alcohol Avoid heavy intake. Alcohol may further reduce blood pressure, causing dizziness or other symptoms.

Surgery and general anaesthetics Verapamil may need to be stopped before surgery. Discuss this with your doctor or dentist.

PROLONGED USE

No problems expected.

Warfarin

Brand name Marevan
Used in the following combined preparations
None

QUICK REFERENCE
Drug group Anticoagulant drug (p.38)
Overdose danger rating High
Dependence rating Low
Prescription needed Yes
Available as generic Yes

GENERAL INFORMATION
Warfarin is an anticoagulant drug used to prevent blood clots, mainly in areas where blood flow is slowest, particularly in the leg and pelvic veins. Such clots can break off and travel through the bloodstream to the lungs, where they lodge and cause pulmonary embolism. The drug is also used to reduce the risk of clots forming in the heart in people with atrial fibrillation, or after insertion of artificial heart valves. These clots may travel to the brain and cause a stroke.

A widely used oral anticoagulant drug, warfarin requires regular monitoring to ensure proper maintenance dosage. Because its full beneficial effects are not felt for two to three days, a faster-acting drug such as heparin is often used to complement the effects of warfarin at the start of treatment.

The most serious adverse effect of warfarin, as with all anticoagulants, is the risk of excessive bleeding, which is usually the result of excessive dosage.

INFORMATION FOR USERS
Your drug prescription is tailored for you. Do not alter dosage without checking with your doctor.
How taken Tablets.
Frequency and timing of doses Once daily, taken at the same time each day.
Dosage range 10–15mg daily according to age and weight (starting dose); 1–9mg daily, as determined by blood tests (maintenance dose).
Onset of effect Within 24–48 hours, with full effect after several days.
Duration of action 2–3 days.
Diet advice None.

Storage Keep in a closed container in a cool, dry place out of reach of children. Protect from light.
Missed dose Take as soon as you remember. Take the following dose on your original schedule.
Stopping the drug Unless nausea, fever, or vomiting occur, do not stop taking the drug without consulting your doctor; stopping the drug may lead to worsening of the underlying condition.

OVERDOSE ACTION
Seek immediate medical advice in all cases. Take emergency action if severe bleeding or loss of consciousness occur.

POSSIBLE ADVERSE EFFECTS
Bleeding is the most common adverse effect with warfarin. Any bruising, dark stools, dark urine, or bleeding should be reported to your doctor at once. Other adverse effects include abdominal pain, diarrhoea, rash, and hair loss and should be discussed with your doctor. If you experience nausea or vomiting or develop a fever, stop taking the drug and consult your doctor urgently.

INTERACTIONS
General note A wide variety of drugs, such as aspirin; barbiturates; oral contraceptives; cimetidine; diuretics; certain laxatives, antidepressants, and antibiotics interact with warfarin, either by increasing or decreasing the anti-clotting effect. Consult your pharmacist before using over-the-counter medicines.

SPECIAL PRECAUTIONS
Be sure to tell your doctor if:
◆ You have long-term liver or kidney problems.
◆ You have high blood pressure.
◆ You have peptic ulcers.
◆ You bleed easily.
◆ You are taking other medications.
Pregnancy Not usually prescribed. If given in early pregnancy, the drug can cause malformations in the unborn child. Taken near the time of delivery, it may cause the mother to bleed excessively. Discuss with your doctor.
Breast-feeding The drug passes into the breast milk, but at normal doses adverse effects on

the baby are unlikely. Discuss with your doctor.

Infants and children Reduced dose necessary.

Over 60 No special problems.

Driving and hazardous work Use caution. Even minor bumps can cause bad bruises and excessive bleeding.

Alcohol Avoid excessive amounts. Alcohol may increase the effects of this drug.

Surgery and general anaesthetics Warfarin may need to be stopped before surgery. Discuss with your doctor or dentist.

PROLONGED USE

No special problems.

Monitoring Regular blood tests are performed during treatment.

Zalcitabine

Brand name Hivid
Used in the following combined preparations
None

QUICK REFERENCE

Drug group Drug for AIDS and immune deficiency (p.97)
Overdose danger rating Medium
Dependence rating Low
Prescription needed Yes
Available as generic No

GENERAL INFORMATION

Zalcitabine is a nucleoside reverse transcriptase inhibitor – an antiviral drug used in the treatment of HIV (human immunodeficiency virus) which causes AIDS (acquired immunodeficiency syndrome). Zalcitabine interferes with reverse transcriptase, an enzyme that is used by the virus to produce genetic material.

Treatment for HIV is now usually begun with triple therapy, which consists of two nucleoside transcriptase inhibitors and a third drug from another class, such as ritonavir, a protease inhibitor.

This combination can slow down the progress of the infection very effectively if treatment is started before the immune system becomes too badly damaged.

INFORMATION FOR USERS

Your drug prescription is tailored for you. Do not alter dosage without checking with your doctor.
How taken Tablets.
Frequency and timing of doses 3 x daily.
Adult dosage range 2,250 micrograms daily.
Onset of effect Within a few hours. Full beneficial effect may not be felt for several weeks or months.
Duration of action Approximately 8 hours.
Diet advice None.
Storage Keep in a closed container in a cool, dry place out of reach of children.
Missed dose Take as soon as you remember. If your next dose is due within 3 hours, take a single dose now and skip the next.
Stopping the drug Do not stop taking the drug without consulting your doctor;

stopping the drug may lead to worsening of the underlying condition.
Exceeding the dose An occasional unintentional extra dose is unlikely to cause problems. But if you notice any unusual symptoms or if a large overdose has been taken, notify your doctor.

POSSIBLE ADVERSE EFFECTS

Most adverse effects of zalcitabine, such as diarrhoea, constipation, and loss of appetite, are minor. Some effects such as damage to the pancreas, liver, or nerves (which may cause numbness or an unusual sensation) are more serious. Treatment must therefore be closely monitored. If nausea, vomiting, pallor, fatigue, muscle or joint pains, sore throat, fever, or mouth ulcers occur, consult your doctor.

INTERACTIONS

General note A wide range of other drugs may increase the risk of harmful effects with zalcitabine. These include drugs that damage the nerves or pancreas or affect blood production. Do not take any other medications without consulting your doctor or pharmacist.

SPECIAL PRECAUTIONS

Be sure to tell your doctor if:
◆ You have long-term liver or kidney problems.
◆ You have a history of blood disorders.
◆ You have heart problems.
◆ You have had pancreatitis.
◆ You are taking other medications.
Pregnancy Safety in pregnancy not established. Discuss with your doctor.
Breast-feeding Safety in breast-feeding not established. Discuss with your doctor.
Infants and children Not recommended.
Over 60 Not recommended.
Driving and hazardous work Not known problems.
Alcohol Keep consumption low. Excessive consumption increases the risk of liver damage.

PROLONGED USE

There is an increased risk of nerve, liver, and pancreas damage and blood abnormalities with prolonged treatment.

Monitoring Regular blood tests are performed to check blood cell production and liver and pancreas function.

Zanamivir

Brand name Relenza
Used in the following combined preparations
None

QUICK REFERENCE
Drug group Antiviral drug (p.67)
Overdose danger rating Low
Dependence rating Low
Prescription needed Yes
Available as generic No

GENERAL INFORMATION
Zanamivir is a new type of antiviral drug used to treat Influenza (flu), a virus that infects and multiplies in the lungs. The drug works by attacking the virus, preventing it from multiplying and spreading in the lungs.

Flu causes fever, chills, headache, aches and pains. Other symptoms include sore throat, cough, and nasal symptoms. Taken by inhaler, zanamivir, helps to clear these symptoms and may shorten the duration of the illness. There is no benefit, however, if you do not have a fever. Therefore, treatment should begin as soon as possible, and certainly within 48 hours of the onset of symptoms. Zanamivir also reduces the risk of flu being passed on to others if it is taken by people in contact with the virus.

Symptoms usually subside in two to seven days, unless complications such as a chest infection occur. The elderly and those with long-term illnesses, such as chronic lung and heart disease, are at most risk of complications.

Zanamivir should be used with caution by people with asthma because it may provoke wheezing requiring urgent use of a bronchodilator.

INFORMATION FOR USERS
Your drug prescription is tailored for you. Do not alter dosage without checking with your doctor.
How taken Inhaler.

Frequency and timing of doses 2 x daily. Inhale the contents of the blisters one at a time.
Adult dosage range
20mg (4 x 5mg blisters) daily for 5 days.
Onset of effect Within 7 days.
Duration of action Up to 12 hours.
Diet advice None.
Storage Keep in a cool, dry place out of reach of children.
Missed dose Take as soon as you remember. If your next dose is due within 2 hours, take a single dose now and skip the next.
Stopping the drug Unless wheezing or breathlessness occur, do not stop taking the drug without consulting your doctor; symptoms may recur.
Exceeding the dose An occasional unintentional dose is unlikely to cause problems. However, if you notice any unusual symptoms, or if a large overdose has been taken, notify your doctor.

POSSIBLE ADVERSE EFFECTS
Adverse effects are uncommon. Those that occur, such as headache, sore throat, a cough, and nasal symptoms, are similar to signs and symptoms of flu and may therefore sometimes be caused by the influenza virus rather than zanamivir. If you develop wheezing or breathlessness, stop taking the drug and consult your doctor.

INTERACTIONS
Inhaled drugs (e.g., salbutamol and beclometasone) These should be inhaled just before zanamivir is administered.

SPECIAL PRECAUTIONS
Be sure to tell your doctor if:
◆ You have ever had an allergic reaction to zanamivir or lactose monohydrate.
◆ You have a long-term illness.
◆ You have a lung disease such as asthma.
◆ You have poor immunity to infections.
◆ You suffer from asthma.
◆ You are taking other medications.
Pregnancy Safety in pregnancy not established. Discuss with your doctor.
Breast-feeding Safety in breast-feeding not established. Discuss with your doctor.
Infants and children Not recommended.
Over 60 No special problems.

Driving and hazardous work No known problems.
Alcohol No known problems.

PROLONGED USE
This drug should only be used for 5 days and is not prescribed for long-term use.

Zidovudine

Brand name Retrovir
Used in the following combined preparation
Combivir

QUICK REFERENCE
Drug group Drug for AIDS and immune deficiency (p.97)
Overdose danger rating Medium
Dependence rating Low
Prescription needed Yes
Available as generic No

GENERAL INFORMATION
Zidovudine, formerly known as azidothymidine, or AZT, is an antiviral drug used in the treatment of HIV (human immunodeficiency virus) which causes AIDS (acquired immunodeficiency syndrome). Zidovudine is a nucleoside reverse transcriptase inhibitor which interferes with an enzyme used by the virus to produce genetic material.

Treatment for HIV is now usually begun with triple therapy, which consists of two nucleoside transcriptase inhibitors and a third drug from another class, such as ritonavir, a protease inhibitor.

When treatment is started before the immune system is too badly damaged, this combination is very effective in slowing the progress of HIV infection.

INFORMATION FOR USERS
Your drug prescription is tailored for you. Do not alter dosage without checking with your doctor.
How taken Tablets, capsules, liquid, injection.
Frequency and timing of doses 2–5 times daily.
Adult dosage range 0.5–1g daily.
Onset of effect Within 48 hours.
Duration of action About 4 hours.
Diet advice None.

Storage Keep in a tightly closed container in a cool, dry place out of reach of children. Protect from light.
Missed dose Take as soon as you remember. If your next dose is due within 2 hours, take a single dose now and skip the next.
Stopping the drug Do not stop taking the drug without consulting your doctor; symptoms may recur.
Exceeding the dose An occasional unintentional extra dose is unlikely to cause problems. Serious adverse effects from large overdoses are unusual, but notify your doctor.

POSSIBLE ADVERSE EFFECTS
Zidovudine may cause nausea, vomiting, headache, and loss of appetite. The most common serious adverse effect of this drug is anaemia. Symptoms include pallor, fatigue, and shortness of breath. Sore throat and fever are less frequent effects, and result from a decreased number of white blood cells. These problems are the result of reduced blood cell production in the bone marrow. If you experience numbness or an unusual sensation, aching muscles, or insomnia, consult your doctor.

INTERACTIONS
General note A wide range of drugs may increase the risk of harmful effects with zidovudine. These include drugs that act on the kidneys or affect blood production. Do not take other medications without consulting your doctor or pharmacist.
Probenecid Blood levels of zidovudine are increased by probenecid, increasing the risk of toxic effects.

SPECIAL PRECAUTIONS
Be sure to tell your doctor if:
◆ You have long-term liver or kidney problems.
◆ You have had a previous allergic reaction to zidovudine.
◆ You have a history of blood disorders.
◆ You are taking other medications.
Pregnancy Safety in pregnancy not fully established. Discuss with your doctor. Zidovudine may be used during pregnancy to prevent transmission of HIV from mother to baby.

Breast-feeding The drug passes into the breast milk and may affect the baby. Discuss with your doctor.

Infants and children Reduced dose necessary.

Over 60 Reduced dose may be necessary. Increased likelihood of adverse effects.

Driving and hazardous work No special problems.

Alcohol No known problems.

PROLONGED USE

There is an increased risk of serious blood disorders with prolonged use of zidovudine.

Monitoring Regular blood checks are required.

Zopiclone

Brand names Zileze, Zimovane
Used in the following combined preparations
None

QUICK REFERENCE

Drug group Sleeping drug (p.11)
Overdose danger rating Medium
Dependence rating Medium
Prescription needed Yes
Available as generic Yes

GENERAL INFORMATION

Zopiclone is a hypnotic (sleeping drug) used for the short-term treatment of insomnia. Sleep problems can take the form of difficulty in falling asleep, frequent night-time and/or early morning awakenings. Hypnotics are given only when non-drug measures (e.g., avoiding caffeine) have proved ineffective.

Unlike benzodiazepines, zopiclone possesses no anti-anxiety properties, so it may be suited for insomnia that is not accompanied by anxiety – for example, international travel or change in shift work routine.

Hypnotics are intended for occasional use only. Dependence can develop after as little as a week of continuous use. Some doctors may recommend taking the drug intermittently (e.g., three times a week).

INFORMATION FOR USERS

Your drug prescription is tailored for you. Do not alter dosage without checking with your doctor.

How taken Tablets.

Frequency and timing of doses Once daily at bedtime when required.

Dosage range 3.75–7.5mg.

Onset of effect Within 30 minutes.

Duration of action 4–6 hours.

Diet advice None.

Storage Keep in a closed container in a cool, dry place out of reach of children. Protect from light.

Missed dose If you fall asleep without having taken a dose and wake some hours later, do not take the missed dose.

Stopping the drug If you have been taking the drug continuously for less than 1 week, it can be safely stopped as soon as you feel you no longer need it. However, if you have been taking the drug for longer, consult your doctor.

Exceeding the dose An occasional, unintentional extra dose is unlikely to cause problems. Large overdoses may cause prolonged sleep, drowsiness, lethargy, and poor muscle coordination and reflexes. Notify your doctor immediately.

POSSIBLE ADVERSE EFFECTS

The most common *adverse effects* of zopiclone are daytime drowsiness, which normally diminishes after the first few days of treatment, and a bitter taste in the mouth. Dizziness or weakness and nausea or diarrhoea are less common complications. Persistent morning drowsiness or impaired coordination are signs of excessive dose. If you develop amnesia or confusion, stop taking the drug. If you develop a rash, stop taking the drug and seek medical advice.

INTERACTIONS

Sedatives All drugs, including alcohol, that have a sedative effect on the central nervous system are likely to increase the sedative effects of zopiclone. Such drugs include other sleeping and anti-anxiety drugs, antihistamines, antidepressants, opioid analgesics, and antipsychotics.

SPECIAL PRECAUTIONS

Be sure to tell your doctor if:
◆ You have or have had any problems with alcohol or drug misuse/abuse.
◆ You have myasthenia gravis.

◆ You have had epileptic fits.
◆ You have liver or kidney problems.
◆ You are taking other medications.

Pregnancy Not recommended.

Breast-feeding Not recommended.

Infants and children Not recommended.

Over 60 Increased likelihood of adverse effects. Reduced dose may therefore be necessary.

Driving and hazardous work Avoid such activities until you have learned how zopiclone affects you because the drug can cause drowsiness, reduced alertness, and slowed reactions.

Alcohol Avoid excessive amounts. Alcohol increases the sedative effects of this drug.

PROLONGED USE

Intended for occasional use only.

Continuous use of zopiclone – or any other sleeping drug – for as little as one week may cause dependence.

PART 3

DRUG FINDER INDEX

This part of the book consists of a drug finder index, which helps you to find information on specific brand-name drugs and generic substances, as well as directing you to further information about them throughout the book.

DRUG FINDER INDEX

This section contains the names of approximately 2,500 individual drug products and substances. It provides a quick and easy reference for readers interested in finding out about about a specific drug or medication, as well as directing the reader to information about them throughout the book. There is no need for you to know what group a drug belongs to, whether an item is a brand name or generic name, or whether it is a prescription or an over-the-counter drug; all types of drug and the major drug groups are listed.

WHAT IT CONTAINS

The entries are listed alphabetically and include all major generic drugs and many less widely used substances. A broad range of

brand names, as well as many vitamins and minerals, are also included. This comprehensive selection reflects the wide diversity of products available for the treatment and prevention of disease. Inclusion of a drug or product does not imply BMA endorsement, nor does the exclusion of a particular drug or product indicate BMA disapproval.

HOW THE REFERENCES WORK

References are to the pages in Part 2, containing the drug profiles of each principal generic drug, and to the section in Part 1 that describes the relevant drug group, as appropriate. Some entries for generic drugs that do not have a full profile contain a brief description here.

A

abacavir an antiviral drug for HIV/AIDS 97

abciximab an antiplatelet drug 36

Abelcet a brand name for amphotericin 137 (an antifungal 74)

Abidec a brand-name multivitamin 88

abnormal blood clotting, drugs used to prevent 37

acamprosate a drug for alcohol abuse, used in addition to counselling

acarbose an oral antidiabetic 80

Accolate a brand name for zafirlukast (a leukotriene antagonist for asthma 56 and bronchospasm 23)

Accupro a brand name for quinapril (an ACE inhibitor vasodilator 30)

Accuretic a brand name for quinapril (an ACE inhibitor vasodilator 30) with hydrochlorothiazide 250 (a diuretic 30)

acebutolol a beta blocker 28

aceclofenac a non-steroidal anti-inflammatory 48

ACE inhibitors vasodilators 30 used as antihypertensive drugs 34

acemetacin a non-steroidal anti-inflammatory 48

acenocoumarol previously known as nicoumalone (an anticoagulant 36)

Acepril a brand name for captopril 156 (an ACE inhibitor vasodilator 30)

acetazolamide 31 (a carbonic anhydrase inhibitor diuretic 30 and drug for glaucoma 110)

acetomenaphthone a vitamin K substance used with nicotinic acid to treat chilblains

acetylcholine a chemical neurotransmitter that stimulates the parasympathetic nervous system 9 and is used as a miotic 112

acetylcholinesterase inhibitors drugs for dementia 19

acetylcysteine a mucolytic 25

Acezide a brand name for captopril 156 (an ACE inhibitor vasodilator 30) with hydrochlorothiazide 250 (a thiazide diuretic 31)

Achromycin a brand name for tetracycline 381 (an antibiotic 60)

aciclovir 126 (an antiviral 67)

Aci-Jel a brand name for acetic acid (an antiseptic)

acipimox a lipid-lowering drug 35

Acitak a brand name for cimetidine 171 (an anti-ulcer drug 41)

acitretin a drug for psoriasis 120

aclarubicin an anticancer drug 94

acne, drugs for 119

Acnecide a brand name for benzoyl peroxide 148 (a drug for acne 119)

Acnidazil a brand name for benzoyl peroxide 148 (a drug for acne 119) with miconazole 302 (an antifungal 74)

Acnisal a brand name for salicylic acid (a drug for acne 119)

acrivastine an antihistamine 56

Actal a brand-name antacid containing alexitol (an antacid 40)

Actifed Compound a brand name for dextromethorphan (a cough suppressant 25) with pseudoephedrine (a decongestant 24) and triprolidine (an antihistamine 56)

Actifed Expectorant a brand name for guaifenesin (an expectorant 25) with pseudoephedrine (a decongestant 24) and triprolidine (an antihistamine 56)

Actinac a brand-name acne preparation 119 containing chloramphenicol 163, hydrocortisone 251, allantoin, butoxyethyl nicotinate, and sulphur

actinomycin D another name for dactinomycin (an anticancer drug 94)

activated charcoal a substance used in the emergency treatment of poisoning

Acular a brand name for ketorolac (a non-steroidal anti-inflammatory 48)

Acupan a brand name for nefopam (a non-opioid analgesic 10)

Adalat a brand name for nifedipine 315 (an anti-angina drug 33 and antihypertensive 34)

Adalat Retard a brand name for nifedipine 315 (an anti-angina drug 33 and antihypertensive 34)

adapalene a retinoid for acne 119

Adcortyl a brand name for triamcinolone (a corticosteroid 78)

adenosine an anti-arrhythmic 32

ADH (antidiuretic hormone) see vasopressin (a drug for diabetes insipidus 83)

Adipine MR a brand name for nifedipine 315 (a calcium channel blocker 30)

Adizem-XL a brand name for diltiazem 203 (a calcium channel blocker 30)

adrenaline see epinephrine 219 (a bronchodilator 23 and drug for glaucoma 110 and anaphylactic shock)

AeroBec a brand name for beclometasone 146 (a corticosteroid 78)

Aerocrom a brand name for sodium cromoglicate 366 (an anti-allergy drug 56) with salbutamol 361 (a bronchodilator 23)

Aerolin a brand name for salbutamol 361 (a bronchodilator 23)

Afrazine a brand name for oxymetazoline (a topical decongestant 24)

Aggrastat a brand name for tirofiban (a drug for prevention of heart attacks 27)

Ailax a brand name for co-danthramer (a stimulant laxative 43)

Airomir a brand name for salbutamol 361 (a bronchodilator 23)

Akineton a brand name for biperiden (an anticholinergic for parkinsonism 18)

Aknemin a brand name for minocycline 303 (a tetracycline antibiotic 60)

albendazole an anthelmintic 76

alclometasone a topical corticosteroid 116

Alcobon a brand name for flucytosine (an antifungal 74)

Aldactide a brand name for spironolactone (a diuretic 30) with hydroflumethiazide (a diuretic 30)

Aldactone a brand name for spironolactone (a potassium-sparing diuretic 31)

Aldara a brand name for imiquimod (a drug to treat warts)

aldesleukin an anticancer drug 94

Aldomet a brand name for methyldopa 298 (an antihypertensive 34)

alendronate a drug for the treatment of bone disorders 54

alexitol an antacid 40

alfacalcidol vitamin D (a vitamin 88)

AlfaD a brand name for alfacalcidol (a vitamin 88)

alfentanil an anaesthetic 11

alfuzosin an alpha-adrenergic blocker for prostate disorders 108

Algesal a brand name for diethylamine salicylate (a rubefacient)

Algicon a brand name for aluminium hydroxide 129, magnesium carbonate, and potassium bicarbonate (all antacids 40) with magnesium alginate (an antifoaming agent 40)

alginic acid a binding agent in antacids 40

alimemazine previously known as trimeprazine (an antihistamine 56)

Alka-Seltzer a brand-name analgesic 9 and antacid 40 containing aspirin 138, sodium bicarbonate 365, and citric acid

Alkeran a brand name for melphalan (an anticancer drug 94)

allantoin a mild antibacterial 64

Allegron a brand name for nortriptyline (a tricyclic antidepressant 14)

Aller-eze a brand name for clemastine (an antihistamine 56)

allopurinol 127 (a drug for gout 51)

Almodan a brand name for amoxicillin 136 (a penicillin antibiotic 60)

Alomide a brand name for lodoxamide (an anti-allergy drug 56)

alpha blockers vasodilators 30 used for urinary retention 109 and hypertension 34

Alphaderm a brand name for hydrocortisone 251 (a corticosteroid 78) with urea (a hydrating agent)

Alphagan a brand name for brimonidine (a drug for glaucoma 110)

Alphaparin a brand name for certoparin (an anticoagulant 36)

alpha tocopheryl acetate vitamin E (a vitamin 88)

Alphavase a brand name for prazosin (an antihypertensive 34)

Alphosyl a brand-name drug for eczema 121 and psoriasis 120 containing coal tar and allantoin (a mild antibacterial 64)

alprazolam a benzodiazepine anti-anxiety drug 13

alprostadil 128 a prostaglandin used for impotence 106

Altacite Plus a brand name for hydrotalcite (an antacid 40) with dimeticone (an antifoaming agent 40)

alteplase a thrombolytic 38 (also known as tissue plasminogen activator)

altretamine an anticancer drug 94

Alu-Cap a brand name for aluminium hydroxide 129 (an antacid 40)

Aludrox a brand name for aluminium hydroxide 129 (an antacid 40)

Aludrox-SA a brand name for ambutonium bromide (an antispasmodic for irritable bowel syndrome 43) with aluminium hydroxide 129 and magnesium hydroxide 284 (both antacids 40)

aluminium acetate an astringent used for inflammation of the skin or outer ear canal 113; also used in rectal preparations 45

aluminium chloride an antiperspirant

aluminium compounds antacids 40

aluminium hydroxide 129 (an antacid 40)

Alupent a brand name for orciprenaline (a bronchodilator 23)

Alvedon a brand name for paracetamol 325 (a non-opioid analgesic 10)

Alvercol a brand name for sterculia (a bulking agent 42) and alverine (an antispasmodic 43)

alverine an antispasmodic for irritable bowel syndrome 43

amantadine 130 (an antiviral 67 and drug used for parkinsonism 18)

Amaryl a brand name for glimepiride (an oral antidiabetic 80)

AmBisome a brand name for amphotericin 137 (an antifungal 74)

amethocaine see tetracaine (a local anaesthetic 11)

Ametop a brand name for tetracaine (a local anaesthetic 11)

Amias a brand name for candesartan (an angiotensin II inhibitor, an antihypertensive 34)

amifostine a drug to reduce risk of infection in patients taking anticancer drugs 94

amikacin an aminoglycoside antibiotic 60

Amikin a brand name for amikacin (an aminoglycoside antibiotic 60)

Amilamont a brand name for amiloride (a potassium-sparing diuretic 31)

Amil-Co a brand name for amiloride 131 with hydrochlorothiazide 250 (both diuretics 30)

amiloride 131 (a potassium-sparing diuretic 31)

Amilospare a brand name for amiloride 131 (a potassium-sparing diuretic 31)

aminacrine a skin antiseptic 116

aminobenzoic acid an ingredient of sunscreens 123

aminoglutethimide a drug for advanced breast cancer 94 and Cushing's syndrome 78

aminoglycosides 62 (antibiotics 60)

aminophylline a bronchodilator 23 related to theophylline 382

aminosalicylates drugs for inflammatory bowel disease 44

amiodarone 132 (an anti-arrhythmic 32)

amisulpride 133 (an antipsychotic drug 15)

amitriptyline 134 (a tricyclic antidepressant 14)

Amix a brand name for amoxicillin 136 (a penicillin antibiotic 60)

amlodipine 135 (a calcium channel blocker 33)

ammonium chloride a drug that increases urine acidity 108 and speeds excretion of poisons, and is an expectorant 25

amobarbital a barbiturate sleeping drug 11

Amoram a brand name for amoxicillin 136 (a penicillin antibiotic 60)

amorolfine an antifungal 74

amoxapine a tricyclic antidepressant 14

amoxicillin 136 (a penicillin antibiotic 60)

Amoxil a brand name for amoxicillin 136 (a penicillin antibiotic 60)

Amphocil a brand name for amphotericin 137 (an antifungal 74)

amphotericin 137 (an antifungal 74)

ampicillin a penicillin antibiotic 60

amsacrine an anticancer drug 94

Amsidine a brand name for amsacrine (an anticancer drug 94)

Amytal a brand name for amobarbital (a barbiturate sleeping drug 11)

Anabact a brand name for metronidazole 301 (an antibacterial 64)

anabolic steroids 86 (male sex hormones 85)

Anacal a brand-name preparation for haemorrhoids 45 containing heparinoid

Anadin 500 a brand-name analgesic 9 containing aspirin 138

Anadin Extra a brand-name analgesic 9 containing aspirin 138, paracetamol 325, and caffeine

Anadin Paracetamol a brand name for paracetamol 325 (an analgesic 9)

anaesthetics, local 11 (analgesics 9 and in antipruritics 114)

Anaflex a brand name for polynoxylin (an antifungal 74 and antibacterial 64)

Anafranil, Anafranil SR brand names for clomipramine 178 (a tricyclic antidepressant 14)

analgesics 9 (used in labour 107 and to treat menstrual disorders 100)

anastrozole an anticancer drug 94

Anbesol a brand-name topical liquid for mouth ulcers and teething pain, containing lidocaine (a local anaesthetic 11), cetylpyridinium, and chlorocresol (both topical antiseptics 116)

Andrews Antacid a brand name for calcium carbonate and magnesium carbonate (both antacids 40)

androgens see male sex hormones 85

Anethaine a brand name for tetracaine (a local anaesthetic 11)

Angettes a brand-name antiplatelet drug 36 containing aspirin 138

Angilol a brand name for propranolol 345 (a beta blocker 28)

Angiopine MR a brand name for nifedipine 315 (a calcium channel blocker 33)

angiotensin II blockers vasodilators 30 used as antihypertensive drugs 34

Angiozem a brand name for diltiazem 203 (a calcium channel blocker 33)

Angitil SR a brand name for diltiazem 203 (a calcium channel blocker 33)

Anhydrol Forte a brand name for aluminium chloride (an antiperspirant)

anistreplase a thrombolytic 38

Anodesyn a brand-name preparation for haemorrhoids 45 containing allantoin (a mild antibacterial 64), lidocaine (a local anaesthetic 80), and ephedrine 218

Anquil a brand name for benperidol (an antipsychotic 15)

Antabuse a brand name for disulfiram 206 (an alcohol abuse deterrent)

antacids 40

antazoline an antihistamine 56

Antepsin a brand name for sucralfate 370 (an ulcer-healing drug 41)

anthelmintic drugs 76

Anthisan a brand name for mepyramine (an antihistamine cream 56)

anti-D immunoglobulin a drug used to prevent sensitization to Rhesus antigen

anti-angina drugs 33

anti-anxiety drugs 13

anti-arrhythmics 32

antibacterial drugs 64 (used for ear disorders 113 and in anti-infective skin preparations 116)

antibiotics 60

antibiotics, uses of (table) 61

anticancer drugs 94 (used as immunosuppressant drugs 96)

anticholinergics drugs for parkinsonism 18, as bronchodilators 23, and for urinary incontinence 108

anticoagulants 37 (drugs that affect blood clotting 36)

anticonvulsant drugs 16

antidepressants 14 (used as sleeping drugs 11, in premenstrual syndrome 100, and for urinary incontinence 108)

antidiabetic drugs 80

antidiarrhoeal drugs 42

antidiuretic hormone (ADH) see vasopressin (a drug for diabetes insipidus 83)

anti-emetics 21

antifibrinolytic drugs 36

antifoaming agents 40

antifungal drugs 74

antifungal drug, choice of (table) 75

antihaemophilic factor a blood protein used to promote blood clotting in haemophilia 36

antihistamines 56

antihistamines, comparison of (table) 58

antihypertensive drugs 34

anti-infective skin preparations 116

antimalarial drugs 73

antimanic drugs 16

antiplatelet drugs 37 (drugs that affect blood clotting 36)

Antipressan a brand name for atenolol 140 (a beta blocker 28)

antiprotozoal drugs 71

antipruritics 114

antipsychotic drugs 15

antirheumatic drugs 50

antiseptics 116

antispasmodics 43 (antidiarrhoeal drugs 42 and drugs for urinary incontinence 108)

antituberculous drugs 65

anti-ulcer drugs 41

antiviral drugs 67

Antizol a brand name for fomepizole (an antidote for ethylene glycol poisoning)

Anturan a brand name for sulphinpyrazone (a drug for gout 51)

Anugesic-HC a brand-name preparation for haemorrhoids 45 containing hydrocortisone 251, benzyl benzoate, bismuth, Peru balsam, pramocaine, and zinc oxide

Anusol a brand-name preparation for haemorrhoids 45 containing zinc oxide, bismuth, and Peru balsam

apomorphine a drug used to treat Parkinson's disease 18

APP a brand name for homatropine (an antispasmodic 43), with bismuth (an anti-ulcer drug 41), calcium carbonate, magnesium carbonate, magnesium trisilicate, and aluminium hydroxide 129 (all antacids 40)

apraclonidine a drug for glaucoma 110

Apresoline a brand name for hydralazine (an antihypertensive 34)

Aprinox a brand name for bendroflumethiazide 147 (a thiazide diuretic 31)

aprotinin an antifibrinolytic 36 used to promote blood clotting

Aprovel a brand name for irbesartan 262 (an angiotensin II inhibitor, an antihypertensive 34)

Apsin a brand name for phenoxymethylpenicillin 329 (a penicillin antibiotic 60)

Apsolol a brand name for propranolol 345 (a beta blocker 28 and anti-anxiety drug 13)

Apstil a brand name for diethylstilbestrol 201 (a female sex hormone 86)

AquaBan a brand name for caffeine with ammonium chloride as a mild diuretic 30

Aquadrate a brand name for urea (a hydrating agent)

Arava a brand name for leflunomide (an antirheumatic drug 50)

Aredia a brand name for pamidronate (a drug for bone disorders 54)

argipressin synthetic vasopressin (a drug for diabetes insipidus 83)

Aricept a brand name for donepezil 208

Aridil a brand name for amiloride 131 with furosemide 239 (both diuretics 30)

Arpicolin a brand name for procyclidine 340 (a drug for parkinsonism 18)

Arpimycin a brand name for erythromycin 222 (an antibiotic 60)

Arret a brand name for loperamide 280 (an antidiarrhoeal 42)

Artane a brand name for trihexyphenidyl (a drug for parkinsonism 18)

Arthrofen a brand name for ibuprofen 254 (an analgesic 9 and non-steroidal anti-inflammatory 48)

Arthrosin a brand name for naproxen 311 (a non-steroidal anti-inflammatory 48 and drug for gout 51)

Arthrotec a brand-name antirheumatic drug containing diclofenac 197 with misoprostol 306

Arthroxen a brand name for naproxen 311 (a non-steroidal anti-inflammatory 48 and drug for gout 51)

articaine a local anaesthetic 11

artificial tear preparations drugs affecting the pupil 112

Arythmol a brand name for propafenone (an anti-arrhythmic 32)

Asacol a brand name for mesalazine 293 (a drug for ulcerative colitis 44)

Ascabiol a brand name for topical benzyl benzoate (an antiparasitic 118)

ascorbic acid vitamin C (a vitamin 88)

Asendis a brand name for amoxapine (a tricyclic antidepressant 14)

Asilone a brand name for aluminium hydroxide 129 and magnesium oxide (both antacids 40) with dimeticone (an antifoaming agent 40)

Asmaven a brand name for salbutamol 361 (a bronchodilator 23)

asparaginase a drug for leukaemia 94

Aspav a brand-name analgesic 9 containing aspirin 138 and papaveretum

aspirin 138 (a non-opioid analgesic 10 and antiplatelet drug 36)

Aspro Clear a brand name for soluble aspirin 138 (a non-opioid analgesic 10)

Atarax a brand name for hydroxyzine (an anti-anxiety drug 13)

Atenix a brand name for atenolol 140 (a beta blocker 28)

atenolol 140 a beta blocker 28

Ativan a brand name for lorazepam (a benzodiazepine anti-anxiety drug 13 and sleeping drug 11)

atorvastatin 141 (a lipid-lowering drug 35)

atovaquone an antiprotozoal 71 and antimalarial 73

atracurium a drug used to relax the muscles in general anaesthesia

atropine 142 (an anticholinergic for irritable bowel syndrome 43 and a mydriatic 112)

Atrovent a brand name for ipratropium bromide 261 (a bronchodilator 23)

Audicort a brand-name anti-infective ear preparation 113 containing benzocaine, neomycin, and triamcinolone (a corticosteroid 78)

Augmentin a brand name for amoxicillin 136 (a penicillin antibiotic 60) with clavulanic acid (a substance that increases the effectiveness of amoxicillin)

auranofin an antirheumatic 50

Aureocort a brand name for chlortetracycline (a tetracycline antibiotic 60) with triamcinolone (a corticosteroid 78)

Aureomycin a brand name for chlortetracycline (a tetracycline antibiotic 60)

aurothiomalate an antirheumatic 50

Avloclor a brand name for chloroquine 165 (an antimalarial 73 and antirheumatic 50)

Avomine a brand name for promethazine 343 (an antihistamine 56 and anti-emetic 21)

Axid a brand name for nizatidine (an anti-ulcer drug 41)

Axsain a brand name for capsaicin (a rubefacient)

Azactam a brand name for aztreonam (an antibiotic 60)

Azamune a brand name for azathioprine 143 (an antirheumatic 50 and immunosuppressant 96)

azapropazone a non-steroidal anti-inflammatory 48

azatadine an antihistamine 56

azathioprine 143 (an antirheumatic 50 and immunosuppressant 96)

azelaic acid an antibacterial 64 (a drug for acne 119)

azelastine an antihistamine 56

azidothymidine zidovudine 402 (an antiviral for HIV infection and AIDS 97)

azithromycin an antibiotic 60

azlocillin a penicillin antibiotic 60

aztreonam an antibiotic 60

AZT zidovudine 402 (an antiviral for HIV infection and AIDS 97)

B

bacitracin an antibiotic 60

baclofen 145 (a muscle relaxant 52)

Baclospas a brand of baclofen 145 (a muscle relaxant 52)

Bactroban a brand name for mupirocin (an antibacterial for skin infections 116)

balsalazide a drug for ulcerative colitis 44

Bambec a brand name for bambuterol (a sympathomimetic bronchodilator 23)

bambuterol a sympathomimetic bronchodilator 23

Baratol a brand name for indoramin 257 (an antihypertensive 34)

barbiturates 12 (sleeping drugs 11)

basiliximab an immunosuppressant 96

Baxan a brand name for cefadroxil (a cephalosporin antibiotic 60)

Baycaron a brand name for mefruside (a thiazide-like diuretic 30)

Bazuka a brand-name preparation for verrucas containing salicylic acid (a keratolytic 119) and lactic acid

becaplermin a drug for healing skin ulcers

Beclazone a brand name for beclometasone 146 (a corticosteroid 78)

Becloforte a brand name for beclometasone 146 (a corticosteroid 78)

beclometasone 146 (a corticosteroid 78)

Becodisks a brand of beclometasone 146 (a corticosteroid 78)

Beconase a brand name for beclometasone 146 (a corticosteroid 78)

Becosym a brand-name vitamin B complex preparation (a vitamin 88)

Becotide Rotacaps a brand name for beclometasone 146 (a corticosteroid 78)

Beechams Coughcaps a brand name for dextromethorphan (a cough suppressant 25)

Beechams Pills a brand name for aloin (a stimulant laxative 43)

Beechams Powders a brand name for paracetamol 325 (a non-opioid analgesic 10) and pseudoephedrine (a decongestant 24)

Beechams Powders Capsules a brand name for paracetamol 325 (a non-opioid analgesic 10) with phenylephrine (a decongestant 24) and caffeine (a stimulant 19)

belladonna an antispasmodic anticholinergic for irritable bowel syndrome 43

Bendrofluazide see bendroflumethiazide 147

bendroflumethiazide 147 previously known as bendrofluazide (a thiazide diuretic 31)

Benemid a brand name for probenecid (a drug for gout 51)

Benoral a brand name for benorilate (a non-steroidal anti-inflammatory 48)

benorilate a non-steroidal anti-inflammatory 48

benperidol an antipsychotic 15

benserazide a drug used to enhance the effect of levodopa 273 (a drug for parkinsonism 18)

Benylin a brand name for diphenhydramine (an antihistamine 56) with menthol (an alcohol) and, in some preparations, codeine 183 (an opioid analgesic 11)

benzalkonium chloride a skin antiseptic 116

Benzamycin a brand name for erythromycin 222 (an antibiotic 60) and benzoyl peroxide 148 (a drug for acne 119)

benzhexol see trihexyphenidyl (a drug for parkinsonism 18)

benzocaine a local anaesthetic 11

benzodiazepines 12 (sleeping drugs 11 and anti-anxiety drugs 13)

benzoin tincture a resin used in inhalations for sinusitis and nasal congestion 24

benzoyl peroxide 148 (a drug for acne 119 and fungal skin infections 74)

benzthiazide a thiazide diuretic 31

benztropine an anticholinergic for parkinsonism 18

benzydamine an analgesic 9 used in mouthwash and throat spray

benzyl benzoate an antiparasitic 118

benzylpenicillin a penicillin antibiotic 60

beractant a drug to mature the lungs of premature babies

Berkatens a brand name for verapamil 396 (an anti-angina drug 33 and anti-arrhythmic 32)

Berkolol a brand name for propranolol 345 (a beta blocker 28)

Berkozide a brand name for bendroflumethiazide 147 (a thiazide diuretic 31)

Berotec a brand name for fenoterol (a sympathomimetic bronchodilator 23)

Beta-Adalat a brand name for nifedipine 315 (an anti-angina drug 33 and antihypertensive 34) with atenolol 140 (a beta blocker 28)

beta blockers 28

Betacap a brand name for betamethasone 150 (a corticosteroid 78)

Beta-Cardone a brand name for sotalol 368 (a beta blocker 28)

beta-carotene vitamin A (a vitamin 88 and food additive)

Betadine a brand name for povidone-iodine (a skin antiseptic 116)

Betaferon a brand name for interferon beta 259 (a drug for multiple sclerosis 52)

Betagan a brand name for levobunolol (a beta blocker 28 and drug for glaucoma 110)

betahistine 149 (a drug for Ménière's disease 21)

Betaloc a brand name for metoprolol 300 (a beta blocker 28)

betamethasone 150 (a corticosteroid 78)

Beta-Prograne a brand name for propranolol 345 (a beta blocker 28)

betaxolol a beta blocker 28 also used in glaucoma 110

bethanechol a parasympathomimetic for urinary retention 108 and paralytic ileus

Betim a brand name for timolol 386 (a beta blocker 28)

Betnelan a brand name for betamethasone 150 (a corticosteroid 78)

Betnesol a brand name for betamethasone 150 (a corticosteroid 78)

Betnesol-N a brand name for betamethasone 150 (a corticosteroid 78) with neomycin (an aminoglycoside antibiotic 60)

Betnovate a brand name for betamethasone 150 (a corticosteroid 78)

Betnovate-C a brand name for betamethasone 150 (a corticosteroid 78) with clioquinol (an anti-infective 116)

Betnovate-N a brand name for betamethasone 150 (a corticosteroid 78) with neomycin (an aminoglycoside antibiotic 60)

Betnovate-Rectal a brand-name preparation for haemorrhoids containing betamethasone 150, lidocaine (a local anaesthetic 11), and phenylephrine (a decongestant 24)

Betoptic a brand-name drug for glaucoma 110 containing betaxolol

Bettamousse a brand name for betamethasone 150 (a corticosteroid 78)

bezafibrate 151 (a lipid-lowering drug 35)

Bezalip-Mono a brand name for bezafibrate 151 (a lipid-lowering drug 35)

bicalutamide an anticancer drug 94

BiNovum a brand-name oral contraceptive 101 containing ethinylestradiol 226 and norethisterone 316

Bioplex a brand-name drug for mouth ulcers containing carbenoxolone

Bioral a brand-name drug for mouth ulcers containing carbenoxolone

Biorphen a brand name for orphenadrine 322 (a drug for parkinsonism 18)

biotin 90 (a vitamin 88)

biperiden an anticholinergic for parkinsonism 18

bisacodyl a stimulant laxative 43

Bismag a brand name for sodium bicarbonate 365 with magnesium carbonate (both antacids 40)

bismuth a metal given in compound form for gastric and duodenal ulcers 41 and haemorrhoids 45

BiSoDol a brand name for sodium bicarbonate 365 with calcium carbonate and magnesium carbonate (all antacids 40)

Blemix a brand name for minocycline 303 (a tetracycline antibiotic 60)

bleomycin a cytotoxic antibiotic for cancer 94

Blocadren a brand name for timolol 386 (a beta blocker 28)

blood clotting, drugs that affect 36

blood clotting, drugs to promote 37

Bocasan a brand-name antimicrobial mouthwash 64 containing sodium perborate

bone disorders, drugs for 54

Bonefos a brand name for sodium clodronate for low blood calcium in cancer patients 94

Bonjela a brand name for choline salicylate (a drug similar to aspirin 138)

Bonjela pastilles a brand name for pastilles for mouth ulcers containing lidocaine (a local anaesthetic 11) and aminacrine (a skin antiseptic 116)

Boots Nirolex Lozenges a cough suppressant containing dextromethorphan and menthol

Botox a brand name for botulinum toxin (a muscle relaxant 52)

botulinum toxin a muscle relaxant 52

Bradosol a brand name for benzalkonium chloride (an antiseptic 116)

Brasivol a brand-name abrasive paste for acne 119

bretylium tosilate an anti-arrhythmic 32

Brevinor a brand-name oral contraceptive 101 containing ethinylestradiol 226 and norethisterone 316

Bricanyl a brand name for terbutaline 379 (a bronchodilator 23 and drug used in premature labour 106)

brimonidine a drug for glaucoma 110

Britaject a brand name for apomorphine (a drug for Parkinson's disease 18)

Broflex a brand name for trihexyphenidyl (a drug for parkinsonism 18)

Brolene a brand name for propamidine isethionate (an antibacterial 64) for eye infections

bromazepam a benzodiazepine anti-anxiety drug 13

bromocriptine 152 (a pituitary agent 83 and drug for parkinsonism 18)

brompheniramine an antihistamine 56

bronchodilators 23

Bronchodil a brand name for reproterol (a bronchodilator 23)

Brufen, Brufen Retard brand names for ibuprofen 254 (a non-steroidal anti-inflammatory 48)

Buccastem a brand name for prochlorperazine 339 (an anti-emetic 21)

buclizine an antihistamine 56 and anti-emetic 21 used for motion sickness

budesonide 153 (a corticosteroid 78)

bulk-forming agents substances used as antidiarrhoeals 42 and laxatives 43

bumetanide 154 (a loop diuretic 31)

bupivacaine a long-lasting local anaesthetic 11 used in labour 106

buprenorphine an opioid analgesic 11

Burinex a brand name for bumetanide 154 (a loop diuretic 31)

Burinex A a brand name for bumetanide 154 (a loop diuretic 31) with amiloride 131 (a potassium-sparing diuretic 31)

Burinex K a brand name for bumetanide 154 (a loop diuretic 31) with potassium

BurnEze a brand name for benzocaine (a local anaesthetic 11)

Buscopan a brand name for hyoscine 252 (an antispasmodic for irritable bowel syndrome 43)

buserelin a drug for menstrual disorders 100

Buspar a brand name for buspirone (an anti-anxiety drug 13)

buspirone a non-benzodiazepine anti-anxiety drug 13

busulfan an alkylating agent for certain leukaemias 94

Butacote a brand name for phenylbutazone (a non-steroidal anti-inflammatory 48)

butobarbital a barbiturate sleeping drug 11

butoxyethyl nicotinate a vasodilator 30

butyrophenones antipsychotic drugs 15 and anti-emetics 21

C

cabergoline a drug to treat infertility 105 or to stop milk production in women who do not want to breast-feed

Cacit a brand name for calcium carbonate (a mineral 91)

Cafergot a brand name for ergotamine 221 (a drug for migraine 20) with caffeine (a stimulant 19)

caffeine a stimulant 19 in coffee, tea, and cola, added to some analgesics 9

Calabren a brand name for glibenclamide 243 (an oral antidiabetic 80)

Caladryl a brand name for diphenhydramine (an antihistamine 56) with calamine lotion (an antipruritic 114)

calamine a substance containing zinc carbonate (an antipruritic 114) used to soothe irritated skin

Calcicard CR a brand of diltiazem 203 (an antihypertensive 34 and anti-angina drug 33)

Calcichew a brand name for calcium carbonate (calcium, a mineral 91)

calciferol vitamin D (a vitamin 88)

Calcijex a brand name for calcitriol (a vitamin 88)

Calciparine a brand of heparin 249 (an anticoagulant 36)

calcipotriol 156 (a drug for psoriasis 120)

calcitonin a drug for bone disorders 54

calcitonin (salmon) previously known as salcatonin (a drug for bone disorders 54)

calcitriol vitamin D (a vitamin 88)

calcium a mineral 91

calcium acetate calcium (a mineral 91)

calcium carbonate a calcium salt (a mineral 91) used as an antacid 40

calcium channel blockers vasodilators 30 used as anti-arrhythmics 32, anti-angina drugs 33, and antihypertensives 34

calcium chloride calcium (a mineral 91)

calcium folinate folinic acid salt used to reduce side effects of methotrexate 296

calcium gluconate calcium (a mineral 91)

Calcium Resonium a drug to lower the amount of potassium in the blood

Calcort a brand name for deflazacort (a corticosteroid 78, 116)

Calgel a brand-name teething gel containing lidocaine (a local anaesthetic 11) and cetylpyridinium (an antibacterial 64)

Calimal a brand name for chlorphenamine 166 (an antihistamine 56)

Calmurid HC a brand-name substance for eczema 121 containing hydrocortisone 251, lactic acid, and urea

Calpol a brand name for paracetamol 325 (a non-opioid analgesic 10)

Calsynar a brand name for calcitonin (salmon) (a drug for bone disorders 54)

CAM a brand name for ephedrine 218 (a bronchodilator 23)

Camcolit a brand name for lithium 278 (a drug for mania 16)

camphor a topical antipruritic 114

Campral EC a brand name for acamprosate (a drug for alcohol abuse)

Campto a brand name for irinotecan (an anticancer drug 94)

candesartan an angiotensin II inhibitor, an antihypertensive 34

Canesten a brand name for clotrimazole 181 (an antifungal 74)

Canesten HC a brand name for clotrimazole 181 (an antifungal 74) with hydrocortisone 251 (a corticosteroid 78)

canrenoate a potassium-sparing diuretic 31

Capastat a brand name for capreomycin sulphate (an antituberculous drug 65)

Capoten a brand name for captopril 156 (an ACE inhibitor vasodilator 30)

Capozide a brand name for captopril 156 (an ACE inhibitor vasodilator 30) with hydrochlorothiazide 250 (a thiazide diuretic 31)

capreomycin an antituberculous drug 65

Caprin a brand name for aspirin 138 (a non-opioid analgesic 10 and antiplatelet drug 36)

capsaicin a rubefacient

captopril 156 (an ACE inhibitor vasodilator 30)

Carace a brand name for lisinopril 277 (an ACE inhibitor vasodilator 30)

Carace Plus a brand-name preparation containing lisinopril 277 (an ACE inhibitor vasodilator 30) and hydrochlorothiazide 250 (a thiazide diuretic 31)

carbachol a drug used for its miotic effect in glaucoma 110 and parasympathomimetic effect in urinary retention 108

Carbalax a brand name for sodium acid phosphate (a laxative 43) and sodium bicarbonate 365 (an antacid 40)

carbamazepine 158 (an anticonvulsant 16 and antipsychotic 15)

carbaryl 159 (an antiparasitic 118 for head lice infestation)

Carbellon a brand name for magnesium hydroxide 284 (an antacid 40 and laxative 43) with charcoal (an adsorbent) and peppermint oil (both substances for bowel spasm 43)

carbenoxolone an anti-ulcer drug 41

carbidopa a substance that enhances the therapeutic effect of levodopa 273 (a drug for parkinsonism 18)

carbimazole 160 (an anti-thyroid drug 82)

carbocisteine a mucolytic 25

Carbo-Dome a brand name for coal tar (a substance for psoriasis 120)

carboplatin an anticancer drug 94

carboprost a drug to control bleeding after childbirth 106

Cardene a brand name for nicardipine (a calcium channel blocker 33)

Cardilate MR a brand name for nifedipine 315 (a calcium channel blocker 33)

Cardinol a brand name for propranolol 345 (a beta blocker 28)

cardioselective drugs a type of beta blocker 28

Cardura a brand name for doxazosin 212 (a sympatholytic antihypertensive 34)

Carisoma a brand name for carisoprodol (a muscle relaxant 52 related to meprobamate, an anti-anxiety drug 13)

carisoprodol a muscle relaxant 52 related to meprobamate (an anti-anxiety drug 13)

carmustine an alkylating agent for Hodgkin's disease and solid tumours 94

carnitine an amino acid used as a nutritional supplement 88

Carnitor a brand name for carnitine (an amino acid used as a nutritional supplement 88)

carteolol a beta blocker 28 for glaucoma 110 and angina 33

carvedilol a beta blocker 28

Carylderm a brand name for carbaryl 159 (an antiparasitic 118 for head lice infestation)

cascara a stimulant laxative 43

castor oil a stimulant laxative 43

Catapres a brand name for clonidine (an antihypertensive 34 and drug for migraine 20)

Catarrh-Ex a brand-name decongestant 24 containing pseudoephedrine and paracetamol 325 (a non-opioid analgesic 10)

Caverject a brand name for alprostadil 128 (a prostaglandin used for impotence 106)

Cedocard a brand name for isosorbide dinitrate 264 (a nitrate vasodilator 30 and anti-angina drug 33)

cefaclor a cephalosporin antibiotic 60

cefadroxil a cephalosporin antibiotic 60

cefalexin 161 (a cephalosporin antibiotic 60)

cefamandole a cephalosporin antibiotic 60

cefazolin a cephalosporin antibiotic 60

cefixime a cephalosporin antibiotic 60

cefodizime a cephalosporin antibiotic 60

cefotaxime a cephalosporin antibiotic 60

cefoxitin a cephalosporin antibiotic 60

cefpirome a cephalosporin antibiotic 60

cefpodoxime a cephalosporin antibiotic 60

cefprozil a cephalosporin antibiotic 60

cefradine a cephalosporin antibiotic 60

Cefrom a brand name for cefpirome (a cephalosporin antibiotic 60)

ceftazidime a cephalosporin antibiotic 60

ceftriaxone a cephalosporin antibiotic 60

cefuroxime a cephalosporin antibiotic 60

Cefzil a brand name for cefprozil (a cephalosporin antibiotic 60)

Celance a brand name for pergolide (a drug for parkinsonism 18)

celecoxib a COX-2 inhibitor 49 (a non-steroidal anti-inflammatory drug 48)

Celectol a brand name for celiprolol (a beta blocker 28)

Celevac a brand name for methylcellulose 297 (a laxative 43 and antidiarrhoeal 42)

celiprolol a beta blocker 28

Cellcept a brand name for mycophenolate mofetil (an immunosuppressant 96)

cephalosporins 62 (antibiotics 60)

Ceporex a brand name for cefalexin 161 (a cephalosporin antibiotic 60)

Cerebrovase a brand name for dipyridamole 205 (an antiplatelet drug 36)

Cerezyme a brand name for imiglucerase (an enzyme for enzyme replacement therapy)

certoparin an anticoagulant 36

Cerumol a brand-name preparation for ear-wax removal 113

cetirizine 162 (an antihistamine 56)

cetrimide a skin antiseptic 116

cetrorelix a drug for infertility 105

Cetrotide a brand name for cetrorelix (a drug for infertility 105)

cetylpyridinium (a topical skin antiseptic 116)

Chemotrim a brand name for co-trimoxazole 189 (an antibacterial 64)

Chendol a brand name for chenodeoxycholic acid (a drug for gallstones 46)

Chimax a brand name for flutamide 236 (an anticancer drug 94)

Chloractil a brand name for chlorpromazine 167 (a phenothiazine antipsychotic 15 and anti-emetic 21)

chloral hydrate a sleeping drug 11

chlorambucil an anticancer drug 94 used for chronic lymphocytic leukaemia and lymphatic and ovarian cancers, and as an immunosuppressant 96 for rheumatoid arthritis 50

chloramphenicol 163 (an antibiotic 60)

chlordiazepoxide 164 (a benzodiazepine anti-anxiety drug 13)

chlorhexidine a skin antiseptic 116

chlormethine previously known as mustine (a drug for Hodgkin's disease 94)

Chloromycetin a brand name for chloramphenicol 163 (an antibiotic 60)

chloroquine 165 (an antimalarial 73 and antirheumatic 50)

chlorothiazide a thiazide diuretic 31

chloroxylenol a skin antiseptic 116

chlorphenamine 166 previously known as chlorpheniramine (an antihistamine 56)

chlorpheniramine see chlorphenamine 166

chlorpromazine 167 (a phenothiazine antipsychotic 15 and anti-emetic 21)

chlorpropamide a drug for diabetes 80

chlortalidone a thiazide diuretic 31

chlortetracycline a tetracycline antibiotic 60

choline salicylate a drug similar to aspirin 138 used in pain-relieving mouth gels 9

choline theophyllinate a xanthine bronchodilator 23

chorionic gonadotrophin 169 (a drug for infertility 105)

chromium a mineral 91

Cicatrin a brand name for bacitracin (an antibacterial 64) with neomycin (an antibiotic 60)

ciclosporin 170 (an immunosuppressant 96)

cidofovir an antiviral for cytomegalovirus 67 in AIDS 97

Cidomycin a brand name for gentamicin 241 (an aminoglycoside antibiotic 60)

cilastatin an enzyme inhibitor used to make imipenem (an antibiotic 60) more effective

cilazapril an ACE inhibitor vasodilator 30

Cilest a brand-name oral contraceptive containing ethinylestradiol 226 and norgestimate

cimetidine 171 (an anti-ulcer drug 41)

Cinaziere a brand name of cinnarizine 172 (an antihistamine anti-emetic 21)

cinchocaine a local anaesthetic 11

cinnarizine 172 (an antihistamine anti-emetic 21)

Cinobac a brand name for cinoxacin (a urinary tract antibiotic 60)

cinoxacin a urinary tract antibiotic 60

Cipramil a brand name for citalopram 175 (an antidepressant 14)

ciprofibrate a lipid-lowering drug 35

ciprofloxacin 173 (an antibiotic 60)

Ciproxin a brand name for ciprofloxacin 173 (an antibacterial 64)

cisatracurium a drug used to relax the muscles in general anaesthesia

cisplatin 174 (an anticancer drug 94)

citalopram 175 (an antidepressant 14)

Citanest a brand name for prilocaine (a local anaesthetic 11)

Citramag a brand name for magnesium citrate (an osmotic laxative 43)

cladribine an anticancer drug 94

clarithromycin a macrolide antibiotic 60

Clarityn a brand name for loratadine 281 (an antihistamine 56)

clavulanic acid a substance given with amoxicillin 136 (a penicillin antibiotic 60) to make it more effective

clemastine an antihistamine 56

Clexane a brand name for enoxaparin (a low-molecular-weight heparin 249, an anticoagulant 36)

Climagest a brand-name preparation for menopausal symptoms 86 containing estradiol 224 and norethisterone 316

Climaval a brand-name preparation for menopausal symptoms 86 containing estradiol 224

Climesse a brand-name preparation for menopausal symptoms 86 containing estradiol 224 and norethisterone 316

clindamycin a lincosamide antibiotic 60

Clinitar a brand name for coal tar (a clindamycin a lincosamide antibioticsubstance used for psoriasis 120 and dandruff 122)

Clinoril a brand name for sulindac (a non-steroidal anti-inflammatory 48)

clioquinol an antibacterial 64 and antifungal 74 for outer-ear infections 113

clobazam a benzodiazepine anti-anxiety drug 13

clobetasol 176 (a topical corticosteroid 116)

clobetasone a topical corticosteroid 116

Cloburate a brand name for clobetasone (a topical corticosteroid 116)

clodronate an anticancer drug 94

clofazimine a drug for leprosy 65

clomethiazole a non-benzodiazepine, non-barbiturate sleeping drug 11

Clomid a brand name for clomifene 177 (a drug for infertility 105)

clomifene 177 (a drug for infertility 105)

clomipramine 178 (a tricyclic antidepressant 14)

clonazepam 179 (a benzodiazepine anticonvulsant 16)

clonidine an antihypertensive 34 and drug for migraine 20

clopamide a thiazide diuretic 31

clopidogrel 180 (an antiplatelet drug 36)

Clopixol a brand name for zuclopenthixol (an antipsychotic 15)

cloral betaine a sleeping drug 11

clorazepate a benzodiazepine anti-anxiety drug 13

Clotam a brand name for tolfenamic acid (a drug for migraine 20)

clotrimazole 181 (an antifungal 74)

clozapine 182 (an antipsychotic 15)

Clozaril a brand name for clozapine 182 (an antipsychotic 15)

coal tar a substance for psoriasis 120 and eczema 121

co-amilofruse a generic product containing amiloride 131 with furosemide 239 (both diuretics 30)

co-amilozide a generic product containing amiloride 131 with hydrochlorothiazide 250 (both diuretics 30)

co-amoxiclav a generic product containing amoxicillin 136 (a penicillin antibiotic 60) with clavulanic acid (a substance that increases the effectiveness of amoxicillin)

Cobadex a brand name for hydrocortisone 251 (a corticosteroid 78) and dimeticone (an anti-foaming agent 40)

Cobalin-H a brand name for hydroxocobalamin (a vitamin 88)

co-beneldopa a generic product containing levodopa 273 (a drug for parkinsonism 18) with benserazide (a drug that enhances the effect of levodopa)

Co-Betaloc a brand name for hydrochlorothiazide 250 (a thiazide diuretic 31) with metoprolol 300 (a beta blocker 28)

cocaine a local anaesthetic 11

co-careldopa a generic product containing carbidopa with levodopa 273 (both drugs for parkinsonism 18)

co-codamol a generic product containing codeine 183 with paracetamol 325 (both analgesics 9)

co-codaprin a generic product containing aspirin 138 with codeine 183 (both analgesics 9)

Codafen Continus a brand name for codeine 183 (an opioid analgesic 11) and ibuprofen 254 (a non-steroidal anti-inflammatory 48)

Codalax a brand name for co-danthramer (a stimulant laxative 43)

co-danthramer a generic product containing dantron with poloxamer (both stimulant laxatives 43)

co-danthrusate a generic product containing dantron with docusate (both stimulant laxatives 43)

codeine 183 (an opioid analgesic 11, cough suppressant 25, and antidiarrhoeal 42)

co-dergocrine mesylate a vasodilator 30 used to improve blood flow to the brain in senile dementia

Codis a brand name for aspirin 138 with codeine 183 (both analgesics 9)

co-dydramol a generic product containing paracetamol 325 with dihydrocodeine (both analgesics 9)

co-fluampicil a generic product containing flucloxacillin with ampicillin (both penicillin antibiotics 60)

co-flumactone a generic product containing hydroflumethiazide with spironolactone (both diuretics 30)

Cogentin a brand name for benztropine (an anticholinergic for parkinsonism 18)

Colazide a brand name for balsalazide (a drug for ulcerative colitis 44)

colchicine 184 (a drug for gout 51)

cold cream an antipruritic 114

cold cures 26 (drugs to treat coughs 25)

colecalciferol vitamin D (a vitamin 88)

colestipol a lipid-lowering drug 35

colestyramine 186 (a lipid-lowering drug 35)

colfosceril palmitate a drug to mature the lungs of premature babies

Colifoam a brand name for hydrocortisone 251 (a corticosteroid 78)

colistimethate the injection form of colistin (an antibiotic 60)

colistin an antibiotic 60

collodion a substance that dries to form a sticky film, protecting broken skin 116

Colofac a brand name for mebeverine 285 (an antispasmodic for irritable bowel syndrome 43)

Colomycin a brand name for colistin (an antibiotic 60)

Colpermin a brand name for peppermint oil (a substance for indigestion 40 and spasm of the bowel 43)

co-magaldrox a generic product containing aluminium hydroxide 129 with magnesium hydroxide 284 (both antacids 40)

combined analgesics 10

Combivent a brand-name inhaler containing salbutamol 361 and ipratropium bromide 261 (both bronchodilators 23)

Combivir a brand-name preparation containing lamivudine 270 and zidovudine 402 (antivirals 67 used for HIV/AIDS 97)

co-methiamol a generic product containing paracetamol 325 and methionine (an antidote to paracetamol poisoning)

Comixco a brand name for co-trimoxazole 189 (an antibacterial 64 and antiprotozoal 71)

Compound W a brand-name keratolytic 119 for warts, containing salicylic acid

Comtess a brand name for entacapone (a drug for parkinsonism 18)

Concavit a brand-name multivitamin 88

Concordin a brand name for protriptyline (a tricyclic antidepressant 14)

Condyline a brand name for podophyllotoxin (a drug for genital warts 67)

conjugated estrogens 187 (a female sex hormone 86 and drug for bone disorders 54)

Conotrane a brand name for benzalkonium chloride (a skin antiseptic 116) with dimeticone (a base for skin preparations 116)

Contac 400 a brand name for chlorphenamine 166 (an antihistamine 56) with phenylpropanolamine 330 (a decongestant 24)

Contac Cough Caps a brand name for dextromethorphan (a cough suppressant 25)

Contimin a brand name for oxybutynin 323 (an anticholinergic and antispasmodic for urinary disorders 108)

contraceptives 101

Convulex a brand name for sodium valproate 367 (an anticonvulsant 16)

co-phenotrope a generic product containing diphenoxylate 204 with atropine 142

copper a mineral 91

co-prenozide a generic product containing oxprenolol (a beta blocker 28) with cyclopenthiazide 190 (a thiazide diuretic 31)

co-proxamol 188 (an opioid analgesic 11)

Coracten a brand name for nifedipine 315 (an anti-angina drug 33 and antihypertensive 34)

Cordarone X a brand name for amiodarone 132 (an anti-arrhythmic 32)

Cordilox a brand name for verapamil 396 (an anti-angina drug 33 and anti-arrhythmic 32)

Corgard a brand name for nadolol (a beta blocker 28)

Corgaretic a brand name for bendroflumethiazide 147 (a thiazide diuretic 31) with nadolol (a beta blocker 28)

Corlan a brand name for hydrocortisone 251 (a corticosteroid 78)

Coro-Nitro a brand name for glyceryl trinitrate 245 (an anti-angina drug 33)

Corsodyl a brand-name mouthwash and oral gel containing chlorhexidine (an antiseptic 116)

corticosteroids 78 (used as bronchodilators 23, immunosuppressants 96, allergy treatments 58, antipruritics 114, anti-infective skin preparations 116, and treatments for eczema 121)

corticosteroids for rheumatic disorders 51

corticosteroids, topical see topical corticosteroids 116

corticotropin a pituitary hormone 83

cortisol an old name for hydrocortisone 251

cortisone a corticosteroid 78

Cortisyl a brand name for cortisone (a corticosteroid 78)

Cosalgesic a brand name for co-proxamol 188 (an opioid analgesic 11)

co-simalcite a generic product containing hydrotalcite (an antacid 40) with dimeticone (an antifoaming agent 40)

Cosopt a brand-name preparation containing dorzolamide 209 and timolol 386 (drugs for glaucoma 110)

co-tenidone a generic product containing atenolol 140 (a beta blocker 28) with chlortalidone (a thiazide diuretic 31)

co-triamterzide a generic product containing hydrochlorothiazide 250 with triamterene 392 (both diuretics 30)

co-trimoxazole 189 (an antibacterial 64 and antiprotozoal 71)

coughs, drugs to treat 25

Coversyl a brand name for perindopril (an ACE inhibitor vasodilator 30)

COX-2 inhibitors 49 (non-steroidal anti-inflammatory drugs 48)

Cozaar a brand name for losartan 282 (an antihypertensive 34)

Cozaar-Comp a brand-name preparation containing losartan 282 and hydrochlorothiazide 250 (a product for high blood pressure 34)

Cream of Magnesia a brand-name for magnesium hydroxide 284 (an antacid 40 and laxative 43)

Cremalgin a brand name topical preparation for muscular pain relief containing glycol salicylate, methyl nicotinate, and capsicum oleoresin

Creon a brand name for pancreatin (a preparation of pancreatic enzymes 46)

crisantaspase an anticancer drug 94

Crixivan a brand name for indinavir (an antiviral for HIV/AIDS 97)

Cromogen a brand name for sodium cromoglicate 366 (an anti-allergy drug 56)

cromoglicate 366 an anti-allergy drug 56

crotamiton an antipruritic 114 and antiparasitic 118 for scabies

Crystapen a brand name for penicillin G (a penicillin antibiotic 60)

Cupanol a brand name for paracetamol 325 (a non-opioid analgesic 10)

Cuplex a brand-name wart preparation containing copper acetate, lactic acid, and salicylic acid

Cuprofen a brand name for ibuprofen 254 (a non-steroidal anti-inflammatory 48)

Curatoderm a brand name for tacalcitol (a drug for psoriasis 120)

Cutivate a brand name for fluticasone 237 (a corticosteroid 78)

cyanocobalamin vitamin B_{12} (a vitamin 88)

Cyclimorph a brand name for morphine 308 (an opioid analgesic 11) with cyclizine (an anti-emetic 21)

cyclizine an antihistamine 56 used as an anti-emetic 21

cyclobenzaprine a muscle relaxant 52

Cyclodox a brand name for doxycycline 214 (a tetracycline antibiotic 60)

Cyclogest a brand name for progesterone (a female sex hormone 86)

cyclopenthiazide 190 (a thiazide diuretic 31)

cyclopentolate an anticholinergic mydriatic 112

cyclophosphamide 191 (an anticancer drug 94)

Cyclo-Progynova a brand name for estradiol 224 with levonorgestrel 276 (both female sex hormones 86)

cycloserine an antibiotic 60 for tuberculosis 65

Cyklokapron a brand name for tranexamic acid (an antifibrinolytic used to promote blood clotting 36)

Cymalon a brand-name preparation for cystitis 108 containing sodium bicarbonate 365, citric acid, sodium citrate, and sodium carbonate

Cymevene a brand name for ganciclovir (an antiviral 67)

cyproheptadine an antihistamine 56 used to stimulate the appetite 19

Cyprostat a brand name for cyproterone acetate (a synthetic sex hormone used for acne 119 and cancer of the prostate 94)

cyproterone a synthetic sex hormone used for acne 119, cancer of the prostate 94, and male sexual disorders 85

Cystoleve a brand name for sodium citrate (used for cystitis 108)

Cystopurin a brand name for potassium citrate (used for cystitis 108)

Cystrin a brand name for oxybutynin 323 (an anticholinergic and antispasmodic for urinary disorders 108)

cytarabine a drug for leukaemia 94

Cytotec a brand name for misoprostol 306 (an anti-ulcer drug 41)

cytotoxic anticancer drugs 94

D

dacarbazine a drug for malignant melanoma and cancer of soft tissues 94

daclizumab an immunosuppressant 96

dactinomycin a cytotoxic antibiotic for cancer 94

Daktacort a brand name for hydrocortisone 251 (a corticosteroid 78) with miconazole 302 (an antifungal 74)

Daktarin a brand name for miconazole 302 (an antifungal 74)

Dalacin C a brand name for clindamycin (a lincosamide antibiotic 60)

dalfopristin an antibiotic 60

Dalivit a brand-name multivitamin 88

Dalmane a brand name for flurazepam (a benzodiazepine sleeping drug 11)

dalteparin a type of heparin 249 (an anticoagulant 36)

danaparoid an anticoagulant 36

danazol 193 (a drug for menstrual disorders 100)

dandruff, drugs for 122

Daneral-SA a brand name for pheniramine (an antihistamine 56)

Danol a brand name for danazol 193 (a drug for menstrual disorders 100)

Dantrium a brand name for dantrolene (a muscle relaxant 52)

dantrolene a muscle relaxant 52

dantron a stimulant laxative 43

Daonil a brand name for glibenclamide 243 (an oral antidiabetic 80)

dapsone an antibacterial 64

Daraprim a brand name for pyrimethamine 348 (an antimalarial 73)

daunorubicin a cytotoxic antibiotic (an anticancer drug 94)

Day Nurse a brand name for dextromethorphan (a cough suppressant 25) with paracetamol 325 (a non-opioid analgesic 10) and phenylpropanolamine 330 (a decongestant 24)

DDAVP a brand name for desmopressin 194 (a pituitary hormone 83)

debrisoquine an antihypertensive 34

Decadron a brand name for dexamethasone 195 (a corticosteroid 78)

Deca-Durabolin-100 a brand name for nandrolone (an anabolic steroid 85)

De-capeptyl sr a brand name for triptorelin (an anticancer drug 94)

decongestants 24

deflazacort a corticosteroid 78, 116

Delfen a brand name for nonoxinol "9" (a spermicidal agent 101)

Deltacortril Enteric a brand name for prednisolone 337 (a corticosteroid 78)

Deltastab a brand name for prednisolone 337 (a corticosteroid 78)

demeclocycline a tetracycline antibiotic 60

dementia, drugs for 19

Demix a brand of doxycycline 214 (a tetracycline antibiotic 60)

De-Nol a brand name for bismuth (a substance

for gastric and duodenal ulcers 41)

Dentomycin a brand name for minocycline 303 (a tetracycline antibiotic 60)

Depixol a brand name for flupentixol 234 (an antipsychotic 15 and antidepressant 14)

Depo-Medrone a brand name for methyl-prednisolone (a corticosteroid 78)

Deponit a brand name for glyceryl trinitrate 245 (an anti-angina drug 33)

Depo-Provera a brand name for medroxyprogesterone 286 (a female sex hormone 86)

Depostat a brand name for gestonerone (a progestogen 86)

Dequacaine a brand name for benzocaine (a local anaesthetic 11) with dequalinium (an antibacterial 64)

Dequadin a brand name for dequalinium (an antibacterial 64)

dequalinium an antibacterial 64 used for mouth infections

Derbac-M a brand-name shampoo containing malathion 285 (an anti-parasitic 118)

Dermacort a brand-name preparation for hydrocortisone cream 251

Dermidex Cream a brand-name topical preparation for skin irritation containing chlorobutanol, lignocaine, cetrimide, and alcloxa

Dermovate a brand name for clobetasol 176 (a topical corticosteroid 116)

Dermovate-NN a brand name for nystatin 317 (an antifungal 74) with clobetasol 176 (a topical corticosteroid 116) and neomycin (an aminoglycoside antibiotic 60)

desferrioxamine an antidote for iron overdose

desflurane a general anaesthetic

desirudin an anticoagulant 36

desmopressin 194 (a pituitary hormone 83 used for diabetes insipidus 80)

desogestrel a progestogen 86

desoxymetasone a topical corticosteroid 116

Destolit a brand name for ursodeoxycholic acid (a drug for gallstones 46)

Dete clo a brand name for tetracycline 381 with chlortetracycline and demeclocycline (all tetracycline antibiotics 60)

Detrunorm a brand name for propiverine (a drug for urinary frequency 108)

Detrusitol a brand name for tolterodine 389 (an anticholinergic and antispasmodic for

urinary disorders 108)

Dettol a brand-name liquid skin antiseptic 116 containing chloroxylenol

dexamethasone 195 (a corticosteroid 78)

dexamfetamine an amfetamine

Dexa-Rhinaspray a brand name for dexamethasone 195 (a corticosteroid 78) with neomycin (an aminoglycoside antibiotic 60) and tramazoline (a nasal decongestant 24)

Dexedrine a brand name for dexamfetamine (an amfetamine)

dexketoprofen a non-steroidal anti-inflammatory 48

dextromethorphan a cough suppressant 25

dextromoramide an opioid analgesic 11

dextropropoxyphene a constituent of co-proxamol 188 (an opioid analgesic 11)

DF 118 a brand name for dihydrocodeine (an opioid analgesic 11)

DHC Continus a brand name for dihydrocodeine (an opioid analgesic 11)

Diabetamide a brand name for glibenclamide 243 (an oral antidiabetic 80)

diabetes, drugs used in 80

Diabinese a brand name for chlorpropamide (an oral antidiabetic 80)

Dialar a brand of diazepam 196 (a benzodiazepine anti-anxiety drug 13, muscle relaxant 52, and anticonvulsant 16)

Diamicron a brand name for gliclazide 244 (an oral antidiabetic 80)

diamorphine 308 (an opioid analgesic 11)

Diamox a brand name for acetazolamide (a carbonic anhydrase inhibitor diuretic 30)

Dianette a brand name for cyproterone acetate (a synthetic sex hormone used for acne 119) with ethinylestradiol 226 (a female sex hormone 86)

Diarphen a brand name for diphenoxylate 204 (an opioid antidiarrhoeal 42) with atropine 142

Diarrest a brand-name antidiarrhoeal 42 containing dicycloverine 199 and codeine 183

Diasorb a brand name for loperamide 280 (an antidiarrhoeal 42)

Diazemuls a brand name for diazepam 196 (a benzodiazepine anti-anxiety drug 13, muscle relaxant 52, and anticonvulsant 16)

diazepam 196 (a benzodiazepine anti-anxiety drug 13, muscle relaxant 52, and anticonvulsant 16)

diazoxide an antihypertensive 34 also used for hypoglycaemia 80

dibromopropamidine an antibacterial agent 64

diclofenac 197 (a non-steroidal anti-inflammatory 48)

Dicloflex a brand name for diclofenac 197 (a non-steroidal anti-inflammatory 48)

Diclomax Retard a brand name for diclofenac sodium 197 (a non-steroidal anti-inflammatory 48)

dicobalt edetate an antidote for cyanide poisoning

Diconal a brand name for dipipanone (an opioid analgesic 11)

dicyclomine see dicycloverine 199

dicycloverine 199 previously known as dicyclomine (a drug for irritable bowel syndrome 42)

Dicynene a brand name for etamsylate (an antifibrinolytic used to promote blood clotting 36)

didanosine 200 (an antiviral drug for HIV infection and AIDS 97)

Didronel a brand name for etidronate 228 (a drug for bone disorders 54)

Didronel PMO a brand name for etidronate 228 (a drug for bone disorders 54) and calcium carbonate

dienestrol a female sex hormone 86 applied as a cream for vaginal dryness

diethylamine salicylate a rubefacient

diethylcarbamazine an anthelmintic 76

diethylstilbestrol 201 previously known as stilboestrol (a female sex hormone 86)

diethyltoluamide (DEET) a mosquito repellent

Differin a brand name for adapalene a retinoid for acne 119

Difflam a brand name for benzydamine (an analgesic 9)

Diflucan a brand name for fluconazole 232 (an antifungal 74)

diflucortolone a topical corticosteroid 116

diflunisal a non-steroidal anti-inflammatory 48

Digibind an antidote for digoxin overdose

digitalis drugs drugs for heart disorders 27

digitoxin a digitalis drug 27

digoxin 202 (a digitalis drug 27)

dihydrocodeine an opioid analgesic 11

dihydroergotamine a drug for migraine 20

dihydrotachysterol vitamin D (a vitamin 88)

Dijex a brand name for didanosine 200 (an

antiviral drug for HIV infection and AIDS 97)

diloxanide furoate an antiprotozoal 71 for amoebic dysentery

diltiazem 203 (an antihypertensive 34 and calcium channel blocker 33)

Dilzem a brand name for diltiazem 203 (a calcium channel blocker 33)

dimenhydrinate an antihistamine 56 used as an anti-emetic 21

dimercaprol an antidote for heavy metal poisoning

dimethyl sulfoxide a drug to treat bladder inflammation

dimeticone a silicone-based substance used in barrier creams 116 and as an antifoaming agent 40

Dimetriose a brand name for gestrinone (a drug for menstrual disorders 100)

Dimotane a brand name for brompheniramine (an antihistamine 56)

Dimotapp a brand name for phenylephrine with phenylpropanolamine 330 (both decongestants 24) and brompheniramine (an antihistamine 56)

Dindevan a brand name for phenindione (an oral anticoagulant 36)

dinoprostone a prostaglandin used to terminate pregnancy 106

dinoprost a prostaglandin used to terminate pregnancy 106

Diocalm a brand-name antidiarrhoeal 42 containing attapulgite and morphine 308

Diocalm Ultra a brand name for loperamide 280 (an antidiarrhoeal 42)

Dioctyl a brand name for docusate (a stimulant laxative 43)

Dioderm a brand name for hydrocortisone 251 (a corticosteroid 78)

Dioralyte a brand name for rehydration tablets containing sodium bicarbonate 365, glucose, potassium chloride, and sodium chloride

Dioralyte Relief a brand name for rehydration powder containing sodium chloride, potassium chloride, and sodium citrate

Diovol a brand-name antacid 40 containing aluminium hydroxide 129, magnesium hydroxide 284, and dimeticone

Dipentum a brand name for olsalazine (a drug for ulcerative colitis 44)

diphenhydramine an antihistamine 56, anti-emetic 21, and antipruritic 114 diphenoxylate 204 (An opioid antidiarrhoeal 42)

diphenylpyraline an antihistamine 56

dipipanone an opioid analgesic 11

dipivefrine a sympathomimetic for glaucoma 110

Diprobase a brand-name emollient preparation 114

Diprosalic a brand-name skin preparation containing betamethasone 150 (a corticosteroid 78) and salicylic acid (a keratolytic 119)

Diprosone a brand name for betamethasone 150 (a corticosteroid 78)

dipyridamole 205 (an antiplatelet drug 36)

Dirythmin SA a brand name for disopyramide (an anti-arrhythmic 32)

Disipal a brand name for orphenadrine 322 (a drug for parkinsonism 18)

disopyramide an anti-arrhythmic 32

Disprin a brand name for soluble aspirin 138 (a non-opioid analgesic 10)

Disprin Extra a brand-name soluble analgesic 9 containing aspirin 138 and paracetamol 325

Disprol a brand name for paracetamol 325 (a non-opioid analgesic 10)

Distaclor MR a brand name for cefaclor (a cephalosporin antibiotic 60)

Distalgesic a brand name for co-proxamol 188 (an opioid analgesic 11)

Distamine a brand name for penicillamine (an antirheumatic 50)

distigmine a parasympathomimetic for urinary retention 108 and myasthenia gravis 53

disulfiram 206 (an alcohol abuse deterrent)

dithranol a drug for psoriasis 120

Dithrocream a brand name for dithranol (a drug for psoriasis 120)

Ditropan a brand name for oxybutynin 323 (an anticholinergic and antispasmodic for urinary disorders 108)

Diumide-K Continus a brand name for furosemide 239 (a loop diuretic 31 and antihypertensive 34) with potassium

diuretics 30

Diurexan a brand name for xipamide (a thiazide diuretic 31)

Dixarit a brand name for clonidine (a drug for migraine 20)

dobutamine a drug for heart failure and shock

docetaxel an anticancer drug 94

docusate a faecal softener, stimulant laxative

43, and ear-wax softener 113

Do-Do tablets a brand-name bronchodilator 23 and decongestant 24 containing ephedrine 218, theophylline 382, and caffeine

Dolmatil a brand name for sulpiride 133 (an antipsychotic 15)

Dolobid a brand name for diflunisal (a non-steroidal anti-inflammatory 48)

Doloxene a brand name for dextropropoxyphene (an opioid analgesic 11)

Domical a brand name for amitriptyline 134 (a tricyclic antidepressant 14)

domperidone 207 (an anti-emetic 21)

donepezil 208 a drug for dementia 19

dopamine-boosting drugs drugs for parkinsonism 18

dopamine a drug for heart failure, kidney failure, and shock

dopexamine a drug for heart failure

Doralese a brand name for indoramin 257 (an antihypertensive 34)

dornase alfa a drug for cystic fibrosis 46

dorzolamide 209 a carbonic anhydrase inhibitor for glaucoma 110

Dostinex a brand name for cabergoline (a drug to treat infertility 105)

dosulepin 210 previously known as dothiepin (a tricyclic antidepressant 14)

Dothapax a brand name for dosulepin 210 (a tricyclic antidepressant 14)

dothiepin see dosulepin 210 (a tricyclic antidepressant 14)

Dovonex a brand name for calcipotriol 156 (a drug for psoriasis 120)

doxapram a respiratory stimulant 19

doxazosin 212 (a sympatholytic antihypertensive 34)

doxepin a tricyclic antidepressant 14

doxorubicin 213 (a cytotoxic anticancer drug 94)

doxycycline 214 (a tetracycline antibiotic 60)

doxylamine an antihistamine 56

Doxylar a brand name for doxycycline 214 (a tetracycline antibiotic 60)

Dozic a brand name for haloperidol 248 (a butyrophenone antipsychotic 15)

Dramamine a brand name for dimenhydrinate (an antihistamine 56 used as an anti-emetic 21)

Drapolene a brand name for benzalkonium chloride with cetrimide (both skin antiseptics 116)

Driclor a brand name for aluminium chloride (an antiperspirant)

Dristan Nasal Spray a brand name for oxymetazoline hydrochloride (a topical decongestant 24) with chlorphenamine 166 (an antihistamine 56)

Drogenil a brand name for flutamide 236 (an anticancer drug 94)

Droleptan a brand name for droperidol (a butyrophenone antipsychotic 15)

droperidol a butyrophenone antipsychotic 15

Dryptal a brand name for furosemide 239 (a loop diuretic 31 and antihypertensive 34)

Dulco-Lax a brand name for bisacodyl (a stimulant laxative 43)

Duofilm a brand-name wart preparation containing lactic acid, salicylic acid, and collodion 116

Duovent a brand name for fenoterol with ipratropium bromide 261 (both bronchodilators 23)

Duphalac a brand name for lactulose 270 (a laxative 43)

Duphaston, Duphaston HRT a brand name for dydrogesterone 215 (a female sex hormone 86)

Duragel a brand name for nonoxinol "11" (a spermicidal agent 101)

Durogesic a brand name for fentanyl (an opioid analgesic 11)

Duromine a brand name for phentermine (an appetite suppressant 19)

Dutonin a brand name for nefazodone (an antidepressant 14)

Dyazide a brand name for hydrochlorothiazide 250 with triamterene 392 (both diuretics 30)

dydrogesterone 215 (a female sex hormone 86)

Dynese a brand name for magaldrate (an antacid 40)

Dysman a brand name for mefenamic acid 287 (a non-steroidal anti-inflammatory 48)

Dyspamet a brand name for cimetidine 171 (an anti-ulcer drug 41)

Dysport a brand name for botulinum toxin (used as a muscle relaxant 52)

Dytac a brand name for triamterene 392 (a potassium-sparing diuretic 31)

Dytide a brand name for benzthiazide with

triamterene 392 (both diuretics 30)

E

ear disorders, drugs for 113

Earex a brand-name preparation for ear-wax removal 113

Ebufac a brand name for ibuprofen 254 (a non-steroidal anti-inflammatory 48)

Econacort a brand name for econazole (an antifungal 74) with hydrocortisone 251 (a corticosteroid 78)

econazole an antifungal 74

Economycin a brand name for tetracycline 381 (an antibiotic 60)

Ecostatin a brand name for econazole (an antifungal 74)

ecothiopate a drug for glaucoma 110

eczema, treatments for 121

Edronax a brand name for reboxetine (an antidepressant 14)

edrophonium a drug for diagnosis of myasthenia gravis 53

Efalith a brand-name ointment for dermatitis 116, 121, containing lithium succinate 278 and zinc sulphate

Efamast a brand name for gamolenic acid 241

efavirenz an antiviral for HIV/AIDS 97

Efcortelan a brand name for hydrocortisone 251 (a corticosteroid 78)

Efcortesol a brand name for hydrocortisone 251 (a corticosteroid 78)

Efexor a brand name for venlafaxine 395 (an antidepressant 14)

Effercitrate a brand name for potassium (a mineral 91)

eformoterol (formoterol) a sympathomimetic bronchodilator 23

Elantan a brand name for isosorbide mononitrate 264 (a nitrate vasodilator 30 and anti-angina drug 33)

Elavil a brand name for amitriptyline 134 (a tricyclic antidepressant 14)

Eldepryl a brand name for selegiline (a drug for parkinsonism 18)

Electrolade brand-name oral rehydration salts with potassium chloride, sodium chloride, sodium bicarbonate 365, and glucose

Elleste Duet a brand-name preparation for menopausal symptoms 86 containing estradiol 224 and norethisterone 316

Elleste Solo a brand name for estradiol 224 (an oestrogen 86)

Elocon a brand name for mometasone 307 (a topical corticosteroid 116)

Eloxatin a brand name for oxaliplatin an anticancer drug 94

Eltroxin a brand name for levothyroxine 384 (a thyroid hormone 82)

Eludril a brand name for chlorhexidine (an antiseptic)

Elyzol a brand name for metronidazole 301 (an antibacterial 64 and antiprotozoal 71)

Emblon a brand name for tamoxifen 375 (an anticancer drug 94)

Emcor a brand name for bisoprolol (a beta blocker 28)

Emeside a brand name for ethosuximide 227 (an anticonvulsant 16)

Emflex a brand name for acemetacin (a non-steroidal anti-inflammatory 48)

Eminase a brand name for anistreplase (a thrombolytic 38)

Emla a brand-name local anaesthetic 11 containing lidocaine and prilocaine

emollients 115 (in antipruritic prepartions 114 and treatments for eczema 121)

enalapril 217 (a vasodilator 30 and antihypertensive 34)

En-De-Kay a brand name for fluoride (a mineral 91)

Endoxana a brand name for cyclophosphamide 191 (an anticancer drug 94)

enflurane a general anaesthetic

ENO's a brand-name antacid 40 containing sodium bicarbonate 365, sodium carbonate, and citric acid

enoxaparin a type of heparin 249 (an anticoagulant 36)

enoximone a drug for heart failure 27

entacapone a drug for parkinsonism 18

Entocort CR a brand name for budesonide 153 (a corticosteroid 78)

Epanutin a brand name for phenytoin 331 (an anticonvulsant 16)

ephedrine 218 (a bronchodilator 23 and decongestant 24)

epidural anaesthesia used for pain relief in labour 107

Epilim a brand name for sodium valproate 367 (an anticonvulsant 16)

epinephrine 219 (a bronchodilator 23 and drug for glaucoma 110 and anaphylactic shock). Also known as adrenaline

EpiPen a brand name for epinephrine 219 (an anti-allergy drug 56)

epirubicin a cytotoxic anticancer drug 94

Epivir a brand name for lamivudine 270 an antiviral 67 used for HIV/AIDS 97

epoetin 220 (a kidney hormone 78 used for anaemia due to kidney failure). Also known as erythropoietin

Epogam a brand name for gamolenic acid 241 (a drug for eczema 121)

epoprostenol a prostaglandin used for its vasodilator effects 30

Eppy a brand name for epinephrine 219 (a drug for glaucoma 110)

Eprex a brand name for epoetin 220 (a kidney hormone 78 used for anaemia due to kidney failure)

eptifibatide a drug for prevention of heart attacks 27

Equagesic a brand name for aspirin 138 with ethoheptazine (both analgesics 9) and meprobamate (an anti-anxiety drug 13)

ergocalciferol vitamin D (a vitamin 88)

ergometrine a uterine stimulant 106

ergotamine 221 (a drug for migraine 20)

Erwinase a brand name for crisantaspase (an anticancer drug 94)

Erycen a brand name for erythromycin 222 (an antibiotic 60)

Erymax a brand name for erythromycin 222 (an antibiotic 60)

Erythrocin a brand name for erythromycin 222 (an antibiotic 60)

Erythromid a brand name for erythromycin 230 (an antibiotic 60)

erythromycin 222 (an antibiotic 60)

Erythroped a brand name for erythromycin 222 (an antibiotic 60)

erythropoietin 220 (a kidney hormone 78 used for anaemia due to kidney failure). Also known as epoetin

Eskamel a brand name for resorcinol (a drug for acne 119) with sulphur (a topical antibacterial 64 and antifungal 74)

Eskornade a brand name for phenylpropanolamine 330 (a decongestant 24) with diphenylpyraline (an antihistamine 56)

esmolol a beta blocker 28

Estracombi a brand-name preparation for menopausal symptoms 86 containing estradiol 224 and norethisterone 316

Estraderm TTS a brand name for estradiol 224 (an oestrogen 86)

estradiol 224 (an oestrogen 86)

estramustine an alkylating agent for cancer of the prostate 94

Estrapak a brand-name preparation for menopausal symptoms 86 containing estradiol 224 and norethisterone 316

Estring a brand-name vaginal ring for menopausal symptoms 86 containing estradiol 224

estriol an oestrogen 86

estrone an oestrogen 86

estropipate an oestrogen 86

etacrynic acid a loop diuretic 31

etamsylate an antifibrinolytic used to promote blood clotting 36

ethambutol 225 (an antituberculous drug 65)

ethinylestradiol 226 (a female sex hormone 86 and oral contraceptive 101)

ethoheptazine an opioid analgesic 11

ethosuximide 227 (an anticonvulsant 16)

etidronate 228 (a drug for bone disorders 54)

etodolac a COX-2 inhibitor 49 (a non-steroidal anti-inflammatory drug 48)

etomidate a drug for induction of general anaesthesia

etonorgestrel a progestogen 86

etoposide a drug for cancers of the lung, lymphatic system, and testes 94

etynodiol a progestogen (a female sex hormone 86)

Eucardic a brand name for carvedilol (an antihypertensive 34)

Euglucon a brand name for glibenclamide 243 (an oral antidiabetic 80)

Eugynon 30 a brand-name oral contraceptive 101 containing ethinylestradiol 226 and levonorgestrel 276

Eumovate a brand name for clobetasone (a topical corticosteroid 116)

Eurax a brand name for crotamiton (an antipruritic 114)

Eurax-Hydrocortisone a brand name for hydrocortisone 251 (a corticosteroid 78) with crotamiton (an antipruritic 114)

Evista a brand name for raloxifene 353 (an anti-oestrogen sex hormone antagonist 86 for osteoporosis 54)

Evorel a brand name for estradiol 224 (an oestrogen 86)

Exelderm a brand name for sulconazole (an antifungal 74)

Exelon a brand name for rivastigmine 359 a drug for dementia 19

Ex-Lax a brand name for senna (a stimulant laxative 43)

Exocin a brand name for ofloxacin (an antibiotic 60)

expectorants 26 (drugs to treat coughs 25)

Expulin a brand-name cough preparation 25 containing chlorphenamine 166, menthol, pholcodine, and pseudoephedrine

Expulin Decongestant a brand-name decongestant 24 with chlorphenamine 166, ephedrine 218, and menthol

Exterol brand-name ear drops for wax removal 113 containing urea

F

factor VIIa a blood extract to promote blood clotting 36

factor VIII a blood extract to promote blood clotting 36

factor IX a blood extract to promote blood clotting 36

famciclovir an antiviral 67

famotidine an anti-ulcer drug 41

Famvir a brand name for famciclovir (an antiviral 67)

Fansidar a brand-name antimalarial 73 containing pyrimethamine 348 and sulfadoxine

Farlutal a brand name for medroxyprogesterone 286 (a female sex hormone 86)

Fasigyn a brand name for tinidazole (an antibacterial 64)

Faverin a brand name for fluvoxamine (an antidepressant 14)

Fectrim a brand name for co-trimoxazole 189 (an antibacterial 64)

Fefol a brand name for folic acid 90 (a vitamin 88) with iron (a mineral 91)

felbinac 230 a non-steroidal anti-inflammatory 48

Feldene a brand name for piroxicam 333 (a non-steroidal anti-inflammatory 48 and drug for gout 51)

felodipine a calcium channel blocker 33

felypressin a vasoconstrictor 27 used in dentistry

female sex hormones 86 (drugs for infertility 105, menstrual disorders 100, and in oral contraceptives 101)

Femapak a brand-name preparation for menopausal symptoms 86 containing estradiol 224 and dydrogesterone 215

Femara a brand name for letrozole (an anticancer drug 94)

Fematrix a brand name for estradiol 224 (an oestrogen 86)

Femeron a brand name for miconazole 302 (an antifungal 74)

Femigraine a brand-name drug for migraine containing aspirin 138 (a non-opioid analgesic 10) with cyclizine (an anti-emetic 21)

Feminax a brand-name analgesic 9 for dysmenorrhoea containing paracetamol 325, codeine 183, hyoscine 252, and caffeine

Femodene a brand-name oral contraceptive 101 containing ethinylestradiol 226 and gestodene

Femodette a brand-name oral contraceptive 101 containing gestodene and ethinylestradiol 226

Femoston a brand-name preparation for menopausal symptoms 86 containing estradiol 224 and dydrogesterone 215

FemSeven a brand name for estradiol 224 (an oestrogen 86)

Femulen a brand-name oral contraceptive 101 containing etynodiol diacetate

Fenbid a brand name for ibuprofen 254 (a non-steroidal anti-inflammatory 48)

fenbufen a non-steroidal anti-inflammatory 48

Fenbuzip a brand name for fenbufen (a non-steroidal anti-inflammatory 48)

fenofibrate a lipid-lowering drug 35

Fenoket a brand name for ketoprofen 268 (a non-steroidal anti-inflammatory 48)

fenoprofen a non-steroidal anti-inflammatory 48

Fenopron a brand name for fenoprofen (a non-steroidal anti-inflammatory 48)

fenoterol a sympathomimetic bronchodilator 23

Fentamox a brand name for tamoxifen 375 (an anticancer drug 94)

fentanyl an opioid analgesic 11 used in general anaesthesia and labour 106

Fentazin a brand name for perphenazine (an antipsychotic 15 and anti-emetic 21)

fenticonazole an antifungal drug 74

Feospan a brand name for iron (a mineral 91)

Ferfolic SV a brand name for folic acid 90 (a vitamin 88) and ferrous gluconate (a mineral 91)

ferric ammonium citrate iron (a mineral 91)

Ferrograd a brand name for iron (a mineral 91)

Ferrograd C a brand name for iron (a mineral 91) with vitamin C (a vitamin 88)

Ferrograd Folic a brand name for folic acid 90 (a vitamin 88) with iron (a mineral 91)

ferrous fumarate iron (a mineral 91)

ferrous gluconate iron (a mineral 91)

ferrous glycine sulphate iron (a mineral 91)

ferrous sulphate iron (a mineral 91)

Fersaday a brand name for iron (a mineral 91)

Fersamal a brand name for iron (a mineral 91)

fexofenadine an antihistamine 56

fibrates lipid-lowering drugs 35

fibrinolysin a thrombolytic enzyme used to break down blood clots 36 and to aid healing of skin ulcers 41

fibrinolytics see thrombolytics 38 (drugs that affect blood clotting 36)

Fibro-vein a brand name for sodium tetradecyl sulphate (a drug for varicose veins)

Filair a brand name for beclometasone 146 (a corticosteroid 78)

filgrastim 230 (a blood growth stimulant)

finasteride 231 (a drug for benign prostatic hypertrophy, a urinary disorder 108)

Flagyl a brand name for metronidazole 301 (an antibacterial 64 and antiprotozoal 71)

Flamatrol a brand name for piroxicam 333 (a non-steroidal anti-inflammatory 48 and drug for gout 51)

Flamazine a brand name for silver sulfadiazine (a topical antibacterial 64)

flavoxate a urinary antispasmodic 108

flecainide an anti-arrhythmic 32

Flexin Continus a brand name for indometacin (a non-steroidal anti-inflammatory 48)

Flixonase a brand name for fluticasone 237 (a corticosteroid 78)

Flixotide a brand name for fluticasone 237 (a corticosteroid 78)

Flomax MR a brand name for tamsulosin 376 (an alpha-blocking drug for prostate disorders 108)

Florinef a brand name for fludrocortisone (a corticosteroid 78)

Floxapen a brand name for flucloxacillin (a penicillin antibiotic 60)

Fluanxol a brand name for flupentixol 234 (an antipsychotic 15 used in depression 14)

flucloxacillin a penicillin antibiotic 60

fluconazole 232 (an antifungal 74)

flucytosine an antifungal 74

fludarabine an anticancer drug 94

fludrocortisone a corticosteroid 78

fludroxycortide previously known as flurandrenolone (a topical corticosteroid 116)

flumazenil an antidote for benzodiazepine overdose

flumetasone a corticosteroid 78

flunisolide a corticosteroid 78

flunitrazepam a benzodiazepine sleeping drug 11

fluocinolone a topical corticosteroid 116

fluocinonide a topical corticosteroid 116

fluocortolone a topical corticosteroid 116

Fluor-a-day a brand name for fluoride (a mineral 91)

fluorescein a drug used to stain the eye before examination

fluoride a mineral 91

Fluorigard a brand name for fluoride (a mineral 91)

fluorometholone a corticosteroid 78 for eye disorders

fluorouracil an anticancer drug 94

fluoxetine 233 (an antidepressant 14)

flupentixol 234 (an antipsychotic 15 used in depression 14)

fluphenazine an antipsychotic 15 used in depression 14

flurandrenolone see fludroxycortide (a topical corticosteroid 116)

flurazepam a benzodiazepine sleeping drug 11

flurbiprofen a non-steroidal anti-inflammatory 48

Flurex a brand name for paracetamol 325 (a non-opioid analgesic 10) with phenylephrine (a decongestant 24) and dextromethorphan (a cough suppressant 25)

flutamide 236 an anticancer drug 94

fluticasone 237 (a corticosteroid 78)

fluvastatin a lipid-lowering drug 35

fluvoxamine an antidepressant 14

FML a brand name for fluorometholone (a corticosteroid 78)

folate sodium folic acid 90 (a vitamin 88)

folic acid 90 (a vitamin 88)

folinic acid a vitamin 88

follicle-stimulating hormone (FSH) a natural hormone for infertility 105

follitropin alfa a drug for infertility 105

follitropin beta a drug for infertility 105

fomepizole an antidote for ethylene glycol poisoning

Foradil a brand name for formoterol (a bronchodilator 23)

formestane a drug for breast cancer 94

formoterol previously known as eformoterol (a bronchodilator 23)

Fortagesic a brand name for pentazocine (an opioid analgesic 11) and paracetamol 325)

Fortovase a brand name for saquinavir (an antiviral for HIV/AIDS 97)

Fortral a brand name for pentazocine (an opioid analgesic 11)

Fortum a brand name for ceftazidime (a cephalosporin antibiotic 60)

Fosamax a brand name for alendronate (a drug for bone disorders 54)

foscarnet an antiviral 67

Foscavir a brand name for foscarnet (an antiviral 67)

fosfestrol a female sex hormone 86 and anticancer drug 94

fosinopril 238 (an ACE inhibitor vasodilator 30)

Fragmin a brand name for dalteparin (a low-molecular-weight heparin 249 used as an anticoagulant 36)

framycetin a topical aminoglycoside antibiotic 60 for ear, eye, and skin infections

frangula a mild stimulant laxative 43

Franol a brand-name bronchodilator 23 containing ephedrine 218 and theophylline 382

Frisium a brand name for clobazam (a benzodiazepine anti-anxiety drug 13)

Froben a brand name for flurbiprofen (a non-steroidal anti-inflammatory drug 48)

Froop a brand name for furosemide 239 (a loop diuretic 31)

Fru-Co a brand name for amiloride 131 with furosemide 239 (both diuretics 30)

Frumil a brand name for amiloride 131 with furosemide 239 (both diuretics 30)

frusemide see furosemide 239

Frusene a brand name for furosemide 239 with

triamterene 392 (both diuretics 30)

FSH follicle-stimulating hormone (a natural hormone for infertility 105)

Fucibet a brand name for betamethasone 150 (a corticosteroid 78) with fusidic acid (an antibiotic 60)

Fucidin a brand name for fusidic acid (an antibiotic 60)

Fucidin H a brand name for fusidic acid (an antibiotic 60) and hydrocortisone 251 (a corticosteroid 78)

Fucithalmic a brand name for fusidic acid (an antibiotic 60)

Fulcin a brand name for griseofulvin (an antifungal 74)

Full Marks a brand name for phenothrin (a topical antiparasitic 118)

Fungilin a brand name for amphotericin 137 (an antifungal 74)

Fungizone a brand name for amphotericin 137 (an antifungal 74)

Furadantin a brand name for nitrofurantoin (an antibacterial 64)

Furamide a brand name for diloxanide furoate (an antiprotozoal 71)

furosemide previously known as frusemide 239 (a loop diuretic 31)

fusidic acid an antibiotic 60

Fybogel a brand name for ispaghula (a bulk-forming agent used as a laxative 43 and antidiarrhoeal 42)

Fynnon Calcium Aspirin a brand name for aspirin 138 (an analgesic 9), calcium carbonate (a mineral 91), and sodium sulphate (an osmotic laxative 43)

G

gabapentin an anticonvulsant 16

Gabitril a brand name for tiagabine (an anticonvulsant 16)

Galcodine a brand name for codeine 183 (a cough suppressant 25)

Galenphol a brand name for pholcodine (a cough suppressant 25)

Galfer a brand name for iron (a mineral 91)

Galfer FA a brand name for folic acid 90 (a vitamin 88) with iron (a mineral 91)

gallamine a drug used to relax the muscles in general anaesthesia

gallstones, drug treatment for 46

Galpseud a brand name for pseudoephedrine (a sympathomimetic decongestant 24)

Gamanil a brand name for lofepramine 279 (a tricyclic antidepressant 14)

gamma globulin an immune globulin 68

gamolenic acid 241 (an extract of evening primrose used for breast pain and eczema 121)

ganciclovir an antiviral 67

Ganda a brand-name preparation for glaucoma 110 containing epinephrine 219 and guanethidine

Garamycin a brand name for gentamicin 241 (an aminoglycoside antibiotic 60)

Gardenal a brand name for phenobarbital 327 (a barbiturate anticonvulsant 16)

Gastrobid Continus a brand name for metoclopramide 299 (a gastrointestinal motility regulator and anti-emetic 21)

Gastrocote a brand-name antacid 40 containing aluminium hydroxide 129, sodium bicarbonate 365, magnesium trisilicate, and alginic acid

Gastroflux a brand name for metoclopramide 299 (a gastrointestinal motility regulator and anti-emetic 21)

Gastromax a brand name for metoclopramide 299 (a gastrointestinal motility regulator and anti-emetic 21)

Gaviscon a brand-name antacid 40 containing aluminium hydroxide 129, sodium bicarbonate 365, magnesium trisilicate, and alginic acid

Gelcosal a brand-name preparation for eczema 121 and psoriasis 120 containing coal tar and salicylic acid

Gelcotar a brand name for coal tar (used for dandruff 122, eczema 121, and psoriasis 120)

gemcitabine an anticancer drug 94

gemeprost a drug used in labour 106

gemfibrozil a lipid-lowering drug 35

Genotropin a brand name for somatropin (a synthetic pituitary hormone 83)

gentamicin 241 (an aminoglycoside antibiotic 60)

gentian mixture, acid and alkaline an appetite stimulant 19

Genticin a brand name for gentamicin 241 (an aminoglycoside antibiotic 60)

Gentisone HC a brand name for gentamicin 241 (an aminoglycoside antibiotic 60) with hydrocortisone 251 (a corticosteroid 78)

gestodene a progestogen 86 and oral contraceptive 101

Gestone a brand name for progesterone (a female sex hormone 86)

gestonerone previously known as gestronol (a progestogen 86)

gestrinone a drug for menstrual disorders 100

Glandosane a brand name for artificial saliva

glaucoma, drugs for 110

glibenclamide 243 (an oral antidiabetic 80)

Glibenese a brand name for glipizide (an oral antidiabetic 80)

gliclazide 244 (an oral antidiabetic 80)

glimepiride an oral antidiabetic 80

glipizide an oral antidiabetic 80

gliquidone an oral antidiabetic 80

GlucaGen a brand name for glucagon (a drug for hypoglycaemia 80)

glucagon a pancreatic hormone for hypoglycaemia 80

Glucamet a brand name for metformin 294 (an oral antidiabetic 80)

Glucobay a brand name for acarbose (an oral antidiabetic 80)

Glucophage a brand name for metformin 294 (an oral antidiabetic 80)

Glurenorm a brand name for gliquidone (an oral antidiabetic 80)

glutaraldehyde a topical preparation for treating warts

Glutarol a brand name for glutaraldehyde (a topical wart preparation)

glycerol a drug used to reduce pressure inside the eye 110, and an ingredient in cough mixtures 25, skin preparations 116, laxative suppositories 43, and ear-wax softening drops 113

glyceryl trinitrate 245 (an anti-angina drug 33)

glycopyrronium bromide an anticholinergic used in general anaesthesia

Glytrin a brand name for glyceryl trinitrate 245 (an anti-angina drug 33)

gold a metal used medically for rheumatoid arthritis 50

gold-based drugs a type of antirheumatic drug 50

Golden Eye a brand name for propamidine isethionate (an antibacterial 64)

gonadorelin a drug for infertility 105

gonadotrophin, chorionic 169 (a drug for infertility 105)

Gopten a brand name for trandolapril (an antihypertensive 34)

goserelin 246 (a female sex hormone 86 and anticancer drug 94, also used for menstrual disorders 100 and infertility 105)

gout, drugs for 51

gramicidin an aminoglycoside antibiotic 60 for eye, ear, and skin infections

Graneodin a brand name for gramicidin with neomycin (both aminoglycoside antibiotics 60)

granisetron an anti-emetic 21

Gregoderm a brand name for hydrocortisone 251 (a corticosteroid 78) with nystatin 317 (an antifungal 74), neomycin (an aminoglycoside antibiotic 60), and polymyxin B (an antibiotic 60)

griseofulvin an antifungal 74

Grisovin a brand name for griseofulvin (an antifungal 74)

growth hormone somatropin (a pituitary hormone 83)

GTN 300mcg a brand name for glyceryl trinitrate 245 (an anti-angina drug 33)

guaifenesin an expectorant 25

guanethidine an antihypertensive 34 also used for glaucoma 110

Guanor Expectorant a brand-name cough preparation 25 containing diphenhydramine, ammonium chloride, and menthol

Guarem a brand name for guar gum (a drug used to control blood glucose levels 80)

guar gum a drug used to control blood glucose levels 80

Gyno-Daktarin a brand name for miconazole 302 (an antifungal 74)

Gynol II a brand name for nonoxinol "9" (a spermicidal agent 101)

Gyno-Pevaryl a brand name for econazole (an antifungal 74)

H

Haelan a brand name for fludroxycortide (a topical corticosteroid 116)

haem arginate a drug to treat porphyria

hair loss, drugs for 123

Halciderm Topical a brand name for halcinonide (a topical corticosteroid 116)

halcinonide a topical corticosteroid 116

Haldol a brand name for haloperidol 248 (a

butyrophenone antipsychotic 15)

Halfan a brand name for halofantrine (an antimalarial 73)

halibut liver oil a natural fish oil rich in vitamin A and vitamin D (both vitamins 88)

halofantrine an antimalarial 73

haloperidol 248 (a butyrophenone antipsychotic 15)

halothane a gas used to induce general anaesthesia

Halycitrol a brand name for vitamin A with vitamin D (both vitamins 88)

hamamelis an astringent in rectal preparations 45

Hansen's disease, drug treatment for 65

Harmogen a brand name for piperazine oestrogen sulphate (a drug for hormone replacement therapy 86)

Hay-Crom a brand name for sodium cromoglicate 366 (an anti-allergy drug 56)

Haymine a brand name for chlorphenamine 166 (an antihistamine 56) with ephedrine 218 (a bronchodilator 23 and decongestant 24)

HCG human chorionic gonadotrophin 169 (a drug for infertility 105)

Hedex a brand name for paracetamol 325 (a non-opioid analgesic 10)

Hedex Extra a brand name for paracetamol 325 (a non-opioid analgesic 10) with caffeine

Heliclear a brand-name preparation containing lansoprazole 272, amoxicillin 136, and clarithromycin 60 (an anti-ulcer product 41)

Heminevrin a brand name for clomethiazole (a non-benzodiazepine, non-barbiturate sleeping drug 11)

heparin 249 (an anticoagulant 36)

heparinoid a drug applied topically to reduce inflammation of the skin 116

Hep-Flush a brand name for heparin 249 (an anticoagulant 36)

heroin diamorphine (an opioid analgesic 11)

Herpid a brand name for idoxuridine (an antiviral 67)

hexachlorophene a skin antiseptic 116

Hexalen a brand name for altretamine (an anticancer drug 94)

hexamine another name for methenamine (a drug for urinary tract infections 108)

hexetidine an antiseptic 116

Hexopal a brand name for nicotinic acid (a vasodilator 30)

Hibitane a brand name for chlorhexidine (a skin antiseptic 116)

Hioxyl a brand name for hydrogen peroxide (an antiseptic 116)

Hiprex a brand name for hexamine (a drug for urinary tract infections 108)

Hirudoid a brand name for heparinoid (a topical anti-inflammatory 116)

Histalix a brand-name cough preparation 25 containing diphenhydramine, ammonium chloride, and menthol

HIV and AIDS, drugs for 97

Hivid a brand name for zalcitabine 400 (an antiviral for HIV infection and AIDS 97)

homatropine a mydriatic 112

Honvan a brand name for fosfestrol (a female sex hormone 86 and anticancer drug 94)

hormone content of common oral contraceptives (table) 102

hormone replacement therapy (HRT) 87 (female sex hormones 86 and for bone disorders 54

hormones 78 (male sex hormones 85, female sex hormones 86, for infertility 105, for menstrual disorders 100, in oral contraceptives 101, and for acne 119

Hormonin a brand name for estradiol 224 (a female sex hormone 86)

HRT see hormone replacement therapy 87

Humalog a brand name for insulin 258 lispro (a very quick-acting drug for diabetes 80)

Human Actrapid a brand name for insulin 258 (a drug for diabetes 80)

Human Insulatard a brand name for insulin 258 (a drug for diabetes 80)

human menopausal gonadotrophins also known as menotrophin (a drug for infertility 105)

Human Mixtard a brand name for insulin 258 (a drug for diabetes 80)

Human Monotard a brand name for insulin 258 (a drug for diabetes 80)

Human Ultratard a brand name for insulin 258 (a drug for diabetes 80)

Human Velosulin a brand name for insulin 258 (a drug for diabetes 80)

Humatrope a brand name for somatropin (a pituitary hormone 83, a synthetic pituitary hormone 83)

Humulin a brand name for insulin 258 (a drug for diabetes 80)

Hyalase a brand name for hyaluronidase (helps injections to penetrate tissues)

hyaluronidase helps injections to penetrate tissues

Hycamtin a brand name for topotecan (an anticancer drug 94)

Hydergine a brand name for co-dergocrine mesylate (a vasodilator 30)

hydralazine an antihypertensive 34

hydrochlorothiazide 250 (a thiazide diuretic 31)

hydrocortisone 251 (a corticosteroid 78 and antipruritic 114)

Hydrocortistab a brand name for hydrocortisone 251 (a corticosteroid 78)

Hydrocortone a brand name for hydrocortisone 251 (a corticosteroid 78)

hydroflumethiazide a thiazide diuretic 31

hydrogen peroxide an antiseptic mouthwash 116

hydromorphone an opioid analgesic 11

HydroSaluric a brand name for hydrochlorothiazide 250 (a thiazide diuretic 31)

hydrotalcite an antacid 40

hydroxocobalamin vitamin B_{12} (a vitamin 88)

hydroxyapatite a drug to treat bone disorders 54

hydroxycarbamide previously known as hydroxyurea (a drug for chronic myeloid leukaemia 94)

hydroxychloroquine an antimalarial 73 and antirheumatic drug 50

hydroxyprogesterone a progestogen 86 used to prevent miscarriage

hydroxyurea see hydroxycarbamide (a drug for leukaemia 94)

hydroxyzine an anti-anxiety drug 13

Hygroton a brand name for chlortalidone (a thiazide diuretic 31)

hyoscine 252 (a drug for irritable bowel syndrome 43 and a drug for affecting the pupil 112)

Hypotears a brand name for polyvinyl alcohol (artificial tears 112)

Hypovase a brand name for prazosin (an antihypertensive 34)

hypromellose a substance in artificial tear preparations 112

Hypurin a brand name for insulin 258 (a drug for diabetes 80)

Hytrin a brand name for terazosin (an alpha blocker 34)

I

Ibugel a brand name for ibuprofen 254 (a non-steroidal anti-inflammatory 48)

Ibuleve a brand-name gel for muscular pain relief containing ibuprofen 254 (a non-steroidal anti-inflammatory 48)

ibuprofen 254 (a non-opioid analgesic 10 and non-steroidal anti-inflammatory 48)

Ibuspray a brand name for ibuprofen 254 (a non-steroidal anti-inflammatory 48)

ichthammol a substance used in skin preparations for eczema 121

idarubicin a cytotoxic antibiotic (an anticancer drug 94)

idoxuridine an antiviral 67

ifosfamide an anticancer drug 94

Ikorel a brand name for nicorandil (an anti-angina drug 33)

Ilosone a brand name for erythromycin 222 (an antibiotic 60)

Ilube a brand name for acetylcysteine (a mucolytic 25) with hypromellose (a substance in artificial tear preparations 112)

Imbrilon a brand name for indometacin (a non-steroidal anti-inflammatory 48 and drug for gout 51)

Imdur a brand name for isosorbide mononitrate 264 (a nitrate vasodilator 30 and anti-angina drug 33)

imidapril an ACE inhibitor vasodilator 30

imiglucerase an enzyme for enzyme replacement therapy

Imigran a brand name for sumatriptan 373 (a drug for migraine 20)

imipenem an antibiotic 60

imipramine 255 (a tricyclic antidepressant 14 and drug for urinary disorders 108)

imiquimod a drug to treat warts

Immukin a brand name for interferon gamma 259 (an antiviral 67)

immunization, travel see travel immunization (table) 71

immunoglobulin a preparation injected to prevent infectious diseases 68

Immunoprin a brand name for azathioprine 143 (an antirheumatic 50 and immunosuppressant 96)

immunosuppressant drugs 96 (used as antirheumatic drugs 50)

Imodium a brand name for loperamide 280 (an antidiarrhoeal 42)

Implanon a brand name for etonorgestrel (a progestogen 86)

impotence, drugs for 106 (drugs for infertility 105)

Imuran a brand name for azathioprine 143 (an antirheumatic 50 and immunosuppressant 96)

incontinence (urinary), drugs for 108

indapamide 256 (a thiazide-like diuretic 30)

Inderal a brand name for propranolol 345 (a beta blocker 28)

Inderal-LA a brand name for propranolol 345 (a beta blocker 28)

Inderetic a brand name for bendroflumethiazide 147 (a thiazide diuretic 31) with propranolol 345 (a beta blocker 28)

Inderex a brand name for bendroflumethiazide 147 (a thiazide diuretic 31) with propranolol 345 (a beta blocker 28)

indinavir an antiviral for HIV/AIDS 97

Indocid a brand name for indometacin (a non-steroidal anti-inflammatory 48 and drug for gout 51)

Indocid-R a brand name for indometacin (a non-steroidal anti-inflammatory 48 and drug for gout 51)

Indolar a brand name for indometacin (a non-steroidal anti-inflammatory 48 and drug for gout 51)

indometacin a non-steroidal anti-inflammatory 48 and drug for gout 51

Indomod a brand name for indometacin (a non-steroidal anti-inflammatory 48 and drug for gout 51)

indoramin 257 an antihypertensive 34 and drug for urinary disorders 108

inducing labour, drugs for 106

Infacol a brand name for dimeticone (an antifoaming agent 40)

Infadrops a brand name for paracetamol 325 (a non-opioid analgesic 10)

infertility, drugs for 105

inflammatory bowel disease, drugs for 44

Innohep a brand name for tinzaparin (a low-molecular-weight heparin 249 used as an anticoagulant 36)

Innovace a brand name for enalapril 217 (a vasodilator 30 and antihypertensive 34)

Innozide a brand name for enalapril 217 (a vasodilator 30 and antihypertensive 34)

inosine pranobex an antiviral 67

inositol a drug related to nicotinic acid (a vasodilator 30, lipid-lowering drug 35, and vitamin supplement)

Inoven a brand name for ibuprofen 254 (an analgesic 9 and non-steroidal anti-inflammatory 48)

Insulatard a brand name for insulin 258 (a drug for diabetes 80)

insulin 258 (a drug for diabetes 80)

insulin lispro a type of insulin 258 (a drug for diabetes 80)

Intal a brand name for sodium cromoglicate 366 (an anti-allergy drug 56)

integrilin a brand name for eptifibatide (a drug for prevention of heart attacks 27)

interferon 259 (an antiviral 67 and anticancer drug 94)

Intralgin a brand-name topical gel containing benzocaine (a local anaesthetic 11) for muscle strains and sprains

Intron-A a brand name for interferon 259 (an antiviral 67 and anticancer drug 94)

Invirase a brand name for saquinavir (an antiviral for HIV/AIDS 97)

iodine a mineral 91

Ionamin a brand name for phentermine (an appetite suppressant 19)

Ionax a brand-name treatment for acne 119

Ionil T a brand-name dandruff shampoo 122 containing benzalkonium chloride, coal tar, and salicylic acid

Iopidine a brand name for apraclonidine (a drug for glaucoma 110)

ipecacuanha a drug used to induce vomiting in drug overdose and poisoning, also used as an expectorant 25

Ipral a brand name for trimethoprim 393 (an antibacterial 64)

ipratropium bromide 261 (a bronchodilator 23)

irbesartan 262 (an angiotensin II inhibitor, an antihypertensive 34)

irinotecan an anticancer drug 94

iron a mineral 91

irritable bowel syndrome, drugs for 43

Ismelin a brand name for guanethidine (an antihypertensive 34 also used for glaucoma 110)

Ismo a brand name for isosorbide mononitrate

264 (a nitrate vasodilator 30 and anti-angina drug 33)

isocarboxazid an MAOI antidepressant 14

isoconazole an antifungal 74

isoflurane a volatile liquid inhaled as a general anaesthetic

Isogel a brand name for ispaghula (a laxative 43 and antidiarrhoeal 42)

Isoket a brand name for isosorbide dinitrate 264 (a nitrate vasodilator 30 and anti-angina drug 33)

isometheptene mucate a drug for migraine 20

isoniazid 263 (an antituberculous drug 65)

isophane insulin a type of insulin 258 (a drug for diabetes 80)

isoprenaline a bronchodilator 23

Isopto Alkaline a brand name for hypromellose (a substance in artificial tear preparations 112)

Isopto Atropine a brand name for atropine 142 (an anticholinergic mydriatic 112) with hypromellose (a substance in artificial tear preparations 112)

Isopto Carbachol a brand name for carbachol eye drops (a miotic for glaucoma 110)

Isopto Carpine a brand name for pilocarpine 332 (a miotic for glaucoma 110) with hypromellose (a substance in artificial tear preparations 112)

Isopto Frin brand-name eye drops containing phenylephrine and hypromellose (a substance in artificial tear preparations 112) for minor eye irritation and redness

Isopto Plain a brand name for hypromellose eye drops (a substance in artificial tear preparations 112)

Isordil a brand name for isosorbide dinitrate 264 (a nitrate vasodilator 30 and anti-angina drug 33)

isosorbide dinitrate 264 (a nitrate vasodilator 30 and anti-angina drug 33)

isosorbide mononitrate 264 (a nitrate vasodilator 30 and anti-angina drug 33)

Isotrate a brand name for isosorbide mononitrate 264 (a nitrate vasodilator 30 and anti-angina drug 33)

isotretinoin 265 (a drug for acne 119)

Isotrex a brand name for isotretinoin 265 (a drug for acne 119)

ispaghula a bulk-forming agent for constipation 43 and diarrhoea 42

isradipine a calcium channel blocker 33

Istin a brand name for amlodipine 135 (a calcium channel blocker 33)

itraconazole an antifungal 74

ivermectin an anthelmintic 76

J

Jectofer a brand name for iron (a mineral 91)

Joy-rides a brand name for hyoscine 252 (used to prevent motion sickness 21)

K

Kabikinase a brand name for streptokinase 369 (a thrombolytic 38)

Kalspare a brand name for triamterene 392 with chlortalidone (both diuretics 30)

Kalten a brand name for amiloride 131 with hydrochlorothiazide 250 (both diuretics 30) and atenolol 140 (a beta blocker 28)

Kamillosan an ointment 116 containing chamomile used for treating nappy rash, sore nipples, and chapped skin

kanamycin an aminoglycoside antibiotic 60

Kannasyn a brand name for kanamycin (an aminoglycoside antibiotic 60)

kaolin an adsorbent used as an antidiarrhoeal 42

Kapake a brand name for paracetamol 325 (a non-opioid analgesic 10)

Karvol a brand name for menthol (a decongestant inhalant 24)

Kay-Cee-L a brand name for potassium (a mineral 91)

Kefadol a brand name for cefamandole (a cephalosporin antibiotic 60)

Keflex a brand name for cefalexin 161 (a cephalosporin antibiotic 60)

Kefzol a brand name for cefazolin (a cephalosporin antibiotic 60)

Kelfizine W a brand name for sulfametopyrazine (a sulphonamide antibacterial 64)

Kemadrin a brand name for procyclidine 340 (an anticholinergic for parkinsonism 18)

Kemicetine a brand name for chloramphenicol 163 (an antibiotic 60)

Kenalog a brand name for triamcinolone (a corticosteroid 78)

Kentene a brand name for piroxicam 333 (a

non-steroidal anti-inflammatory 48 and drug for gout 51)

Keral a brand name for dexketoprofen (a non-steroidal anti-inflammatory 48)

Kerlone a brand name for betaxolol (a beta blocker 28)

ketamine a drug used to induce general anaesthesia

Ketocid a brand name for ketoprofen 268 (a non-steroidal anti-inflammatory 48)

ketoconazole 267 (an antifungal 74)

ketoprofen 268 (a non-steroidal anti-inflammatory 48)

ketorolac a non-steroidal anti-inflammatory 48 used as an analgesic 9

ketotifen a drug similar to sodium cromoglicate 366 for allergies and asthma 56

Ketovail a brand name for ketoprofen 268 (a non-steroidal anti-inflammatory 48)

Ketovite a brand-name vitamin supplement 88

Ketozip XL a brand name for ketoprofen 268 (a non-steroidal anti-inflammatory 48)

Klaricid a brand name for clarithromycin (an antibiotic 60)

Klean-prep a brand-name osmotic laxative 43

Kliofem a brand-name product for menopausal symptoms 86 containing estradiol 224 and norethisterone 316

Kloref a brand-name potassium supplement (a mineral 91)

Kolanticon a brand name for aluminium hydroxide 129 and magnesium oxide (both antacids 40) with dicycloverine 199 (an anticholinergic antispasmodic 43) and dimeticone (an antifoaming agent 40)

Konakion a brand name for phytomenadione (vitamin K)

Konsyl a brand name for ispaghula (a bulk-forming agent for constipation 43 and diarrhoea 42)

Kwells a brand name for hyoscine 252 (used to prevent motion sickness 21)

Kytril a brand name for granisetron (an anti-emetic 21)

L

labetalol a beta blocker 28

Labosept brand-name throat pastilles containing dequalinium (an antibacterial 64)

labour, drugs used in 106

lacidipine a calcium channel blocker 33

Lacri-Lube a brand-name eye ointment for dry eyes 112

lactic acid an ingredient in preparations for warts, emollients 116, and pessaries

lactitol an osmotic laxative 43

Lactugal a brand name for lactulose 270 (a laxative 43)

lactulose 270 (a laxative 43)

Ladropen a brand name for flucloxacillin (a penicillin antibiotic 60)

Lamictal a brand name for lamotrigine 271 (an anticonvulsant 16)

Lamisil a brand name for terbinafine 378 (an antifungal 74)

lamivudine 270 (an antiviral 67 used for HIV/AIDS 97)

lamotrigine 271 (an anticonvulsant 16)

Lamprene a brand name for clofazimine (a drug for leprosy 65)

Lanoxin a brand name for digoxin 202 (a digitalis drug 27)

Lanoxin-PG a brand name for digoxin 202 (a digitalis drug 27)

lanreotide an anticancer drug 94

lansoprazole 272 an anti-ulcer drug 41

Laractone a brand name for spironolactone (a potassium-sparing diuretic 31)

Larafen a brand name for ketoprofen 268 (a non-steroidal anti-inflammatory 48)

Larapam a brand name for piroxicam 333 (a non-steroidal anti-inflammatory 48 and drug for gout 51)

Largactil a brand name for chlorpromazine 167 (a phenothiazine antipsychotic 15 and anti-emetic 21)

Lariam a brand name for mefloquine 289 (an antimalarial 73)

Lasikal a brand name for furosemide 239 (a loop diuretic 31) with potassium (a mineral 91)

Lasilactone a brand name for furosemide 239 with spironolactone (both diuretics 30)

Lasix a brand name for furosemide 239 (a loop diuretic 31)

Lasma a brand name for theophylline 382 (a bronchodilator 23)

Lasonil a brand name for heparinoid (a topical anti-inflammatory 116)

Lasoride a brand name for amiloride 131 (a potassium-sparing diuretic 31) with furosemide 239 (a loop diuretic 31 and antihypertensive 34)

Lassar's Paste a skin preparation for psoriasis 120 containing dithranol, zinc oxide, and salicylic acid

latanoprost a drug for glaucoma 110

laxatives 43

Laxoberal a brand name for sodium picosulfate (a stimulant laxative 43)

Laxose a brand name for lactulose 270 (a laxative 43)

Ledclair a brand name for sodium calcium edetate (an antidote for poisoning with lead and heavy metals)

Lederfen a brand name for fenbufen (a non-steroidal anti-inflammatory 48)

Lederfolin a brand name for folinic acid (a vitamin 88)

Ledermycin a brand name for demeclocycline (a tetracycline antibiotic 60)

Lederspan a brand name for triamcinolone (a corticosteroid 78)

leflunomide an antirheumatic drug 50

Lemsip a brand name for paracetamol 325 (a non-opioid analgesic 10) with phenylephrine (a decongestant 24), chlorphenamine 166 (an antihistamine 56), and caffeine

Lenium a brand-name dandruff shampoo 122 containing selenium (a mineral 91)

lenograstim a blood growth stimulant

Lentard MC a brand name for insulin 258 (a drug for diabetes 80)

Lentaron a brand name for formestane (a drug for breast cancer 94)

Lentizol a brand name for amitriptyline 134 (a tricyclic antidepressant 14)

lepirudin an anticoagulant 36

lercanidipine a calcium channel blocker 33

Lescol a brand name for fluvastatin (a lipid-lowering drug 35)

letrozole an anticancer drug 94

Leucovorin see calcium folinate 88

Leukeran a brand name for chlorambucil (an anticancer drug 94)

leukotriene antagonists 58 (treatments for allergy 56)

leuprorelin a drug for menstrual disorders 100

levamisole an anthelmintic 76

levobunolol a beta blocker 28 and drug for glaucoma 110

levocabastine a topical antihistamine 116

levodopa 273 (a drug for parkinsonism 18)

levofloxacin 275 (an antibacterial 64)

levomepromazine previously known as methotrimeprazine (an antipsychotic 15)

levonorgestrel 276 (a female sex hormone 86 and oral contraceptive 101)

levothyroxine previously known as thyroxine 384 (a thyroid hormone 82)

Librium a brand name for chlordiazepoxide 164 (a benzodiazepine anti-anxiety drug 13)

lidocaine previously known as lignocaine (a local anaesthetic 11, anti-arrhythmic 32, and antipruritic 114)

lignocaine see lidocaine

Li-liquid a brand name for lithium 278 (a drug for mania 16)

lincosamides 62 (antibiotics 60)

lindane a topical antiparasitic 118

Lingraine a brand name for ergotamine 221 (a drug for migraine 20)

Lioresal a brand name for baclofen 145 (a muscle relaxant 52)

liothyronine a thyroid hormone 82

Lipantil a brand name for fenofibrate (a lipid-lowering drug 35)

lipid-lowering drugs 35

Lipitor a brand name for atorvastatin 141 (a lipid-lowering drug 35)

Lipostat a brand name for pravastatin 336 (a cholesterol-lowering agent 35)

liquid paraffin a lubricating agent used as a laxative 43 and in artificial tear preparations 112

Liquifilm Tears brand-name eye drops containing polyvinyl acetate (artificial tears 112)

liquorice a substance for peptic ulcers 41

lisinopril 277 (an ACE inhibitor vasodilator 30)

Liskonum a brand name for lithium 278 (a drug for mania 16)

lisuride a drug for parkinsonism 18

Litarex a brand name for lithium 278 (a drug for mania 16)

lithium 278 (an antimanic drug 16)

Livial a brand name for tibolone 385 (a female sex hormone 86)

Livostin a brand name for levocabastine (an antihistamine 56)

Locabiotal a brand name for fusafungine (an antibacterial 64 and anti-inflammatory agent 48)

48)

local anaesthetics 11 (analgesics 9)

Loceryl a brand name for amorolfine (an antifungal 74)

Locoid a brand name for hydrocortisone 251 (a corticosteroid 78)

Locorten-Vioform a brand name for clioquinol (an anti-infective skin preparation 116) with flumetasone (a corticosteroid 78)

Lodine SR a brand name for etodolac (a non-steroidal anti-inflammatory 48)

Iodoxamide an anti-allergy drug 56

Loestrin 20 a brand-name oral contraceptive 101 containing ethinylestradiol 226 and norethisterone 316

lofepramine 279 (a tricyclic antidepressant 14)

Logynon a brand-name oral contraceptive 101 containing ethinylestradiol 226 and levonorgestrel 276

Lomexin a brand name for fenticonazole (an antifungal 74)

Lomotil a brand-name antidiarrhoeal 42 containing atropine 142 and diphenoxylate 204

lomustine an alkylating agent for Hodgkin's disease 94

Loniten a brand name for minoxidil 305 (an antihypertensive 34)

loop diuretics 31

Loperagen a brand name for loperamide 280 (an antidiarrhoeal 42)

loperamide 280 (an antidiarrhoeal 42)

Lopid a brand name for gemfibrozil (a lipid-lowering drug 35)

loprazolam a benzodiazepine sleeping drug 11

Lopresor a brand name for metoprolol 300 (a cardioselective beta blocker 28)

loratadine 281 (an antihistamine 56)

lorazepam a benzodiazepine anti-anxiety drug 13 and sleeping drug 11

lormetazepam a benzodiazepine sleeping drug 11

losartan 282 (an antihypertensive 34)

Losec a brand name for omeprazole 320 (an anti-ulcer drug 41)

Lotriderm a brand-name product containing betamethasone 150 (a corticosteroid 78) and clotrimazole 181 (an antifungal 74)

Loxapac a brand name for loxapine (an antipsychotic 15)

loxapine an antipsychotic 15

Luborant a brand name for artificial saliva

Ludiomil a brand name for maprotiline (an antidepressant 14)

Lugol's solution an iodine solution for an overactive thyroid gland 82

Lustral a brand name for sertraline (an antidepressant 14)

luteinizing hormone (LH) an infertility drug 105

Lyclear a brand name for permethrin 327 (a topical antiparasitic 118)

lymecycline a tetracycline antibiotic 60

M

Maalox a brand-name antacid containing aluminium hydroxide 129 and magnesium hydroxide 284

Maalox Plus a brand-name antacid containing aluminium hydroxide 129, magnesium hydroxide 284, and dimeticone

Mabthera a brand name for rituximab (an anticancer drug 94)

Macrobid a brand name for nitrofurantoin (an antibacterial 64)

Macrodantin a brand name for nitrofurantoin (an antibacterial 64)

macrolides 62 (a class of antibiotic 60)

Madopar a brand name for levodopa 273 (a drug for parkinsonism 18) with benserazide (a drug that enhances the effect of levodopa)

Magnapen a brand name for ampicillin with flucloxacillin (both penicillin antibiotics 60)

magnesium a mineral 91

magnesium alginate an antifoaming agent 40

magnesium carbonate an antacid 40

magnesium citrate an osmotic laxative 43

magnesium compounds antacids 40

magnesium hydroxide 284 (an antacid 40 and laxative 43)

magnesium oxide an antacid 40

magnesium sulphate an osmotic laxative 43

magnesium trisilicate an antacid 40

malathion 285 (an antiparasitic 118 for head lice and scabies infestation)

male sex hormones 85 (drugs for infertility 105)

Malix a brand name for glibenclamide 243 (an oral antidiabetic 80)

Maloprim a brand-name antimalarial 73 containing dapsone and pyrimethamine 348

Manerix a brand name for moclobemide (a

ible MAOI antidepressant 14)

Manevac a brand name for ispaghula (a bulk-forming agent 40) with senna (a stimulant laxative 43)

mannitol an osmotic diuretic 31

MAOIs see monoamine oxidase inhibitors 14

maprotiline an antidepressant 14

Marcain a brand name for bupivacaine (a local anaesthetic 11 used in labour 106)

Marevan a brand name for warfarin 398 (an anticoagulant 36)

Marvelon a brand-name oral contraceptive 101 containing ethinylestradiol 226 and desogestrel

Masnoderm a brand name for clotrimazole 181 (an antifungal 74)

Maxalt a brand name for rizatriptan (a drug for migraine 20)

Maxepa a brand name for concentrated fish oils (used to reduce fats in the blood 35)

Maxidex a brand name for dexamethasone 195 (a corticosteroid 78) with hypromellose (a substance in artificial tear preparations 112)

Maxitrol a brand name for dexamethasone 195 (a corticosteroid 78) with hypromellose (a substance used in artificial tear preparations 112) and neomycin and polymyxin B (both antibiotics 60)

Maxivent a brand name for salbutamol 361 (a bronchodilator 23)

Maxolon a brand name for metoclopramide 299 (a gastrointestinal motility regulator and anti-emetic 21)

Maxtrex a brand name for methotrexate 296 (an antimetabolite anticancer drug 94)

MCR-50 a brand name for isosorbide mononitrate 264 (a nitrate vasodilator 30 and anti-angina drug 33)

MCT Oil used to treat cystic fibrosis

mebendazole an anthelmintic 76

mebeverine 285 (an antispasmodic for irritable bowel syndrome 43)

meclozine an antihistamine 56 used for travel sickness

mecysteine a mucolytic for coughs 25

Medijel a brand name for a pain-relieving mouth gel containing lidocaine (a local anaesthetic 11) and aminacrine (a skin antiseptic 116)

Medinex a brand name for diphenhydramine (an antihistamine 56)

Medinol a brand name for paracetamol 325 (a

non-opioid analgesic 10)

Medised a brand name for paracetamol 325 (a non-opioid analgesic 10) with promethazine 343 (an antihistamine 56 and anti-emetic 21)

Medrone a brand name for methylprednisolone (a corticosteroid 78)

medroxyprogesterone 286 (a female sex hormone 86 and anticancer drug 94)

mefenamic acid 287 (a non-steroidal anti-inflammatory 48)

mefloquine 289 (an antimalarial 73)

Mefoxin a brand name for cefoxitin (a cephalosporin antibiotic 60)

mefruside a thiazide-like diuretic 30

Megace a brand name for megestrol 290 (a female sex hormone 86 and anticancer drug 94)

megestrol 290 (a female sex hormone 86 and anticancer drug 94)

melatonin a hormone 78

Melleril a brand name for thioridazine 383 (a phenothiazine antipsychotic 15)

meloxicam 291 a non-steroidal anti-inflammatory drug 48 and non-opioid analgesic 10

melphalan an alkylating agent for multiple myeloma 94

menadiol vitamin K (a vitamin 88)

meningitis, drugs for 64

Menorest a brand name for estradiol 224 (an oestrogen 86)

menotrophin also known as human menopausal gonadotrophins (a drug for infertility 105)

menstrual disorders, drugs used to treat 100

menthol an alcohol from mint oils used as an inhalation and topical antipruritic 114

mepacrine an antiprotozoal 71 (for giardiasis)

mepivacaine a local anaesthetic 11

meprobamate an anti-anxiety drug 13

meptazinol an opioid analgesic 11

Meptid a brand name for meptazinol (an opioid analgesic 11)

mequitazine an antihistamine 56

Merbentyl a brand name for dicycloverine 199 (a drug for irritable bowel syndrome 43)

mercaptopurine 292 (an anticancer drug 94)

Mercilon a brand-name oral contraceptive 101 containing ethinylestradiol 226 and desogestrel

Merocaine Lozenges a brand-name preparation for sore throat and minor mouth infections, containing benzocaine (a local anaesthetic 11) and cetylpyridinium (a topical antiseptic 116)

Merocet a brand name for cetylpyridinium (a topical antiseptic 116)

mesalazine 293 (a drug for ulcerative colitis 44)

mesna a drug used to protect the urinary tract from damage caused by some anticancer drugs 94

mesterolone a male sex hormone 85

Mestinon a brand name for pyridostigmine 347 (a drug for myasthenia gravis 53)

mestranol an oestrogen 86 and oral contraceptive 101

metaraminol a drug used to treat hypotension (low blood pressure)

Metenix-5 a brand name for metolazone (a thiazide-like diuretic 30)

metformin 294 (a drug for diabetes 80)

methadone 295 (an opioid used as an analgesic 9 and to treat heroin dependence)

Methadose a brand name for methadone 295 (an opioid used as an analgesic 9 and to ease heroin withdrawal)

Metharose a brand name for methadone 295 (an opioid used as an analgesic 9 and to ease heroin withdrawal)

methenamine a drug for urinary tract infections 108

Methex a brand name for methadone 295 (an opioid used as an analgesic 9 and to ease heroin withdrawal)

methionine an antidote for paracetamol 325 poisoning

methocarbamol a muscle relaxant 52

methohexital a barbiturate used to induce general anaesthesia

methotrexate 296 (an antimetabolite anticancer drug 94)

methotrimeprazine see levomepromazine (an antipsychotic 15)

methoxamine a drug used to treat hypotension (low blood pressure)

methoxsalen a drug for psoriasis 120

methylcellulose 297 (a laxative 43, antidiarrhoeal 42, and artificial tear preparation 112)

methyldopa 298 (an antihypertensive 34)

methylphenidate a drug used to treat hyperactivity in children

methylphenobarbital a barbiturate anticonvulsant 16

methylprednisolone a corticosteroid 78

methyl salicylate a topical analgesic 9 for muscle and joint pain

methysergide a drug to prevent migraine 20

metipranolol a beta blocker 28 for glaucoma 110

metirosine a drug for phaeochromocytoma (a tumour of the adrenal glands 94)

metoclopramide 299 (a gastrointestinal motility regulator and anti-emetic 21)

metolazone a thiazide-like diuretic 30

Metopirone a brand name for metyrapone (a diuretic 30)

metoprolol 300 a beta blocker 28

Metosyn a brand name for fluocinonide (a topical corticosteroid 116)

Metrodin a brand name for urofollitropin (a drug for pituitary disorders 83)

Metrogel a brand name for topical metronidazole 301 (an antibacterial 64)

Metrolyl a brand name for metronidazole 301 (an antibacterial 64 and antiprotozoal 71)

metronidazole 301 (an antibacterial 64 and antiprotozoal 71)

Metrotop a brand name for topical metronidazole 301 (an antibacterial 64)

metyrapone a diuretic 30 used to reduce fluid retention in Cushing's disease

mexiletine an anti-arrhythmic 32

Mexitil a brand name for mexiletine (an anti-arrhythmic 32)

mianserin an antidepressant 14

miconazole 302 (an antifungal 74)

Microgynon 30 a brand-name oral contraceptive 101 containing ethinylestradiol 226 and levonorgestrel 276

Micronor a brand-name oral contraceptive 101 containing norethisterone 316

Microval a brand-name oral contraceptive 101 containing levonorgestrel 276

Mictral a brand-name drug for urinary tract infections 108 containing nalidixic acid (an antibacterial 64) and sodium bicarbonate 365 (an antacid 40)

Midamor a brand name for amiloride 131 (a potassium-sparing diuretic 31)

midazolam a benzodiazepine 11 used as premedication

Midrid a brand-name drug for migraine 20 containing paracetamol 325 and isometheptene mucate

mifepristone a drug used during labour 106

ugs used for 20

Migraleve a brand-name drug for migraine 20 containing codeine 183, paracetamol 325, and buclizine

Migranal a brand name for dihydroergotamine (a drug for migraine 20)

Migravess a brand-name drug for migraine 20 containing aspirin 138 and metoclopramide 299

Migril a brand-name drug for migraine 20 containing ergotamine 221, caffeine, and cyclizine

Milk of Magnesia a brand name for magnesium hydroxide 284 (an antacid 40 and laxative 43)

Milpar a brand-name laxative 43 containing magnesium hydroxide 284 and liquid paraffin

milrinone a drug used for its vasodilator effects 30

mineral requirements 91

minerals 91

minerals, main food sources of (table) 92

Minihep a brand name for heparin 249 (an anticoagulant 36)

Minims Atropine a brand name for atropine 142 (a mydriatic 112)

Minims Chloramphenicol a brand name for chloramphenicol 163 (an antibiotic 60)

Minims Cyclopentolate a brand name for cyclopentolate (an anticholinergic mydriatic 112)

Minims Gentamicin a brand name for gentamicin 241 (an aminoglycoside antibiotic 60)

Minims Phenylephrine a brand name for phenylephrine (a decongestant 24)

Minims Pilocarpine a brand name for pilocarpine 332 (a miotic for glaucoma 110)

Minims Prednisolone a brand name for prednisolone 337 (a corticosteroid 78)

Minitran a brand name for glyceryl trinitrate 245 (an anti-angina drug 33)

Minocin a brand name for minocycline 303 (a tetracycline antibiotic 60)

minocycline 303 (a tetracycline antibiotic 60)

Minodiab a brand name for glipizide (an oral antidiabetic 80)

minoxidil 305 (an antihypertensive 34)

Mintec a brand name for peppermint oil (a substance for irritable bowel syndrome 43)

Mintezol a brand name for tiabendazole (an anthelmintic 76)

Minulet a brand-name oral contraceptive 101 containing ethinylestradiol 226 and gestodene

miotics drugs affecting the pupil 112 and for glaucoma 110

Mirapexin a brand name for pramipexole (a drug for parkinsonism 18)

Mirena an intrauterine contraceptive device 101 containing levonorgestrel 276 (a female sex hormone 86)

mirtazapine an antidepressant 14

misoprostol 306 (an anti-ulcer drug 41)

Mistamine a brand name for mizolastine an antihistamine 56

mitobronitol an anticancer drug 94

mitomycin a cytotoxic antibiotic for breast and stomach cancer 94

mitoxantrone previously known as mitozantrone (an anticancer drug 94)

mitozantrone see mitoxantrone

mivacurium a drug used to relax muscles during general anaesthesia

Mixtard a brand name for insulin 258 (a drug for diabetes 80)

mizolastine an antihistamine 56

Mizollen a brand name for mizolastine (an antihistamine 56)

Mobic a brand name for meloxicam 291 (a non-steroidal anti-inflammatory drug 48 and non-opioid analgesic 10)

Mobiflex a brand name for tenoxicam (a non-steroidal anti-inflammatory 48)

moclobemide a reversible MAOI antidepressant 14

modafinil a drug for narcolepsy 19

Modalim a brand name for ciprofibrate (a lipid-lowering drug 35)

Modaplate a brand name for dipyridamole 205 (an antiplatelet drug 36)

Modecate a brand name for fluphenazine (an antipsychotic 15)

Moditen a brand name for fluphenazine (an antipsychotic 15)

Modrasone a brand name for alclometasone (a topical corticosteroid 116)

Modrenal a brand name for trilostane (an adrenal antagonist used for Cushing's syndrome (an adrenal disorder 78) and for breast cancer 94

Moducren a brand-name antihypertensive 34 containing amiloride 131, hydrochlorothiazide 250, and timolol 386

Moduret-25 a brand name for amiloride 131 with hydrochlorothiazide 250 (both diuretics 30)

Moduretic a brand name for amiloride 131 with hydrochlorothiazide 250 (both diuretics 30)

moexipril an ACE inhibitor vasodilator 30

Mogadon a brand name for nitrazepam (a benzodiazepine sleeping drug 11)

molgramostim a blood growth stimulant

Molipaxin a brand name for trazodone 391 (an antidepressant 14)

molybdenum a mineral 91 required in minute amounts in the diet, poisonous if ingested in large quantities

mometasone 307 a topical corticosteroid 116

Monit a brand name for isosorbide mononitrate 264 (a nitrate vasodilator 30 and anti-angina drug 33)

monoamine oxidase inhibitors (MAOIs) a type of antidepressant 14

Mono-Cedocard a brand name for isosorbide mononitrate 264 (a nitrate vasodilator 30 and anti-angina drug 33)

Monoclate-P a brand name for factor VIII (a blood extract used to promote blood clotting 37)

Monocor a brand name for bisoprolol (a beta blocker 28)

Monoparin, Monoparin CA brand names for heparin 249 (an anti-coagulant 36)

monosulfiram an antiparasitic 118 for scabies

Monotrim a brand name for trimethoprim 393 (an antibacterial 64)

Monovent a brand name for terbutaline 379 (a bronchodilator 23 and drug for premature labour 106)

Monozide 10 a brand name for bisoprolol (a beta blocker 28) with hydrochlorothiazide 250 (a thiazide diuretic 31)

Monphytol a brand-name antifungal 74 for athlete's foot

montelukast 308 a leukotriene antagonist for asthma 56 and bronchospasm 23

moracizine an anti-arrhythmic agent 32

morphine 308 (an opioid analgesic 11)

Motens a brand name for lacidipine (a calcium channel blocker 33)

Motifene a brand name for diclofenac 197 (a non-steroidal anti-inflammatory drug 48)

Motilium a brand name for domperidone 207

(an anti-emetic 21)

Motipress a brand name for fluphenazine (an antipsychotic 15) with nortriptyline (a tricyclic antidepressant 14)

Motival a brand name for fluphenazine (an antipsychotic 15) with nortriptyline (a tricyclic antidepressant 14)

Motrin a brand name for ibuprofen 254 (a non-steroidal anti-inflammatory 48)

Movelat a brand-name topical preparation 116 containing mucopolysaccharide and salicylic acid

Movicol an osmotic laxative 43

moxisylyte previously known as thymoxamine (a drug used to reduce pupil size after examination 112 and as a vasodilator 30 to improve blood supply to the limbs)

moxonidine 310 (a centrally acting antihypertensive 34)

MST Continus a brand name for morphine 308 (an opioid analgesic 11)

Mucaine a brand-name antacid 40 containing aluminium hydroxide 129, magnesium hydroxide 284, and oxetacaine

Mucodyne a brand name for carbocisteine (a mucolytic decongestant 25)

Mucogel a brand-name antacid 40 containing aluminium hydroxide 129 and magnesium hydroxide 284

mucolytics drugs to treat coughs 25

Mu-Cron Tablets a brand name for phenylpropanolamine 330 (a decongestant 24) with paracetamol 325 (a non-opioid analgesic 10)

Multiparin a brand name for heparin 249 (an anticoagulant 36)

mupirocin an antibacterial for skin infections 116

muscle relaxants 52 (used in labour 106 as uterine muscle relaxants 107)

mustine see chlormethine (a drug for Hodgkin's disease 94)

MXL a brand name for morphine sulphate 308 (an opioid analgesic 11)

Myambutol a brand name for ethambutol 225 (an antituberculous drug 65)

myasthenia gravis, drugs used for 53

Mycil Gold a brand name for clotrimazole 181 (an antifungal 74)

Mycobutin a brand name for rifabutin (an antituberculous drug 65)

mycophenolate mofetil an immunosuppressant drug 96

nd name for undecanoate acid
(an antifungal 74)

Mydriacyl a brand name for tropicamide (a mydriatic 112)

mydriatics drugs affecting the pupils 112

Mydrilate a brand name for cyclopentolate (an anticholinergic mydriatic 112)

Myelobromol a brand name for mitobronitol (an anticancer drug 94)

Myocrisin a brand name for sodium aurothiomalate (an antirheumatic 50)

Myotonine a brand name for bethanechol (a parasympathomimetic for urinary retention 108)

Mysoline a brand name for primidone 338 (an anticonvulsant 16)

N

nabilone an anti-emetic 21 derived from marijuana for nausea and vomiting induced by anticancer drugs 94

nabumetone a non-steroidal anti-inflammatory 48

nadolol a beta blocker 28

nafarelin a drug for menstrual disorders 100

naftidrofuryl 311 a vasodilator 30

nalbuphine an opioid analgesic 11

Nalcrom a brand name for sodium cromoglicate 366 (an anti-allergy drug 56)

nalidixic acid an antibacterial 64

naloxone an antidote for opioid poisoning

nandrolone an anabolic steroid 85

Napratec a brand name for an antirheumatic drug containing naproxen 311 (a non-steroidal anti-inflammatory 48 and drug for gout 51) and misoprostol 306 (an anti-ulcer drug 41)

Naprosyn a brand name for naproxen 311 (a non-steroidal anti-inflammatory 48 and drug for gout 51)

naproxen 311 (a non-steroidal anti-inflammatory 48 and drug for gout 51)

Naramig a brand name for naratriptan (a drug for migraine 20)

naratriptan a drug for migraine 20

Narcan a brand name for naloxone (an antidote for opioid poisoning)

Nardil a brand name for phenelzine (an MAOI antidepressant 14)

Naropin a brand name for ropivacaine (local anaesthetic 11)

Narphen a brand name for phenazocine (an opioid analgesic 11)

Naseptin a brand name for chlorhexidine (a skin antiseptic 116) with neomycin (an aminoglycoside antibiotic 60)

Nasonex a brand name for mometasone 307 (a topical corticosteroid 116)

Natrilix a brand name for indapamide 256 (a thiazide-like diuretic 30)

Navidrex a brand name for cyclopenthiazide 190 (a thiazide diuretic 31)

Navispare a brand name for cyclopenthiazide 190 with amiloride 131 (both diuretics 30)

Navoban a brand name for tropisetron (an anti-emetic 21)

Nebcin a brand name for tobramycin (an aminoglycoside antibiotic 60)

Nebilet a brand name for nebivolol (a beta blocker 28 antihypertensive 34)

nebivolol a beta blocker 28 antihypertensive 34

nedocromil a drug similar to sodium cromoglicate 366 used to prevent asthma attacks

nefazodone an antidepressant 14

nefopam a non-opioid analgesic 10

Negram a brand name for nalidixic acid (an antibacterial 64)

nelfinavir an antiviral for HIV/AIDS 97

Neo-Bendromax a brand of bendroflumethiazide 147 (a thiazide diuretic 31)

Neogest a brand name for norgestrel (a female sex hormone 86)

Neo-Mercazole a brand name for carbimazole 160 (an antithyroid drug 82)

neomycin an aminoglycoside antibiotic 60 used in ear drops 113

Neo-NaClex a brand name for bendroflumethiazide 147 (a thiazide diuretic 31)

Neo-NaClex-K a brand name for bendroflumethiazide 147 (a thiazide diuretic 31) with potassium

Neoral a brand name for ciclosporin 170 (an immunosuppressant 96)

NeoRecormon a brand name for epoetin 220 (a kidney hormone 78)

Neosporin a brand name for gramicidin with neomycin and polymyxin B (all antibiotics 60)

neostigmine a drug for myasthenia gravis 53

Neotigason a brand name for acitretin (a drug

for psoriasis 120)

Nephril a brand name for polythiazide (a thiazide diuretic 31)

Nericur a brand name for benzoyl peroxide 148 (a drug for acne 119)

Nerisone a brand name for diflucortolone (a topical corticosteroid 116)

nervous system stimulants 19

Netillin a brand name for netilmicin (an aminoglycoside antibiotic 60)

netilmicin an aminoglycoside antibiotic 60

Neulactil a brand name for pericyazine (an antipsychotic 15)

Neupogen a brand name for filgrastim 230 (a blood growth stimulant)

Neurontin a brand name for gabapentin (an anticonvulsant 16)

Neutrexin a brand name for trimetrexate (an antimicrobial for pneumocystis pneumonia in AIDS 71)

niacinamide also known as nicotinamide (a vitamin 88)

niacin nicotinic acid (a vitamin 88)

nicardipine a calcium channel blocker 33

niclosamide an anthelmintic 76 for tapeworm infestation

nicorandil 313 (an anti-angina drug 33)

Nicorette a brand name for nicotine given as a drug for relief of smoking withdrawal symptoms

nicotinamide a B vitamin (a vitamin 88)

nicotine 314 (a nervous system stimulant 19)

Nicotinell a brand name for nicotine given as a drug for relief of smoking withdrawal symptoms

nicotinic acid a vasodilator 30, lipid-lowering drug 35, and vitamin 88

nicotinyl alcohol tartrate niacin (a vitamin 88)

nicoumalone see acenocoumarol (an anticoagulant 36)

nifedipine 315 (a calcium channel blocker 33)

Niferex a brand name for iron (a mineral 91)

Night Nurse a brand-name preparation for relief of cold symptoms, containing paracetamol 325 (a non-opioid analgesic 10) with promethazine 343 (an antihistamine 56 and anti-emetic 21)

nikethamide a respiratory stimulant 19

nimodipine a calcium channel blocker 33

Nindaxa a brand name for indapamide 256 (a thiazide-like diuretic 30)

Nipent a brand name for pentostatin (an anticancer drug 94)

nisoldipine a calcium channel blocker 33

nitrates vasodilators 30 used as anti-angina drugs 33

nitrates vasodilators 30

nitrazepam a benzodiazepine sleeping drug 11

Nitrocine a brand name for glyceryl trinitrate 245 (an anti-angina drug 33)

Nitro-Dur a brand name for glyceryl trinitrate 245 (an anti-angina drug 33)

nitrofurantoin an antibacterial 64

Nitrolingual a brand name for glyceryl trinitrate 245 (an anti-angina drug 33)

Nitronal a brand name for glyceryl trinitrate 245 (an anti-angina drug 33)

nitroprusside antihypertensive 34

nitrous oxide an anaesthetic gas

Nivaquine a brand name for chloroquine 165 (an antimalarial 73 and antirheumatic 50)

Nivemycin a brand name for neomycin (an aminoglycoside antibiotic 60)

nizatidine an anti-ulcer drug 41

Nizoral a brand name for ketoconazole 267 (an antifungal 74)

Nolvadex a brand name for tamoxifen 375 (an anticancer drug 94)

Nolvadex Forte a brand name for tamoxifen 375 (an anticancer drug 94)

non-cardioselective drugs a type of beta blocker 28

non-nucleoside reverse transcriptase inhibitors 98 (drugs for HIV and AIDS 97)

non-opioid analgesics 10

nonoxinol "9" (a spermicidal agent 101)

non-steroidal anti-inflammatory drugs (NSAIDs) 48 (analgesics 10 used for menstrual disorders 100 and as antirheumatic drugs 50)

nontocog alfa a synthetic form of factor IX to promote blood clotting 36

Nootropil a brand name for piracetam (an anticonvulsant 16)

noradrenaline see norepinephrine

Norditropin a brand name for somatropin (a synthetic pituitary hormone 83)

norepinephrine previously known as noradrenaline (a drug similar to epinephrine 219 used to raise blood pressure during anaphylactic shock)

norethisterone 316 (a female sex hormone 86 and oral contraceptive 101)

norfloxacin an antibiotic 60

Norgalax a brand name for docusate (a

stimulant laxative 43)

norgestimate an oral contraceptive 101

Norgeston a brand-name oral contraceptive 101 containing levonorgestrel 276

norgestrel a progestogen 86

Noriday a brand-name oral contraceptive 101 containing norethisterone 316

Norimin a brand-name oral contraceptive 101 containing ethinylestradiol 226 and norethisterone 316

Norimode a brand name for loperamide 280 (an antidiarrhoeal 42)

Norinyl-1 a brand-name oral contraceptive 101 containing norethisterone 316 and mestranol

Noristerat a brand-name injectable contraceptive 101 containing norethisterone 316 (a female sex hormone 86)

Normacol Plus a brand name for frangula with sterculia (both laxatives 43)

Normax a brand name for dantron and docusate (both laxatives 43)

Normosang a brand name for haem arginate (a drug to treat porphyria)

Norplant a brand name for levonorgestrel 276 (a female sex hormone 86)

Norprolac a brand name for quinagolide (a drug used for infertility 105)

nortriptyline a tricyclic antidepressant 14

Norvir a brand name for ritonavir (an antiviral for HIV/AIDS 97)

NovoNorm a brand name for repaglinide 356 an oral antidiabetic 80

Nozinan a brand name for methotrimeprazine (an antipsychotic 15)

NSAIDs see non-steroidal anti-inflammatory drugs 48

Nubain a brand name for nalbuphine (an opioid analgesic 11)

nucleoside reverse transcriptase inhibitors 98 (drugs for HIV and AIDS 97)

Nuelin a brand name for theophylline 382 (a bronchodilator 23)

Nulacin a brand-name antacid 40 containing calcium carbonate, magnesium carbonate, magnesium trisilicate, and magnesium oxide

Nupercainal a brand name for cinchocaine (a local anaesthetic 11)

Nurofen a brand name for ibuprofen 254 (a non-opioid analgesic 10 and non-steroidal anti-inflammatory 48)

Nurofen Plus a brand name for ibuprofen 254 (a non-steroidal anti-inflammatory drug 48) with codeine 183 (an opioid analgesic 11)

Nu-Seals Aspirin a brand name for aspirin 138 (a non-opioid analgesic 10 and antiplatelet drug 36)

Nutraplus a brand name for urea (an emollient)

Nutrizym GR a brand name for pancreatin (a preparation of pancreatic enzymes 46)

Nuvelle a brand name for estradiol 224 and levonorgestrel 276 (both female sex hormones 86)

Nycopren a brand name for naproxen 311 (a non-steroidal anti-inflammatory 48 and drug for gout 51)

Nylax a brand-name stimulant laxative 43

Nystadermal a brand name for nystatin 317 (an antifungal 74) with triamcinolone (a corticosteroid 78)

Nystaform a brand name for nystatin 317 (an antifungal 74) with chlorhexidine (a skin antiseptic 116)

Nystaform-HC a brand name for hydrocortisone 251 (a corticosteroid 78) with nystatin 317 (an antifungal 74) and chlorhexidine (a skin antiseptic 116)

Nystamont a brand name for nystatin 317 (an antifungal 74)

Nystan a brand name for nystatin 317 (an antifungal 74)

nystatin 317 (an antifungal 74)

Nytol a brand-name preparation for sleep disturbance containing diphenhydramine (an antihistamine 56)

O

Occlusal a brand name for salicylic acid (a wart remover)

Octapressin a brand name for felypressin (a vasoconstrictor 27 used in dentistry)

octocog alfa a synthetic form of factor VIII to promote blood clotting 36

octoxinol a spermicidal agent 101

octreotide a synthetic pituitary hormone 83 used to relieve symptoms of cancer of the pancreas 94

Ocufen a brand name for flurbiprofen (a non-steroidal anti-inflammatory 48)

Ocusert Pilo a brand name for pilocarpine 332

(a miotic for glaucoma 110)

Odrik a brand name for trandolapril (an ACE inhibitor vasodilator 30)

Oestrifen a brand name for tamoxifen 375 (an anticancer drug 94)

Oestrogel a brand name for estradiol 224 (an oestrogen 86)

oestrogen a female sex hormone 86

oestrogens synthetic female sex hormones 86

ofloxacin an antibiotic 60

Oilatum Emollient a brand-name bath additive containing liquid paraffin for dry skin conditions

Oilatum Gel a brand name for a shower gel containing liquid paraffin for dry skin conditions

olanzapine 319 (an antipsychotic 15)

Olbetam a brand name for acipimox (a lipid-lowering drug 35)

olsalazine a drug for ulcerative colitis 44

omeprazole 320 (an anti-ulcer drug 41)

Oncovin a brand name for vincristine (an anticancer drug 94)

ondansetron 321 (an anti-emetic 21)

One-Alpha a brand name for alfacalcidol (a vitamin 88)

Opilon a brand name for moxisylyte (a vasodilator 30)

opioid analgesics 11 (used for pain relief in labour 107)

opioids antidiarrhoeal drugs 42

opium tincture morphine 308 (an opioid analgesic 11)

Opticrom a brand name for sodium cromoglicate 366 (an anti-allergy drug 56)

Optimine a brand name for azatadine (an antihistamine 56)

Optrex Eye Lotion a brand-name preparation containing witch hazel (an astringent)

Opumide a brand name for indapamide 256 (a thiazide-like diuretic 30)

Orabase a brand-name ointment to protect the skin or mouth from damage

Orabet a brand name for metformin 294 (a drug for diabetes 80)

oral contraceptives 101 (used for acne 119)

oral contraceptives, hormone content of common (table)102

Oraldene a brand name antiseptic mouthwash containing hexetidine

Oramorph a brand name for morphine 308 (an

Orap a brand name for pimozide (an antipsychotic 15)

orciprenaline a sympathomimetic used as a bronchodilator 23

Orelox a brand name for cefpodoxime (a cephalosporin antibiotic 60)

Orgaran a brand name for danaparoid (an anticoagulant 36)

Orimeten a brand name for aminoglutethimide (an anticancer drug 94)

Orlept a brand name for sodium valproate 367 (an anticonvulsant 16)

orlistat 321 (an anti-obesity drug 88)

Orovite a brand-name multivitamin 88

orphenadrine 322 (an anticholinergic muscle relaxant 52 and drug for parkinsonism 18)

Ortho-Creme a brand name for nonoxinol "9" (a spermicidal agent 101)

Ortho-Dienoestrol a brand name for dienestrol (a female sex hormone 86)

Orthoforms a brand name for nonoxinol "9" (a spermicidal agent 101)

Ortho-Gynest a brand name for estriol (an oestrogen 86)

Orudis a brand name for ketoprofen 268 (a non-steroidal anti-inflammatory 48)

Oruvail a brand name for ketoprofen 268 (a non-steroidal anti-inflammatory 48)

Osmolax a brand name for lactulose 270 (a laxative 43)

osmotic diuretics 31

osmotic laxatives 43

Ossopan a brand name for hydroxyapatite (a calcium supplement used to treat bone disorders 54)

Ostram a brand name for calcium phosphate (a mineral 91)

Otomize a brand name for dexamethasone 195 (a corticosteroid 78) and neomycin (an aminoglycoside antibiotic 60)

Otosporin a brand name for hydrocortisone 251 (a corticosteroid 78) with neomycin and polymyxin B (both antibiotics 60)

Otrivine-Antistin a brand name for antazoline (an antihistamine 56) with xylometazoline (a decongestant 24)

Otrivine a brand name for xylometazoline (a decongestant 24)

Ovestin a brand name for estriol (an oestrogen 86)

Ovex a brand name for mebendazole (an

anthelmintic 76)

Ovran a brand-name oral contraceptive 101 containing ethinylestradiol 226 and levonorgestrel 276

Ovranette a brand-name oral contraceptive 101 containing ethinylestradiol 226 and levonorgestrel 276

Ovysmen a brand-name oral contraceptive 101 containing ethinylestradiol 226 and norethisterone 316

oxaliplatin an anticancer drug 94

oxazepam a benzodiazepine anti-anxiety drug 13

oxerutin a drug used to treat peripheral vascular disease 30

oxetacaine a local anaesthetic 11 used with antacids 40 for reflux oesophagitis

oxitropium a bronchodilator 23

Oxivent a brand name for oxitropium (a bronchodilator 23)

oxpentifylline see pentoxifylline (a vasodilator 30 used to improve blood flow to the limbs in peripheral vascular disease)

oxprenolol a beta blocker 28

oxybenzone a sunscreen 123

oxybuprocaine a local anaesthetic 11

oxybutynin 323 (an anticholinergic and antispasmodic for urinary disorders 108)

oxycodone an opioid analgesic 11

oxymetazoline a topical decongestant 24 also used for ear disorders 113

Oxymycin a brand name for oxytetracycline (a tetracycline antibiotic 60)

oxypertine an antipsychotic 15

oxytetracycline a tetracycline antibiotic 60

oxytocin a uterine stimulant 106

P

paclitaxel an anticancer drug 94

painkillers see analgesics 9

Paldesic a brand name for paracetamol 325 (a non-opioid analgesic 10)

Palfium a brand name for dextromoramide (an opioid analgesic 11)

palivizumab an antiviral drug 67

Palladone a brand name for hydromorphone (an opioid analgesic 11)

Paludrine a brand name for proguanil 341 (an antimalarial 73)

Pamergan P100 a brand name for pethidine (an opioid analgesic 11) with promethazine 343 (an antihistamine 56 and anti-emetic 21)

pamidronate a drug for bone disorders 54

Panadeine a brand name for paracetamol 325 (a non-opioid analgesic 10) with codeine 183

Panadol a brand name for paracetamol 325 (a non-opioid analgesic 10)

Panadol Extra a brand name for paracetamol 325 (a non-opioid analgesic 10) with caffeine

Panadol Ultra a brand name for paracetamol 325 with codeine 183 (both analgesics 9)

Panaleve a brand name for paracetamol 325 (a non-opioid analgesic 10)

Pancrease a brand name for pancreatin (a preparation of pancreatic enzymes 46)

pancreatic enzymes 47

pancreatin a preparation of pancreatic enzymes 46

Pancrex a brand name for pancreatin (a preparation of pancreatic enzymes 46)

pancuronium a muscle relaxant 52 used during general anaesthesia

Panoxyl a brand name for benzoyl peroxide 148 (a drug for acne 119)

panthenol pantothenic acid (a vitamin 88)

pantoprazole an ulcer healing drug 41

pantothenic acid (a vitamin 88)

papaveretum an opioid analgesic 11

papaverine a muscle relaxant 52

Papulex a brand name for nicotinamide (a drug for acne 119)

paracetamol 325 (a non-opioid analgesic 10)

Paracodol a brand-name analgesic 9 containing codeine 183 and paracetamol 325

Paradote a brand-name analgesic 9 containing paracetamol 325 and methionine (an antidote for paracetamol poisoning)

Parake a brand-name analgesic 9 containing codeine 183 and paracetamol 325

paraldehyde an anticonvulsant 16 used for status epilepticus

Paramax a brand-name migraine drug 20 containing paracetamol 325 and metoclopramide 299

Paramol a brand name for paracetamol 325 with dihydrocodeine (both analgesics 9)

Paraplatin a brand name for carboplatin (an anticancer drug 94)

parasites (skin), drugs to treat 118

Pariet a brand name for rabeprazole (an anti-ulcer drug 41)

parkinsonism, drugs for 18

Parlodel a brand name for bromocriptine 152 (a pituitary agent 83 and drug for parkinsonism 18)

Parmid a brand name for metoclopramide 299 (a gastrointestinal motility regulator and anti-emetic 21)

Parnate a brand name for tranylcypromine (an MAOI antidepressant 14)

paromomycin an antiprotozoal 71

Paroven a brand name for oxerutin (a drug used to treat peripheral vascular disease 30)

paroxetine 326 (an antidepressant 14)

Partobulin a brand name for anti-D immunoglobulin (a drug used to prevent sensitization to Rhesus antigen)

Parvolex a brand name for acetylcysteine (a mucolytic 25)

Pavacol-D a brand name for pholcodine (a cough suppressant 25)

Penbritin a brand name for ampicillin (a penicillin antibiotic 60)

penciclovir an antiviral drug 67

Pendramine a brand name for penicillamine (an antirheumatic 50)

penicillamine an antirheumatic 50

penicillins 62 (antibiotics 60)

penicillin G see benzylpenicillin (a penicillin antibiotic 60)

penicillin V see phenoxymethylpenicillin 329 (a penicillin antibiotic 60)

Pentacarinat a brand name for pentamidine (an antiprotozoal 71)

pentamidine an antiprotozoal 71

Pentasa a brand name for mesalazine 293 (a drug for ulcerative colitis 44)

pentazocine an opioid analgesic 11

pentostatin an anticancer drug 94

pentoxifylline previously known as oxpentifylline (a vasodilator 30 used to improve blood flow to the limbs in peripheral vascular disease)

Pepcid a brand name for famotidine (an anti-ulcer drug 41)

peppermint oil a substance for indigestion and bowel spasm 43

Peptimax a brand name for cimetidine 171 (an anti-ulcer drug 41)

Pepto-Bismol a brand-name preparation for diarrhoea 42 and upset stomach 40 containing bismuth

Percutol a brand name for glyceryl trinitrate 245 (an anti-angina drug 33)

Perdix a brand name for moexipril (an ACE inhibitor vasodilator 30)

Perfan a brand name for enoximone (a drug for heart failure 27)

pergolide a drug for parkinsonism 18

Pergonal a brand name for menotrophin (a drug for infertility 105)

Periactin a brand name for cyproheptadine (an antihistamine 56 used as an appetite stimulant 19)

pericyazine an antipsychotic 15

Perinal a brand name for hydrocortisone 251 (a corticosteroid 78) with lidocaine (a local anaesthetic 11)

perindopril an ACE inhibitor vasodilator 30

permethrin 327 a topical antiparasitic 118

Peroxyl a brand of hydrogen peroxide antiseptic mouthwash 116

perphenazine an antipsychotic 15 and anti-emetic 21

Persantin a brand name for dipyridamole 205 (an antiplatelet drug 36)

Peru balsam an antiseptic 116 for haemorrhoids 45

pethidine an opioid analgesic 11 and drug used in labour 106

Pevaryl a brand name for econazole (an antifungal 74)

phenazocine an opioid analgesic 11

phenelzine an MAOI antidepressant 14

Phenergan a brand name for promethazine 343 (an antihistamine 56 and anti-emetic 21)

phenindione an oral anticoagulant 36

pheniramine an antihistamine 56

phenobarbital 327 (a barbiturate anticonvulsant 16)

phenol an antiseptic used in throat lozenges and sprays 116

phenothiazines anti-emetics 21

phenothrin a topical antiparasitic 118 for head and pubic lice infestation

phenoxybenzamine a drug for phaeochromocytoma (a tumour of the adrenal glands 94)

phenoxymethylpenicillin 329 (a penicillin antibiotic 60)

Phensic a brand-name analgesic 9 containing

aspirin 138 and caffeine

phentermine an appetite suppressant 19

phentolamine an antihypertensive 34

phenylbutazone a non-steroidal anti-inflammatory 48

phenylephrine a decongestant 24

phenylpropanolamine 330 (a decongestant 24)

phenytoin 331 (an anticonvulsant 16)

Phimetin a brand name for cimetidine 171 (an anti-ulcer drug 41)

pHiso-Med a brand name for chlorhexidine (a skin antiseptic 116)

pholcodine a cough suppressant 25

phosphorus a mineral 91

Phyllocontin Continus a brand name for aminophylline 382 (a bronchodilator 23)

Physeptone a brand name for methadone 295 (an opioid used as an analgesic 10 and to ease heroin withdrawal)

Physiotens a brand name for moxonidine 310 (a centrally acting antihypertensive 34)

Phytex a brand-name antifungal 74 containing salicylic acid

phytomenadione natural vitamin K (a vitamin 88)

Picolax a brand name for sodium picosulfate and magnesium citrate (both laxatives 43)

pilocarpine 332 (a miotic for glaucoma 110)

pimozide an antipsychotic 15

pindolol a beta blocker 28

piperacillin a penicillin antibiotic 60

piperazine an anthelmintic 76

piperonal a head-lice repellent

pipotiazine palmitate an antipsychotic 15

Pipril a brand name for piperacillin (a penicillin antibiotic 60)

piracetam an anticonvulsant 16

pirenzepine an anticholinergic for peptic ulcers 41

Piriton a brand name for chlorphenamine 166 (an antihistamine 56)

piroxicam 333 (a non-steroidal anti-inflammatory 48 and drug for gout 51)

Pirozip a brand name for piroxicam 333 (a non-steroidal anti-inflammatory 48 and drug for gout 51)

pituitary disorders, drugs for 83

pizotifen 334 (a drug for migraine 20)

Plaquenil a brand name for hydroxychloroquine (an antimalarial 73 and antirheumatic 50)

Plavix a brand name for clopidogrel 180 (an antiplatelet drug 36)

Plendil a brand name for felodipine (a calcium channel blocker 33)

podophyllin a topical treatment for genital warts

podophyllotoxin a topical treatment for genital warts

podophyllum a topical treatment for warts

poloxamer a stimulant laxative 43

Polyfax a brand name for bacitracin with polymyxin B (both antibiotics 60)

polymyxin B an antibiotic 60

polynoxylin an antifungal 74 and antibacterial 64

polystyrene sulphonate a drug to remove excess potassium from the blood

Polytar a brand name for coal tar (a substance used for eczema 121, psoriasis 120, and dandruff 122)

polythiazide a thiazide diuretic 31

Polytrim a brand-name antibacterial 64 containing trimethoprim 393 and polythiazide a thiazide diureticpolymyxin B

polyvinyl alcohol an ingredient of artificial tear preparations 112

Ponstan a brand name for mefenamic acid 287 (a non-steroidal anti-inflammatory 48)

Poractant alfa a drug to mature the lungs of premature babies

Pork Insulatard a brand name for insulin 258 (a drug for diabetes 80)

Pork Mixtard a brand name for insulin 258 (a drug for diabetes 80)

Posalfilin a brand name for podophyllum with salicylic acid (both drugs for warts)

postcoital contraception 105

potassium a mineral 91

potassium bicarbonate an antacid 40

potassium channel openers vasodilators 30 used as anti-angina drugs 33

potassium chloride potassium (a mineral 91)

potassium citrate a drug for cystitis that reduces the acidity of urine 108

potassium clavulanate a preparation of clavulanic acid (a substance given with amoxicillin 136 to make it more effective)

potassium hydroxyquinolone sulphate an agent with antibacterial 64, antifungal 74, and deodorant properties, used for skin infections 116 and acne 119

potassium iodide a drug used for an overactive thyroid before surgery 82

potassium permanganate a skin antiseptic 116

potassium-sparing diuretics 31

povidone-iodine a skin antiseptic 116

Pragmatar a brand-name preparation for eczema 121, psoriasis 120, and dandruff 122 containing coal tar, salicylic acid, and sulphur

pralidoxime mesylate an antidote for organophosphorus poisoning

pramipexole a drug for parkinsonism 18

pramocaine a local anaesthetic 11

pravastatin 336 a cholesterol-lowering agent 35

Praxilene a brand name for naftidrofuryl 311 (a vasodilator 30)

praziquantel an anthelmintic 76 for tapeworm infestation

prazosin an antihypertensive 34 also used to relieve urinary obstruction 108

Precortisyl a brand name for prednisolone 337 (a corticosteroid 78)

Predenema a brand name for prednisolone 337 (a corticosteroid 78)

Predfoam a brand name for prednisolone 337 (a corticosteroid 78)

Prednesol a brand name for prednisolone 337 (a corticosteroid 78)

prednisolone 337 (a corticosteroid 78)

Predsol a brand name for prednisolone 337 (a corticosteroid 78)

Predsol-N a brand name for prednisolone 337 (a corticosteroid 78) with neomycin (an aminoglycoside antibiotic 60)

Pregaday a brand name for folic acid 90 (a vitamin 88) with iron (a mineral 910

Pregnyl a brand name for chorionic gonadotrophin 169 (a drug for infertility 105)

Premarin a brand name for conjugated estrogens 187 (a female sex hormone 86)

Premique a brand-name preparation for menopausal symptoms 86 containing conjugated estrogens 187 with medroxyprogesterone 286

Prempak-C a brand-name drug for menopausal symptoms 86 containing conjugated estrogens 187 and norgestrel

Prepadine a brand name for dosulepin 210 (a tricyclic antidepressant 14)

Prescal a brand name for isradipine (a calcium channel blocker 33)

Preservex a brand name for aceclofenac (a non-steroidal anti-inflammatory 48)

Prestim a brand name for bendroflumethiazide

147 (a thiazide diuretic 31) with timolol 386 (a beta blocker 28)

Priadel a brand name for lithium 278 (a drug for mania 16)

prilocaine a local anaesthetic 11

Primalan a brand name for mequitazine (an antihistamine 56)

primaquine an antimalarial 73 and antiprotozoal 71

Primaxin a brand name for imipenem (an antibiotic 60) with cilastatin (used to make imipenem more effective)

primidone 338 (an anticonvulsant 16)

Primolut N a brand name for norethisterone 316 (a female sex hormone 86)

Primoteston Depot a brand name for testosterone 380 (a male sex hormone 85)

Primperan a brand name for metoclopramide 299 (a gastrointestinal motility regulator and anti-emetic 21)

Prioderm a brand name for malathion 285 (a topical antiparasitic 118)

Pripsen a brand name for piperazine (an anthelmintic 76) with senna (a stimulant laxative 43)

Pro-Banthine a brand name for propantheline (an anticholinergic antispasmodic for irritable bowel syndrome 43 and urinary incontinence 108)

probenecid a uricosuric for gout 51

procainamide an anti-arrhythmic 32

procaine benzylpenicillin a penicillin antibiotic 60

procaine a local anaesthetic 11

procarbazine a drug for lymphatic cancers and small-cell cancer of the lung 94

prochlorperazine 339 (a phenothiazine anti-emetic 21 and antipsychotic 15)

Proctofoam HC a brand name for hydrocortisone 251 (a corticosteroid 78) with pramocaine (a local anaesthetic 11)

Proctosedyl a brand name for hydrocortisone 251 (a corticosteroid 78) with cinchocaine (a local anaesthetic 11)

procyclidine 340 (an anticholinergic for parkinsonism 18)

Profasi a brand name for chorionic gonadotrophin 169 (a drug for infertility 105)

Proflex a brand name for ibuprofen 254 (a non-steroidal anti-inflammatory 48)

progesterone a female sex hormone 86

progestogens synthetic female sex hormones 86

Prograf a brand name for tacrolimus (an immunosuppressant 96)

proguanil 341 (an antimalarial 73)

Progynova a brand name for estradiol 224 (an oestrogen 86)

Progynova TS a brand name for estradiol 224 (an oestrogen 86)

Proluton Depot a brand name for hydroxyprogesterone (a progestogen 86 used to prevent miscarriage)

promazine 342 (a phenothiazine antipsychotic 15)

promethazine 343 (an antihistamine 56 and anti-emetic 21)

Prominal a brand name for methylphenobarbital (a barbiturate anticonvulsant 16)

Propaderm a brand name for beclometasone 146 (a corticosteroid 78)

propafenone an anti-arrhythmic 32

Propain a brand-name analgesic 9 containing codeine 183, diphenhydramine, paracetamol 325, and caffeine

propamidine isethionate an antibacterial 64 for eye infections

Propanix a brand name for propranolol 345 (a beta blocker 28 and anti-anxiety drug 13)

propantheline an anticholinergic anti-spasmodic for irritable bowel syndrome 43 and urinary incontinence 108

Propine a brand name for dipivefrine (a sympathomimetic for glaucoma 110)

propiverine a drug for urinary frequency 108

Pro-Plus a brand name for caffeine (a stimulant 19)

propofol an anaesthetic agent 9

propranolol 345 (a beta blocker 28 and anti-anxiety drug 13)

propylthiouracil 346 (an antithyroid drug 82)

Proscar a brand name for finasteride 231 (a drug for benign prostatic hypertrophy)

Prostap SR a brand name for leuprorelin (a drug for menstrual disorders 100)

Prostigmin a brand name for neostigmine (a drug for myasthenia gravis 53)

protamine an antidote for heparin 249

protease inhibitors 98 (drugs for HIV and AIDS 97)

Prothiaden a brand name for dosulepin 210 (a tricyclic antidepressant 14)

protirelin a drug to test thyroid function 82

Protium a brand name for pantoprazole (an ulcer healing drug 41)

protriptyline a tricyclic antidepressant 14

Provera a brand name for medroxyprogesterone 286 (a female sex hormone 86)

Provigil a brand name for modafinil (a drug for narcolepsy 19)

Pro-Viron a brand name for mesterolone (a male sex hormone 85)

proxymetacaine a local anaesthetic 11

Prozac a brand name for fluoxetine 233 (an antidepressant 14)

Proziere a brand name for prochlorperazine 339 (a phenothiazine anti-emetic 21)

pseudoephedrine a sympathomimetic decongestant 24

psoriasis, drugs for 120

Psorin a brand-name drug for psoriasis 120 containing dithranol, coal tar, and salicylic acid

Pulmicort a brand name for budesonide 153 (a corticosteroid 78)

Pulmozyme a brand name for dornase alfa (a drug for cystic fibrosis 25)

pumactant a drug to mature the lungs of premature babies

pupils, drugs affecting 112

Puri-Nethol a brand name for mercaptopurine 292 (an anticancer drug 94)

Pylorid a brand name for ranitidine bismuth citrate (an anti-ulcer drug 41)

Pyralvex an anti-inflammatory drug for mouth ulcers

pyrazinamide an antituberculous drug 65

pyridostigmine 347 (a drug for myasthenia gravis 53)

pyridoxine a vitamin 88

pyrimethamine 348 (an antimalarial 73)

pyrithione zinc an antimicrobial for dandruff 122

Pyrogastrone a brand name for aluminium hydroxide 129, magnesium trisilicate, and sodium bicarbonate 365 (all antacids 40), carbenoxolone (an anti-ulcer drug 41) and alginic acid (an antifoaming agent 40)

Q

Quellada M a brand name for malathion 285

(an antiparasitic 118)

Questran a brand name for colestyramine 186 (a lipid-lowering drug 35)

quetiapine 350 (an antipsychotic drug 15)

quinagolide a drug for infertility 105

quinapril an ACE inhibitor vasodilator 30

quinidine an anti-arrhythmic drug 32

quinine 351 (an antimalarial 73 and muscle relaxant 52)

Quinocort a brand name for hydrocortisone 251 (a corticosteroid 78) with potassium hydroxyquinoline sulphate (an agent for skin infections 116)

Quinoderm a brand-name preparation for acne 119 containing benzoyl peroxide 148 and potassium hydroxyquinoline sulphate (an agent for skin infections 116)

quinolones 62 (antibiotics 60 and antibacterials 64)

Quinoped a brand-name antifungal 74 containing benzoyl peroxide 148 and potassium hydroxyquinoline sulphate (an agent for skin infections 116)

quinupristin an antibiotic 60

R

rabeprazole an anti-ulcer drug 41

Radian B a brand-name topical preparation rabeprazole an anti-ulcer drugfor muscle aches and sprains

raloxifene 353 (an anti-oestrogen sex hormone antagonist 86 used for osteoporosis 54)

raltitrexed an anticancer drug 94

ramipril 354 (an ACE inhibitor vasodilator 30)

ranitidine 355 (an anti-ulcer drug 41)

ranitidine bismuth citrate an anti-ulcer drug 41

Rapilysin a brand name for reteplase (a thrombolytic 38)

Rapitard MC a brand name for insulin 258 (a drug for diabetes 80)

Rapitil a brand name for nedocromil (an anti-allergy drug 56)

Rappell a brand name for piperonal (a head-lice repellent)

Rastinon a brand name for tolbutamide 387 (a drug for diabetes 80)

razoxane a cytotoxic anticancer drug 94

reboxetine an antidepressant 14

rectal and anal disorders, drugs for 45

Redoxon a brand name for vitamin C (a

vitamin 88)

Refludan a brand name for lepirudin (an anticoagulant 36)

Refolinon a brand name for folinic acid (a vitamin 88)

Regaine a brand name for minoxidil 305 (for treatment of male pattern baldness 123)

Regranex a brand name for beclapermin (a drug for healing skin ulcers)

Regulan a brand name for ispaghula (a bulk-forming agent used as a laxative 43)

Regulose a brand of lactulose 270 (a laxative 43)

Rehidrat a brand name for oral rehydration salts containing potassium, sodium chloride, sodium bicarbonate 365, and glucose

Relaxit a brand-name lubricant laxative 43

Relenza a brand name for zanamivir 401 (an antiviral drug 67)

Relifex a brand name for nabumetone (a non-steroidal anti-inflammatory 48)

Remedeine a brand name for paracetamol 325 (a non-opioid analgesic 10) with dihydrocodeine (an opioid analgesic 11)

remifentanil a drug used in anaesthesia

Rennie Digestif a brand-name antacid 40 containing calcium carbonate with magnesium carbonate

repaglinide 356 an oral antidiabetic 80

reproterol a bronchodilator 23

Requip a brand name for ropinirole (a drug for parkinsonism 18)

Resolve a brand-name analgesic 9 and antacid 40 with paracetamol 325, sodium bicarbonate 365 , potassium bicarbonate, calcium carbonate, citric acid, and vitamin C

Resonium A a brand name for polystyrene sulphonate (a drug to remove excess potassium from the blood)

resorcinol a keratolytic mainly for acne 119

respiratory stimulants nervous system stimulants 19

Restandol a brand name for testosterone 380 (a male sex hormone 85)

reteplase a thrombolytic 38

Retin-A a brand name for tretinoin (a drug for acne 119)

retinoic acid vitamin A (a vitamin 88)

retinoids vitamin A (a vitamin 88)

retinol vitamin A (a vitamin 88)

Retinova a brand name for tretinoin (a drug

for acne 119)

Retrovir a brand name for zidovudine 402 (an antiviral for HIV infection and AIDS 97)

Revanil a brand name for lisuride (a drug for parkinsonism 18)

Revasc a brand name for desirudin (an anticoagulant 36)

Rheumacin LA a brand name for indometacin (a non-steroidal anti-inflammatory 48 and drug for gout 51)

rheumatic disorders, corticosteroids for 51

Rheumox a brand name for azapropazone (a non-steroidal anti-inflammatory 48)

Rhinocort a brand name for budesonide 153 (a corticosteroid 78)

Rhinolast a brand name for azelastine (an antihistamine 56)

Rhumalgan a brand name for diclofenac 197 (a non-steroidal anti-inflammatory 48)

ribavirin previously known as tribavirin (an antiviral 67, used for certain lung infections in infants and children)

riboflavin a vitamin 88

Ridaura a brand name for auranofin (an antirheumatic 50)

Rideril a brand name for thioridazine 383 (a phenothiazine antipsychotic 15)

rifabutin an antituberculous drug 65

Rifadin a brand name for rifampicin 357 (an antituberculous drug 65)

rifampicin 357 (an antituberculous drug 65)

Rifater a brand name for isoniazid 263 with rifampicin 357 and pyrazinamide (all antituberculous drugs 65)

Rifinah a brand name for isoniazid 263 with rifampicin 357 (both antituberculous drugs 65)

Rilutek a brand name for riluzole (a glutamate inhibitor used to help patients who have sclerosis)

riluzole a glutamate inhibitor used to help patients with sclerosis

Rimactane a brand name for rifampicin 357 (an antituberculous drug 65)

Rimactazid a brand name for isoniazid 263 with rifampicin 357 (both antituberculous drugs 65)

Rimapam a brand name for diazepam 196 (a benzodiazepine anti-anxiety drug 13, muscle relaxant 52, and anticonvulsant 16)

rimexolone a corticosteroid 78

Rimoxallin a brand name for amoxicillin 136 (a penicillin antibiotic 60)

Rimso-50 a brand name for dimethyl sulfoxide (a drug for urinary infection 108)

Rinatec a brand name for ipratropium bromide 261 (a bronchodilator 23)

Rinstead pastilles a brand name for pastilles for mouth ulcers containing chloroxylenol

Risperdal a brand name for risperidone 358 (an antipsychotic 15)

risperidone 358 (an antipsychotic 15)

Ritalin a brand name for methylphenidate (a drug for hyperactivity)

ritodrine a uterine muscle relaxant 106

ritonavir an antiviral for HIV/AIDS 97

rituximab an anticancer drug 94

rivastigmine 359 (a drug for dementia 19)

Rivotril a brand name for clonazepam 179 (a benzodiazepine anticonvulsant 16)

rizatriptan a drug for migraine 20

Roaccutane a brand name for isotretinoin 265 (a drug for acne 119)

Robaxin a brand name for methocarbamol (a muscle relaxant 52)

Robinul a brand name for glycopyrronium bromide (an anticholinergic used in general anaesthesia)

Robinul-Neostigmine a brand name for neostigmine (a drug for myasthenia gravis 53)

Robitussin Dry Cough a brand name for guaifenesin (an expectorant 25)

Rocaltrol a brand name for calcitriol (a vitamin 88)

rocuronium a drug to relax the muscles during general anaesthesia

rofecoxib a COX-2 inhibitor 49 (a non-steroidal anti-inflammatory drug 48)

Roferon-A a brand name for interferon 259 (an antiviral 67 and anticancer drug 94)

Rohypnol a brand name for flunitrazepam (a benzodiazepine sleeping drug 11)

Rommix a brand name for erythromycin 222 (an antibiotic 60)

Ronicol a brand name for nicotinyl alcohol (a form of niacin)

ropinirole a drug for parkinsonism 18

ropivacaine a local anaesthetic 11

Roter a brand-name antacid 40 containing sodium bicarbonate 365, magnesium carbonate, frangula, and bismuth

Rowachol a brand-name preparation of essential oils for gallstones 46

Rowatinex a brand-name preparation to dissolve kidney stones 51 and to treat kidney infections

Rozex a brand name for metronidazole 301 (an antibacterial 64)

Rusyde a brand name for furosemide 239 (a loop diuretic 31)

Rynacrom a brand name for sodium cromoglicate 366 (an anti-allergy drug 56)

Rynacrom Compound a brand name for sodium cromoglicate 366 (an anti-allergy drug 56) with xylometazoline (a decongestant 24)

Rythmodan a brand name for disopyramide (an anti-arrhythmic 32)

S

Sabril a brand name for vigabatrin (an anticonvulsant 16)

Saizen a brand name for somatropin (a synthetic pituitary hormone 83)

Salactol a brand-name wart preparation containing salicylic acid, lactic acid, and collodion 116

Salagen a brand name for pilocarpine 332 (a miotic for glaucoma 110)

Salamol a brand name for salbutamol 361 (a bronchodilator 23)

Salatac a brand-name wart preparation containing salicylic acid, lactic acid, and collodion 116

Salazopyrin a brand name for sulfasalazine 371 (a drug for inflammatory bowel disease 44 and an antirheumatic 50)

Salbulin a brand name for salbutamol 361 (a bronchodilator 23)

salbutamol 361 (a bronchodilator 23 and drug used in labour 106)

salcatonin see calcitonin (salmon) (a drug used for bone disorders 54)

salicylic acid a keratolytic for acne 119, dandruff 122, psoriasis 120, and warts)

Salivace a brand name for artificial saliva

Saliva Orthana a brand name for artificial saliva

Saliveze a brand name for artificial saliva

Salivix a brand name for artificial saliva

salmeterol 362 (a bronchodilator 23)

Salofalk a brand name for mesalazine 293 (a drug for ulcerative colitis 44)

Salzone a brand name for paracetamol 325 (a non-opioid analgesic 10)

Sandimmun a brand name for ciclosporin 170 (an immunosuppressant 96)

Sandocal a brand name for calcium (a mineral 91)

Sando-K a brand name for potassium (a mineral 91)

Sandostatin a brand name for octreotide (a synthetic pituitary hormone 83 used for symptoms of cancer of the pancreas 94)

Sanomigran a brand name for pizotifen 334 (a drug for migraine 20)

saquinavir an antiviral for HIV/AIDS 97

Saventrine a brand name for isoprenaline (a bronchodilator 23)

Savlon a brand name for chlorhexidine with cetrimide (both skin antiseptics 116)

Schering PC4 a brand-name postcoital contraceptive containing ethinylestradiol 226 and levonorgestrel 276

Scheriproct a brand name for prednisolone 337 (a corticosteroid 78) with cinchocaine (a local anaesthetic 11)

Scopoderm TTS a brand-name anti-emetic 21 containing hyoscine 252

Sea-Legs a brand name for meclozine (an antihistamine 56 used to prevent motion sickness 21)

Secadrex a brand name for hydrochlorothiazide 250 (a thiazide diuretic 31) with acebutolol (a beta blocker 28)

secobarbital a barbiturate sleeping drug 11

Seconal Sodium a brand name for secobarbital (a barbiturate sleeping drug 11)

Sectral a brand name for acebutolol (a beta blocker 28)

Securon SR a brand name for verapamil 396 (an anti-angina drug 33 and anti-arrhythmic 32)

Securopen a brand name for azlocillin (a penicillin antibiotic 60)

selective serotonin re-uptake inhibitors (SSRIs) antidepressants 14

selegiline a drug for severe parkinsonism 18

selenium a mineral 91

selenium sulphide a substance for skin inflammation 116 and dandruff 122

Selsun a brand-name dandruff shampoo 122 containing selenium sulphide

Semi-Daonil a brand name for glibenclamide 243 (an oral antidiabetic 80)

Semprex a brand name for acrivastine (an antihistamine 56)

senna a stimulant laxative 43

Senokot a brand name for senna (a stimulant laxative 43)

Septanest a brand name for articaine (a local anaesthetic 11)

Septrin a brand name for co-trimoxazole 189 (an antibacterial 64)

Serc a brand name for betahistine 149 (a drug for Ménière's disease 21)

Serdolect a brand name for sertindole (an antipsychotic 15)

Serenace a brand name for haloperidol 248 (a butyrophenone antipsychotic 15)

Serevent a brand name for salmeterol 362 (a bronchodilator 23)

sermorelin a drug for growth disorders 83

Serophene a brand name for clomifene 177 (a drug for infertility 105)

Seroquel a brand name for quetiapine 350 (an antipsychotic drug 15)

Seroxat a brand name for paroxetine 326 (an antidepressant 14)

sertindole an antipsychotic 15

sertraline an antidepressant 14

Setlers a brand-name antacid 40 containing calcium carbonate and magnesium hydroxide 284

Sevoflurane a general anaesthetic

Sevredol a brand name for morphine 308 (an opioid analgesic 11)

sildenafil 363 (a drug for impotence 106)

silver nitrate a skin disinfectant 116

silver sulfadiazine a topical antibacterial 64 used to prevent infection in burns 116

Simeco a brand name antacid 40 containing aluminium hydroxide 129, dimeticone, magnesium carbonate, and magnesium hydroxide 284

Simplene a brand name for epinephrine 219 (a drug for glaucoma 110)

Simulect a brand name for basiliximab (an immunosuppressant 96)

simvastatin 364 (a lipid-lowering drug 35)

Sinemet 62.5 a brand name for levodopa 273 with carbidopa (both drugs for parkinsonism 18)

Sinequan a brand name for doxepin (a tricyclic antidepressant 14)

Singulair a brand name for montelukast 308 (a leukotriene antagonist for asthma 56 and bronchospasm 23)

Sinthrome a brand name for acenocoumarol (an anticoagulant 36)

Sinutab a brand name for paracetamol 325 (a non-opioid analgesic 10) with phenylpropanolamine 330 (a decongestant 24)

Siopel a brand-name barrier cream containing cetrimide and dimeticone

Skelid a brand name for tiludronic acid (a drug for bone disorders 54)

Skinoren a brand name for azelaic acid (an antibacterial 64, drug for acne 119)

sleeping drugs 11

Slo-Indo a brand name for indometacin (a non-steroidal anti-inflammatory 48 and drug for gout 51)

Slo-Phyllin a brand name for theophylline 382 (a bronchodilator 23)

Slow-Fe a brand name for iron (a mineral 91)

Slow-Fe Folic a brand name for folic acid 90 (a vitamin 88) with iron (a mineral 91)

Slow-K a brand name for potassium (a mineral 91)

Slow-Sodium a brand name for sodium chloride (a mineral 91)

Slozem a brand name for diltiazem 203 (a calcium channel blocker 30)

Sno Phenicol a brand name for eye drops containing chloramphenicol 163 (an antibiotic 60)

Sno Tears a brand name for polyvinyl alcohol (used in artificial tear preparations 112)

soda mint tablets sodium bicarbonate 365 (an antacid 40)

sodium a mineral 91

sodium acid phosphate a laxative 43

sodium aurothiomalate a substance containing gold, an antirheumatic 50

sodium bicarbonate 365 (an antacid 40)

sodium.calcium edetate an antidote for poisoning by lead and other heavy metals

sodium cellulose phosphate an agent used to reduce levels of calcium in the blood

sodium chloride common salt, contains sodium (a mineral 91)

sodium citrate a drug for urinary tract infections 108

sodium clodronate an agent used to treat low blood calcium in cancer patients 94

sodium cromoglicate 366 (an anti-allergy drug 56)

sodium feredetate iron (a mineral 91)

sodium fluoride a mineral 91

sodium fusidate an antibiotic 60

sodium nitroprusside a vasodilator 30

sodium perborate an antiseptic 116

sodium picosulfate a stimulant laxative 43

sodium stibogluconate an antiprotozoal 71

sodium tetradecyl sulphate a drug for treating varicose veins

sodium valproate 367 (an anticonvulsant 16)

Sofradex a brand name for dexamethasone 195 (a corticosteroid 78) with framycetin and gramicidin (both antibiotics 60)

softening agents laxatives 43

Solarcaine a brand name for benzocaine (a local anaesthetic 11) with triclosan (an antimicrobial 116)

Solian a brand name for amisulpride 133, an antipsychotic 15

Solpadeine a brand-name analgesic 9 containing codeine 183, paracetamol 325, and caffeine

Solpadol a brand name for paracetamol 325 (a non-opioid analgesic 10) with codeine 183 (an opioid analgesic 11)

Soltamox a brand name for tamoxifen 375 (an antioestrogen anticancer drug 94)

Solu-Cortef a brand name for hydrocortisone 251 (a corticosteroid 78)

Solu-Medrone a brand name for methylprednisolone (a corticosteroid 78)

Solvazinc a brand name for zinc (a mineral 91)

somatropin a synthetic pituitary hormone 83

Somatuline a brand name for lanreotide (an anticancer drug 94)

Sominex a brand-name sleeping drug 11 containing promethazine 343

Soneryl a brand name for butobarbital (a benzodiazepine sleeping drug 11)

Sorbichew a brand name for isosorbide dinitrate 264 (a nitrate vasodilator 30 and anti-angina drug 33)

Sorbid SA a brand name for isosorbide dinitrate 264 (a nitrate vasodilator 30 and anti-angina drug 33)

sorbitol a sweetening agent used in diabetic foods and included in skin creams as a moisturizer 116

Sorbitrate a brand name for isosorbide dinitrate 264 (a nitrate vasodilator 30 and anti-angina drug 33)

Sotacor a brand name for sotalol 368 (a beta blocker 28)

sotalol 368 (a beta blocker 28)

Sparine a brand name for promazine 342 (a phenothiazine antipsychotic 15)

Spasmonal a brand name for alverine citrate (an antispasmodic for irritable bowel syndrome 43)

spectinomycin an aminoglycoside antibiotic 60

Spectraban a brand name for aminobenzoic acid with padimate-O (both sunscreens 123)

Spiro-Co a brand name for spironolactone and hydroflumethiazide (both diuretics 30)

Spirolone a brand name for spironolactone (a potassium-sparing diuretic 31)

spironolactone a potassium-sparing diuretic 31

Spirospare a brand name for spironolactone (a potassium-sparing diuretic 31)

Sporanox a brand name for itraconazole (an antifungal 74)

Sprilon a brand-name skin preparation containing dimeticone and zinc oxide

SSRIs (selective serotonin re-uptake inhibitors) antidepressants 14

Stabillin-VK a brand name for phenoxymethylpenicillin 329 (a penicillin antibiotic 60)

stanozolol an anabolic steroid 85

Staril a brand name for fosinopril 238 (an ACE inhibitor vasodilator 30)

statins lipid-lowering drugs 35

stavudine an antiviral used to treat HIV infection and AIDS 97

Stelazine a brand name for trifluoperazine (a phenothiazine antipsychotic 15 and anti-emetic 21)

Stemetil a brand name for prochlorperazine 339 (a phenothiazine anti-emetic 21 and antipsychotic 15)

sterculia a bulk-forming agent used as an antidiarrhoeal 42 and laxative 43

steroids see anabolic steroids 86, corticosteroids 78, corticosteroids for rheumatic disorders 51, and topical corticosteroids 116

Ster-Zac a brand name for triclosan (an antimicrobial 116)

Stesolid a brand name for diazepam 196 (a benzodiazepine anti-anxiety drug 13, muscle relaxant 52, and anticonvulsant 16)

Stiedex a brand name for desoxymetasone (a

topical corticosteroid 116)

Stiemycin a brand name for erythromycin 222 (an antibiotic 60)

stilboestrol see diethylstilbestrol 201 (a female sex hormone 86)

Stilnoct a brand name for zolpidem (a sleeping drug 11)

Stimlor a brand name for naftidrofuryl 311 (a vasodilator 30)

stimulant (contact) laxatives 43

stimulants, nervous system 19

stimulants, uterine 106

Strefen a brand name for flurbiprofen (a non steroidal antinflammatory drug 48)

Strepsils a brand-name preparation for mouth and throat infections containing amylmetacresol and dichlorobenzyl alcohol (both antiseptics 116)

Streptase a brand name for streptokinase 369 (a thrombolytic 38)

streptokinase 369 (a thrombolytic 38)

streptomycin an antituberculous drug 65 and aminoglycoside antibiotic 60

Stromba a brand name for stanozolol (an anabolic steroid 85)

Stugeron a brand name for cinnarizine 178 (an antihistamine anti-emetic 21)

Stugeron Forte a brand name for cinnarizine 178 (an antihistamine anti-emetic 21)

sucralfate 370 (an ulcer-healing drug 41)

Sudafed a brand name for pseudoephedrine (a decongestant 24)

Sudafed-Co a brand name for paracetamol 325 (a non-opioid analgesic 10) and pseudoephedrine (a decongestant 24)

Sudafed Expectorant a brand name for guaifenesin (an expectorant 25) with pseudoephedrine (a decongestant 24)

Sudafed SA a brand name for pseudoephedrine (a decongestant 24)

Sudocrem a brand-name skin preparation containing benzyl benzoate and zinc oxide

sulconazole an antifungal 74

Suleo-M a brand name for malathion 285 (a topical antiparasitic 118)

sulfacetamide a sulphonamide antibacterial 64

sulfadiazine a sulphonamide antibacterial 64

sulfadimidine a sulphonamide antibacterial 64

sulfadoxine a drug used with pyrimethamine 348 for malaria 73

sulfamethoxazole a sulphonamide antibacterial 64 combined with trimethoprim in co-trimoxazole 189

sulfametopyrazine a sulphonamide antibacterial 64

sulfasalazine 371 (a drug for inflammatory bowel disease 44 and an antirheumatic 50)

sulfathiazole a sulphonamide antibacterial 64

sulfinpyrazone a drug for gout 51

sulindac a non-steroidal anti-inflammatory 48

Sulparex a brand name for sulpiride 133 (an antipsychotic 15)

sulphonamides antibiotics 60 and antibacterials 64

sulphur a topical antibacterial 64 and anti-fungal 74 for acne 119 and dandruff 122

sulpiride 133 (an antipsychotic 15)

Sulpitil a brand name for sulpiride 133 (an antipsychotic 15)

sumatriptan 373 (a drug for migraine 20)

sunscreens 123

Suprane a brand name for desflurane (a general anaesthetic)

Suprax a brand name for cefixime (a cephalosporin antibiotic 60)

Suprecur a brand name for buserelin (a drug for menstrual disorders 100)

Suprefact a brand name for buserelin (a drug for menstrual disorders 100)

Surgam a brand name for tiaprofenic acid (a non-steroidal anti-inflammatory 48)

Surmontil a brand name for trimipramine (a tricyclic antidepressant 14)

Suscard a brand name for glyceryl trinitrate 245 (an anti-angina drug 33)

Sustac a brand name for glyceryl trinitrate 245 (an anti-angina drug 33)

Sustanon a brand name for testosterone 380 (a male sex hormone 85)

Sustiva a brand name for efavirenz (an antiviral for HIV/AIDS 97)

suxamethonium a muscle relaxant used during general anaesthesia

Symmetrel a brand name for amantadine 130 (an antiviral 67 and drug for parkinsonism 18)

sympathomimetics a type of bronchodilator 23

Synacthen a brand name for tetracosactide (a drug to assess adrenal gland function 83)

Synagis a brand name for palvizumab, an antiviral drug 67

Synalar a brand name for fluocinolone (a topical corticosteroid 116)

Synalar C a brand name for fluocinolone (a

topical corticosteroid 116) with clioquinol (an antiseptic 116)

Synalar N a brand name for fluocinolone (a topical corticosteroid 116) with neomycin (an aminoglycoside antibiotic 60)

Synarel a brand name for nafarelin (a drug for menstrual disorders 100)

Syndol a brand name for codeine 183 and paracetamol 325 (both analgesics 9), with caffeine (a stimulant 19) and doxylamine (an antihistamine 56)

Synflex a brand name for naproxen 311 (a non-steroidal anti-inflammatory 48 and drug for gout 51)

Synphase a brand-name oral contraceptive 101 containing ethinylestradiol 226 and norethisterone 316

Syntaris a brand name for flunisolide (a corticosteroid 78)

Syntocinon a brand name for oxytocin (a uterine stimulant 106)

Syntometrine a brand name for ergometrine with oxytocin (both uterine stimulants 106)

Syscor MR a brand name for nisoldipine (a calcium channel blocker 33)

Sytron a brand name for sodium feredetate (iron, a mineral 91)

T

tacalcitol a drug for psoriasis 120

tacrolimus an immunosuppressant 96

Tagamet a brand name for cimetidine 171 (an anti-ulcer drug 41)

Tambocor a brand name for flecainide (an anti-arrhythmic 32)

Tamofen a brand name for tamoxifen 375 (an anticancer drug 94)

tamoxifen 375 (an anticancer drug 94)

Tampovagan a brand name for diethylstilbestrol 201 (a female sex hormone 86) and lactic acid

tamsulosin 376 (an alpha-blocking drug for prostate disorders 108)

Tanatril a brand name for imidapril (an ACE inhibitor vasodilator 30)

Targocid a brand name for teicoplanin (an antibiotic 60)

Tarivid a brand name for ofloxacin (an antibiotic 60)

Tavanic a brand name for levofloxacin 275 (an antibacterial 64)

Tavegil a brand name for clemastine (an antihistamine 56)

tazarotene a retinoid for psoriasis 120

tazobactam an antibiotic 60

Tazocin a brand name for piperacillin (an antibiotic 60) with tazobactam (a substance that increases the effectiveness of piperacillin)

TCAs see tricyclic antidepressants 14

TCP Liquid a brand-name antiseptic 116 containing phenol, chlorophenol, and 2-iodophenol

tear preparations, artificial see artificial tear preparations 112

Tears Naturale a brand-name artificial tear preparation 112 containing hypromellose

Tegretol a brand name for carbamazepine 158 (an anticonvulsant 16)

teicoplanin an antibiotic 60

Telfast a brand name for fexofenadine (an antihistamine 56)

temazepam 377 (a benzodiazepine sleeping drug 11)

Temgesic a brand name for buprenorphine (an opioid analgesic 11)

Temodal a brand name for temozolomide (an anticancer drug 94)

temozolomide an anticancer drug 94

Tenchlor a brand name for atenolol 140 (a beta blocker 28) with chlortalidone (a thiazide diuretic 31)

Tenif a brand name for atenolol 140 (a beta blocker 28) with nifedipine 315 (an anti-angina drug 33 and antihypertensive 34)

Tenkicin a brand name for phenoxymethylpenicillin 329 (a penicillin antibiotic 60)

Tenoret-50 a brand name for atenolol 140 (a beta blocker 28) with chlortalidone (a thiazide diuretic 31)

Tenoretic a brand name for atenolol 140 (a beta blocker 28) with chlortalidone (a thiazide diuretic 31)

Tenormin a brand name for atenolol 140 (a beta blocker 28)

tenoxicam a non-steroidal anti-inflammatory 48

Tensipine MR a brand name for nifedipine 315 (a calcium channel blocker 33)

Tensium a brand name for diazepam 196 (a benzodiazepine anti-anxiety drug 13 and muscle relaxant 52)

Teoptic a brand name for carteolol (a beta blocker 28 used for glaucoma 110)

terazosin a sympatholytic antihypertensive 34

terbinafine 378 (an antifungal 74)

terbutaline 379 (a sympathomimetic bronchodilator 23 and uterine muscle relaxant 106)

terlipressin a drug similar to vasopressin (a pituitary hormone 83) used to stop bleeding

terminating pregnancy, drugs for 107

Terra-Cortril a brand name for hydrocortisone 251 (a corticosteroid 78) with oxytetracycline (a tetracycline antibiotic 60)

Terra-Cortril Nystatin a brand name for hydrocortisone 251 (a corticosteroid 78) with nystatin 317 (an antifungal 74) and oxytetracycline (a tetracycline antibiotic 60)

Terramycin a brand name for oxytetracycline (a tetracycline antibiotic 60)

Tertroxin a brand name for liothyronine (a thyroid hormone 82)

testosterone 380 (a male sex hormone 85)

tetrabenazine a drug for tremor

Tetrabid a brand name for tetracycline 373 (an antibiotic 60 and antimalarial 73)

tetracaine previously known as amethocaine (a local anaesthetic 11)

tetracosactide a drug similar to corticotropin used to assess adrenal gland function 83

tetracycline 381 (an antibiotic 60 and antimalarial 73)

tetracyclines 62 (antibiotics 60)

Tetralysal 300 a brand name for lymecycline (a tetracycline antibiotic 60)

T-Gel a brand name for coal tar (an agent for dandruff 122 and psoriasis 120)

thalidomide a drug used for Hansen's disease (leprosy) 65

Theo-Dur a brand name for theophylline 382 (a bronchodilator 23)

theophylline 382 (a bronchodilator 23)

Thephorin a brand name for phenindamine (an antihistamine 56)

thiamine a vitamin 88

thiazides 31 (diuretics 30)

thiopental a fast-acting barbiturate used to induce general anaesthesia

thioridazine 383 (a phenothiazine antipsychotic 15)

thiotepa an anticancer drug 94

thrombolytics 38 (drugs that affect blood clotting 36)

thymoxamine see moxisylyte (a drug used to reduce pupil size after examination 112 and as a vasodilator 30 to improve blood supply to the limbs)

thyroid disorders, drugs for 82

thyroid hormones synthetic thyroid hormones used for hypothyroidism 82

thyroxine see levothyroxine 384 (a thyroid hormone 82)

tiabendazole an anthelmintic 76

tiagabine an anti-epileptic 16

tiaprofenic acid a non-steroidal anti-inflammatory 48

tibolone 385 (a female sex hormone 86)

ticarcillin a penicillin antibiotic 60

Ticlid a brand name for ticlopidine (an antiplatelet drug 36)

ticlopidine an antiplatelet drug 36

Tilade a brand name for nedocromil (a bronchodilator 23)

Tildiem a brand name for diltiazem 203 (an anti-angina drug 33)

Tiloryth a brand name for erythromycin 222 (an antibiotic 60)

tiludronic acid a drug for bone disorders 54

Timecef a brand name for cefodizime (a cephalosporin antibiotic 60)

Timentin a brand name for ticarcillin (a penicillin antibiotic 60) with clavulanic acid (a substance that increases the effectiveness of ticarcillin)

Timodine a brand name for hydrocortisone 251 (a corticosteroid 78) with nystatin 317 (an antifungal 74), benzalkonium chloride (an antiseptic 116), and dimeticone (a base for skin preparations 116)

timolol 386 (a beta blocker 28 and drug for glaucoma 110)

Timoptol a brand name for timolol 386 (a beta blocker 28 and drug for glaucoma 110)

Timpron a brand name for naproxen 311 (a non-steroidal anti-inflammatory 48 and drug for gout 51)

Tinaderm-M a brand name for nystatin 317 with tolnaftate (both antifungals 74)

tinidazole an antibacterial 64 and antiprotozoal 71

tinzaparin a type of heparin 249 (an anticoagulant 36)

tioconazole an antifungal 74

tioguanine an anticancer drug for acute leukaemia 94

tirofiban a drug for prevention of heart attacks 27

tissue plasminogen activator see alteplase (a thrombolytic 38)

Titralac a brand name for calcium carbonate (a substance used to reduce blood phosphate levels) and glycine

Tixylix a brand name for promethazine 343 (an antihistamine 56) with pholcodine (a cough suppressant 25)

Tixylix Cough and Cold a brand-name cough suppressant 25 and decongestant 24 containing chlorphenamine 166, pseudoephedrine, and pholcodine

tobramycin an aminoglycoside antibiotic 60

tocopherol vitamin E (a vitamin 88)

tocopheryl vitamin E (a vitamin 88)

Tofranil a brand name for imipramine 255 (a tricyclic antidepressant 14)

Tolanase a brand name for tolazamide (an oral antidiabetic 80)

tolazamide an oral antidiabetic 80

tolbutamide 387 (a drug for diabetes 80)

tolfenamic acid a drug for migraine 20

tolnaftate an antifungal 74

tolterodine 389 (an anticholinergic and antispasmodic for urinary disorders 108)

Topal a brand-name antacid 40 containing aluminium hydroxide 129, magnesium carbonate, and alginic acid

Topamax a brand name for topiramate (an anticonvulsant 16)

topical corticosteroids 116

Topicycline a brand name for tetracycline 381 (an antibiotic 60)

topiramate an anticonvulsant 16

topotecan an anticancer drug 94

Toradol a brand name for ketorolac (a non-steroidal anti-inflammatory 48 used as an analgesic 9)

torasemide a loop diuretic 31

Torem a brand name for torasemide (a loop diuretic 31)

toremifene an anticancer drug 94

Totamol a brand name for atenolol 140 (a beta blocker 28)

Totaretic a brand name for atenolol 140 (a beta blocker 28) with chlortalidone (a thiazide diuretic 31)

tramadol 390 (an analgesic related to codeine 183, an opioid analgesic 11)

Tramake a brand name for tramadol 390 (an opioid analgesic 11)

tramazoline a nasal decongestant 24

Tramil a brand name for paracetamol 325 and caffeine (a stimulant 19)

Tramil 500 a brand name for paracetamol 325 (a non-opioid analgesic 10)

Trandate a brand name for labetalol (a beta blocker 28)

trandolapril an ACE inhibitor vasodilator 30

tranexamic acid an antifibrinolytic used to promote blood clotting 36

Transiderm-Nitro a brand name for glyceryl trinitrate 245 (an anti-angina drug 33)

Transvasin a topical treatment for muscle aches and sprains 52

Tranxene a brand name for clorazepate (a benzodiazepine anti-anxiety drug 13)

tranylcypromine an MAOI antidepressant 14

Trasicor a brand name for oxprenolol (a beta blocker 28)

Trasidrex a brand name for cyclopenthiazide 190 (a thiazide diuretic 31) with oxprenolol (a beta blocker 28)

travel immunization (table) 71

travel vaccinations 70

Travogyn a brand name for isoconazole (an antifungal 74)

Traxam a brand name for felbinac 230 (a non-steroidal anti-inflammatory 48)

trazodone 391 (an antidepressant 14)

Trental a brand name for pentoxifylline (a vasodilator 30)

treosulfan a drug for ovarian cancer 94

tretinoin a drug for acne 119

Tri-Adcortyl a brand name for nystatin 317 (an antifungal 74) with gramicidin and neomycin (both aminoglycoside antibiotics 60) and triamcinolone (a corticosteroid 78)

Triadene a brand-name oral contraceptive 101 containing ethinylestradiol 226 and gestodene

TriamaxCo a brand-name diuretic 30 containing triamterene 392 and hydrochlorothiazide 250

triamcinolone a corticosteroid 78 also used for ear disorders 113

DRUG FINDER INDEX

Triam-Co a brand name for
hydrochlorothiazide 250 with triamterene
392 (both diuretics 30)

triamterene 392 (a potassium-sparing diuretic
31)

Triapin a brand-name preparation containing
felodipine (a calcium channel blocker 33)
and ramipril (an ACE inhibitor vasodilator
30)

tribavirin see ribavirin (an antiviral 67, used
for some lung infections in infants and
children)

triclofos a non-benzodiazepine, non-
barbiturate sleeping drug 11

triclosan a topical antimicrobial 116

tricyclic antidepressants (TCAs) antidepressants 14

Tridestra a brand-name preparation for
menopausal symptoms 86 containing
estradiol 224 and medroxyprogesterone
acetate 286

trientine a drug to eliminate copper from the
liver in Wilson's disease

trifluoperazine a phenothiazine antipsychotic
15 and an anti-emetic 21

Trifyba a brand name for a bulk-forming
laxative 43 containing bran

trihexyphenidyl previously known as benzhexol
(a drug for parkinsonism 18)

tri-iodothyronine see liothyronine (a thyroid
hormone 82)

trilostane an adrenal antagonist used for
Cushing's syndrome (an adrenal disorder
78) and breast cancer 94

trimeprazine see alimemazine (an
antihistamine 56)

trimetaphan a camsylate drug used to lower
blood pressure below normal in surgery

trimethoprim 393 (an antibacterial 64)

trimetrexate an antimicrobial for
pneumocystis pneumonia in AIDS 71

Tri-Minulet a brand-name oral contraceptive
101 containing ethinylestradiol 226 and
gestodene

trimipramine a tricyclic antidepressant 14

Trimogal a brand name for trimethoprim 393
(an antibacterial 64)

Trimopan a brand name for trimethoprim 393
(an antibacterial 64)

Trimovate a brand name for clobetasone (a
topical corticosteroid 116) with nystatin 317
(an antifungal 74) and oxytetracycline (a
tetracycline antibiotic 60)

Trinordiol a brand-name oral contraceptive 101
containing ethinylestradiol 226 and
levonorgestrel 276

TriNovum a brand-name oral contraceptive 101
containing ethinylestradiol 226 with
norethisterone 316

Triogesic a brand name for paracetamol 325 (a
non-opioid analgesic 10) with
phenylpropanolamine 330 (a decongestant
24)

Triominic a brand name for
phenylpropanolamine 330 (a decongestant
24) with pheniramine (an antihistamine 56)

tripotassium dicitratobismuthate a bismuth
compound used to treat peptic ulcer 41

Triprimix a brand name for trimethoprim 393
(an antibacterial 64)

triprolidine an antihistamine 56

Triptafen a brand name for amitriptyline 134
(a tricyclic antidepressant 14) with
perphenazine (an antipsychotic 15)

triptorelin an anticancer drug 94

Trisequens a brand name for estradiol 224 and
estriol (both female sex hormones 86)

trisodium edetate a drug to remove excess
calcium from the blood

Tritace a brand name for ramipril 354 (an ACE
inhibitor vasodilator 30)

Trobicin a brand name for spectinomycin (an
aminoglycoside antibiotic 60)

Tropergen a brand name for diphenoxylate 204
(an antidiarrhoeal 42) and atropine 142

tropicamide a mydriatic 112

tropisetron an anti-emetic 21

Tropium a brand name for chlordiazepoxide
164 (a benzodiazepine anti-anxiety drug 13)

Trosyl a brand name for tioconazole (an
antifungal 74)

Trusopt a brand name for dorzolamide 209 (a
drug for glaucoma 110)

tryptophan an antidepressant 14

Tuinal a brand name for amobarbital with
secobarbital (both barbiturate sleeping drugs 11)

tulobuterol a bronchodilator 23

Tylex a brand-name analgesic 9 containing
codeine 183 and paracetamol 325

Tyrozets a brand name for benzocaine (a local
anaesthetic 11) with tyrothricin (an
antibiotic 60)

U

Ubretid a brand name for distigmine (a parasympathomimetic for urinary retention 108 and myasthenia gravis 53)

Ucerax a brand name for hydroxyzine (an anti-anxiety drug 13)

Ukidan a brand name for urokinase (a thrombolytic 38)

Ultec a brand name for cimetidine 171 (an anti-ulcer drug 41)

Ultiva a brand name for remifentanil (a drug used in anaesthesia)

Ultralanum Plain a brand name for fluocortolone (a topical corticosteroid 116)

Ultraproct a brand name for fluocortolone (a topical corticosteroid 116) with cinchocaine (a local anaesthetic 11)

undecenoic acid an antifungal 74 for athlete's foot

Uniflu a brand name for codeine 183 (an opioid analgesic 11 and cough suppressant 25) with diphenhydramine (an antihistamine 56), paracetamol 325 (a non-opioid analgesic 10), phenylephrine (a decongestant 24), and caffeine (a stimulant 19)

Unigest a brand name for aluminium hydrochloride (an antacid 40) with dimeticone (an antifoaming agent 40)

Unihep a brand name for heparin 249 (an anticoagulant 36)

Uniparin, Uniparin Calcium a brand name for heparin 249 (an anticoagulant 36)

Uniphyllin Continus a brand name for theophylline 382 (a bronchodilator 23)

Uniroid HC a brand name for hydrocortisone 251 (a corticosteroid 78) with cinchocaine (a local anaesthetic 11)

Univer a brand name for verapamil 396 (an anti-angina drug 33 and anti-arrhythmic 32)

urea a topical treatment to moisturize dry skin 114 and soften ear wax 113

Uriben a brand name for nalidixic acid (an antibacterial 64)

urinary disorders, drugs for 108

Urispas a brand name for flavoxate (a urinary antispasmodic 108)

urofollitropin a drug for pituitary disorders 83

urokinase a thrombolytic 38

ursodeoxycholic acid a drug for gallstones 46

Ursofalk a brand name for ursodeoxycholic acid (a drug for gallstones 46)

uterine muscle relaxants drugs used in labour 106

uterine stimulants drugs used in labour 106

Utinor a brand name for norfloxacin (an antibiotic 60)

Utovlan a brand name for norethisterone 316 (a female sex hormone 86)

V

vaccines 68

vaccinations, travel see travel vaccinations 70

vaccinations, common 69

Vagifem a brand name for estradiol 224 (a female sex hormone 86)

Vaginyl a brand name for metronidazole 301 (an antibacterial 64 and antiprotozoal 71)

valaciclovir an antiviral 67

Valclair a brand name for diazepam 196 (a benzodiazepine anti-anxiety drug 13, muscle relaxant 52, and anticonvulsant 16)

Valderma Cream a brand-name preparation for minor skin problems, containing potassium hydroxyquinoline sulphate (an antibacterial 64 and antifungal 74), and chlorocresol (a topical antiseptic 116)

Valium a brand name for diazepam 196 (a benzodiazepine anti-anxiety drug 13, muscle relaxant 52, and anticonvulsant 16)

Vallergan a brand name for trimeprazine (an antihistamine 56)

Valoid a brand name for cyclizine (an antiemetic 21)

valproate an anticonvulsant 16

valproic acid an anticonvulsant 16

valsartan an antihypertensive 34)

Valtrex a brand name for valaciclovir (an antiviral 67)

Vancocin a brand name for vancomycin (an antibiotic 60 for serious infections)

vancomycin an antibiotic 60 for serious infections

Vaqta a brand-name vaccine to protect against viral hepatitis

Varidase a brand-name preparation containing streptokinase 369 (a thrombolytic 38), and streptodornase (a fibrinolytic enzyme) used to treat leg ulcers

Vascace a brand name for cilazapril (an ACE inhibitor vasodilator drug 30)

Vaseline Petroleum Jelly an ointment used to treat dry skin 114

vasodilators 30

Vasogen a brand name barrier cream 116 containing calamine, dimeticone, and zinc oxide

vasopressin a pituitary hormone 83 used to treat diabetes insipidus 80

Vasoxine a brand name for methoxamine (a vasoconstrictor)

Vectavir a brand name for penciclovir (an antiviral 67 used in the treatment of AIDS 97)

vecuronium a muscle-relaxant 52 used in general anaesthesia

Veganin a brand name analgesic containing aspirin 138, paracetamol 325, and codeine 183

Veil a brand name skin preparation 114 to hide scars

Velbe a brand name for vinblastine (an anticancer drug 94)

Velosef a brand name for cefradine (a cephalosporin antibiotic 60)

Velosulin a brand name for insulin 258 (a drug for diabetes 80)

venlafaxine 395 (an antidepressant 14)

Venofer a brand-name iron supplement

Ventmax SR a brand name for salbutamol 361 (a bronchodilator 23 and drug used in labour 106)

Ventodisks a brand name for salbutamol 361 (a bronchodilator 23 and drug used in labour 106)

Ventolin a brand name for salbutamol 361 (a bronchodilator 23 and drug used in labour 106)

Vepesid a brand name for etoposide (an anticancer drug 94)

Veracur a brand name for formaldehyde (a substance for warts)

verapamil 396 (a calcium channel blocker for angina 33 and arrhythmias 32)

Vermox a brand name for mebendazole (an anthelmintic 76)

Verrugon a brand name for salicylic acid (a keratolytic for warts)

Vesagex a brand name antiseptic 116 containing cetrimide

Vesanoid a brand name for tretinoin (a drug for acne 119)

Vexol a brand name for rimexolone (a corticoteroid 78)

Viagra a brand name for sildenafil 363 (a drug for impotence 106)

Viazem XL a brand name for diltiazem (a calcium channel blocker 33 and antihypertensive 34)

Vibramycin, Vibramycin-D brand names for doxycycline 214 (a tetracycline antibiotic 60)

Vicks Cold Care a brand name cold remedy containing paracetamol 325 (a non-opioid analgesic 10), dextromethorphan (a cough suppressant 25), and phenylpropanolamine 330 (a decongestant 24)

Vicks Medinite a brand name cold remedy containing paracetamol 325 (a non-opioid analgesic 10), dextromethorphan (a cough suppressant 25) and pseudoephedrine (a decongestant 24)

Videne a brand name for povidone-iodine (a skin antiseptic 116)

Videx a brand name for didanosine 200 (an antiviral 67 for HIV infection and AIDS 97)

vigabatrin an anticonvulsant 16

Vigam a brand name for human normal immune globulin injection 68

Vigranon B a brand name for vitamin B complex preparation (a vitamin 88)

viloxazine a tricyclic antidepressant 14

vinblastine an anticancer drug 94

vincristine an anticancer drug 94

vindesine an anticancer drug 94

vinorelbine an anticancer drug 94

Vioform-Hydrocortisone a brand name for hydrocortisone 251 (a corticosteroid 78) and clioquinol (an antimicrobial 116)

Vioxx a brand name for rofecoxib (a non-steroidal anti-inflammatory drug 48)

Viracept a brand name for nelfinavir (an antiviral 67 used to treat HIV and AIDS 97)

Viraferon a brand name for interferon alfa 259 (an antiviral 67 used to treat viral hepatitis)

Viramune a brand name for nevirapine (an antiviral 67 used to treat HIV and AIDS 97)

Virazid a brand name for tribavirin (an antiviral 67)

Viridal, Viridal Duo brand names for alprostadil 128 (a prostaglandin used for impotence 106)

Virormone a brand name for testosterone 380 (a male sex hormone 85)

Visclair a brand name for mecysteine (a

mucolytic for coughs 25)

Viscotears a brand-name artificial tears preparation

Viskaldix a brand name for pindolol (a beta blocker 28) and clopamide (a thiazide diuretic 31)

Visken a brand name for pindolol (a beta blocker 28)

Vista-Methasone a brand name for betamethasone 150 (a corticosteroid 78)

Vistide a brand name for cidofovir (an antiviral 67 used for Cytomegalovirus infections in AIDS 97)

vitamin requirements 90

vitamins 88

vitamins, main food sources of (table) 90

vitamin A a vitamin 88

vitamin B Complex see vitamins 88

vitamin B$_1$ another name for thiamine (a vitamin 88)

vitamin B$_2$ another name for riboflavin (a vitamin 88)

vitamin B$_6$ another name for pyridoxine (a vitamin 88)

vitamin B$_{12}$ a vitamin 88

vitamin C another name for ascorbic acid (a vitamin 88)

vitamin D a vitamin 88

vitamin E a vitamin 88

vitamin K a vitamin 88

Vivalan a brand name for viloxazine (a tricyclic antidepressant 14)

Vivapryl a brand name for selegiline (a drug for Parkinsonism 18)

Vivotif a brand name vaccine 68 to protect against typhoid fever

Volmax a brand name for salbutamol 361 (a bronchodilator 23)

Volraman a brand name for diclofenac 197 (a non-steroidal anti-inflammatory 48)

Volsaid Retard a brand name for diclofenac 197 (a non-steroidal anti-inflammatory 48)

Voltarol a brand name for diclofenac 197 (a non-steroidal anti-inflammatory 48)

Voltarol Retard a brand name for diclofenac 197 (a non-steroidal anti-inflammatory 48)

W

warfarin 398 (an anticoagulant 36)

Warticon a brand name for podophyllotoxin (a drug for genital warts)

WaspEze a brand-name aerosol preparation for insect bites and stings containing benzocaine (a local anaesthetic 11) and mepyramine (an antihistamine 56)

Waxsol a brand name for docusate (an ear-wax softener 113)

Welldorm Elixir a brand name for chloral hydrate (non-benzodiazepine, non-barbiturate sleeping drug 11)

Welldorm Tablets a brand name for cloral betaine (a non-benzodiazepine, non-barbiturate sleeping drug 11)

Wellferon a brand name for interferon 259 (an anticancer drug 94)

Wellvone a brand name for atovaquone (an antiprotozoal 71 and antimalarial 73)

Windcheaters a brand-name preparation containing dimeticone (an antifoaming agent 40)

witch hazel an astringent used in topical 116 and rectal preparations 45

Woodward's Gripe Water a brand-name preparation for wind pain in infants containing sodium bicarbonate 365 and dill seed oil

X

Xalatan a brand name for latanoprost (a drug for glaucoma 110)

xamoterol a drug for mild heart failure

Xanax a brand name for alprazolam (a benzodiazepine anti-anxiety drug 13)

xanthines a type of bronchodilator 23

Xatral a brand name for alfuzosin (a drug for prostate disorders 108)

Xenical a brand name for orlistat 321 (an anti-obesity drug 88)

xipamide a thiazide-like diuretic 30

Xylocaine a brand name for lidocaine (a local anaesthetic 11)

xylometazoline a decongestant 24

Xyloproct a brand-name anal preparation 45 containing hydrocortisone 251, aluminium acetate, lidocaine, and zinc oxide

Y

Yomesan a brand name for niclosamide (an anthelmintic 76 for tapeworm infestation)

Yutopar a brand name for ritodrine (a uterine muscle relaxant 106)

Z

Zaditen a brand name for ketotifen (a drug used to prevent asthma 23)

zafirlukast a leukotriene antagonist for asthma 56 and bronchospasm 23

zalcitabine 400 (an antiviral for HIV infection and AIDS 97)

Zamadol a brand name for tramadol 390 (an opioid analgesic 11)

zanamivir 401 an antiviral drug 67

Zanidip a brand name for lercanidipine (a calcium channel blocker 33)

Zantac a brand name for ranitidine 355 (an anti-ulcer drug 41)

Zarontin a brand name for ethosuximide 227 (an anticonvulsant 16)

Zenapax a brand name for daclizumab (an immunosuppressant 96)

Zerit a brand name for stavudine (an antiviral for HIV infection and AIDS 97)

Zestoretic a brand name for lisinopril 277 (an ACE inhibitor vasodilator 30) and hydrochlorothiazide 250 (a diuretic 30)

Zestril a brand name for lisinopril 277 (an ACE inhibitor vasodilator 30)

Ziagen a brand name for abacavir (an antiviral for HIV/AIDS 97)

zidovudine (AZT) 402 (an antiviral for HIV infection and AIDS 97)

Zimovane LS a brand name for zopiclone 403 (a sleeping drug 11)

Zinacef a brand name for cefuroxime (a cephalosporin antibiotic 60)

Zinamide a brand name for pyrazinamide (an antituberculous drug 65)

zinc a mineral 91

Zincomed a brand name for zinc (a mineral 91)

zinc oxide a soothing agent 116

zinc pyrithione an antimicrobial with antibacterial 64 and antifungal 74 properties used for dandruff 122

zinc sulphate zinc (a mineral 91)

Zineryt a brand-name acne preparation 119 containing erythromycin 222 (an antibiotic 60) and zinc (a mineral 91)

Zinga a brand name for nizatidine (an anti-ulcer drug 41)

Zinnat a brand name for cefuroxime (a cephalosporin antibiotic 60)

Zirtek a brand name for cetirizine 162 (an antihistamine 56)

Zispin a brand name for mirtazapine (an antidepressant 14)

Zita a brand name for cimetidine 171 (an anti-ulcer drug 41)

Zithromax a brand name for azithromycin (an antibiotic 60)

Zocor a brand name for simvastatin 364 (a lipid-lowering drug 35)

Zofran a brand name for ondansetron 321 (an anti-emetic 21)

Zoladex a brand name for goserelin 246 (a female sex hormone 86 and anticancer drug 94)

Zoleptil a brand name for zotepine (an antipsychotic 15)

zolmitriptan a drug for migraine 20

zolpidem a sleeping drug 11

Zomacton a brand name for somatropin (a synthetic pituitary hormone 83)

Zomig a brand name for zolmitriptan (a drug for migraine 20)

zopiclone 403 a sleeping drug 11

zotepine an antipsychotic 15

Zoton a brand name for lansoprazole 272 (an anti-ulcer drug 41)

Zovirax a brand name for aciclovir 126 (an antiviral 67)

Z Span a brand name for zinc (a mineral 91)

zuclopenthixol an antipsychotic 15

Zumenon a brand name for estradiol 224 (a female sex hormone 86)

Zydol a brand name for tramadol 390 (an opioid analgesic 11)

Zyloric a brand name for allopurinol 127 (a drug for gout 51)

Zyomet a brand name for metronidazole 301)

Zyprexa a brand name for olanzapine 319 (an antipsychotic 15)